Otology and
Middle Ear Surgery

Otology and Middle Ear Surgery

Editor

Asok K Saha

MS DNB D Ortho MSc MNAMS
Associate Professor
Department of ENT and Head & Neck Surgery
Medical College
Kolkata, West Bengal, India

Foreword

Naresh Panda

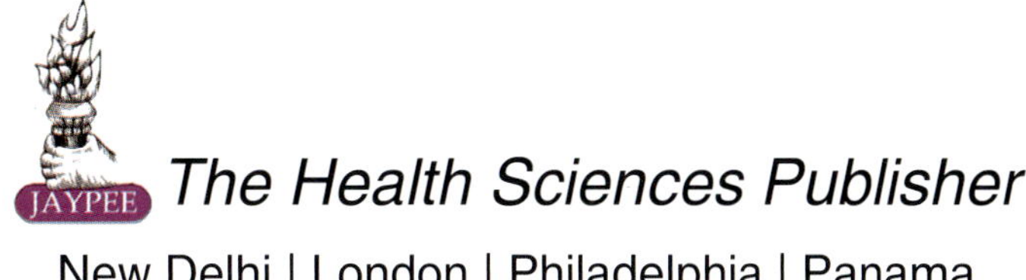

The Health Sciences Publisher

New Delhi | London | Philadelphia | Panama

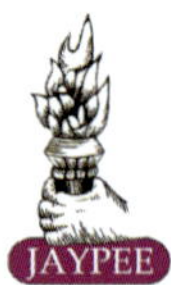 **Jaypee Brothers Medical Publishers (P) Ltd**

Headquarters

Jaypee Brothers Medical Publishers (P) Ltd
4838/24, Ansari Road, Daryaganj
New Delhi 110 002, India
Phone: +91-11-43574357
Fax: +91-11-43574314
Email: jaypee@jaypeebrothers.com

Overseas Offices

J.P. Medical Ltd
83 Victoria Street, London
SW1H 0HW (UK)
Phone: +44 20 3170 8910
Fax: +44 (0)20 3008 6180
Email: info@jpmedpub.com

Jaypee-Highlights Medical Publishers Inc
City of Knowledge, Bld. 235, 2nd Floor, Clayton
Panama City, Panama
Phone: +1 507-301-0496
Fax: +1 507-301-0499
Email: cservice@jphmedical.com

Jaypee Medical Inc
325 Chestnut Street
Suite 412, Philadelphia, PA 19106, USA
Phone: +1 267-519-9789
Email: support@jpmedus.com

Jaypee Brothers Medical Publishers (P) Ltd
17/1-B Babar Road, Block-B, Shaymali
Mohammadpur, Dhaka-1207
Bangladesh
Mobile: +08801912003485
Email: jaypeedhaka@gmail.com

Jaypee Brothers Medical Publishers (P) Ltd
Bhotahity, Kathmandu
Nepal
Phone: +977-9741283608
Email: kathmandu@jaypeebrothers.com

Website: www.jaypeebrothers.com
Website: www.jaypeedigital.com

Inquiries for bulk sales may be solicited at: jaypee@jaypeebrothers.com

Otology and Middle Ear Surgery

First Edition: **2016**

ISBN: 978-93-5250-122-9

Printed at Replika Press Pvt. Ltd.

Dedicated to

My parents, Late Amiya Kumar Saha and Late Shanti Rani Saha;
My in-laws, Late Amarendra Nath Saha and Smt Sabitri Saha;
My sister, Late Chandana Saha; My nieces, Sanchita Saha and Miss Anasuya;
My sons, Dr Anindya and Arnab;
My daughter-in-law, Dr Sananda;
and, specially to my wife Debjani Saha.

Lastly, to my teachers, students and patients
whose invisible blessings helped me to complete this book.

Contributors

Abdul Wadood MS
Senior Resident
Department of Otolaryngology and
Head & Neck Surgery
PGIMER
Chandigarh, India

Anirvan Banerjee FRCS (ORS-HNS), FRCS(ENT) Edin,
MS(ENT), DLO(RCS-Eng)
Consultant ENT Surgeon
Editor ENT News
Middlesborough, UK

Arpit Sharma MS
Senior Resident
Medanta Medicity
Gurgaon, Haryana, India

Asok K Saha MS DNB D Ortho MSc MNAMS
Associate Professor
Department of ENT and Head & Neck Surgery
Medical College
Kolkata, West Bengal, India

Chaturbhuj L Rajak MD (PGIMER), DNB
Consultant Radiologist
Quadra Medical Services Pvt Ltd
Kolkata, West Bengal, India

Dev Roy FRCS (ORS-HNS), FRCS (ENT) Edin, MS(ENT),
DLO(RCS-Eng)
Associate Professor
Department of ENT
Apollo Gleneagles Hospital
Kolkata, West Bengal, India

Enakshi Saha MD
Associate Professor
Department of Anesthesiology and
Critical Care Medicine
Medical College
Kolkata, West Bengal, India

Indranil Chatterjee MASLP
Lecturer (Speech and Hearing)
Department of Audiology
Ali Yavar Jung National Institute for the Hearing
Handicapped
Eastern Regional Center
Kolkata, West Bengal, India

Jaimanti Bakshi MS, DNB, MNAMS
Additional Professor
Department of Otolaryngology and
Head & Neck Surgery
PGIMER
Chandigarh, India

KK Handa MS (PGIMER), DNB, MNAMS
Director
ENT and Head & Neck Surgery
Medanta Medicity
Gurgaon, Haryana
Formerly Associate Professor
Department of ENT AIIMS
New Delhi, India

Foreword

It is my great pleasure to write the foreword of the book 'Otology and Middle Ear Surgery'. The book meets the demand of didactic information and surgical procedures in Otology in a very appealing way. As a teacher, I still cherish the memory of Dr Asok as a resident here at PGIMER, Chandigarh long back. His depth of knowledge and skill of surgery today makes him a successful teacher and a versatile surgeon. The book focuses on otology with an up-to-date information and colorful illustrations. I am confident that the book will be a great asset to students, trainees and practitioners in the field of otology.

Naresh Panda
MS DNB FRCSEd. FAMS
Professor and Head
Department of Otolaryngology
PGIMER
Chandigarh, India

Preface

Genesis of the book *"Otology and Middle Ear Surgery"* arises from the request of my students, both undergraduate and postgraduate, to write a book on ear and ear surgery for helping them during study as well as in clinical practice. Therefore, I decided to write a book that may fulfill their requirements. Most of the chapters are written by me. Some chapters (including chapter 16 to 22) are contributed by my guest authors who are eminent in their fields. I express my deep gratitude to my esteemed contributors who have helped me to bring forth this book. I have tried to cover most of the chapters on otology with an up-to-date information within a single volume. I am hopeful that all the readers of this book will highly benefit by studying sincerely and practicing honestly from this book.

I gratefully acknowledge Dr Sidhartha Das, Clinical tutor, Department of ENT, Calcutta National Medical College, for helping me to take microscopic ear photographs.

I also owe my thanks to Dr Soumik Das, Associate Professor, Department of ENT, Medical College, Kolkata and Dr Avik Basu, one of my bright students for giving their valuable time in proofreading.

I extend my sincere gratitude to my teacher Professor (Dr) Naresh Panda, Head, Department of ENT, PGIMER, Chandigarh and Professor (Dr) Sankar Prasad Bera, Head, Department of ENT, KPC Medical College, Kolkata for their invaluable suggestions.

I also convey my heartiest thanks to Mr Purnendu Roy Chowdhury (MCA) for his immense encouragement and painstaking efforts in bringing out this book in such an excellent form. I feel deeply indebted to all my family members for boosting my morale.

Lastly, I sincerely acknowledge Mr S Hazra, Jaypee Brothers, Kolkata and M/s Jaypee Brothers Medical Publishers (P) Ltd, New Delhi, India for assistance and encouragement in publishing this book.

In spite of my best efforts to make this edition error-free, some printed errors might have gone unnoticed. Thanks are also due to my readers if the same are brought to my notice. Valuable suggestions, criticism and feedback are invited through E-mail to dr.asoksaha@gmail.com from teachers, students and ENT practitioners to enrich this book in future edition.

Asok K Saha

Contents

Anatomy of Ear

Asok K Saha

INTRODUCTION

Ear is divided into three parts:
- External ear
- Middle ear
- Inner ear

External ear comprises:
- Pinna
- External auditory canal (EAC)
- Tympanic membrane (TM).

Pinna: It is a single piece of elastic fibrocartilage covered by skin. The cartilage is continuous with the cartilage of the external auditory canal. This cartilage is absent in lobule and in between the crux of helix and tragus bridged by intrinsic ligament.

Various Land Marks on Pinna (Fig. 1)

Ligaments and muscles of pinna: There are both intrinsic and extrinsic ligaments and muscles.[1]
- Extrinsic ligaments—are two, anterior ligament and posterior ligament those connect the cartilage of pinna to the temporal bone. Anterior ligament attaches tragus and anterior rim of the crus of helix to the root of zygomatic arch. Posterior ligament attaches medial surface of the concha to the lateral surface of the mastoid prominence
- Intrinsic ligaments connect various parts of cartilage within the pinna, one runs between tragus and helix and another between antihelix and inferior portion of helix
- Extrinsic muscles are anterior, posterior and superior auricularis. These muscles arising from auricle are inserted into epicranial aponeurosis and give rise to postauricular myogenic response following auditory stimulation

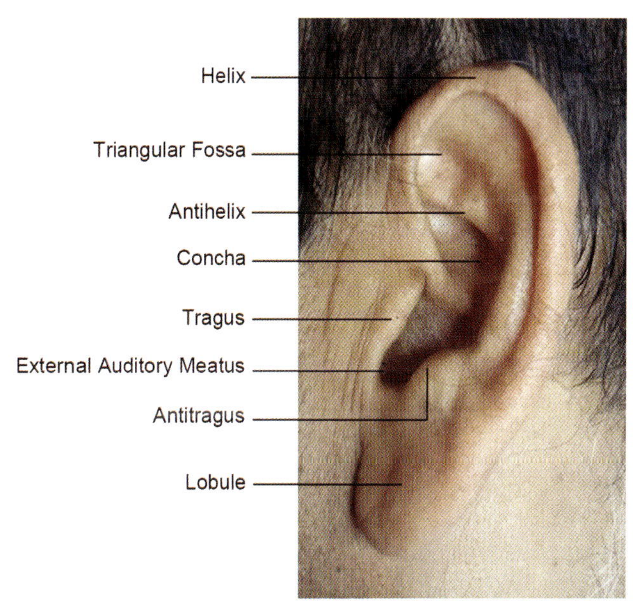

Fig. 1: Landmarks of left pinna

- Intrinsic muscles are helicis major, helicis minor, tragicus and antitragicus. These muscles are small, inconsistent and functionally unimportant
- Both intrinsic and extrinsic muscles are supplied by branches of facial nerve.

Sensory Nerve Supply of Pinna (Fig. 2A)

Lymphatic Drainage (Fig. 2B)

- From posterior surface of pinna lymphatics empty into the lymph nodes of mastoid tip
- From tragus and upper part of the anterior surface of pinna lymphatics drain into the preauricular lymph nodes

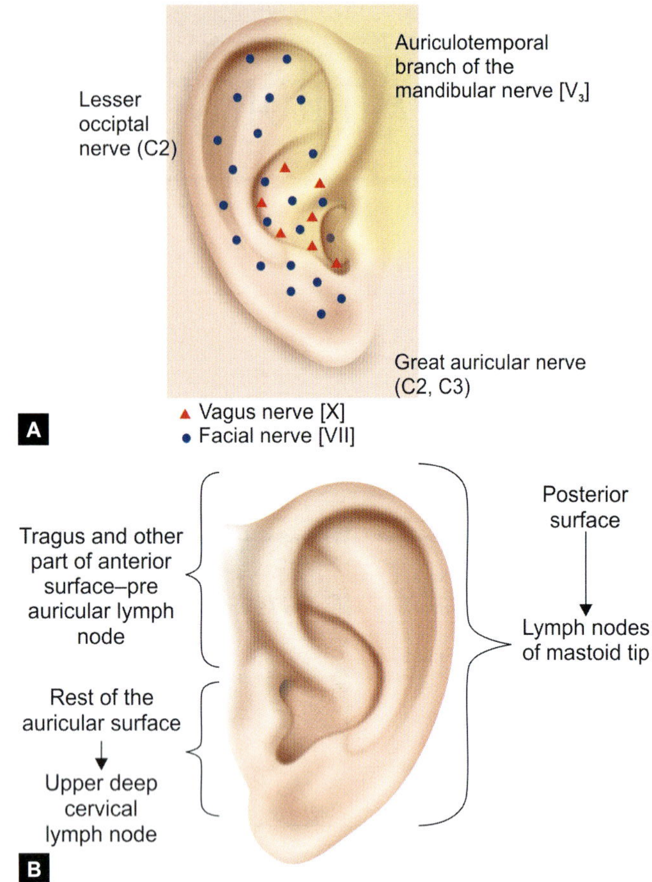

Figs 2A and B: (A) Sensory nerve supply of pinna; (B) Lymphatic drainage

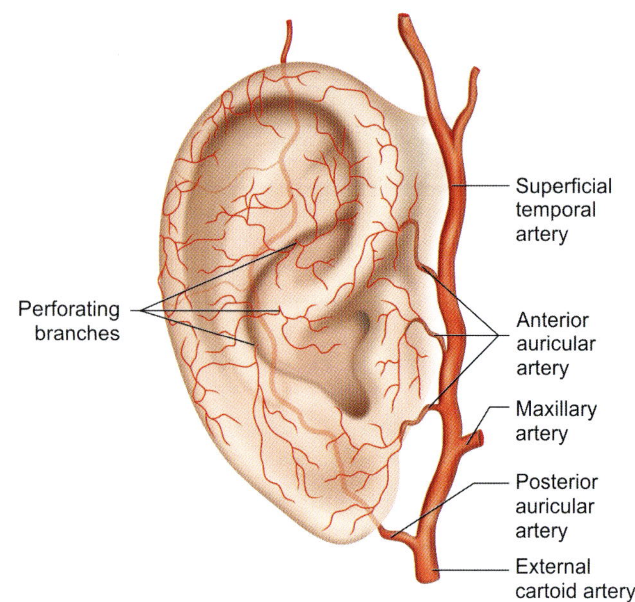

Fig. 3: Blood supply of pinna

- From rest of the auricle the lymphatic drainage is to the upper deep cervical lymph nodes.

Blood Supply (Fig. 3)

- Posterior auricular—branch of external carotid
- Anterior auricular—branch of superficial temporal
- A branch of occipital artery
- Veins are corresponding to arteries. They drain into external jugular and common facial vein.

External Auditory Canal (EAC)

- It extends from concha to tympanic membrane
- Posterior canal walls is 2.5 cm
- Anterior canal wall is 4.0 cm
- Lateral one-third is formed by cartilage which is 8 mm in length
- Medial two-thirds is formed by bone which is 16 mm in length
- At the medial end of bony canal, there is tympanic sulcus which is absent superiorly

- There are two constrictions in EAC—First one is at the junction of the cartilage and bone. Second is at the isthmus (5 mm from TM)
- Two suture lines are present in EAC (canal wall). One is tympanosquamous anteriorly and other one is tympanomastoid posteriorly
- Fissures of Santorini are two deficiencies seen in cartilaginous portion of EAC
- Direction of EAC—Outer part is upward, backward and medially. Inner part is downwards, forwards and medially
- Anterior, inferior and posterior bony walls are formed by tympanic part of temporal bone
- Roof and part of the posterior wall are formed by squamous part of temporal bone
- Skin is very thin and is firmly attached to bone and cartilage of meatus
- Ceruminous glands, sebaceous glands and hairs are present in subcutaneous tissue of cartilaginous part. The ceruminous glands are modified apocrine sweat glands producing cerumen (wax). Both ceruminous and sebaceous glands arise from hair follicles
- Meatal recess is present in anteroinferior part of bony meatus beyond the isthmus. It is the cesspit for discharge and debris
- Foramen of Huschke[2] is a deficiency present in anteroinferior part of bony canal in children (up to four years) or sometimes in adult. It transmits infection to and from parotid.

Blood Supply of EAC

Arterial blood supply comes from branches of external carotid artery.

- Superficial temporal artery
- Maxillary artery
- Posterior auricular artery

Venous drainage—It drains into external jugular vein, maxillary vein and pterygoid plexus.

Lymphatic Drainage

It follows that of pinna.

Nerve Supply

- Anterior and superior wall are supplied by auriculotemporal, branch of mandibular nerve
- Posterior and inferior wall are supplied by auricular branch of vagus (Arnold's nerve)
- Posterior wall is supplied by facial nerve.

Relationship of EAC

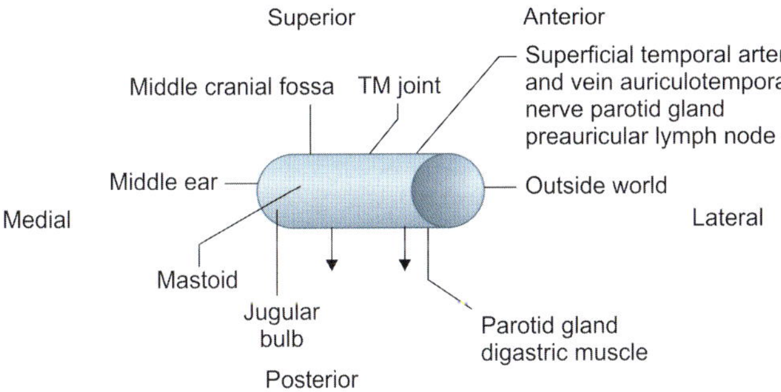

Tympanic Membrane (TM)

It separates EAC from middle ear.
- It is nearly oval in shape. Its largest diameter is 9–10 mm (Vertical). Shortest diameter is 8–9 mm (anteroposterior)
- Total surface area is 85 sq. mm. Vibrating surface area is 55 sq. mm
- It is placed at an angle of 55 degree with the floor of the meatus
- It is semitransparent, pearly gray in color
- It is weighing nearly 12–14 mg
- Its thickness is 0.1–0.15 mm.

Peripheral Part of TM (Fig. 4)

It is thickened to form fibrocartilagenous ring attached to tympanic sulcus at the medial end of EAC. The sulcus is deficit superiorly. From the ends of this notch the anterior and posterior malleolar folds are prolonged to lateral process of the malleus.

TM above the anterior and posterior malleolar fold is pars flaccida. TM below these folds is pars tensa. TM is convex towards the middle ear cavity. The point of greatest convexity of TM at the tip of malleus is umbo.

Layers of TM
- Outer (Cuticular layer) is stratified epithelium.
- Intermediate (Fibrous layer) is radial, circular and parabolic.
- Inner (Mucosa) is ciliated columnar epithelium.

Arterial Supply of the TM

- Cuticular layer is supplied by deep auricular branch of maxillary artery and stylomastoid branch of posterior auricular artery
- Middle and mucosal layer are supplied by tympanic branch of maxillary artery and twigs from the middle meningeal artery.

Venous Drainage of TM

- Superficial part is drained into external jugular vein
- Deep part is drained into transverse sinus and dural vein and venous plexus around Eustachian Tube.

Nerve Supply to TM

- Anterior portion is supplied by auriculotemporal branch of mandibular, which is the branch of trigeminal
- Posterior portion is supplied by auricular branch of vagus
- Medial surface is supplied by tympanic branch of glossopharyngeal (Jacobson's nerve).

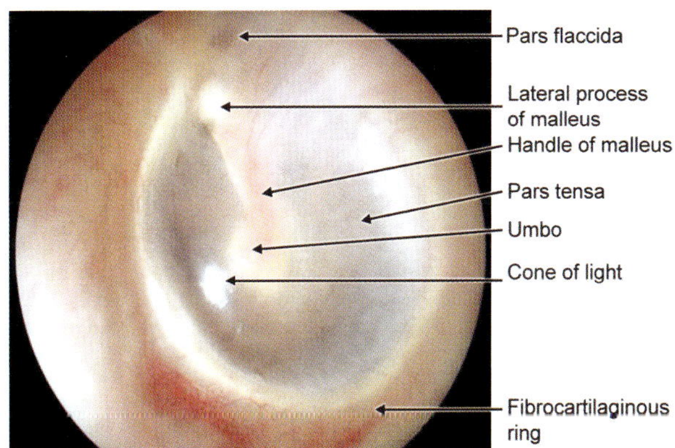

Fig. 4: Left tympanic membrane (lateral aspect)

Middle Ear (Fig. 5)

- Middle ear cleft comprises of:
    - → Tympanic cavity—It has four walls/roof/floor.
    - → Eustachian tube.
    - → Mastoid air cell system.
- It is lined by mucous membrane
- It is filled with air.

Middle ear is biconcave irregular space. It has three parts:
- → Epitympanum that is lying above pars tensa.
- → Mesotympanum that is opposite to pars tensa.
- → Hypotympanum is lying below the level of pars tensa.

Epitympanum or attic is the portion of middle ear which lies above the level of short process of malleus. It lies within a fan-shaped dehiscence in the tympanic bone known as notch of Rivinus; it is bounded as roof by tegmen tympani formed by petrosal and squamous portion of the temporal bone, anterior boundary by tympanosquamous suture line, posterior boundary by tympanomastoid suture line, laterally by pars flaccida and scutum (outer attic wall) and medial wall by portion of medial wall of mesotympanum lying above the level of facial canal.

Contents of epitympanum are—
- Head of malleus
- Body of incus
- Associated ligaments/mucosal folds.

The cog is a bony ridge hanging from the tegmen just anterior to the head of malleus. It lies immediately above and slightly posterior to the processus cochleariformis. It divides anterior epitympanum from rest of the epitympanum.

Anterior epitympanum is also known as supratubal recess which is a common site for attic cholesteatoma and also site for its recurrence.

Portion of tympanic membrane forming lateral wall of epitympanum (Pars flaccida) is more prone to form retractions due to negative middle ear pressure because:
- The middle layer of dense collagen present in Pars tensa is absent here
- The fibrous annulus of the tympanic membrane departs from its bony sulcus at the anterior and posterior spines which sends off fibrous bands to meet the neck of malleus.

The epitympanum communicates with the mesotympanum via to small openings between various mucosal folds—anterior isthmus tympani and posterior isthmus tympani—these are discussed later.

Mesotympanum: It is the portion of the middle ear which lies between horizontal planes drawn at the top and bottom of edges of the tympanic membrane. Its contents are—stapes, long process of Incus, oval and round window. Eustachian tube exits from anterior aspect of mesotympanum. Two crescent-shaped racess extend posteriorly from mesotympanam. These are—
- Facial racess (lateral)—is situated between tympanic membrane and facial nerve
- Sinus tympanum (medial)—is present between facial nerve and medial wall of the tympanum.

Hypotympanum: It is the portion of middle ear cavity which lies below the level of the bony ear canal. It is an irregular bony groove rarely associated with cholesteatoma. At times if its floor is dehiscent then the jugular bulb may be exposed. In hypotympanam, a thin plate of bone occupying the skull base where internal carotid runs anteriorly and the internal jugular vein turns posteriorly is called Crotch or jugulocarotid spine. Following these vessels jugular bulb is exposed and IX, X, XI CN are found in proximity to the multiple openings of inferior petrosal sinus.[3]

Protympanum: It is the portion of middle ear around the tympanic orifice of the Eustachian tube. It lies inferior to the canal for tensor tympani. Internal-carotid artery usually covered by thin bone passes medial and inferior to the bony Eustachian tube.

Dimension of Middle Ear

- Vertical length is 15 mm
- Anteroposterior is 15 mm
- Transverse diameter above 6 mm and below 4 mm.

It communicates with nasopharynx anteriorly through Eustachian tube and mastoid posteriorly through Aditus opening.

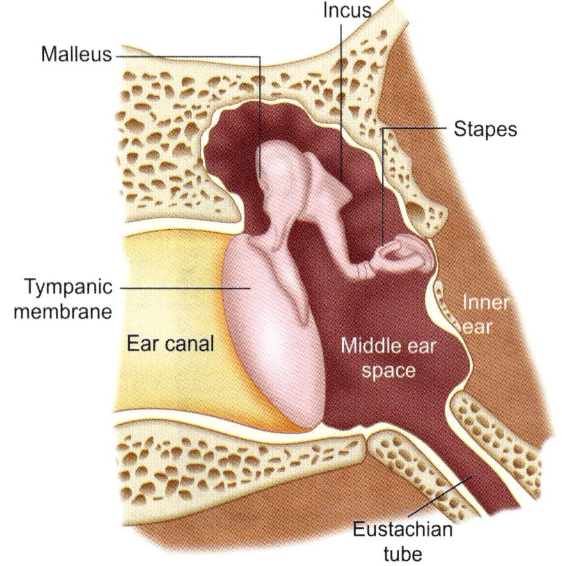

Fig. 5: Parts of middle ear

Tympanic Cavity

Relations—
- Laterally tympanic membrane
- Posteriorly mastoid antrum
- Medially lateral wall of internal ear
- Anteriorly Eustachian tube opening.

Roof: It is the tegmen tympani that separates tympanic cavity from middle cranial fossa. It has petrosquamous suture through which infection may be transmitted to the superior petrosal sinus by venous spread.

Floor: It is a thin convex plate of bone that separates the tympanic cavity from superior bulb of internal jugular vein. Near the medial wall, it has an aperture for tympanic branch of glossopharyngeal nerve (passage of Jacobson's nerve).

Lateral Wall of Tympanic Cavity

Lateral wall *of tympanic cavity is formed by*

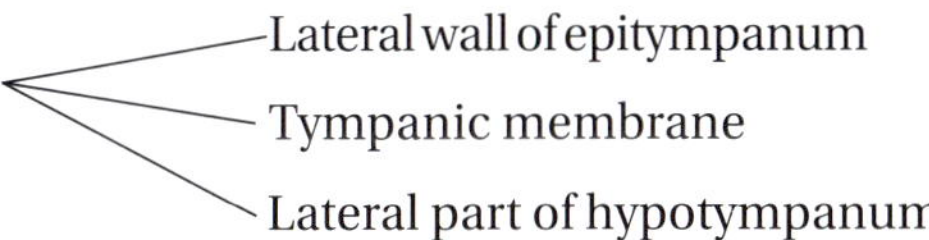

Medial surface of lateral wall has three holes in bone.
1. Posterior canaliculus for chorda tympani: It is present at the angle of junction between posterior and lateral wall of the cavity immediately behind the TM and on a level with the upper end of handle of malleus. It is a small canal which descends in front of the facial nerve canal and opens into it 6 mm above the stylomastoid foramen. Through this opening chorda tympani nerve and branch of stylomastoid artery enter the tympanic cavity.
2. Petrotympanic fissure: It is situated anteriorly just above the attachment of tympanic membrane. It is a 2 mm deep slit and it lodges anterior process, anterior ligament of malleus and anterior tympanic branch of maxillary artery.
3. Anterior canaliculus for chorda tympani (canal of Huguier): It is placed at the medial end of petrotympanic fissure. Through this chorda tympani leaves the tympanic cavity (Fig. 6).

Medial Wall of Tympanic Cavity (Lateral Wall of Internal Ear) (Fig. 7)

Prominent structures are Promontory/Fenestra vestibuli (oval window)/Fenestra cochleae (round window)/Facial nerve canal prominence/processus cochleariformis.
- Promontory: A rounded elevation that is caused by lateral projection of the basal turn of cochlea. It is

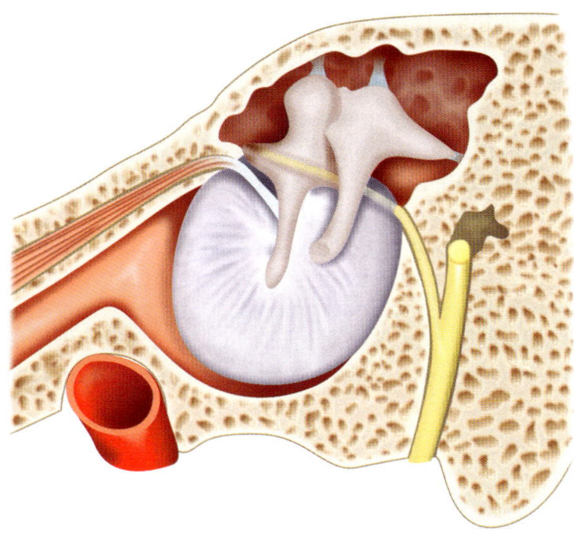

Fig. 6: Anterior and posterior canaliculi with chorda tympani

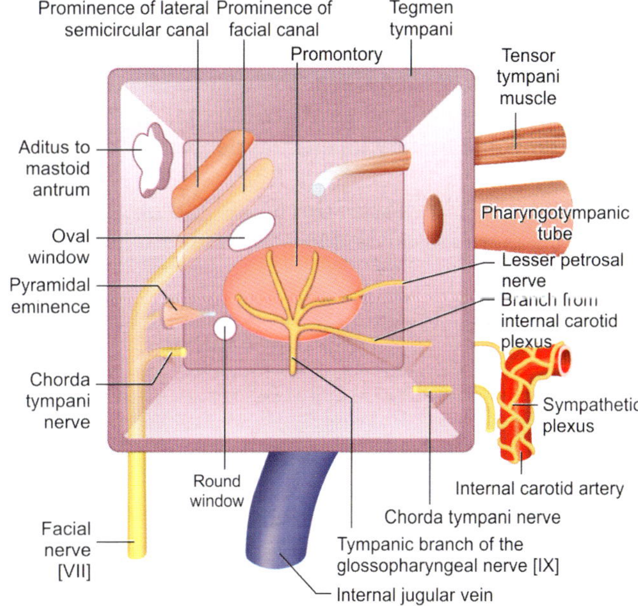

Fig. 7: Structures on the medial wall of middle ear

furrowed by grooves containing nerves of tympanic plexus. A depression behind the promontory is sinus tympani that indicates the position of the ampulla of the posterior semicircular canal
- Fenestra vestibuli (Oval window): A reniform (kidney-shaped) opening between tympanic cavity and inner ear. It is situated posterosuperior to promontory. It is occupied by stapes foot plate. Stapes foot plate is attached to the margins of fenestra by annular ligament. Its size is 3.25 x 1.75 mm

- Fenestra cochleae (round window): It is situated below and behind the fenestra vestibule. It lies completely under the cover of the overhanging edge of the promontory in a deep hollow. It opens from tympanic cavity to scala tympani of the cochlea. It is covered by the membrane of round window (secondary tympanic membrane). Its size is 2.3 mm in largest diameter and 1.87 mm in shortest diameter
- Prominence of facial canal: It traverses the medial wall of tympanic cavity from front to backwards. It is located above the oval window where it forms the second genu
- Processus cochleariformis: It is a hook like projection lying anterior to oval window for tendon of tensor tympani
- Lateral semicircular canal: It is rounded eminence in the medial wall, situated above and behind the prominence of facial nerve canal.

Anterior Wall of Tympanic Cavity

Anterior wall of tympanic cavity consists of a thin plate of bone that separates the middle ear cavity from internal carotid artery. The upper portion of this plate of bone is smaller than the lower portion. This plate is pierced by one or more tympanic branches of the internal carotid artery and accompanying superior and inferior caroticotympanic nerves that carry sympathetic fibers. The small upper portion of anterior wall has two openings—upper one for canal of tensor tympani and lower one for the Eustachian tube opening.

Posterior Wall of Tympanic Cavity

Posterior wall of tympanic cavity is wider above than below. Main structures are—
- Aditus to antrum of mastoid
- Pyramid
- Fossa incudis
- Opening for exit of chorda tympani nerve.

Aditus: It is the opening between epitympanic recess and mastoid antrum.

Pyramidal eminence: It is hollow. It contains stapedius muscles. It is situated immediately behind the fenestra vestibule and in front of vertical portion of facial canal.

Fossa incudis: It is a small depression in the lower and posterior part of the epitympanic recess containing short process of incus.

Posterior tympanum: It is the posterior part of the mesotympanum and common site for cholesteatoma.

Posterior tympanum is divided into four sinuses in relation to second genu, vertical segment of facial nerve and pyramidal eminence. The sinuses, lateral to the facial nerve are facial recess and lateral sinus. The sinuses that are medial to the facial nerve are posterior tympanic sinus and sinus tympani.[4]

Facial recess: It is also called supra pyramidal recess. It is a collection of air cells lying lateral to the facial nerve. It is bounded medially by vertical part of facial nerve, laterally by chorda tympani, superiorly by fossa incudis and anterolaterally by tympanic membrane (Fig. 8).

Importance of facial recess: Direct access can be made through this into the middle ear without disturbing posterior canal wall (posterior tympanotomy can be done through facial recess) (Fig. 10).

Lateral sinus: It lies inferior to the pyramidal eminence lateral to facial nerve and medial to annulus.

Posterior tympanic sinus: It lies medial to the facial nerve and pyramidal eminence, superior to the ponticulus and posterior to the footplate (Fig. 11).

Sinus tympani: It is a deep recess medial to the pyramid and vertical part of the facial nerve. It is bounded by subiculum below and ponticulus above (Fig. 9).

Subiculum: It a bony ridge that separates the round window from oval window by posterior extension of promontory.

Ponticulus: It is a spicule of bone that leaves the promontory above subiculum and runs to the pyramid in the posterior wall of the cavity.[5]

Mastoid Antrum (Fig. 12)

- It is an air sinus in the petrous part of temporal bone
- It communicates with the attic through the aditus.

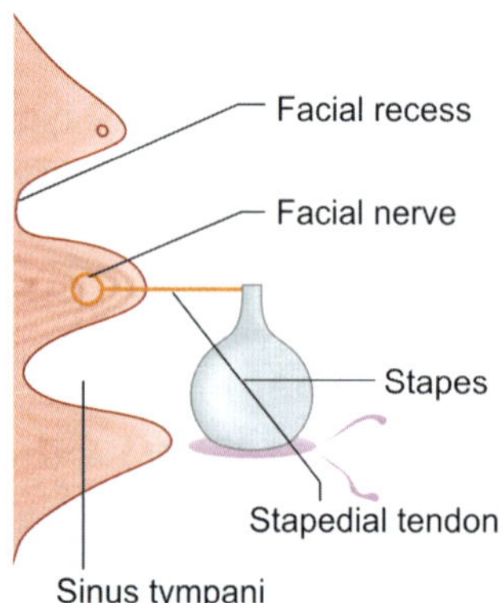

Fig. 8: Facial recess and sinus tympani

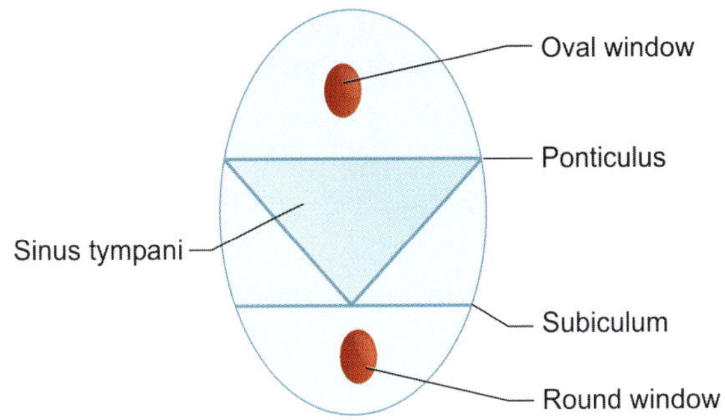

Fig. 9: Sinus tympani in relation to oval and round window

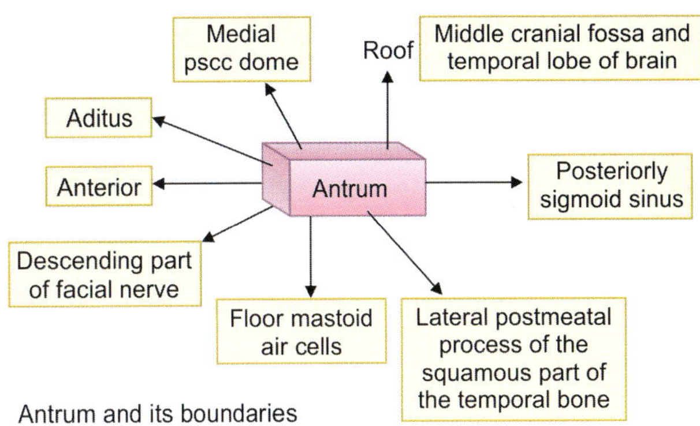

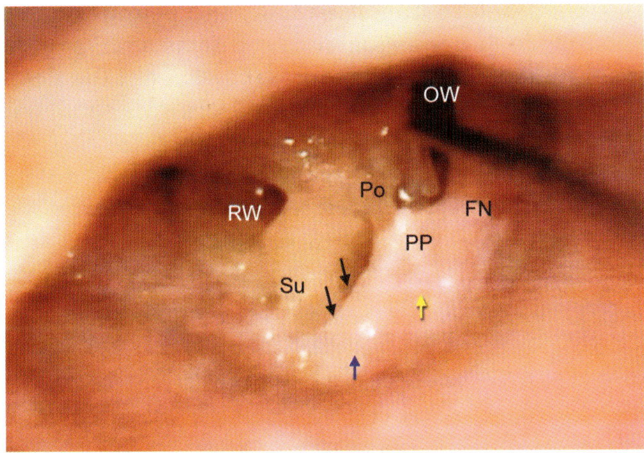

Fig. 10: Two sinuses lateral to the facial nerve—facial recess and lateral sinus

Abbreviations: Yellow arrow, facial recess; blue arrow, lateral sinus; FN, facial nerve; PP, pyramidalis process; Po, ponticulus; Su, sobiculum; OW, oval window; RW, round window. (From surgical techniques in chronic otitis media and otosclerosis, text and atlas, Agadurappa Mahadevaiah and Bhavin Parikh, second edition, 2011, p-7)

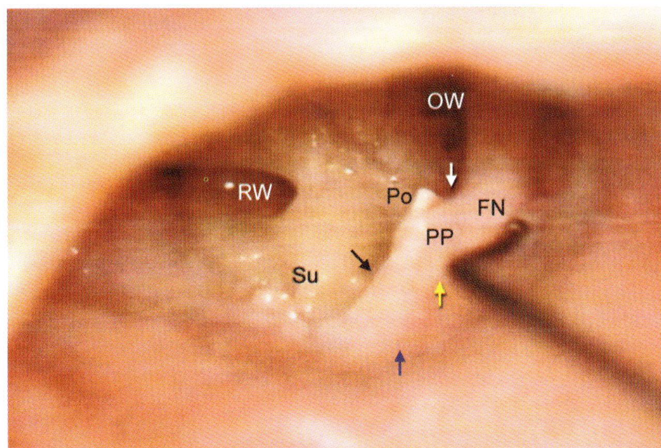

Fig. 11: Two sinuses medial to the facial nerve—posterior tympanic sinus and sinus tympani

Abbreviations: White arrow, posterior tympanic sinus; black arrow, sinus tympani; FN, facial nerve; PP, pyramidalis process; Po, ponticulus; Su, sobiculum; OW, oval window; RW, round window. (From surgical techniques in chronic otitis media and otosclerosis, text and atlas, Agadurappa Mahadevaiah and Bhavin Parikh, second edition, 2011, p-7)

Antrum and its Boundaries

Thickness of lateral wall at birth is ~2 mm and in adult is ~12–15 mm. The size of the mastoid antrum at birth is more or less equal to the size in adult. But it lies at a higher level (with respect to External meatus) than in adult.

Macewen's Triangle (Suprameatal Triangle) (Fig. 13)

Boundary
- Above—suprameatal crest
- Anteroinferionly—posterosuperior margin of external auditory canal (EAC)
- Posteriorly—vertical tangent to external auditory canal (EAC)
- Surface marking of antrum is the suprameatal triangle/cymba concha
- Capacity of mastoid antrum in adult is 1 mL. Each of its diameters is about 10 mm.

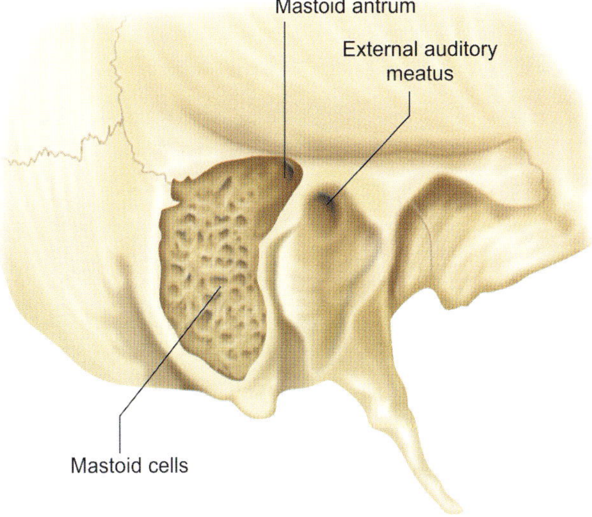

Fig. 12: Mastoid antrum, mastoid cells and EAC

Trautmann's Triangle (Fig. 14)

It is bounded by:
- Sigmoid sinus posteriorly
- Bony labyrinth anteriorly
- Superior petrosal sinus superiorly.

It is the landmark for entry into the posterior cranial fossa.

Infection into the posterior cranial fossa can spread through this triangle.

Solid Angle

It is the solid bone medial to the antrum in the angle formed by the three semicircular canals (Fig. 15).

Antrum Threshold Angle

It is bounded above by horizontal semicircular canal (HSCC) and fossa incudis—
- Laterally by chorda tympani nerve
- Medially by descending part of VII nerve.

Arcuate eminence: It is seen in superior surface of petrous bone. Underneath this eminence superior semicircular canal lies.

Donaldson's line: It is the surgical landmark for endolymphatic Surgery (Fig. 16).

It is derived by extending the plane of lateral semicircular canal, so that it bisects the posterior semicircular canal and contacts the posterior fossa dura; Endolymphatic sac is inferior to this line.[6]

Korner's Septum (Figs 17A and B)

Mastoid develops from squamous and petrous bones. Persistence of petrosquamous suture as a bone plate separating superficial squamosal cells from the deep petrosal cells is the Korner's septum. It forms a false bottom of mastoid antrum.

Surgical importance—it may cause difficulty in locating the antrum and deeper cells, leading to incomplete removal

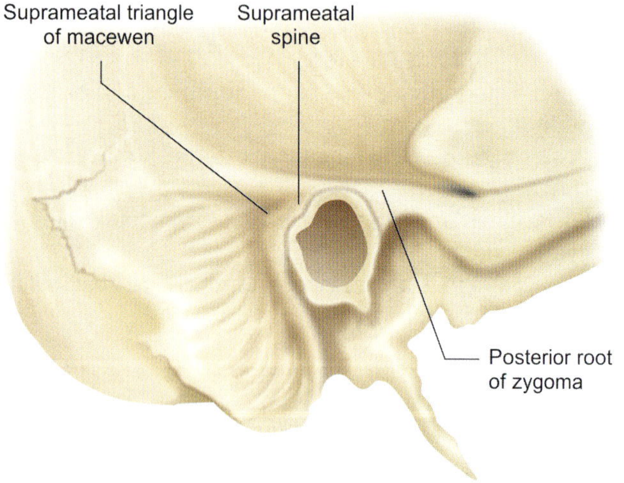

Fig. 13: Macewen's triangle

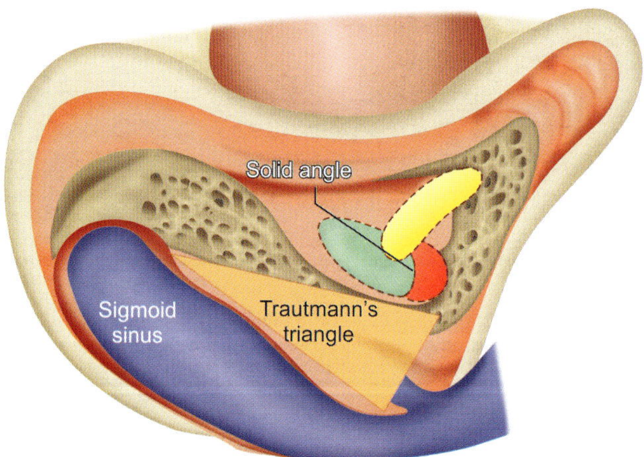

Fig. 15: Solid angle

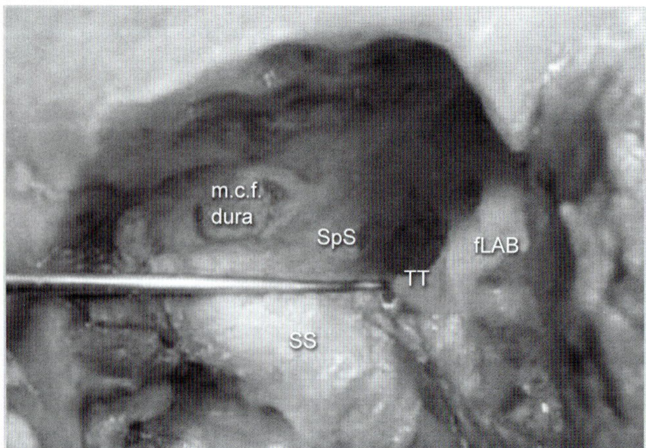

Fig. 14: Trautmann's triangle

Abbreviations: SS, sigmoid sinus; LAB, bony labyrinth; TT, trautmann's triangle; SPS, superior petrosal sinus; mcf dura, middle cranial fossa dura

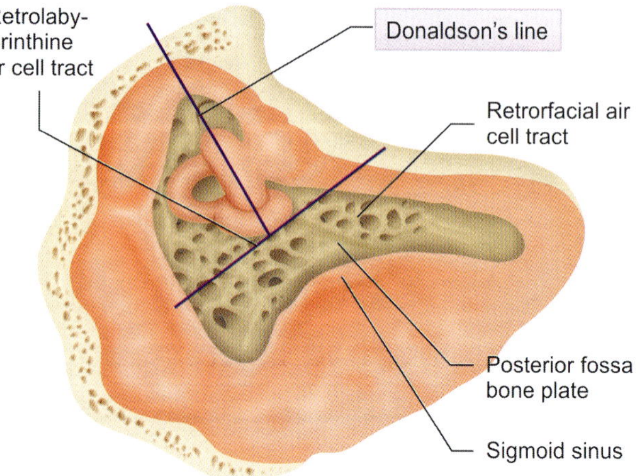

Fig. 16: Donaldson's line

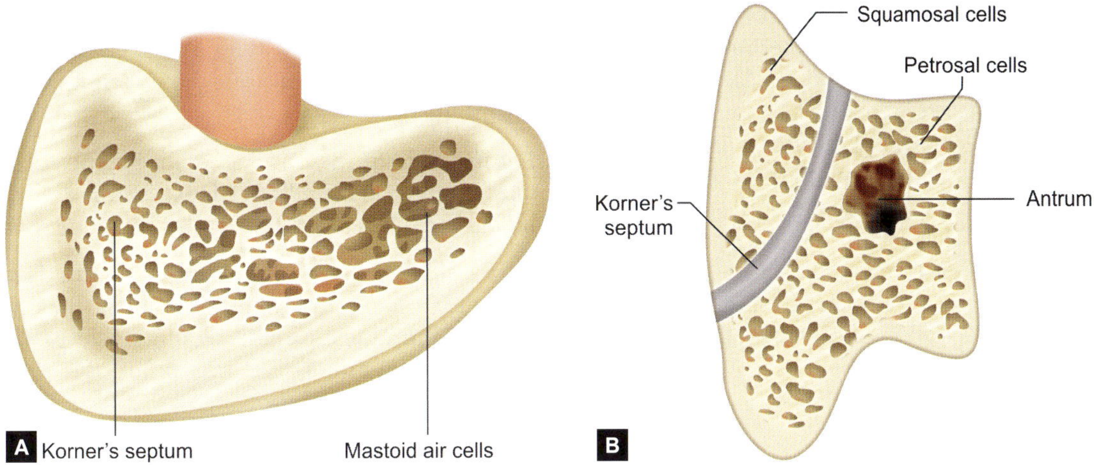

Figs 17A and B: (A) Korner's septum; (B) Petrosquamosal suture persisting as a bony plate (Korner's septum)

of disease at mastoidectomy. To reach the mastoid antrum the Korner's septum is to be removed.

Types of Mastoid Antrum (Figs 18A and B)

- Well-pneumatized or cellular (80%)—there are present many group of cells like tip cells, dural cells, perisinus cells, sinodural angle cells, retrofacial cells and zygomatic cells
- Sclerotic (20%) or acellular—there are present few or no cells
- Mixed (Diploeic)—mastoid consists of narrow spaces and a few air cells
- Extent of pneumatization depends on
  - Eustachian tube function (Tumarkin's theory)
  - Environment, hereditary (Diamart)
  - Infantile otitis media (Wittmark).

Pneumatization begins in the first year and is completed by 4–6 years of age.

Eustachian tube: It is also called auditory tube or pharyngotympanic tube that connects the nasopharynx to the middle ear. It is named after the anatomist Bartolomeo Eustachi of 16th century (Fig. 19).

It is 36 mm long → 12 mm bony
→ 24 mm cartilaginous

Greatest diameter is at pharyngeal orifice and narrowest part (Isthmus) is at the junction of the bony and cartilaginous portions. It is directed downwards, forwards and medially.

It forms an angle of 45⁰ with sagittal plane and 30⁰ with the horizontal plane.

Bony part: It extends from anterior wall of tympanic cavity to the angle of junction of squamous and petrous portions of temporal bone. Medially, it is related to the carotid canal. Tympanic end of the tube measures about 5 mm × 2 mm, situated in the anterior wall of the middle ear, slightly above the level of the floor.

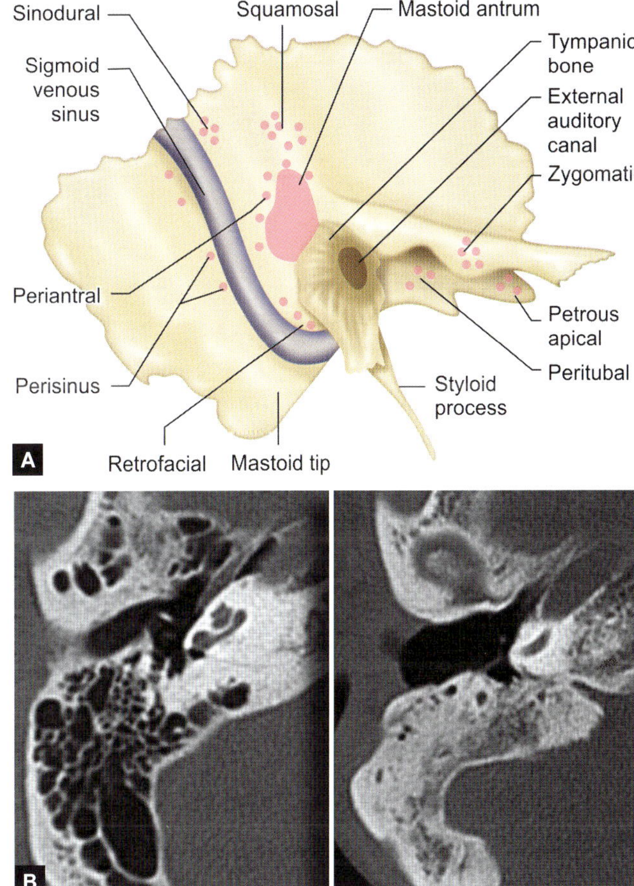

Figs 18A and B: (A) Mastoid air cells; (B) Normal pneumatization (left) and a completely sclerotic mastoid (right)

Cartilaginous part: Cartilage lies more in posteromedial wall of the tube. The gap is completed by fibrous membrane. It opens in the lateral wall of nasopharynx between petrous part of temporal bone and greater wings of sphenoid bone and raises an elevation called torus tubarius, 1–1.25 cm behind the posterior end of inferior terbinate. It is lined with ciliated columnar epithelium (Fig. 20).

Three muscles are related to the tube—tensor veli palatini (dilator tubae muscle), levator veli palatini and salpingopharyngeus. Tube is opened secondary to the voluntary contraction of tensor veli palatini which is attached to the lateral lamina of the tube and levator veli palatini which runs inferior and parallel to the cartilaginous part of the tube forming a bulk under the medial lamina that pushes upwards and medially during contraction.

Thus, it helps the tensor veli palatini muscles in assisting the opening of the tube (Figs 21A to C). Exact function of salpingopharyngeus muscles for opening of the tube is uncertain.

Elastin hinge: It is the cartilage at the junction of medial and lateral lamina at the roof rich in elastin fibers. By its recoil it makes the tube close when dilator is not in function.

Ostmann's pad of fat: It is a mass of fatty tissue related laterally to the membranous part of cartilaginious tube. It keeps the tube closed in resting position and thereby protecting the middle ear from reflux of nasopharyngeal secretions.

Mucosa of Eustachian tube: It is lined by pseudostratified ciliated columnar epithelium interspersed with goblet cells.

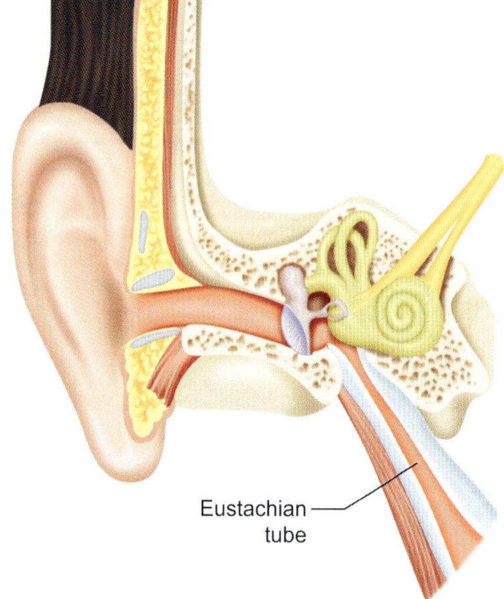

Fig. 19: Eustachian tube

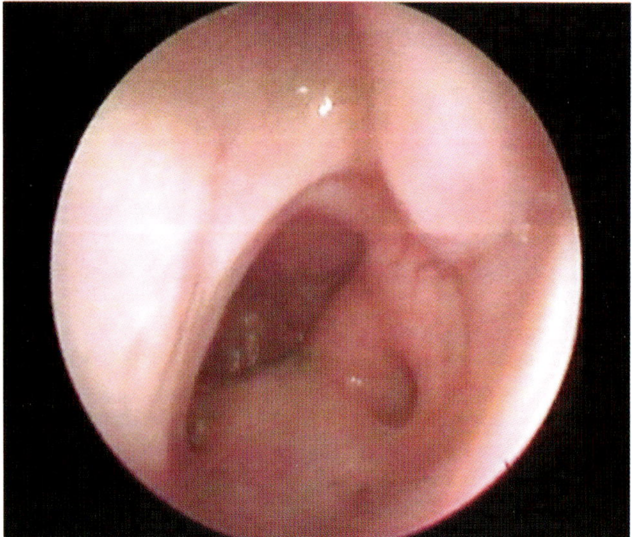

Fig. 20: Endoscopic view of pharyngeal opening of Eustachian tube in nasopharynx

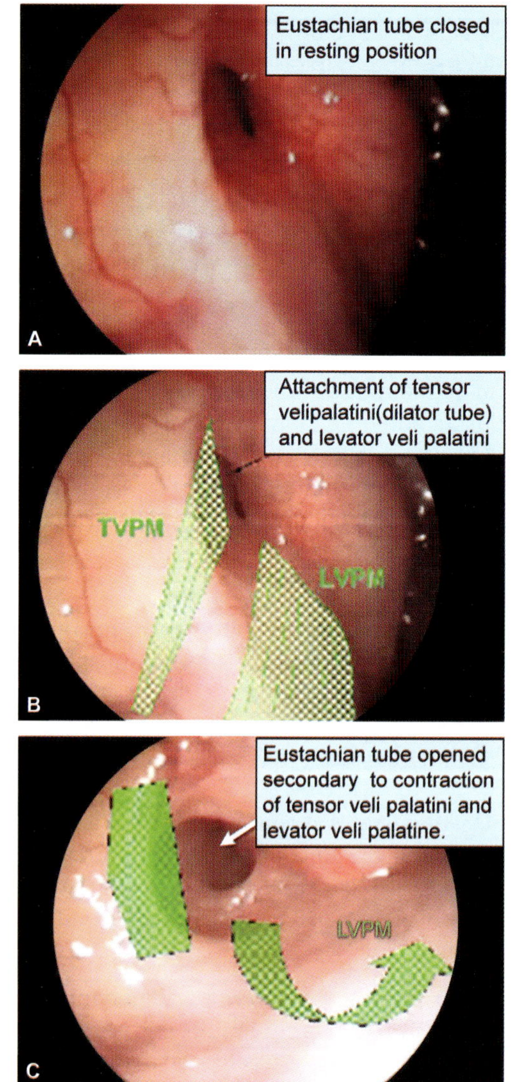

Figs 21A to C: Endoscopic view of Eustachian tube function and muscles related to the tube

Submucosa in cartilaginous part is rich in seromucinous glands. The cilia beat in the direction of nasopharynx to drain middle ear secretion into nasopharynx.

Nerve supply of Eustachian tube: Sensory and secretomotor supply are largely by tympanic branch of CN IX. Pharyngeal orifice is innervated through CN XI in about 50% of cases and maxillary portion of the CN V through pharyngeal branch of Pterygopalatine ganglion in other 50%. Tensor veli palatini and tensor tympani are supplied by mandibular branch of CN V. Levetor veli palatini and salpingopharyngeus are supplied by cranial part of CN XI through vagus.

Function of Eustachian Tube

- Ventilation and pressure equalization (Primary function)—Under normal circumstances Eustachian tube remains closed but it opens to ventilate the middle ear and to prevent damage by equalizing pressure between the middle ear and the atmosphere. Opening of Eustachian tube takes place during the act of deglutition. From mesotympanum air passes to attic, aditus ad antrum and mastoid air cells. Increase or decrease in middle ear pressure affects hearing by decreasing motion of tympanic membrane and osiscles of the ear. Eustachian tube opens periodically and equalizes the ear pressure on both sides of the tympanic membrane; closing of Eustachian tube protects the middle ear from unwanted pressure fluctuation and loud sound
- Drainage of middle ear secretion (Secondary function)—Eustachian tube drains mucus from the middle ear towards nasopharynx by cilliary clearance thus preventing infection from ascending to the middle ear. High pressure in the nasopharynx during forceful nose blowing and close nose swallowing may force nasopharyngeal secretion in the middle ear (Figs 22A and B).

In the newborn child Eustachian tube is—
- 1/2 the size of an adult
- Direction is more horizontal
- Pharyngeal opening is on a level with the palate
- No tubal elevation near the pharyngeal opening.

Ossicles are Malleus, Incus and Stapes

Malleus: It is—
- Shaped like mallet (Fig. 23)
- 8–9 mm long/ largest ossicle
- Weighing 23–25 mg
- Head/neck/three processes:
    - Manubrium (handle)
    - Anterior process
    - Lateral process
    - Head is situated in epitympanic recess. It articulates posteriorly with Incus
    - Neck—narrow part just below the head. It gives rise to the three processes

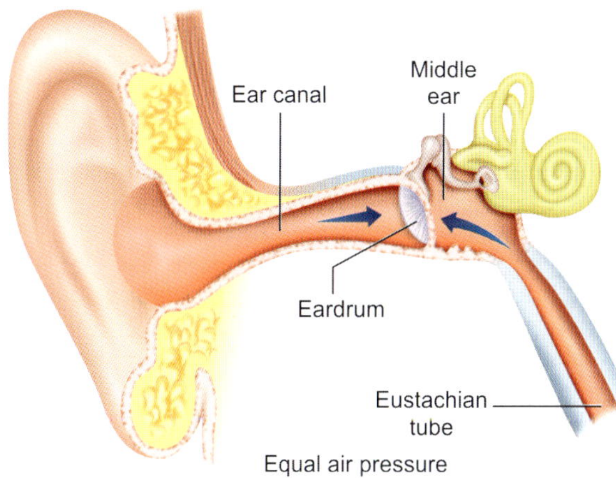

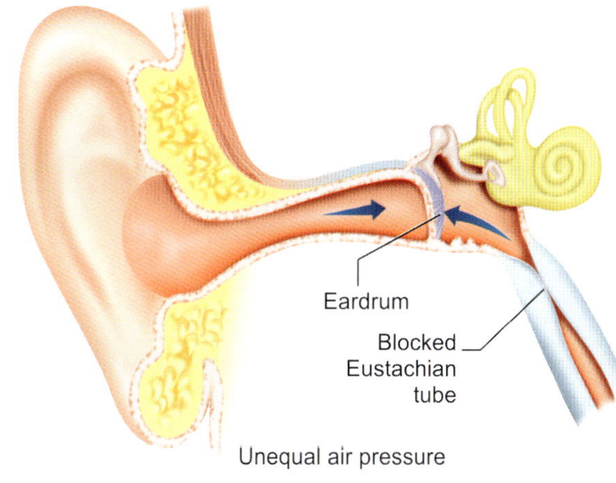

Figs 22A and B: Eustachian tube physiology

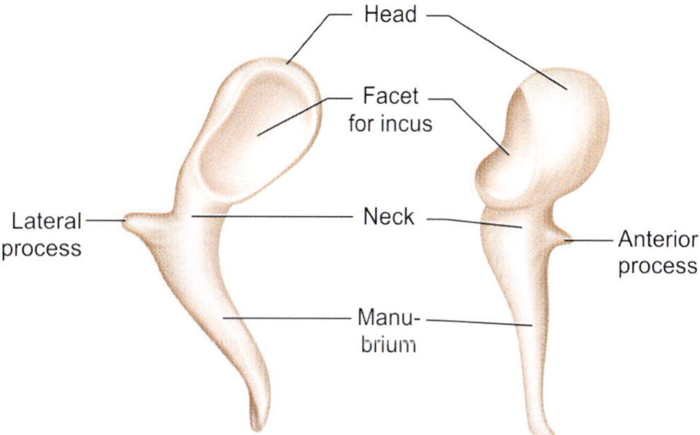

Fig. 23: The left malleus (posterior and medial view)

- Manubrium (Handle)—directed downwards, medially and backwards. Lateral margin is attached to TM. Medial surface upper end gives the insertion of tensor tympani
- Anterior process is directed forwards from neck. It is connected to petrotympanic fibers by ligamentous fibers
- Lateral process is directed laterally. It gives attachment to the anterior and posterior malleolar folds.

Incus: It is—

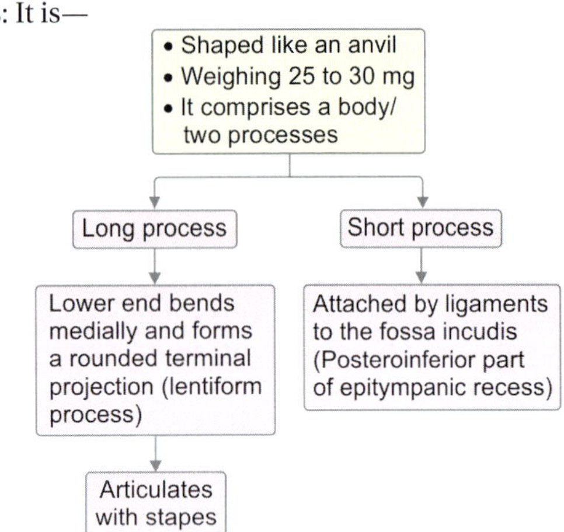

The long process descends vertically, behind and parallel to the handle of the malleus (Fig. 24).

The short process projects posteriorly and is attached by ligamentous fiber to the fossa incudis.

Stapes: It is—
- Shortest bone of the body
- Weighing 2.5–3 mg
- It comprises a head/neck/two limbs/a base

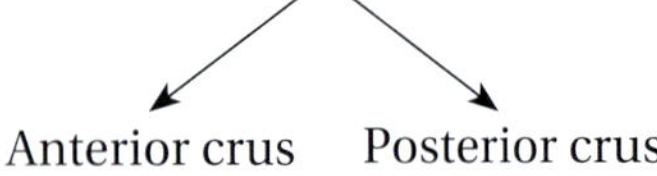

- Head—articulates with the lenticular process of Incus
- Stapedius tendon is inserted into the posterior part of the neck and upper part of the posterior crus

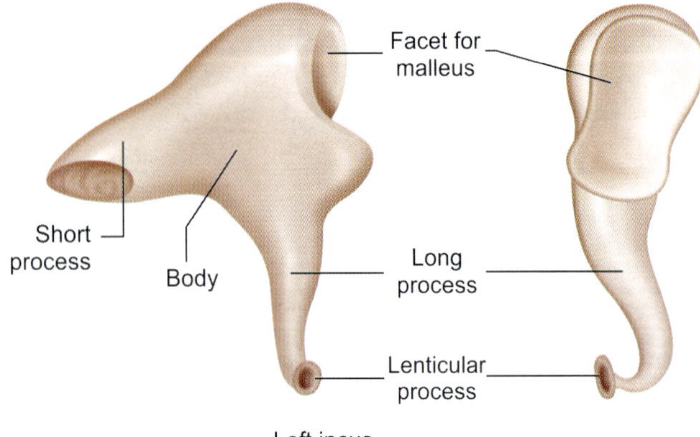

Fig. 24: Left incus (medial and anterior view)

- Anterior crus is thinner and less curved (than the posterior)
- Posterior crus is thicker and more curved
- Footplate lies in the fenestera vestibule
- It is attached to the oval window by the annular ligament
- Long axis is almost horizontal (Fig. 25).

The ossicles conduct sound energy from the tympanic membrane to the oval window and then to the inner ear fluid.

All the ossicles are supplied by branches of anterior, inferior and posterior tympanic arteries.

Muscles of tympanic cavity—There are two muscles:
- Tensor tympani
- Stapedius.

Tensor tympani: This muscle is contained in a bony canal above the bony part of the Eustachian tube. It arises from the cartilaginous part of the Eustachian tube and adjacent part of greater wing of sphenoid. It passes backwards and forms a tendon which bends laterally around the processus cochleariformis and is attached to the handle of malleus near its root.

Nerve Supply—It develops from the first arch and is supplied by branch of nerve to medial pterygoid (branch of mandibular nerve ← branch of trigeminal nerve).

Functions—It tenses the tympanic membrane.

Stapedius: It arises from a conical cavity in pyramidal eminence. The tendon passes forwards and is inserted into the posterior surface of neck of stapes.

Nerve Supply—It is second arch muscle and supplied by a branch of CN VII.

Action—In response to loud sound the muscles contracts exerting a protective dampening effect before vibration reach the inner ear. Paralysis of stapedius results in hyperacusis.

Blood supply of middle ear: It is supplied by 7 arteries. Two major vessels—
- Anterior tympanic, branch of Maxillary artery which supplies tympanic membrane

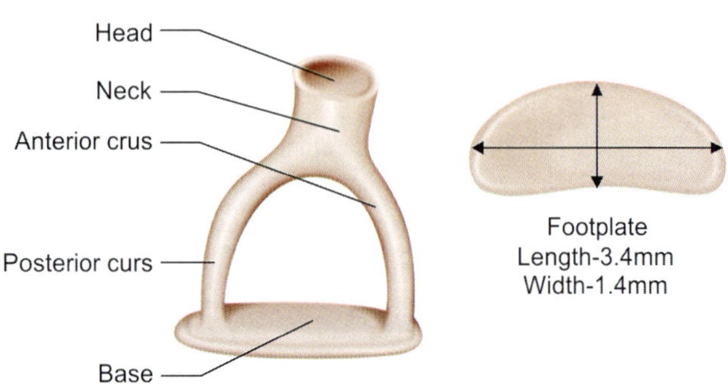

Fig. 25: Left stapes (superior view) and views of footplate from vestibule

- Posterior tympanic, branch of stylomastoid which is a branch of posterior auricular. It supplies middle ear and mastoid air cells.

Five Minor Vessels
- Petrosal branch of middle meningeal artery (runs along greater petrosal nerve)
- Superior tympanic branch of middle meningeal artery runs along canal for tensor tympani muscle
- Branch of artery of the pterygoid canal (runs along Eustachian tube)
- Caroticotympanic branch of internal carotid artery
- Inferior tympanic branch of ascending pharyngeal.

Veins are drain into—
- Pterygoid venous plexus
- Superior petrosal sinus.

Lymphatics:
- From middle ear drain into retropharyngeal and parotid nodes
- From Eustachian tube drain into retropharyngeal group.

Nerve supply: Middle ear is supplied by the nerves from the tympanic plexus which lies on the promontory.

It is formed by the tympanic branch of glossopharyngeal and caroticotympanic nerves from carotid plexus of the sympathetic.

It carries secretomotor fibers for parotid gland.

Course of secretomotor fibers to parotid: Inferior salivary nucleus → CN IX → tympanic branch →tympanic plexus → lesser petrosal nerve → otic ganglion → auriculotemporal nerve → parotid gland.

Section of tympanic branch of glossopharyngeal nerve can be carried out in middle ear in cases of Frey's syndrome.

Mastoid antrum is supplied by meningeal branch of mandibular nerve.

Mucosal folds of the middle ear[7]: The mucosa of the tympanic cavity is called tunica mucosa cavi tympani.

It lines the bony walls of the tympanic cavity and extends to cover the ossicles, muscles, ligaments and nerves—like the peritoneum covers the viscera in the abdomen, raising several folds and dividing the middle ear into various compartments.

Middle ear contains only air; all the structures lie outside the mucus membrane.

The mucosa is continuous anteriorly with mucosa of Eustachian tube and posteriorly with that of mastoid antrum and mastoid air cells.

The mucosa has a nonciliated simple epithelium. In its anterior and inferior part is ciliated columnar epithelium. Its posterior part is cuboidal type.

Anterior malleolar fold—It is reflected from the tympanic membrane over the anterior process and ligament of malleus as well as adjacent portion of the chorda tympani nerve.

Posterior malleolar fold—stretches between handle of malleus and the posterior tympanic wall. It surrounds the lateral ligament of the malleus and posterior part of chorda tympani nerve.

Each of these folds presents inferiorly a concave free border. Between the folds and tympanic membrane are two blind pouches, i.e. the anterior and posterior pouches of vonTröltsch. These are also called as anterior and posterior recesses of tympanic membrane.

Anterior pouch of von Tröltsch—It is a shallow pouch between tympanic membrane and anterior malleolar fold (Fig. 26A).

Posterior pouch of von Tröltsch — It is the blind pouch between tympanic membrane and posterior malleolar fold. It possesses superior, medial and lateral wall but is opened inferiorly towards posterior mesotympanum. Inferior edge of posterior malleolar fold contains the chorda tympani (Fig. 26B).

Prussak's space: Also called the superior recess of the tympanic membrane. This is closed pocket that lies between the pars flaccida of the TM and the neck of the malleus (Fig. 27).

Relations:
- Laterally—Pars flaccida of TM
- Medially—Neck of malleus
- Inferiorly—Lateral process of malleus and anterior and posterior malleolar folds
- Superiorly—Lateral malleolar fold.

Importance of Prussack's space

Epitympanic cholesteatomas originate in Prussack's space.

Cholesteatomas from Prussack's space may extend via three possible routes.

1. Posterior route (most common)—Cholesteatoma penetrates the superior incudal space lateral to the body of the incus

    ↓

    Cholesteatoma penetrates aditus ad antrum

    ↓

    Cholesteatoma gains access to mastoid

2. Inferior route—through posterior pouch of von Tröeltsch. This allows cholesteatoma to descend in the posterior masotympanum in the region of the stapes/RW/ST and FR.

3. Anterior extension (less common)—penetration anterior to head of malleus, it involves anterior tympanum. Downward growth involves the anterior mesotympanum and supratubal recess via anterior pouch of von Tröeltsch.

Incudal fold—It passes from the roof of the tympanic cavity to the body and short lymph of the incus.

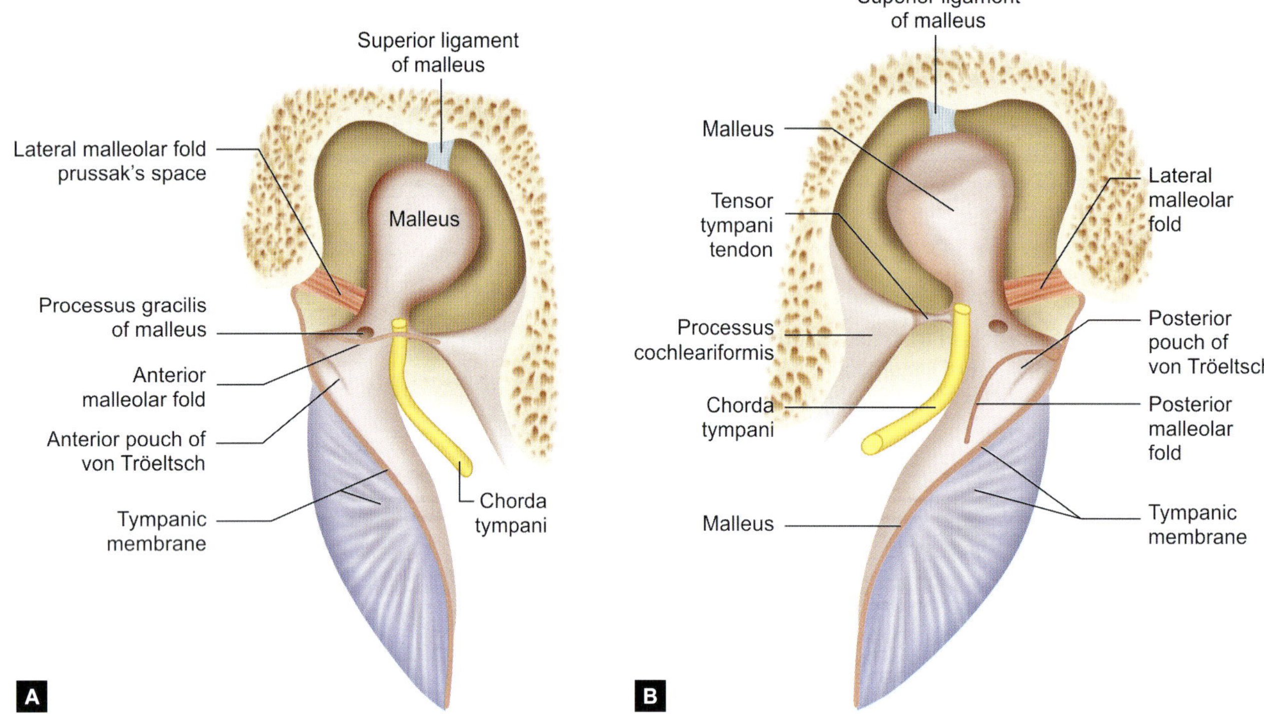

Figs 26A and B: (A) Anterior pouch of von Tröeltsch viewed from anterior aspect; (B) Posterior pouch of von Tröeltsch viewed from posterior aspect

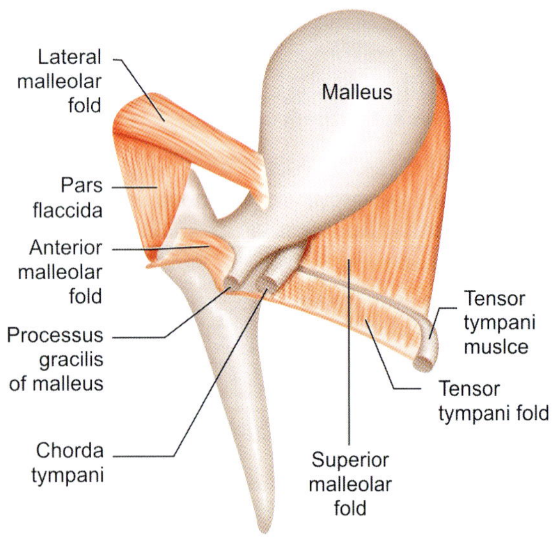

Fig. 27: Prussack's space viewed from front

The body, short process of incus, head of malleus and incudal fold completely separate off a lateral cupular portion (pars cupularis) of the epitympanic recess.

Stapedial folds[8]—Five folds are recognized that stretches from the posterior wall of the tympanic cavity and surrounds the stapes. These are:

1. Obturatoria stapedis that stretches between the two limbs of the suprastructure.
2. Anterior stapedial folds between the promontory and the anterior crus.
3. Posterior stapedial between the promontory and the posterior crus.
4. Plica stapedis between the pyramidal eminence and the posterior crus.
5. Superior stapedial folds that stretch from the long crus of incus to either crus of the stapes or from facial canal to the crura.

Tympanic Diaphragm

It is a series of mucosal folds and suspensory ligaments nearly separate the mesotympanum from epitympanum and mastoid (Figs 28A and B).

Major components of the partitions are:

- Malleus head/incus body
- Lateral and medial incudal folds
- Anterior and lateral malleolar folds
- Tensor tympani fold.

Only two narrow passage, anterior and posterior tympanic isthmuses, breach this diaphragm (Fig. 29).

Anterior isthmus tympani—larger and more consistent opening of the two, lies medial to the body of the incus and passes between the stapes and tensor tympani tendon.

Posterior isthmus tympani—It lies between medial incudal fold and posterior tympanic wall. When there is

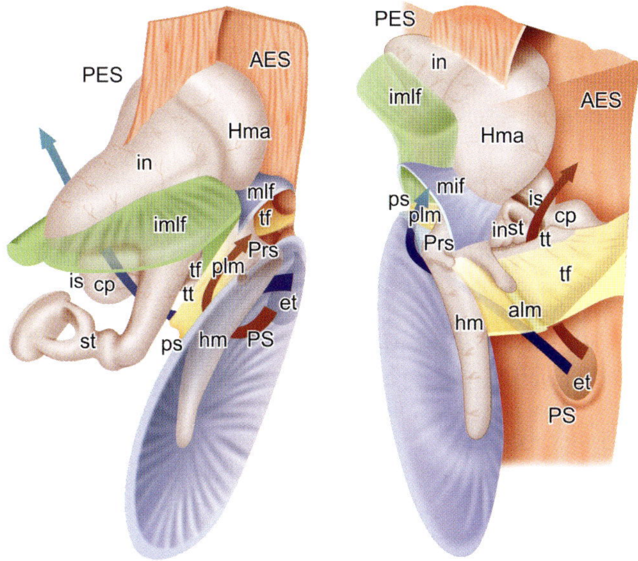

Figs 28A and B: (A) A schematic drawing representing the two independent aeration routes of the epitympanum. The major aeration route (red arrow) passing through the isthmus for the large upper unit (epitympanic compartments, antrum and mastoid cells); (B) The second independent aeration route (yellow arrow) for the smaller lower unit (Prussak's space) passing through the posterior pouch between the tympanum and the posterior malleolar ligamental fold

Abbreviations: PES, posterior epitympanic space; AES, anterior epitympanic space; in, incus; Hma, malleus head; imlf, incudo malleolar lateral fold; mlf, malleolar lateral fold; is, tympanic isthmus; st, stapes; cp, cochleariform process; et, eustachian tube; pml, posterior malleolar ligament; aml, anterior malleolar ligament; tf, tensor fold; PS, protympanic space; tt, tensor tympani; Prs, Prussak space; hm, malleus handle; ps, posterior spine

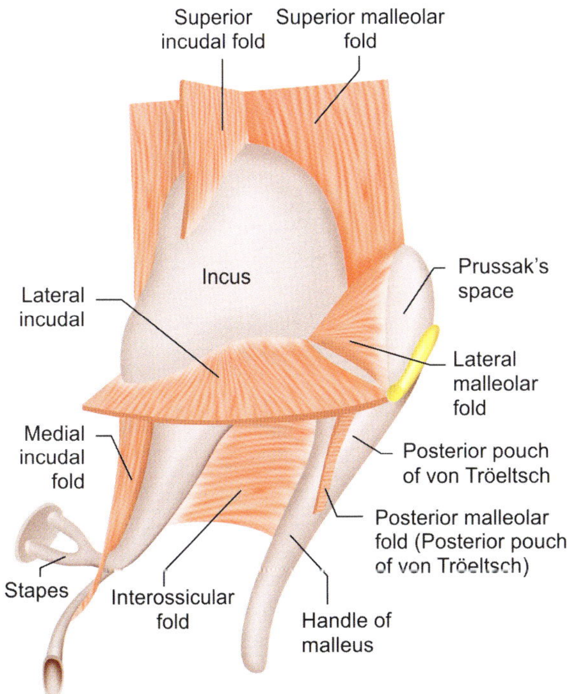

Fig. 29: Right middle ear (posterosuperior and lateral view)

no medial incudal fold, the tympanic isthmus is a single passage way. When tensor tympani fold is incomplete an additional large connection between the anterior attic and mesotympanum is present (<10% of ear).

Clinical Importance of Tympanic Diaphragm (Fig. 30)

- It resists spread of epitympanic cholesteatoma to the mesotympanum and vice versa
- The tympanic isthmi and aditus are important for aeration of mastoid. If they are blocked by disease (cholesteatoma/granulation/tympanosclerosis/oedema), negative pressure develops in mastoid followed by exudation, cholesteatoma, granulation or chronic infection, etc.

INNER EAR (LABYRINTH)

- It is important organ of hearing and balance
- It consists of a bony and a membranous labyrinth
- The membranous labyrinth is filled with a clear fluid called endolymph while the place between the membranous and bony labyrinth is filled with perilymph.

Bony Labyrinth (Fig. 31)

- Vestibule
- Semicircular canals (SCCs)
- Cochlea.

Vestibule

It is the central part of bony labyrinth, ovoid in shape (5 mm × 3 mm). Its lateral wall has the oval window (fenestra vestibuli). Inside its medial wall, there are two recesses, a spherical recess containing saccule and an elliptical recess lodging utricle. Below the elliptical recess, there is an opening of aqueduct of vestibule or endolymphatic duct. Posterior part of vestibule has five openings of three

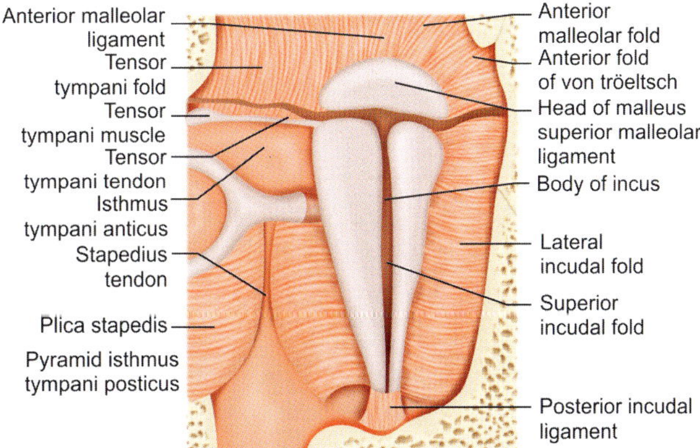

Fig. 30: Tympanic diaphragm (attic folds)

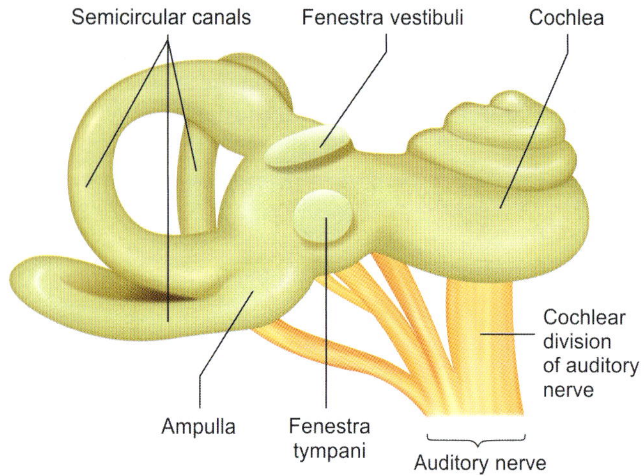

Fig. 31: Bony labyrinth

semicircular canals. Medial wall of vestibule is related to the internal auditory meatus (IAM).

Semicircular Canals (SCCs)

There are three semicircular canals—lateral, posterior and superior. All are about 0.8 mm in diameter. They lie in plane at right angle to one another. The posterior SCC is 18–22 mm long, superior SCC is 15–20 mm long, lateral SCC is 12–15 mm long.

Each canal has an ampulated end, opening independently into vestibule and nonampulated ends of posterior and superior canals unite to form a common channel—the crus commune. The three canals open into vestibule by five openings.

- Superior semicircular canal: It is placed transverse to the long-axis of petrous temporal bone and its upward convexity forms the arcuate eminence.
- Posterior semicircular canal: It runs parallel to the posterior surface of the petrous bone.
- Lateral semicircular canal: It lies 30 degrees to the horizontal plane; hence after 30 degrees flexion of head the lateral canal becomes horizontal.
- Superior semicircular canal of one side is parallel to the posterior semicircular canal of other side.

Cochlea

Bony cochlea is a coiled tube making 2.5 to 2.75 turns round a central pyramid of bone called modiolus. It measures 35 mm (long) × 5 mm (base to apex) and 9 mm across its base.

Apex of cochlea points towards anterosuperior part of medial wall of middle ear cavity (Figs 32A and B).

Base of cochlea points towards the fundus of the internal auditory meatus.

An osseous spiral lamina (a thin plate of bone) projects from the modular like the thread of a screw. It divides the cochlear canal into upper scala vestibule and lower scala tympani. Both the scalae are continous with each other at the apex of the cochlea through helicotrema.

Bony labyrinth contains perilymph resembling cerebrospinal fluid in its composition.

Scala vestibule is closed by footplate of stapes separating it from air-filled middle ear.

Scala tympani is closed by secondary tympanic membrane (round window). It is also connected with subarachnoid space through aqueduct of cochlea.

Membranous Labyrinth (Fig. 33)

- It lies within bony labyrinth
- It is filled with endolymphatic fluid
- Vestibulocochlea nerve fibers are distributed in the walls of membranous labyrinth

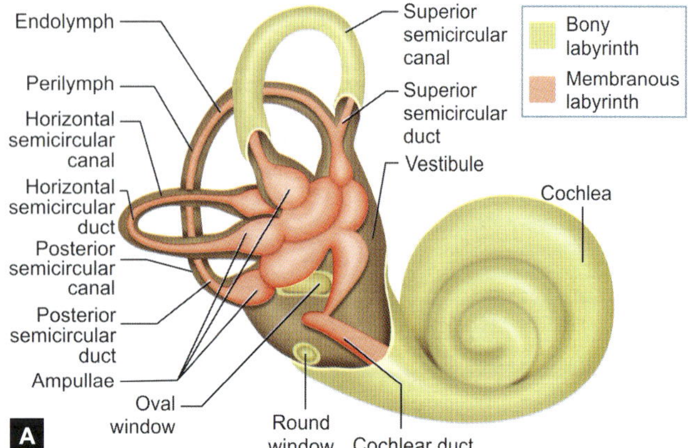

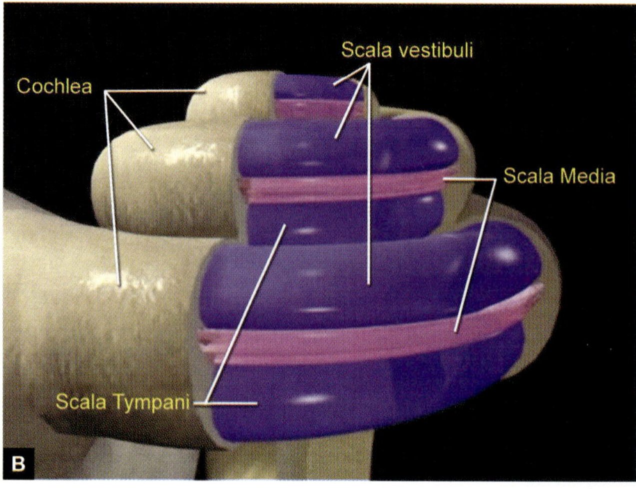

Figs 32A and B: (A) Medial wall of right bony labyrinth after removal of lateral wall; (B) Structure of cochlear canal after removal of bony wall

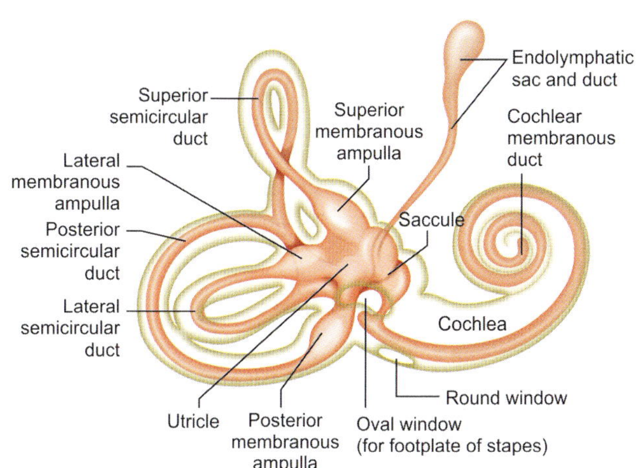

Fig. 33: Membranous labyrinth of right side

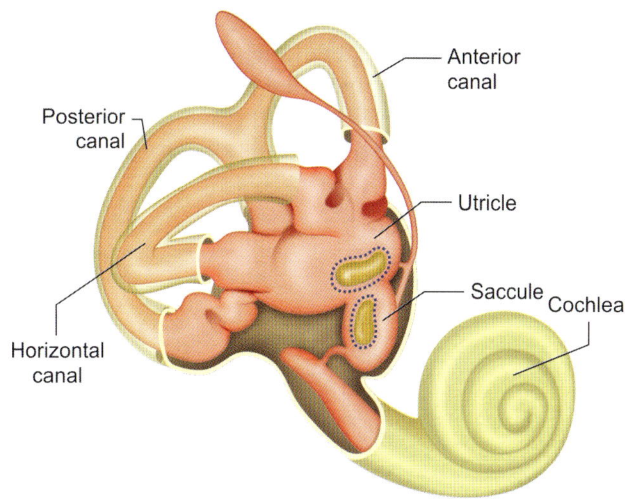

Fig. 34: Parts of membranous labyrinth

- It is separated from bony labyrinth by perilymphatic fluid.

Parts of Membranous Labyrinth (Fig. 34)

- Utricle
- Saccule
- Semicircular ducts
- Endolymphatic duct and sac
- Cochlear duct.

Utricle: It is an irregular oblong structure, larger than saccule. It is 2–5 mm in diameter. It occupies elliptical recess of bony vestibule (posterosuperior part). It receives five openings of three semicircular ducts. It is also connected to the saccule through utriculosaccular duct. A thick area of sensory epithelium of 3 mm × 2 mm is called utricular macula present in the lateral wall and adjoining floor. It is innervated by utricular fibers of vestibular nerve. It is concerned with linear acceleration and deacceleration.

Saccule: It is globular in shape, lies anterior to utricle. It is 1 to 1.5 mm in diameter. It occupies the spherical recess of bony vestibule and opposite the stapes foot plate. It is connected to the utricle through a 'Y-shaped' tube to endolymphatic duct and sac. It is also connected anteriorly to the basal end of cochlear duct by ductus reuniens. Its anterior wall has a 1 mm square thickening of sensory epithelium- macula which is set at right angle to the utricular macula. Its exact function is not known. It probably detects the linear acceleration such as gravity and straight line motion.

Semicircular ducts: They are three in number, corresponding exactly to the three bony canals. They open into utricle by five orifices, one being common to the medial end of superior and posterior duct. The ampulated end of each duct has a thickened ridge of neuroepithelium called crista ampullaris.

Crista ampullaris is the sensitive organ to the movement of endolymph. It responds to pressure changes of endolymph (while maculae response to gravitational changes).

Structures of Utricle, Saccule and Semicircular Ducts

- Each has three layers
- External layer—fibrous
- Middle layer—vascular connective tissue
- Internal layer—simple epithelium, it varies from squamous to cuboidal with a basement membrane having light and dark cells.

Structure of Crista Ampullaries

- It is the receptor organ of semicircular duct
- It is a crest of sensory epithelia supported on a mound of connective tissue and lies at a right angle to the longitudinal axis of the canal.

  The cilia of sensory hair cells project into a bulbous gelatinous mass, the cupula. Cupula extends from the surface of the crista to the ceiling of the ampulla forming a water tight swing door cell that moves with the endolymph. The gelatinous mass of cupula consists of polysaccharides. It contains canals into which the cilia of sensory cell project (Fig. 35).

Sensory Epithelium

It comprises hair cells and supporting cells of Hensen showing microvilli on upper ends. Hair cells are of two types (Fig. 36):

- Type I—It is flasked-shaped with single large cup-like nerve terminal at the base.
- Type II—It is cylindrical with multiple nerve terminals at the base.

Apical surface of both cells carry a long hair called Kinocilium (thicker) and a number of other cilium (40 to 100) called stereocilia or modified microvilli. Movement of stereocilia towards the Kinocilium results depolarization and away from the Kinocilium results hyperpolarization.

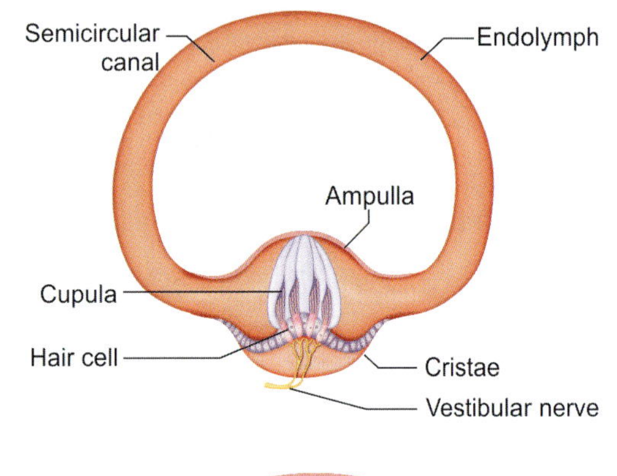

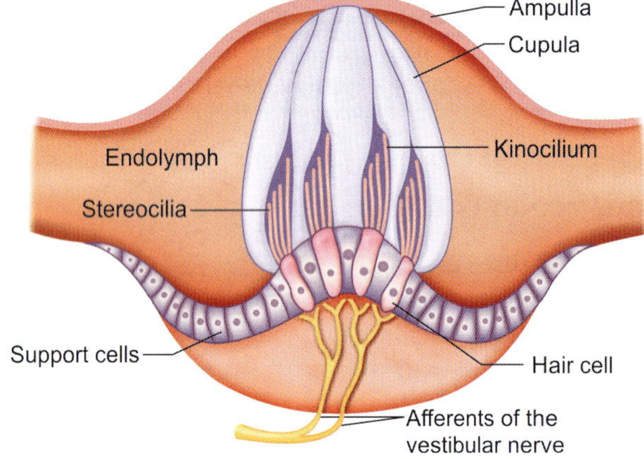

Fig. 35: Cut section of ampulla of semicircular canal

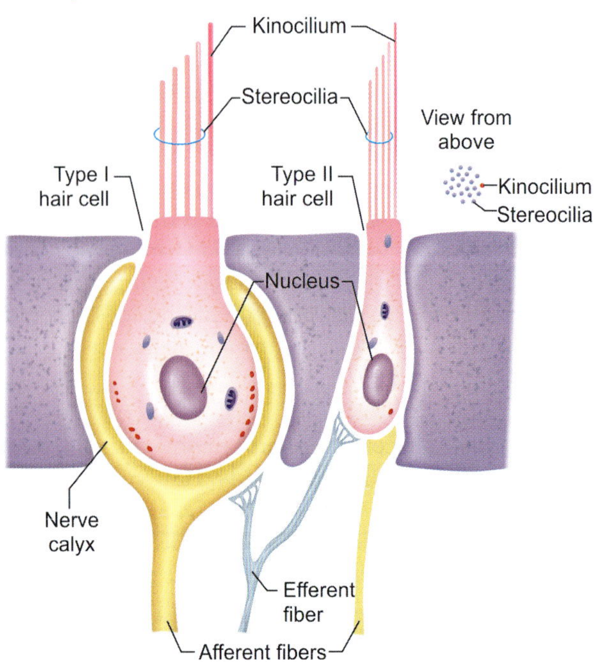

Fig. 36: Hair cells of semicircular canal

Semicircular Canal System

It is sensitive to angular acceleration of head. As head is rotated, endolymph within the duct tends to remain stationary in space because of inherent inertia. The resultant flow of endolymph with respect to the duct is resisted by elasticity of the gelatinous ampulla which becomes deflected resulting in bending of hair cells (Fig. 37).

Structure of Macula

It is the small area of sensory epithelium less than 1 mm square. It is found on the floor of utricle in a horizontal plane and on the anterior wall of saccule in the vertical plane. Macula has two parts:

- A sensory neuroepithelium made up of type I and type II cells
- Statoconial membrane, composed of small calcium carbonate crystals (otoconia) embedded in a mucopolysaccharide gel. The cilia of the hair cells project into the gelatinous layer. Position of statochonial membrane related to sensory epithelium varies according to the magnitude and direction of the force acting upon it. Shearing force between the structures results in the bending of hair cells embedded in the statoconial membrane (Figs 38A and B).

The linear, gravitational and head tilt movements cause displacement of otolithic membrane and thus stimulates hair cells which lie in different planes.

Vestibular Aqueduct and its Clinical Significant (Figs 39A and B)

- It is bony canal in temporal bone
- It carries endolymphatic duct containing endolymph
- It extends from vestibule (utricle and saccule) to endolymphatic sac, terminating in epidural space

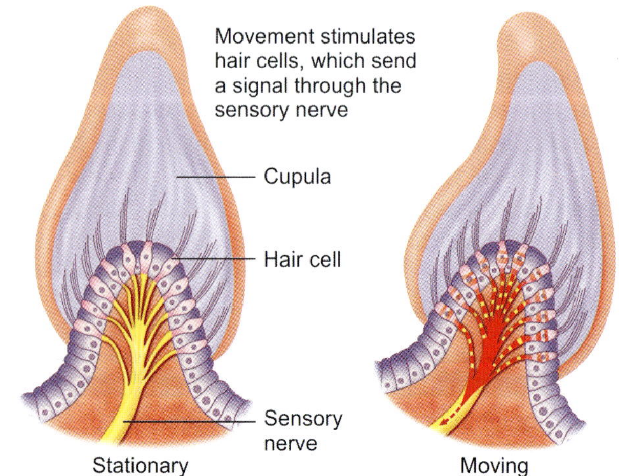

Fig. 37: Cupula is deflected as head is rotated resulting in bending of hair cells

- Its function is not known. It is thought to involve pressure regulation of membranous vestibule.

Enlarge Vestibular Aqueduct

- Predisposes to sensory neural hearing loss
- It is associated with Pendred's syndrome and anatomic deficits of cochlear modiolus.

Cochlear Aqueduct (Fig. 40)

- It is bony canal that connects the scala tympani (containing perilymph) to subarachnoid space (containing cerebrospinal fluid).
- The function is not known. It is thought to be involved in fluid and pressure regulation of the bony labyrinth.

Cochlear Duct

It lies within the bony cochlea (Fig. 41A). Bony cochlea has three compartments:

- Scala vestibuli
- Scala tympani
- Scala media or membranous cochlea (also called cochlear duct)—It is blind coiled tube connected to the saccule by ductus reuniens. It is triangular in cross section. It has three wall formed by:
  - The basilar membrane stretches from spiral lamina to the spiral ligament. It has two zones: zona arcuata (supported by sensory area of the cochlea called organ of corti. It has a length of 35 mm and width 0.21 to 0.36 mm), zona pectinata

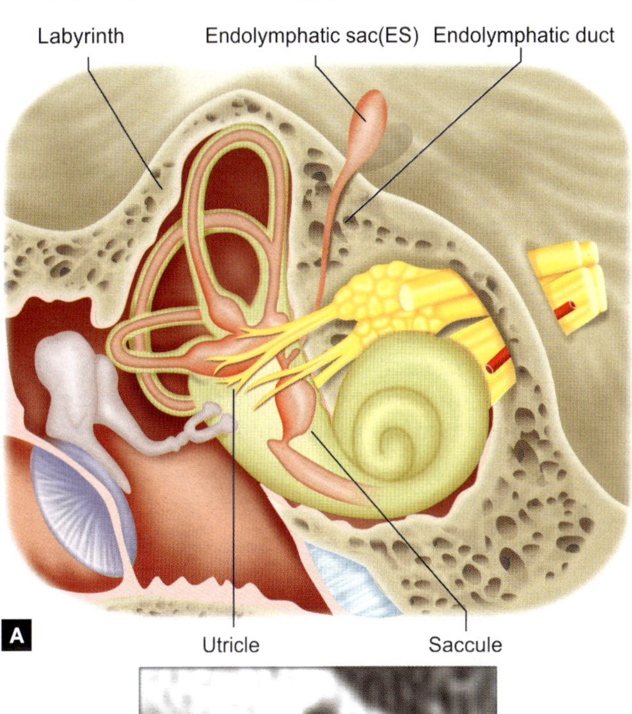

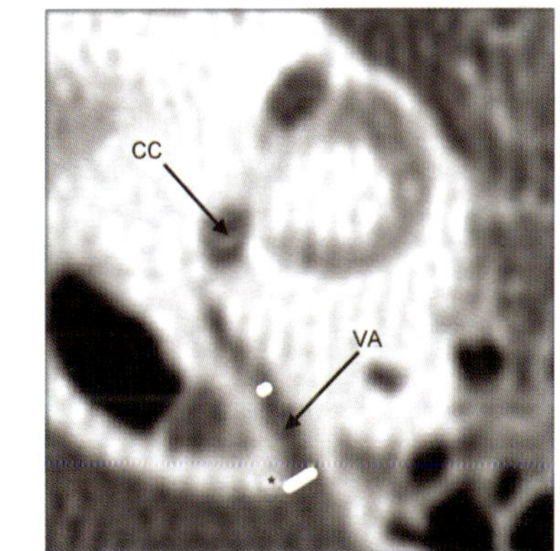

Figs 39A and B: (A) Vestibular aqueduct with endolymphatic duct ending to endolymphatic sac in epidural space; (B) Axial CT of temporal bone showing vestibular aqueduct (VA) and crus commune (CC)

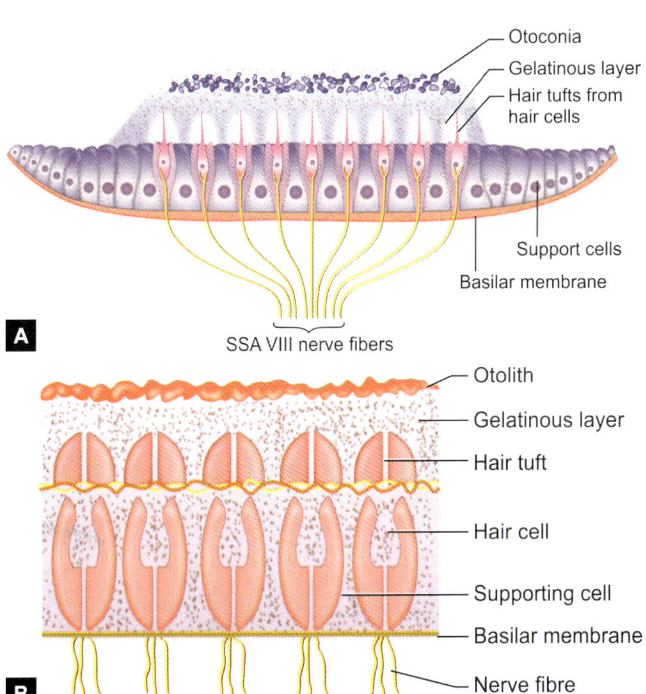

Figs 38A and B: (A) Macula of utricle and saccule; (B) Otolith organ

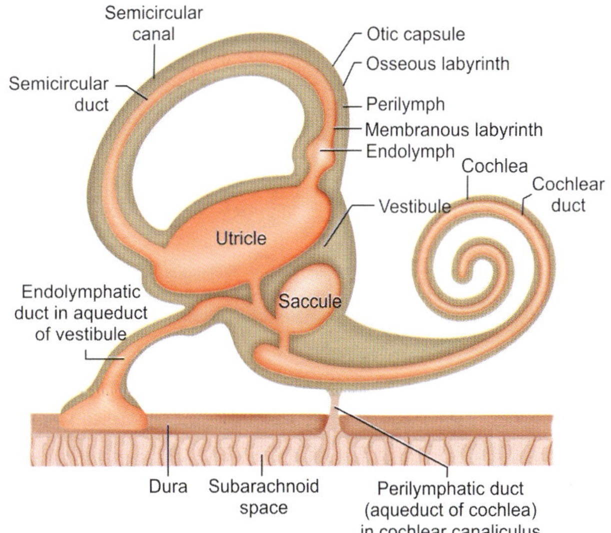

Fig. 40: Cochlear aqueduct

– The Reissner's membrane (vestibular membrane)—It lies over the basilar membrane below the scala vestibule

– The stria vascularis—It contains vacular epithelium. It is concerned with secretion of endolymph.

Organ of Corti (Fig. 41B)

- It is the sense organ of hearing.
- It is situated on the basilar membrane.
- Important components are:
  – Tunnel of corti—It is formed by inner rod cells (6000) and outer rods (4000). It contains corti lymph resembling perilymph. Its exact function is not known.

– Hair cells—These are important receptor cells of hearing. They transduce sound energy into electrical energy. Inner hair cells form a single row (3500) which is richly supplied by afferent cochlear fibers and important in the transmission of auditory impulses, carrying information from hair cells to brain. Outer hair cells (12,000) are arranged in three to four layers which receive efferent innervations from olivary complex, carrying information from brain to hair cells and modulating the function of inner hair cells.

Supporting Cells

Deiter's cells—It is situated between outer hair cells giving support to outer hair cells.

Cells of Hansen (lie outside the Deiter's cell).

Tectorial membrane—It is gelatinous matrix with delicate fibers. It overlies the organ of corti. Shearing force between hair cell and tectorial membrane produces the stimulus to hair cells.

Blood Supply of Labyrinth (Flowchart 1)

Apical regions of modiolus are drained by anterior spiral vein and basal regions drain into posterior spiral vein. This too spiral veins join with anterior and posterior branches of vestibular vein to form vein of cochlear aqueduct that empties into jugular bulb (Fig. 42).

Anterior part of vestibular labyrinth is drained by anterior vestibular vein that becomes the labyrinthine vein

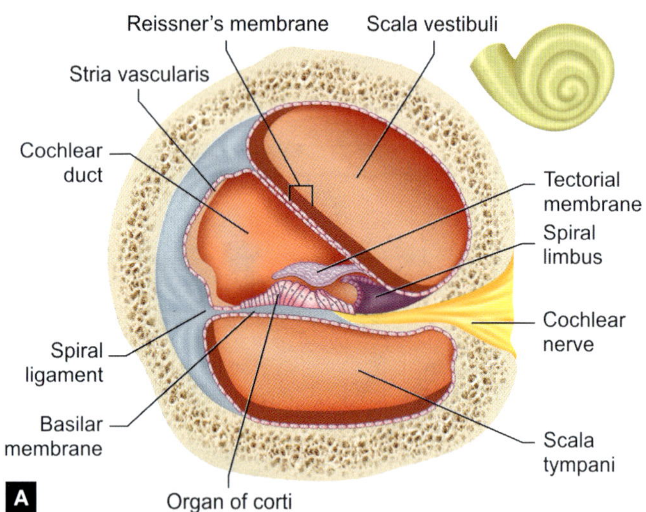

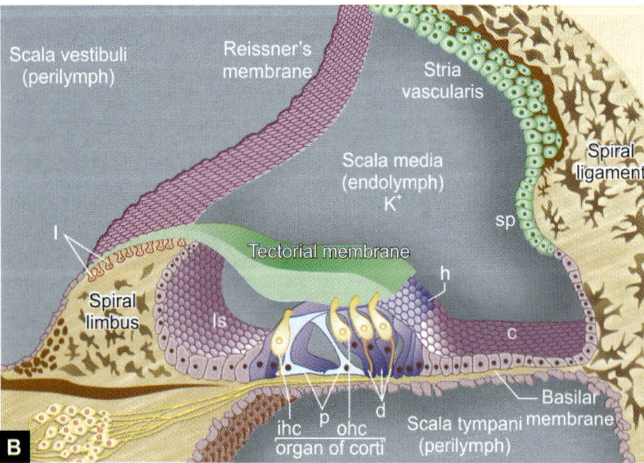

Figs 41A and B: (A) Cut section of bony cochlea; (B) Organ of corti: (sp) spiral prominence, (i) interdental cells, pillar cells (p), cells of Deiters (d), cells of Hansen (h), epithelial cells of the inner sulcus (is), inner hair cells (ihc) and the triple row of outer hair cells (ohc)

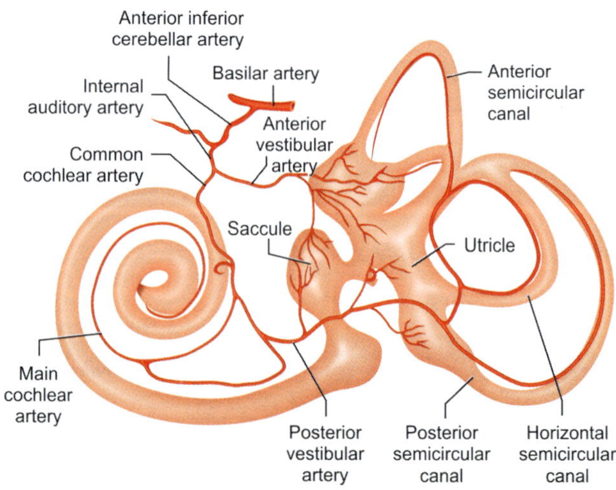

Fig. 42: Blood supply of labyrinth

Flowchart 1: Blood supply of labyrinth

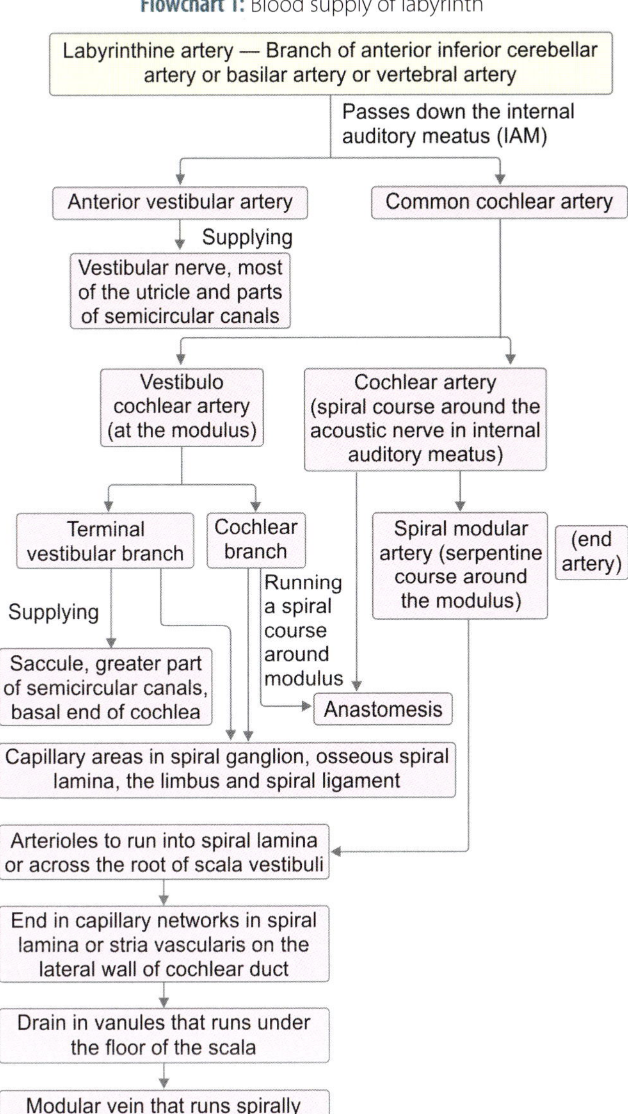

accompanying the labyrinthine artery ends in the superior petrosal sinus. Posterior part of the vestibular labyrinthine is drained by vein of vestibular aqueduct alongside the endolymphatic duct that empties in sigmoid sinus.

Key Points

Blood supply to the inner ear is independent of blood supply to middle ear and bony otic capsule. There is no cross circulation between the two.

Blood supply to cochlea and vestibular labyrinth is segmental—independent ischemic damage can occur to these organs.

Tracing of Neural Sound Pathway from Cochlea to Brain (Fig. 43)

Hair cells are innervated by dendrites of bipolar cells of spiral ganglion situated in Rosenthal's canal (canal along the osseous spiral lamina):

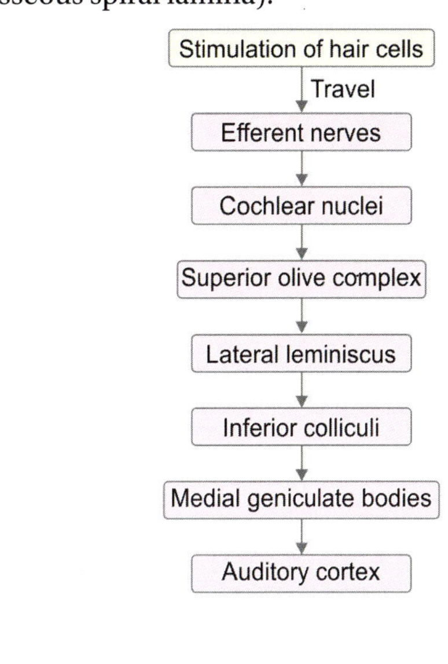

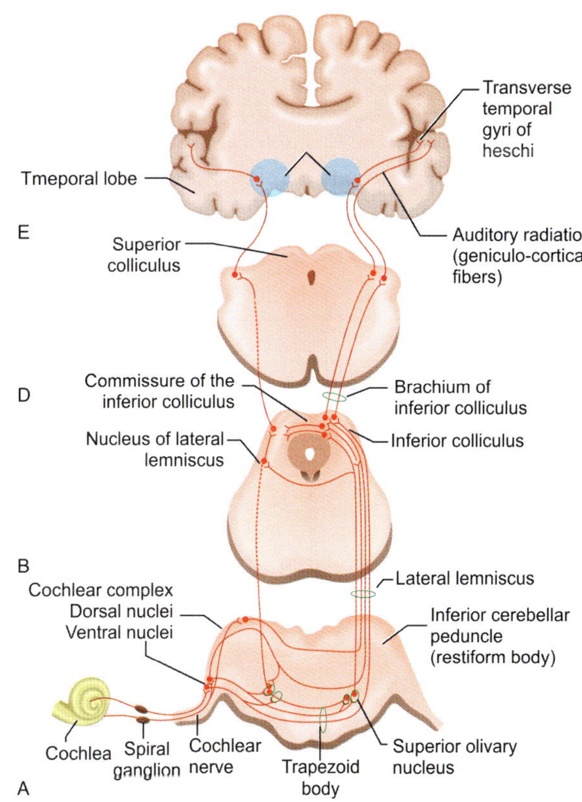

Fig. 43: Auditory pathway from the right cochlea

At the level of superior olivary complex and above—there is significant crossover between left and right sides. Remember mnemonic *E.coli*—MA

- Vestibulocochlear nerve :
  The VIII nerve divides deep in IAM (Internal acoustic meatus) into two:

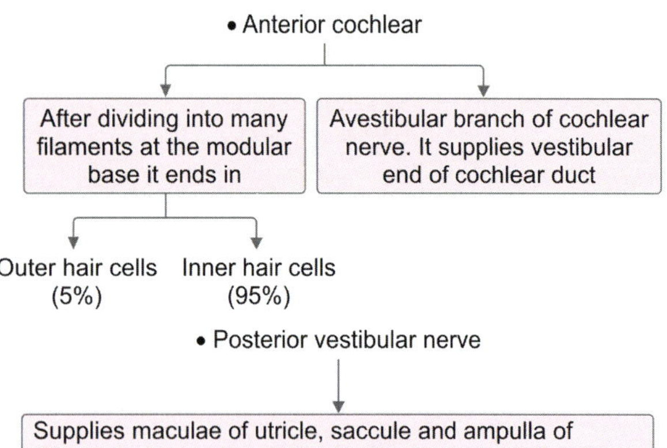

Key Points

Firing patterns of semicircular ducts upon stimulation:
- The neural fibers from each canal fire at a basal rate
- In the horizontal canal displacement of hair cells stereocillia toward the vestibule (ampullopetal) increases the firing rate whereas displacement away from the vestibule (ampullofugal) decreases the rate. Opposite situation exists in posterior and superior canals.

Development of Ear

Each part of ear develops independently and the deformity of one does not usually presuppose deformity of another.

Pinna

In the 5th week of intrauterine life pinna develops from the growth of mesenchymal tissue of first and second branchial arches that forms six hillocks of His.[1] Around the primitive meatus these auricular hillocks fuse to form the definite pinna which is gradually translocated from the side of the neck to a more cranial and lateral site by the end of third month.

Differentiation of Pinna (Fig. 44)[9]

- First branchial arch:
  - First hillock—tragus
  - Second hillock—crus of helix
  - Third hillock—helix

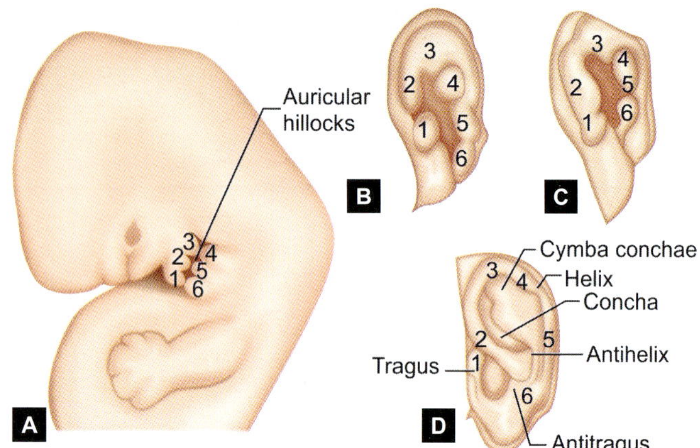

Figs 44A to D: Development of pinna: (A) Six auricular hillocks of His around the dorsal end of first branchial cleft (6 weeks embryo). (B to D) Progressive fusion of hillocks and formation of pinna (12 weeks)

- Second branchial arch:
  - Fourth hillock—antihelix
  - Fifth hillock—antitragus
  - Sixth hillock—lobule and lower helix.

External Auditory Canal (EAC)

It develops from the first branchial cleft of ectodermal origin during the 5th week of embryonic development. At the beginning of 3rd month a meatal plug forms at the bottom of the cleft. During the 7th month, the plug disappears resulting in canalization and creation of EAC. Epithelial lining contributes to the development of the definite Tympanic membrane.[10]

Tympanic Membrane

It develops from three germinal layers:
- Ectoderm—forming the outer epithelial layer
- Mesoderm—forming the middle fibrous layer
- Entoderm—forming the inner mucosal layer.

Middle ear: Develops from first branchial pouch that elongates to form the tubotympanic recess. Tubotympanic recess gives rise to tympanic cavity, Eustachian tube and mastoid air cells. The ossicles begin to condense from mesenchyme of the first and second pharyngeal arches in the 7th week. Middle ear muscles begin forming in the 9th week (Figs 45A and B).

Branchial arch derivatives in the middle ear:
- 1st branchial arch:
  - Mechel's cartilage −>malleus, incus
  - Mesoderm −>tensor tympani muscle.
- 2nd branchial arch:
  Reichert's cartilage −>stapes
  Mesoderm −> stapedius muscle.

*Footplate of stapes and annular ligament are derived from otic capsule.

Ossicles[11] assume to function with attaching malleus to tympanic membrane and stapes to oval window by 9 months. Sound is transmitted from tympanic membrane to cochlea via ossicular chain and then transduced into neural impulses via organ of corti.

Facial nerve is a nerve of second branchial arch. The developing nerve divides the blastema (condensation of second arch mesenchymal cells) into stapes, interhyale (stapedius muscle picasa) and laterohyale (precursor of the posterior wall of the middle ear) by the 4.5 weeks. The intraosseous course of the nerve is dependent on this bony expansion.

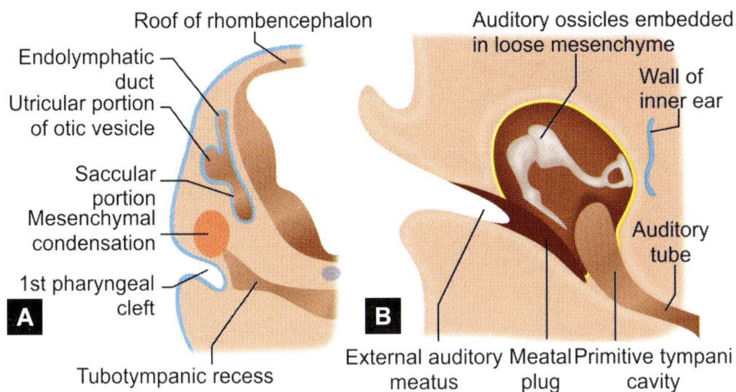

Figs 45A and B: (A) Cross-section showing tubotympanic recess, first pharyngeal cleft and mesenchymal condensation with ossicular development (7th weeks embryo); (B) Middle ear with cartilaginous precursors of ossicles, primitive tympanic membrane and external auditory canal resulting from extension of meatal plug to the tympanic cavity (9th week embryo)

Inner Ear

Membranous Labyrinth

- In the 3rd week, a thickening of surface ectoderm on each side of rhombencephalon (hindbrain) called otic placode develops; later it is shifting caudally to the level of the 2nd branchial arch
- In the 4th week, each otic placodes invaginates to form an otic pit which in term forming otic vesicle. Otic vesicle is the precursor of the definitive membranous labyrinth differentiating into three parts:
  - Dorsomedial elongated endolymphatic part forming endolymphatic duct and sac
  - Central expanded utricular part forming utricle and three semicircular ducts arising from utricular diverticula in the 7th week
  - Ventral conical saccular part forming saccule, cochlear duct (that coils about 2.5 turns) and ductus reunions (connecting saccule and cochlear duct) in the 5th week (Fig. 46).

Organ of Corti is innervated by spiral ganglion, its fibers forming cochlear branch of CN VIII that synapses to medial geniculate body. Macula of the utricle and saccule and cristae of three semicircular canals are innervated by the vestibular ganglion, its fibers forming vestibular branch of CN VIII (Figs 47A to D).

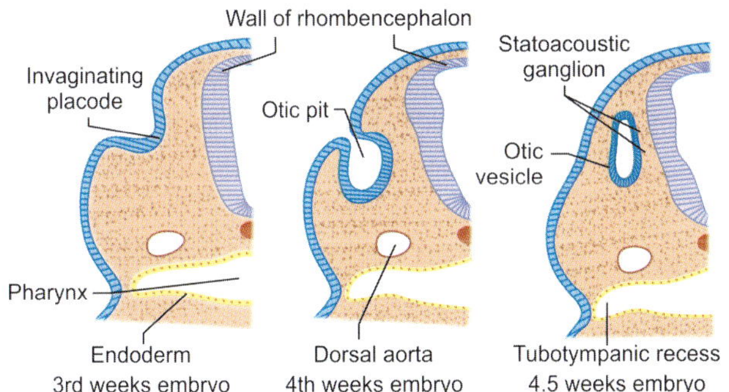

Fig. 46: Transverse section through rhombencephalon showing otic placode invaginating to form otic pit that forms otic vesicle—the precursor of membranous labyrinth

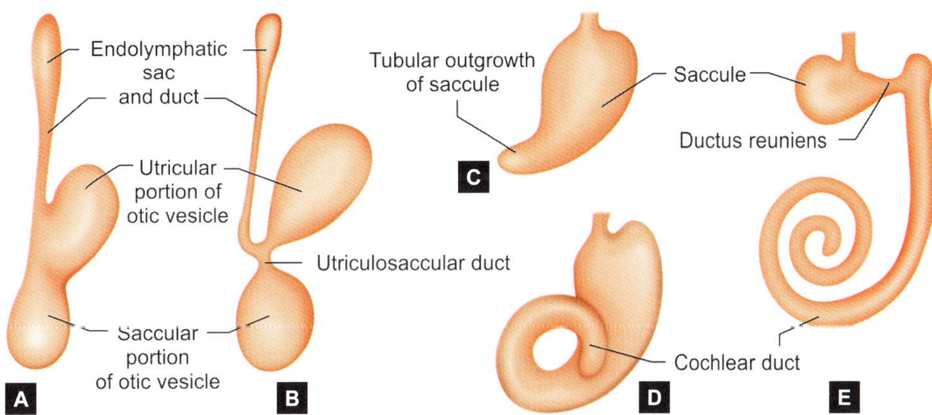

Figs 47A to E: Otocyst showing development of utricle, saccule and cochlear duct

Bony Labyrinth

In the 9th week, otic vesicle induces mesenchyme of membranous labyrinth to chondrify forming cartilaginous otic capsule that undergoes vacuolization forming perilymphatic space around the membranous labyrinth. The otic capsule subsequently ossifies to form bony labyrinth by 23rd weeks.

Modular Regulation[12]

Most of the gene responsible for the regulation of inner ear formation and its morphogenesis are members of the homeobox gene family, such as *Pax, Msx* and *Otx* homeobox genes. The development of inner ear structure, such as the cochlea is regulated by *D1x5/D1x6, Otx1/Otx2* and *Pax2* which in turn are controlled by the master gene *Shh. Shh* is secreted by notochord.[13]

REFERENCES

1. Anthony Wright. Anatomy and ultra structure of the inner ear. Basic sciences, Scott Brown's otolaryngology. 5th edition. 1987. p 1-46.
2. Tony Wright. Anatomy and Development of the ear and hearing. Disease of the ear edited by Harold Ludman & Tony Wright. 6th edition. 2006. p-9
3. Ralph A Nelson. Temporal bone surgical dissection manual, 1st edition, Los Angles: Published by House Ear Institute. 1982. p 41-4.
4. Agadurappa Mahadevaiah, Bhavin Parikh. Surgical techniques in chronic otitis media and otosclerosis, Text and Atlas. 2nd edition. 2011. p 6-7.
5. Lt Col BS Tuli et al. Text book of ear, nose and throat, 1st edition. 2005. p 11-20.
6. Aina Julianna Gulya. Anatomy of the ear and temporal bone, Glasscock-Shambough Surgery of ear, 5th edition. 2007. p 35-57.
7. Proctor B. The development of the middle ear spaces and their surgical significance. Journal of laryngology and otology. 1964;78:631-49.
8. Proctor B. Chronic otitis media and mastoiditis chapter 29, Otolaryngology Vol II– Paparella, 3rd edition. 1991. p1355-6.
9. www.wikilectures. eu/index.php/development of the ear- Cached16 Feb 2012.
10. Langman's Medical embryology, Jan Langman(author), TW Sadler (editor).
11. The developing human: Clinically oriented Embryology. 9e, Keith L Moore, M.Sc, Ph.D, FIAC, FRSM, FAAA(author), T.V.N Persaud MD, Ph.D, DSc, FRCPath(Lond), FAAA(author), Mark G Torchia, M.Sc, Ph.D (author).
12. http://download.videohelp.com/visualis.net/devt.html.
13. Chatterjee A, Kraus S, Lufkin P, Thomas (2010). A symphony of inner ear developmental control genes. Retrieved April 20. 2013.

Physiology of Hearing

Asok K Saha

INTRODUCTION

Hearing is important to develop language for communication and to determine the unseen sound sources for location. Normal hearing is a process involving—

Sound as a stimulus

↓

Conduction of stimulus to sensory organs of hearing

↓

Sensory transduction of stimulus at organs of hearing

↓

Neural transmission of the signal

↓

Central auditory processing of the signal at the brain.[1]

Physics and Sound

Sound is a subjective sensation generated from a vibrating system that causes waves of alternating compression (dense molecule) and rarefraction (loose molecule) of an elastic medium.

- It travels faster in denser medium in waveform
- Displacement of air molecule lags by one fourth of a cycle
- The simple sound is sinusoidal wave or pure tone.

Basic relation is $P = RV$, where P = Pressure of the sound wave, V = Velocity of the air molecules, R = Impedance which is the function of the medium in which the sound is traveling.

Physical Dimensions of Sound

- Intensity
- Frequency
- Complexity.

Whereas Perceptual Dimensions

- Loudness
- Pitch
- Timbre.

Intensity

It refers to the strength of the sound, i.e. power transmitted by sound wave through a unit area and is an average taken over a whole cycle. It is dependent on pressure and velocity.

Intensity = (Peak pressure × Peak velocity)/2. The factor 2 is a function of the shape of the waveform. Displacement produced by sound wave varies in inverse proportion to the frequency, if intensity is constant. Therefore, for a constant intensity, low-frequency vibrations produce greater displacements.[2]

Measurement of root mean square (RMS)[3] helps to eliminate the shape of waveform out of equation. Calculation is done by taking the value of the pressure/ or velocity at each moment in the waveform, squaring it and averaging all the squared values over the waveform. Finally, the square root is taken of the average. RMS values are helpful as relationship of intensity, pressure and velocity reserves over all the shapes of the waveform.

Intensity = RMS pressure²/2R

= RMS velocity² × R

Decibel: It is the unit used to measure the intensity of a sound. It is named after Alexander Graham Bell, the inventor of the telephone. It is 1/10th of a bel.

1 bel = Log of intensity of sound/intensity of a standard sound

dB = 10 log₁₀ Im/Iref

Im = Measure intensity

Iref = reference intensity

The range of human hearing is 0–120 dB.

Decibel (dB) scale for sound pressure level (SPL)

0 dB = 0.0002 dyne/cm^2 (threshold)

120 dB= 200 dyne/cm^2 (limit)

A difference of 1 dB is the minimum perceptible change in volume of the sound (Table 1).

The decibel scale has the following characteristics:

- It is logarithmic and incorporates a ratio
- It is not linear (i.e. an increase from 1 to 3 dB is not equal to an increase from 5 to 7dB)
- It is relative measure (i.e. 0 dB does not indicate the absence of sound)
- It is expressed with different reference levels.

Frequency

Frequency refers to the number of cycles (complete oscillations) of a vibrating body per unit of time. The psychoacoustic equivalent of frequency is pitch. Pitch becomes higher when the frequency of sound increases (Fig. 1).

Hertz (Hz): It is the unit used to measure frequency (also called cycles per second or CPS). It is named after German scientist Heinrich Rudolph Hertz.

Human ear is able to hear from 20–20,000 Hz. Dogs hear above 20,000 Hz (Supersonic). Bats hear below 20 Hz (Subsonic).

Frequency range is measured in octave bands (octave scale), i.e. each frequency is double the previous one, i.e. 250, 500, 1000, 2000, 4000 Hz, etc.

Amplitude of sound waves refers the intensity of sound, hence the loudness.

Human ear is sensitive to sound over a wide range of amplitude 0.0002–200 dyne/cm^2.

Complexity of Sound

Pure tone—It is the simple periodical regular sound of single frequency (Fig. 2).

Tone: Tone may have different amplitudes but same frequency.

Complex sound: It has more than one frequency.

Fourier Analysis—An analysis of a complex sound into its constituent sinusoids is known as Fourier analysis. The analysis of waveforms into sine waves (Sinusoids) rather than into any other waveforms is useful as:

- Any realistic waveforms can be made out of sums of sinusoids
- Sinusoidal sound waves behave in a simple way in many complex environments (e.g. EAC, or middle ear)
- Cochlea itself seems to perform Fourier analysis.

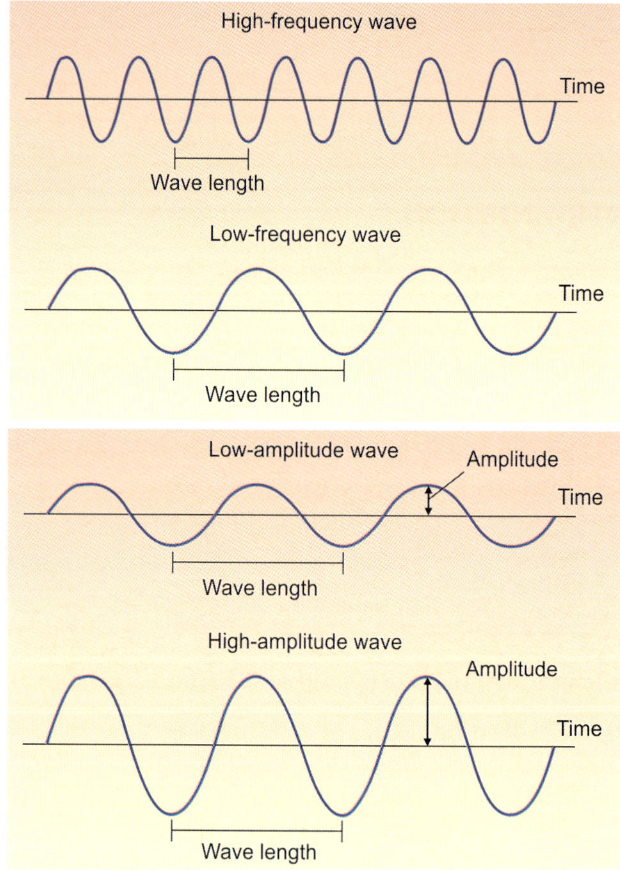

Fig. 1: Frequency and amplitude of the sound wave in ear

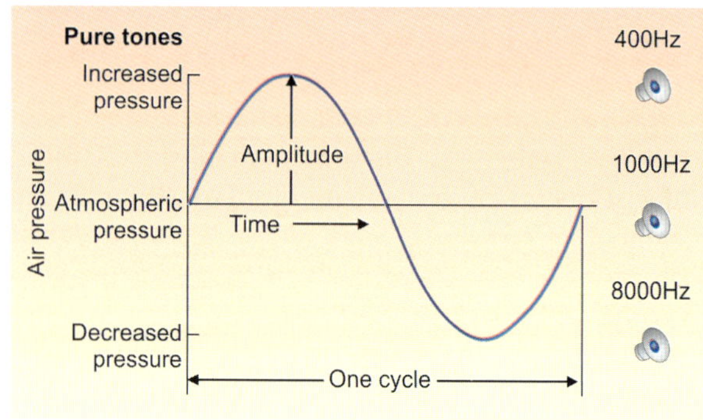

Fig. 2: Pure tone sound

Table 1: Sound pressure of common sound	
dB SPL	**Sound source**
15–20	Whisper
40–60	Conversional speech
60–90	Noisy room
90–120	Loud music or painful noise
> 120	Gun fire
140–180	Jet aircraft engine noise

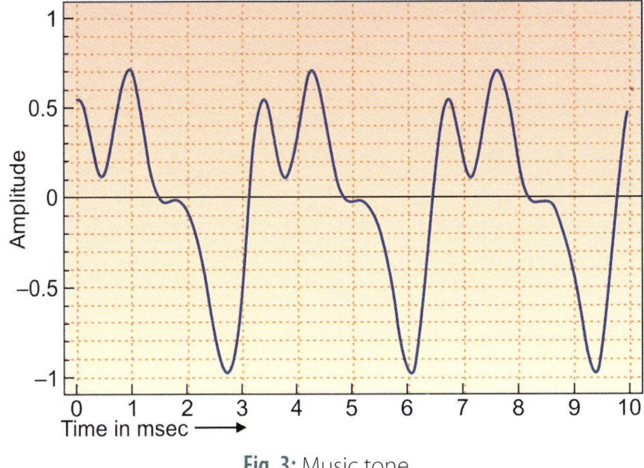

Fig. 3: Music tone

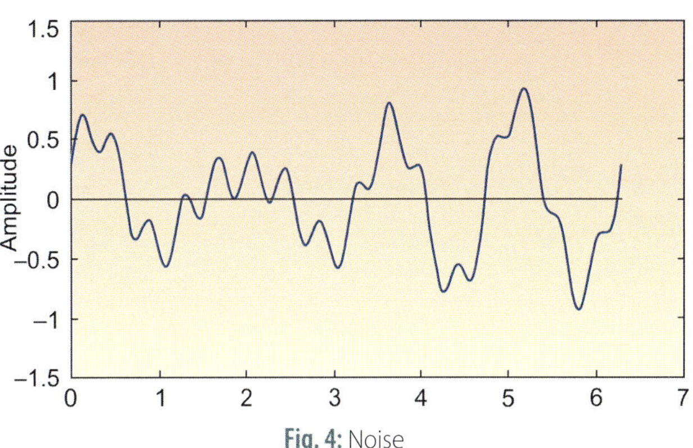

Fig. 4: Noise

Music tone: A fundamental frequency with many harmonics (Fig. 3).

Noise: It is an aperiodic complex sound of no characteristic frequency. It may be white noise, narrow band noise or speech noise (between 500 and 3000 Hz) (Fig. 4).

Timbre of sound is the presence of overtones. It consists of basic frequency and its multiples.

Resonant frequency: It is the frequency at which a mass vibrates with minimum amount of external force.

- External auditory canal (EAC)—3000 Hz
- Middle ear—800 Hz
- Tympanic membrane—800–1600 Hz
- Ossicular chain—500–1200 Hz.

Sound Transmission in the Normal Ear (Figs 5A and B)

Sound waves are collected by the pinna (funnel-shaped), focus into EAC and strikes the tympanic membrane (TM). TM vibrates and moves the ossicles, resulting vibrations of oval window (OW) membrane. Vibrations of OW membrane are transmitted to inner ear fluids in scala vestibuli, scala tympani and scala media (cochlear duct) where hair cells of the organ of corti are stimulated. The hair cells act as transducers, converting mechanical energy into electrical impulses that run along the auditory nerve to binaural auditory processing area.

Acoustic Function of External Ear

- It collects and directs sound waves and acts as a resonator (one end is open and other end is closed)
- It increases the sound pressure at the tympanic membrane in a frequency sensitive way
- It produces a gain of 20 dB at 2500 Hz with less gain at lower and higher frequencies

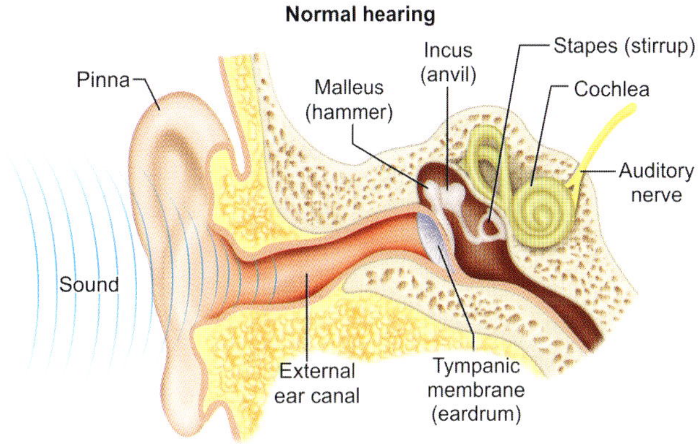

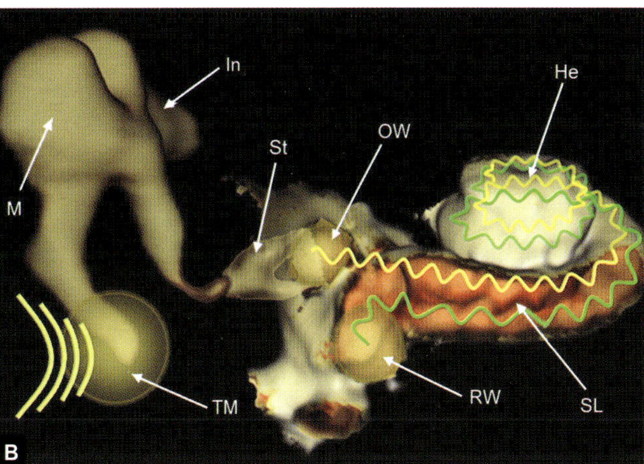

Figs 5A and B: (A) Propagation of sound wave in ear; (B) Normal hearing mechanism

Abbreviations: TM; tympanic membrane, M; malleus, In; incus, St; stapes, OW; oval window, SL; spiral lamina, He; helicotrema, RW; round window

- Total occlusion of the EAC causes hearing loss not more than 40 dB. Ear plugs/ear muffs attenuate sound less than 30 dB

- The impedance of eardrum is about 3–4 times more than air
- About 30% of incident sound energy gets reflected from EAC. EAC cuts off unwanted frequency to help in better speech discrimination.

Acoustic Function of Middle Ear

Impedance is the resistance offered by a medium for propagation of sound. Air is the best medium for transmission of sound because of its low resistance. Water has higher impedance as compared to air. Sound gets reflected when passes through two media of different impedance. Similar thing occurs in the ear. Cochlear fluids have impedance equaling to the impedance of sea water (1.5×10^6 N.sec/m³).

When sound in air travels to the sea water 99.9% of sound energy is reflected and 0.1% is transmitted. Similar thing happens while sound goes to cochlear fluid from air resulting about 22–30 dB loss. Nature has compensated for this loss of sound energy by interposition of middle ear (ME). ME helps to convert the low-pressure high displacement vibrations of the ear drum into high-pressure low displacement vibrations. This makes suitable to drive the cochlear fluid. This function of the ME is said impedance matching (Acoustic transformer). This is achieved by:

- Role of TM
    - Bekesy postulated that TM vibrates like a stiff plate up to 2 kHz. Inferior edge is flaccid, hence most mobile. About 6 kHz the movement becomes chaotic with reduction in transfer efficiency[4,5]
    - Khanna stated that displacement of malleus is 0.5 times the mean displacement of TM for frequency below 6 kHz.[6]
- The area ratio:
    - The key transformer within the ME is the ratio of the TM (A_{TM}) to stapes foot plate area (A_{FP}); it is 20 times[7]
    - It results in sound pressure applied to inner ear by stapes foot plate 26 dB larger than sound pressure at TM.
- Ossicular lever
    - The ratio of length of manibrium (lm) to long process of incus (li) around the axis of rotation of ossicles is 1.3. It results 2 dB increase in sound pressure applied by stapes to inner ear (Fig. 6)
    - Therefore, theoretical ME sound pressure gain is about 26 dB + 2 dB = 28 dB. But actual or measured ME sound pressure gain in normal temporal bone under physiologic condition is found only about 20 dB near 1000 Hz with longer gain at other frequencies[8]

- This difference between measured and theoretical sound pressure gain is due to:
    - The anatomic transformer model attributes that the entire TM moves as a rigid body. In actual, portion of TM moves differently. At low-frequency entire TM moves with same phase with variable magnitudes. At frequencies above 1000 Hz, the pattern of vibration of TM breaks up into smaller vibrating portions. They vibrate with different phases. This reduces the efficiency of TM as a coupler of sound pressure[9]
    - In actual, TM and ossicular ligament are stretched by forces and pressure to accelerate the mass of ME component. Part of force generated in EAC is lost to move TM and ossicles and is failed to reach the cochlea
    - Air inside the ME cavity also dampens the low frequency sound transmission.
    - Slippage in ossicular system at frequencies above 1000–2000 Hz reduces the motion of the stapes in relation to malleus. This is associated with translocation movement in the rotational axis of the ossicles or flexion in ossicular joints.[10,11] This is happening in reality whereas anatomic transformer model implies ossicular system acting as a rigid body.
- Impedance efficiency
    - Only 50% of sound energy from TM gets transmitted and absorbed in the cochlea. Without middle ear only 3% of the sound energy will be absorbed by

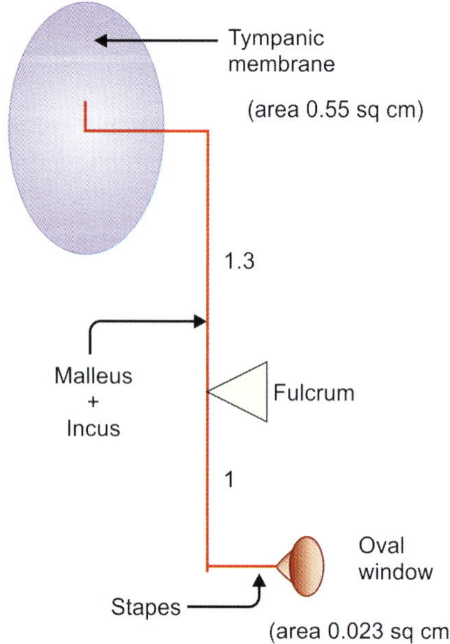

Fig. 6: Area ratio and ossicular lever

the cochlea. Middle ear efficiency is best at 1 KHz. Grommet insertion improves transmission of low-frequency sounds. Endogenous sounds are of low-frequency.

- The effective stimulus to inner ear is the difference of the sound pressure between the oval and round window. The ME maximizes the actual pressure difference by:
  - Tympano-ossicular system—It preferentially increases the sound pressure at the oval window (OW) of inner ear. It results middle ear sound pressure gain
  - Intact TM reduces the sound pressure in tympanic cavity by 10–20 dB compared to pressure in EAC, thereby resulting round window (RW) protection from pressure in the ear canal
  - The presence of air in ME outside the round window permits the free motion of round window in response to the stimulation of inner ear by mobility of stapes footplate.

Phase Difference (Fig. 7)

The cochlea responds to difference in sound pressure between the cochlear windows.[12]

The tympano-ossicular system transforms the sound pressure in ear canal to sound pressure at oval window is termed as ossicular coupling. Motion of TM in response to ear canal sound creates acoustic pressure in the middle ear cavity and stimulates the inner ear. The sound pressures in middle ear that act at the oval window and round window, Pow and PRw respectively are similar but not identical as two windows are separated by few millimeters. The sound pressure difference between the windows is termed as acoustic coupling, ΔP where $\Delta P = P_{ow} - P_{Rw}$.

The total pressure acts at the oval window is $P_s + P_{ow}$, Where P_s = ossicularly coupled stapes sound pressure.

The total pressure acts at the round window is PRw.

The window pressure difference P_{wD} is $P_s + P_{ow} - P_{Rw}$.

Stapes volume velocity (U_s) =

$$\frac{\text{Ossicular coupling } (P_s) + \text{Acoustic coupling } (P_{ow} - P_{rw})}{\text{Stapes–Cochlear input impedance } (Z_{sc})}$$

This equation is used to predict middle ear sound transmission in diseased or reconstructed ear in terms of P_s, ΔP and Z_{SC} (Fig. 8).

This difference depends on the relative magnitude and phase of the individual sound pressures at the two windows. When there is a significant difference in magnitude of the ossicularly and acoustically coupled sound as in normal ear or after successful tympanoplasty, the differences in phase difference have little effect in determining the window pressure difference.

In this specific case, the magnitude of the oval window sound pressure is 10 times (20 dB) greater than the round window sound pressure. The range of possible window pressure difference (P_{wD}) is shown in figure by two sine waves (Fig. 9).

One with an amplitude of 9 representing the difference when the total oval window pressure and the round window pressure are in phase (0° phase difference) and the other with an amplitude of 11 representing the difference when the pressure are out of phase (180° phase difference). Even with this maximum effect of varying the phase difference, the two curves shown in figure are similar in magnitude, within 2 dB of each other. With longer magnitude differences (i.e. 40–60 dB) expected in normal ear and in ears that have undergone successful tympanoplasty phase variations have a negligible effect.

Phase differences can play an important role when ossicular coupling is compromised as in ears with interrupted ossicular chain.

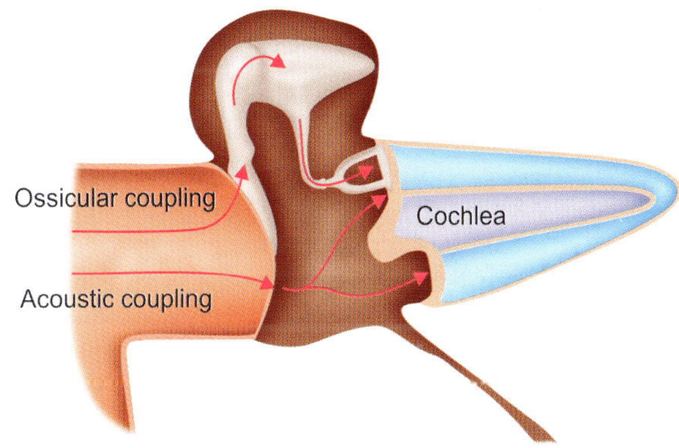

Fig. 7: Schematic showing pathways of ossicular coupling and acoustic coupling

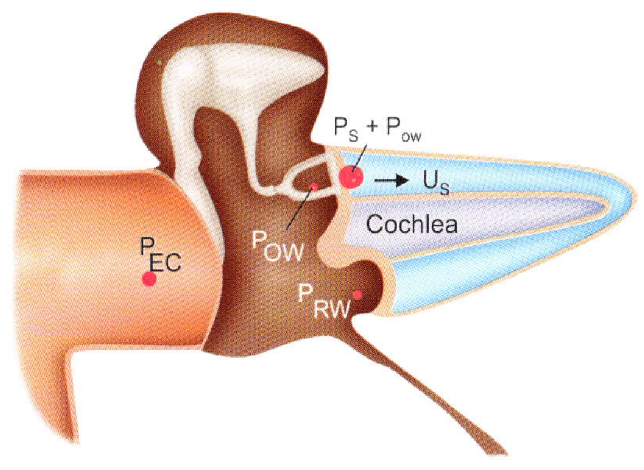

Fig. 8: Schematic showing: P_{EC} = Sound pressure in ear canal; P_{ow} = sound pressure at the oval window; P_{Rw} = sound pressure at the round window; P_s = ossicularly coupled stapes sound pressue; U_s = stapes volume velocity

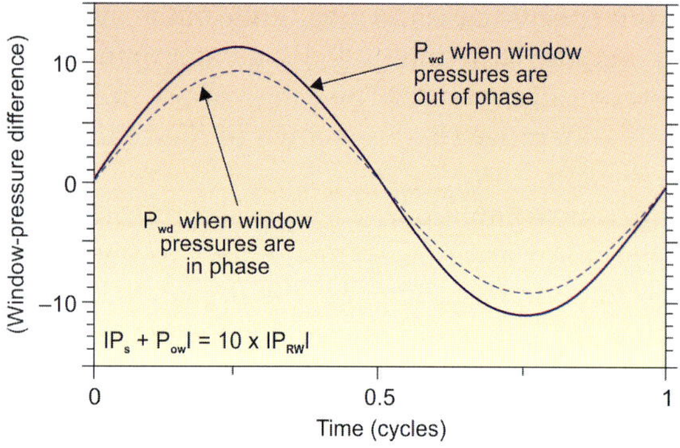

Fig. 9: Schematic showing difference in phase size are of little importance in determining the difference between the two sound pressures when there is significance difference in magnitude between window pressures. The shaded line shows the window pressure difference P_{WD} when the total oval window pressure and round window pressure are in phase, and the result is a P_{WD} wave of amplitude 9 = 10–1. The solid line shows P_{WD} when pressure at two windows is out of phase, and result is P_{WD} wave of amplitude 11 = 10 – (–1)

Diseased Middle Ear Scenario

Sound transmission in diseased or damaged middle ear is different.

When there is ossicular disruption in presence of intact TM, ossicular coupling is lost but sound input to inner ear, Cochlea results from acoustic coupling. Ossicular disruption results in a conductive hearing loss of 60 dB as acoustic coupling is about 60 dB smaller than ossicular coupling.

Loss of TM, malleus and incus losses ossicular coupling but enhances acoustic coupling of about 10–20 dB as compared to normal ear. This is due to loss of the shielding effect of TM which in normal ear attenuates the middle ear sound pressure by 10–20 dB relative to the ear canal sound pressure.[13]

In damaged middle ear, transformer mechanism is lost. Differential pressure level between the two windows is not maintained. Scala vestibule is more soft and pliable than Scala tympani. Differential movement of fluid within Cochlea is still possible.

Bone Conduction

It is the normal route for hearing some components of one's own voice. It is useful in severe conductive heaving loss. Tonndorf[14] described the mechanisms by which a bone vibrator could stimulate the inner ear. The bone conduction mechanisms involve relative motion between the ossicles and inner ear, which is influenced by diseases of the external and middle ears.

Inner ear factors on bone conduction are:

- Differential distortion of bone structures of cochlea (s. vestibuli is larger than s. tympani) resulting movement of cochlear fluids
- Direct vibrations of osseous spiral lamina
- Direct transmission of vibrations from the skull via CSF to the cochlear fluids
- Leaving one window open results in improved sound conduction
- Vibration of skull gets transmission of the ossicles of middle ear
- Inertia of middle ear ossicles does not coincide with inertia of vibrating skull.
  - These accounts of Carhart's notch around 2 kHz.

The middle ear acts as a band pass filter with peak transmission around 1 kHz.

External ear factors on bone conductions are:

- Bone vibrations are conducted through EAC and air within it
- Vibrations escape externally if EAC is open and occlusion of EAC increases bone conduction[15]
- Radiation of sound externally best happens at low-frequencies. Therefore, change with occlusion is greatest at low-frequencies.

Function of Middle Ear Muscles and Joints

Tensor tympani attached to the handle of malleus pulls the malleus medially by 1 mm or more but have little effect on the stapes because of gliding on the incudomalleolar joint (Fig. 10).

Stapedius muscle attached to the posterior aspect of stapes changes the position of the stapes by 1 mm but has little effect on the position of other ossicles because of sliding in the incudostapedial joint.

- The contraction of the two muscles results in increased stiffness of the ossicular chain; hence causes bluntness of low-frequencies
- The consequence of joint induced flexibility decreases in high-frequency response of middle ear
- The stapedius contraction reduces transmission up to 30 dB for low frequencies (<1–2 kHz) and up to 10 dB for high frequencies.

The contraction of the stapedius muscle in response to sound is called acoustic reflex. The whole stapedial reflex arc has 3–4 synapses. Stapedial reflex latency is 6–7 miliseconds (ms).

Sensory Transduction at Organ of Hearing (Fig. 11A)

The scala vestibuli and scala tympani contain perilymph. Scala media contains endolymph. Perilymph space opens

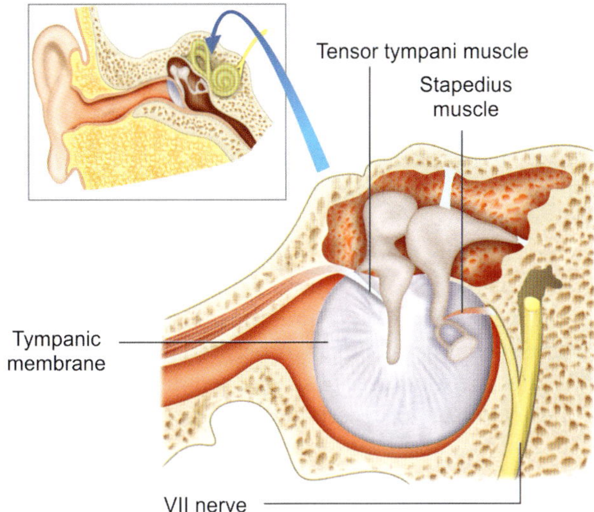

Fig. 10: Attachment of tensor tympani and stapedius muscles

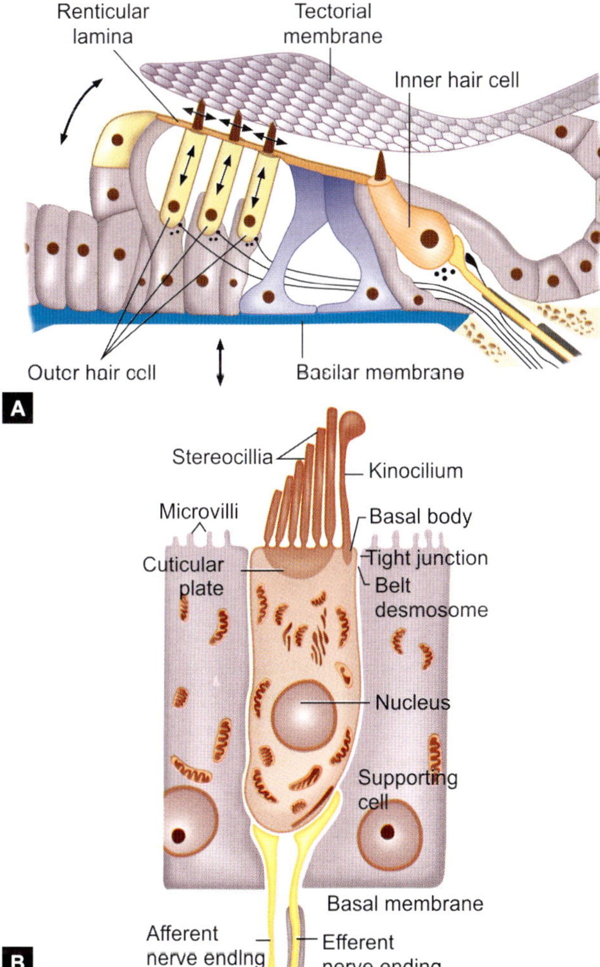

Figs 11A and B: (A)Sensory transduction in inner ear-tectorial membrane picks up sound pressure waves in the inner ear fluids and pushes down on the hairs of the outer hair cells; (B) Stereocilia and receptor hair cells

into CSF via cochlear aqueduct. Endolymphatic space joins endolymphatic sac by endolymphatic duct. The scala vestibuli is separated from scala media by the Reissner's membrane. The Reissner's membrane is very thin and does not obstruct sound transmission from scala vestibule to scala media.

Endolymph is formed by stria vascularis.[16] It has low sodium and high potassium content. Endolymph has positve potential gradient +80 mV (Endocochlear potential). NaK ATPase is responsible for the gradient.

Site of production of perilymph is controversial. View regarding production of perilymph is —

Perilymph from scala vestibuli originates from plasma while perilymph from scala tympani originates from plasma and CSF. Ionic concentration resembles extracellular fluid. Electrical potential of scala tympani is +7 mV and scala vestibuli is +5 mV.

Organ of Corti is the end organ of hearing. It contains—
- Stereocilia and receptor hair cells—3 rows of outer hair cells, 1 row of inner hair cells (Fig. 11B)
- Tectorial and basilar membrane
- Cochlear fluid

The activity of stapes results change in pressure across the basilar membrane; the membrane bends and fluid flows in this space. This causes the inner hair cells stereocilia to move. If the hairs are bending towards the tallest stereocilium, the cell's voltage increases resulting more release of neurotransmitter. Auditory nerves connected to the hair cells increase their activity. If the hair cells are bending away from the tallest stereocilium the cell's voltage decreases resulting less release of neurotransmitter. The auditory nerves connected to the hair cells decrease their activity. The inner hair cells transform the vibration of the basilar membrane into the discharge pattern of the auditory nerve fiber. About 95% of the afferent auditory nerves make contact with inner hair cells. The outer hair cells take part in cochlear micromechanics. It amplifies the motion of basilar membrane. In transduction of basilar membrane into neural activity, outer hair cells have no known role, as very few outer hair cells synapses with auditory nerves. Inside of the outer hair cells have 70 mV.

Basilar membrane is tonotopically organized. Low-frequencies are presented at the apex of the cochlea. High-frequencies are presented near the base of the cochlea (Fig. 12A).

Frequency selectivity of basilar membrane is reflected in the response of the individual nerve fibers (Fig. 12B).

Neural transmission of signal: Auditory nerve fibers transmit different codes to central auditory system. Inner hair cells excite auditory nerves. Single auditory stimulus is always excitatory (Fig. 13).

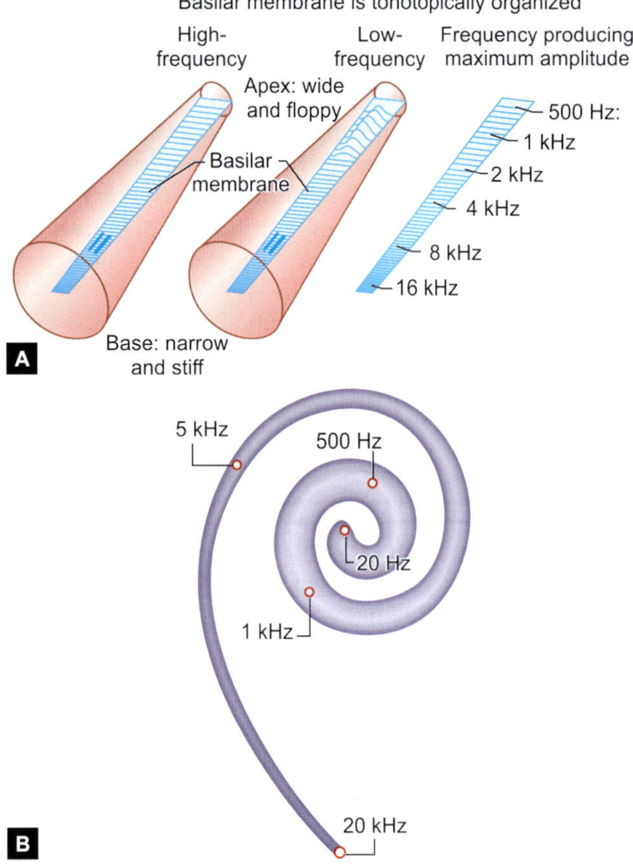

Figs 12A and B: (A) Tontopical organization of basilar membrane; (B) Frequency selectivity of basilar membrane

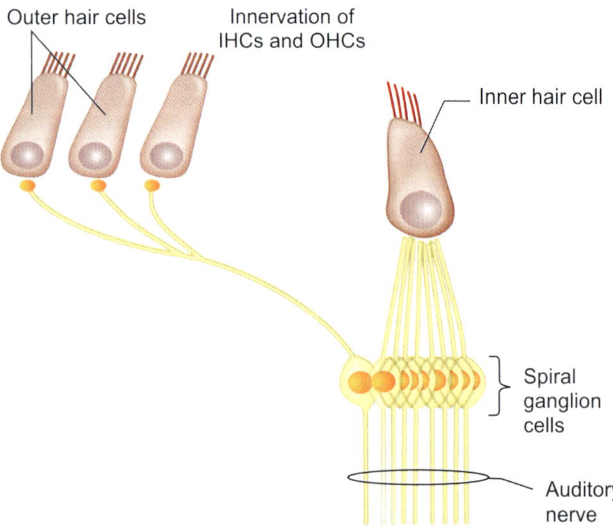

Fig. 13: Neural transmission in auditory nerve

Place code: Basilar membrane separates sound according to their frequencies. It is basis for the place hypothesis for frequency discrimination. It is preserved throughout the auditory nervous system including neurons in the nuclei of the ascending auditory nervous system. These are anatomically organized according to their fiber's characteristic frequency (CF). Place coding provides partial information.

Temporal code: It reflects the frequency of vibration of individual segment of the basilar membrane. The discharges of individual nerve fibers are phase locking and related to waveform of the sound. It is the basis for the temporal hypothesis of frequency discrimination. It imparts an object code that means it informs about the properties of sound.

The two codes for sound are processed in different parts of CNS. They are examples of stream separation.

Central auditory processing of the signal — Classical assending auditory pathway is

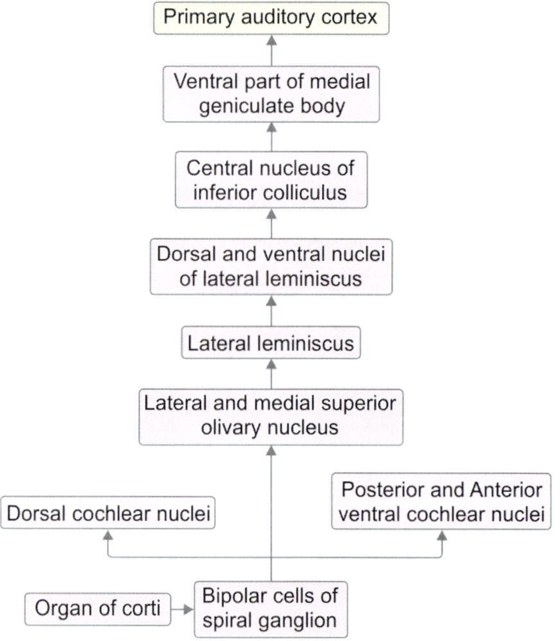

The auditory fibers run via the ipsilateral and contralateral routes. They have multiple decussations. Thus, each ear is represented by both cerebral hemispheres. The primary auditory cortex is situated in superior temporal gyrus (Brodmann's area 41) (Figs 14 and 15).

Theories of Hearing

There are various theories to explain the mechanism of hearing. These are:

- Place theory of Helmholtz
- Telephone theory of Rutherford
- Volley theory of Wever
- Place volley theory of Lawrence
- Traveling wave theory of Bekesy.

Place theory (of Helmholtz): According to Helmholtz, basilar membrane has different segments that are resonated to

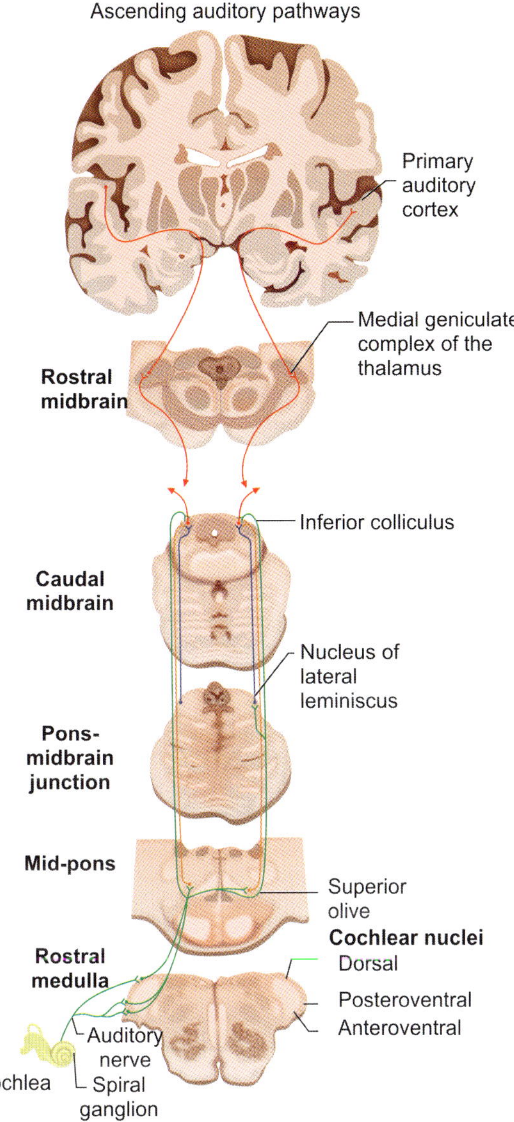

Fig. 14: Central connections of auditory pathways

Volley theory (of Wever): Wever proposed that several neurons acting as a group can fire in response to high-frequency sound, even though none of them can do it individually.

Place Volley theory (of Lawrence): It combines both Volley and Place theory. Lawrence proposed that the higher frequencies are perceived by the place mechanism, while the lower frequencies are perceived by the Telephone mechanism. Intermediate frequencies are heard by both mechanisms.

Traveling wave theory (of Bekesy): Bekesy proposed that the frequency coding takes place at the level of cochlea. High-frequencies are represented towards the base while low-frequencies are closer to apex.

The electrical potential of the cochlea: If an electrode is placed within one of the cochlear scalae or on the wall of the cochlea or in its vicinity electrical potentials are generated in response to acoustic stimulation. The electrical potentials are divided into three components (Fig. 16)—

Cochlear Microphonic (CMP): It is an alternating current (AC) potential that follows the waveform of the stimulus. It is derived from the outer hair cells allowing flow of K^+ through hair cells and producing voltage fluctuations, called cochlear microphonic. The microphonic represents the massed effects of the transducer currents flowing through outer hair cells. Within the cochlea microphonic is essential for mechanically amplifying the traveling wave.

Summating potential (SP): A direct current (DC) shift is seen in the base line of the microphonic. This is the summating potential. It appears as either a positive or negative shift depending on the stimulus conditions. It takes some time to reach the maximum amplitude after the onset of a stimulus. It is generated mainly from outer hair cells and small contribution comes from inner hair cells response. It is superimposed on VIIIth nerve action potential.

Both CM and SP are receptor potentials. They differ from action potential as they are graded rather than all or none phenomenon. They have no latency. They are not propagated and they have no postresponse refractory period.

The Neural potentials: At the starting and ending of the stimulus a series of deflections in negative direction are formed that are called as the neural potentials. The first phase is known as the N1 potential and second smaller phase as the N2 potential. They arise from the massed action potentials in the auditory nerve produced at the beginning of the stimulus and sometimes at the end. The summed effect is thought to be realized as action potentials emerging

different frequencies, resonators dampen slowly and are sharply tuned. This may cause after ringing after cessation of stimulus. This theory fails to explain why a stream of clicks of frequencies ranging from 1220, 1300 and 1400 Hz is heard as 100 Hz.

Telephone theory (of Rutherford): It suggests that the entire cochlea responds as a whole to all frequencies. The sound of all frequencies is transmitted as in telephone cable and frequency analysis is performed at a higher level (brain). Damage of certain portions of cochlea can cause preferential loss of hearing of certain frequencies. This cannot be explained by telephone theory.

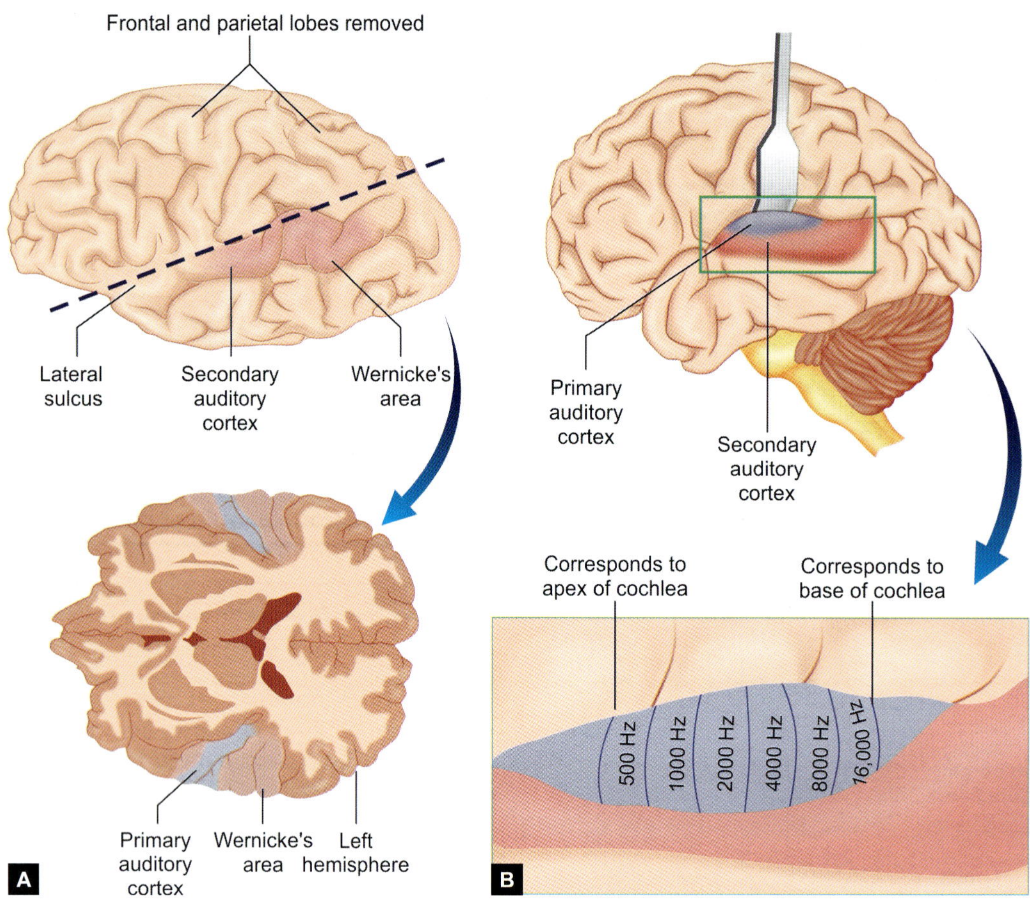

Figs 15A and B: (A) Auditory cortical areas; (B) Central auditory processing

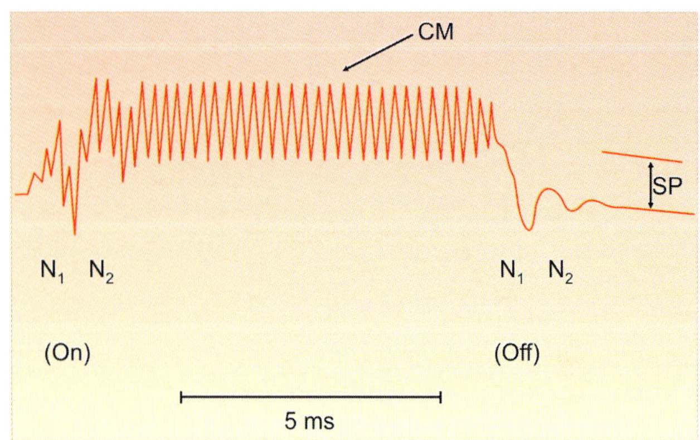

Fig. 16: Electrical response to a tone burst including N$_1$ and N$_2$ neural potentials, cochlear microphonic (CM) and summating potential (SP) (*Souce:* Scott Brown's Otolaryngology, head and neck surgery 7th edition Vol.3 2008 p.3196.)

from internal auditory meatus.[17] It is an all or nonresponse of auditory nerve fibers. Auditory nerves send AP to brain for analysis.

REFERENCES

1. Prof. Hesham Kozou, Physiology of hearing, http://www.Alexorl. Edu.eg
2. Crisbert I. Cualteros, Physiology of hearing http://www.slideshare. com
3. James O Pickles. Physiology of hearing Scott-Brown's Otolaryngology, Head and Neck surgery, 7th edition. 2008;3:3173-201.
4. Von Bekesy. Uber die Messung der Schwingung samplitude der Gehorknochelen mittles einer kapazitiven Sonde. Akvstische Zeitschrift. 1941;6:1-16.
5. Von Bekesy G. Experiments in hearing New York: McGraw Hill, 1960.

6. Khanna SM, Tonndorf J. Tympanic membrane vibration in cats studied by time-averaged holography. Journal of the Acoustical Society of America. 1972;51:1904-20.

7. Wever EG, Lawrence M. Physiological acoustic. Princeton (NJ): Princeton University Press: 1954.

8. Saumil N Merchant, John J Rosowski. Auditory Physiology: Glasscock-Shambaugh, Surgery of the ear, fifth edition. 2003;p.59-80.

9. Tonndorf J, Khanna SM, Funnell ERJ. Interferometric measurement of the amplitude and the phase of tympanic membrane vibrations in cat. Hear Res. 1989;38:1-18.

10. Goode RL, Killion M, Nakamura K, Nishihara S. New knowledge about the function of an improved analog model. Am J Otol. 1994;15:145-54.

11. Guinan JJ, Peake WT. Middle ear characteristics of anesthetized cats. J acoust Joc Am. 1967;41:1237-61.

12. Wever EG, Lawrence M. The acoustic pathway to the cochlea. J Acoust Soc Am. 1950;22:460-7.

13. Saumil N Merchant, Micheal E Raviez, Susan E Voss, William T Peake, John J Rosowski. Middle Ear Mechanisms in normal, diseased and reconstructed ears. Otolaryngology reviews 2000 edited by Vinod H Shah and Prabodh P. Karnik. p. 30-45.

14. Tonndorf J. Bone conduction: studies in experimental animals. Acta Oto-Laringologica Supplementum. 1966;213:1-32.

15. Tonndorf J. Bone Conduction. In Keidel WD. Neff ED (eds). Handbook of sensory physiology. Vol.5/3. Berlin: Springer. 1976;37-84.

16. Wangemann P, Sachacht J. Homeostatic mechanisms in the cochlea. In Dallos P, Popper An, Fay RR (eds). Springer handbook of auditory research, Vol.8. The cochlea. New York: Springer-Verlag. 1996;130-85.

17. Texas DC, Eldredge DH, Davis H. Cochlea responds to acoustic transients: an interpretation of the whole- nerve action potential. Journal of the Acoustical Society of America. 1962;34: 1438-59.

Audiology

Asok K Saha, Indranil Chatterjee

INTRODUCTION

Audiology is the study of hearing and hearing-related disorders.

PURE TONE AUDIOMETRY

- It is a reliable method of testing hearing acuity of a subject only for pure tone sounds
- Hearing threshold at both air and bone are tested at different frequencies and plotted graphically is called a pure tone audiogram
- The parameters of the audiogram are frequency, as measured in cycles per second (Hz) and intensity, as measured in decibels (dB)
- Electronic device that is used here is called an audiometer.

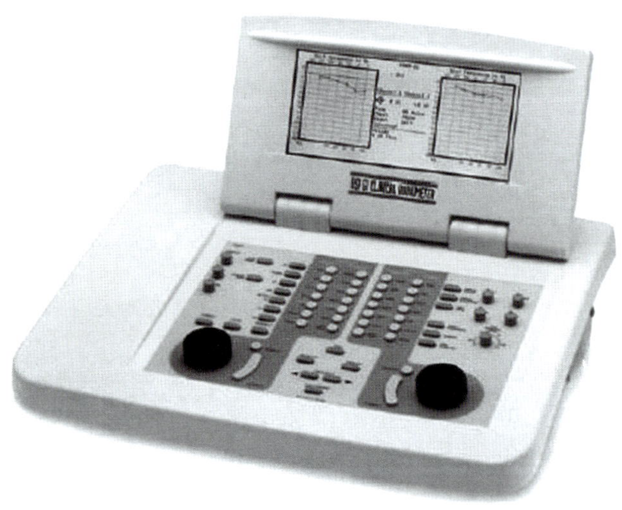

Fig. 1: Audiometer

THE AUDIOMETER

An audiometer produces pure tones of various frequencies, attenuates them to various intensity levels and delivers them to transducers. It also produces **broadband** and **narrowband noise**. In addition, the audiometer serves to attenuate and direct signals from other sources, such as a microphone or compact disc player. There are several types of audiometers, and they are classified primarily by their functions. A pure tone audiometer includes nearly all of the functions that an audiologist might want to use for subjective audiometric assessment (Fig. 1).[1]

Components of an Audiometer

Oscillator: The oscillator generates pure tones, usually at discrete frequencies at the octave and mid-octave frequencies of 125, 250, 500, 750, 1000, 1500, 2000, 3000, 4000, 6000, and 8000 Hz. Some audiometers do not include all of these frequencies; other audiometers extend to higher frequencies. The oscillator is controlled by some form of frequency-selector switch.

Amplifier: It increases pure tone intensity.

Attenuator: The oscillator is controlled by some form of frequency-selector switch. The attenuator controls the intensity level of the signal, usually in 5 dB steps from –10 dB HL to a maximum output level that varies by frequency and transducer type.

Interrupter switch: The interrupter switch controls the duration of the signal that is presented to the patient. It turns the signal on/off without an audible tone.

Transducer: Transducers are the devices that convert the electrical energy from the audiometer into acoustical or vibratory energy. Transducers used for audiometric purposes are earphones, loudspeakers, or bone-conduction vibrators. Earphones are of three varieties, insert, supra-aural, and circumaural. An insert earphone is a small earphone coupled to the ear canal by means of an ear insert, which is made of pliable, soft material used to provide the acoustic coupling between an earphone and the ear canal.

Noise generator: This is a type of oscillator for the generation of different types of noises for audiological masking.

Ear selector: It permits testing of one ear at a time.

Mode selector: It helps to choose the mode of sound production, such as air conduction and bone conduction.
- The testing should be preferably carried out in a sound proof/anechoic chamber.[2] Ambient noise must be below the level that would cause hearing loss in a normal listener
- The typical audiogram is determined by establishing hearing threshold for single frequency sound at 250, 500, 1000, 2000, 4000 and 8000 Hz for air conduction and at 250, 500, 1000, 2000 and 4000 Hz for bone conduction
- Primary speech thresholds are 500, 1000 and 2000 Hz
- Pure tone average (PTA) is obtained by averaging the air conduction hearing level at speech frequencies.

Procedure for Pure Tone Audiometry (Table 1)

Standard test procedure used is Hughson-West lake method. It is slightly modified by Carhart and Jerger[3] which is most commonly used in practice. Here a pure tone signal is presented at a comfortably loud level. Patient responds by raising the hand or pressing a button. Signal intensity is then decreased in 10 dB steps until no response is obtained. Then the intensity is increased in 5 dB steps until the patient responds. This ascending-descending procedure is repeated until the patient responds at a given intensity 2/3 or 3/5 times.
- Threshold: It is the lowest intensity level that a patient can detect 50% of the time

- Patients with HL have audiogram with poorer thresholds (larger numbers in decibels) at the involved frequencies (> 25 dB)
- Normal adult hearing is represented as 0–25 dB
- Air conduction thresholds are measured using ear phones
- Bone conduction thresholds are measured using a bone vibrator placed on the skull (mastoid/forehead)
- Masking of the nontest ear may be required to obtain correct threshold (Table 2).

Method Outlined by ASHA (American Speech and Hearing Association)

The test is started with a 1000 Hz tone and threshold is obtained for various frequencies. The method is obtained as follows in Flowchart 1.

Conductive Hearing Loss (CHL)

Patients with CHL have normal cochlear function. They show normal hearing threshold by bone conduction but poor hearing threshold by air conduction, representing significant air-bone gap (>10 dB) (Fig. 2).

Sensorineural Hearing Loss (SNHL)

Patients with SNHL have both poor air and bone conduction thresholds. The bone conduction level is more than 20 dB HL and the air-bone gap is 10 dB or less (Fig. 3).

Mixed Hearing Loss

Bone conduction is worse (more) than 20 dB but the air–bone gap is 15 dB or more, signifying lesions in both the conductive and the sensorineural apparatus (Fig. 4).

Crossover and Masking

Sound that is presented to the test ear can travel via bone conduction through the head and be perceived in the opposite, nontest ear—this phenomenon is called crossover.

Table 1: PTA categorization of degree of HL[4]	
<25 dB HL	Normal hearing
26–40 dB HL	Mild hearing loss
41–55 dB HL	Moderate hearing loss
56–70 dB HL	Moderately severe hearing loss
71–90 dB HL	Severe hearing loss
>90 dB HL	Profound hearing loss
Pure tone average—It is the patient's ability to hear within speech frequencies.	

Table 2: Audiometric symbol for common use[5]		
Interpretation	**Left ear (Blue)**	**Right ear (Red)**
Unmasked air conduction	X	O
Masked air conduction	□	△
Unmasked bone conduction	>	<
Masked bone conduction	⌐	⌐
No response	↘	↙

Flowchart 1: Method outlined by ASHA (American speech and hearing association)

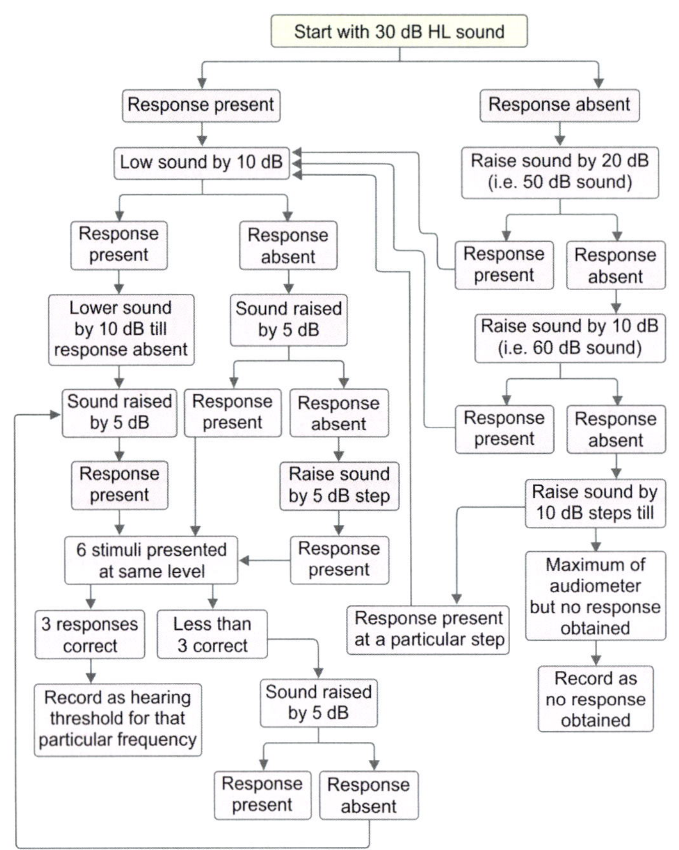

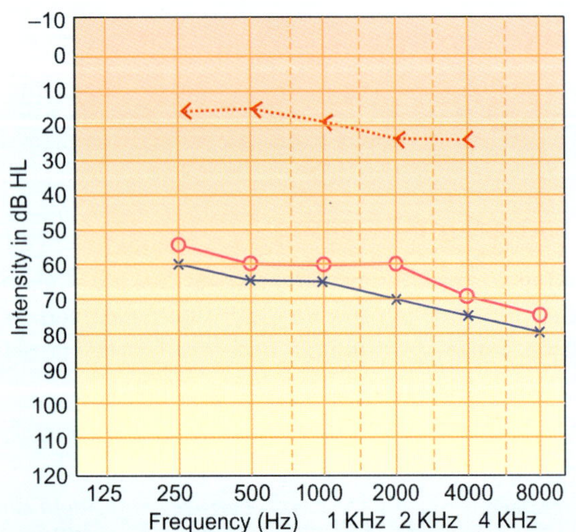

Fig. 2: Pure tone audiogram in conductive hearing loss

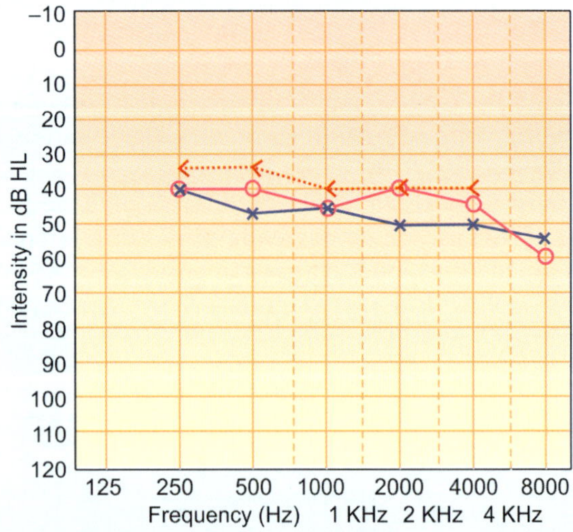

Fig. 3: Pure tone audiogram in sensorineural hearing loss

It may obscure measurement results in the test ear. Therefore, nontested ear must be eliminated from the test.

Interaural attenuation (IA)—The test tone, if loud enough when passing from the test ear to the cochlea of the nontest ear it loses a certain portion of the sound energy. This loss of sound energy is called interaural attenuation. IA values are smaller for lower frequencies than the higher frequency regions.

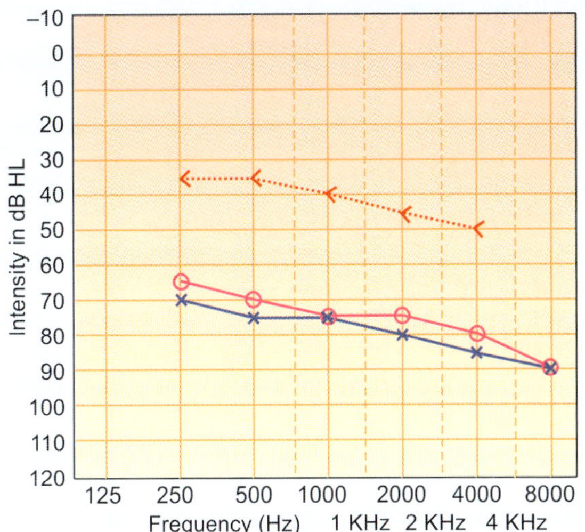

Fig. 4: Pure tone audiogram in mixed hearing loss

- IA of air conduction tone is ~ 40–80 dB
- IA values for bone conducted sound is ~ 0–20 dB (may even be negative)
- Cross-hearing during air conduction should be suspected if—AC (test ear) -BC (nontest ear) > IA
  - Crossover during bone conduction may happen when a difference as little as 0 dB exists between bone conduction thresholds of the two ears
  - Masking is presentation of sound to the nontest ear and serves to prevent the nontest ear from interfering with true sound perception in the test ear.

When to Mask for Air Conduction

When unmasked AC threshold in the test ear exceeds the bone conduction threshold of the nontest ear by ≥40 dB, masking should be done in the nontest ear (IA value for air conduction is ~40 dB).

When to Mask for Bone Conduction

Contralateral ear should be masked when the unmasked bone conduction thresholds demonstrate an apparent air-bone gap of ≥10 dB present in the nontest ear (IA may be 0 dB HL as both cochleae may be stimulated equally).

Masking is usually done using a "narrowband noise" in which the masking noise is centered around the frequency to be masked.

Speech spectrum noise is used for masking during speech frequencies. This is a broadband noise filtered to a band of frequencies is speech spectrum.

The minimum masking sound can be calculated by a formula:

For bone conduction

Minimum masking = Bt + (Am –Bm)

For air conduction

Minimum masking = At -40 + (Am – Bm)

Where Bt = bone conduction threshold in test ear, Am = air conduction threshold in the masked (nontest) ear, Bm = bone conduction threshold in the masked (nontest) ear, At = air conduction threshold in the test ear.

40 is the IA for air conduction.

SPEECH AUDIOMETRY

Patient's ability to hear and understand speech is assessed. It includes:

Speech Reception Thresholds (SRT)[6]

This test is performed to confirm the pure tone threshold findings. A specific set of bisyllabic words known as spondees, are presented to the patient at decreasing intensities. Spondees are two syllable words with equal stress on each syllable, e.g. oatmeal, base ball, sunlight and popcorn.

The SRT is the lowest intensity at which 50% of the words are repeated correctly by the patient. The range of SRT is ± 7 dB of PTA.

Speech Discrimination Score (SDS) or Word Recognition[7]

The speech discrimination test uses word recognition to assess the patient's understanding of speech.

A list of single syllable words (phonetically balanced word, c.g. pin, sin, day, bus) is presented to the patient's each ear separately at 30–40 dB above the SRT (supra threshold level). The patient repeats each word and score is determined according to the percentage of the words that are correctly identified. A list of 50 words is presented with each word valued at 2%, maximum score is 100%.

- Normal people — score is >90%
- In cochlear lesion — SDS is low
- In retrocochlear lesion — the score is very poor
- SDS <80% affects the ability to understand the speech.

Rollover Phenomenon[8]

As the intensity is gradually increased the percentage of correctly identified words gradually increases until a maximum (PB-max) is reached. Any further increase in intensity beyond this gradually lessens the percentage of correctly identified words and PB identification score falls and a minimum score (PB-min) is reached at a very high intensity level.

$$\text{Rollover ratio} = \frac{PB_{max} - PB_{min}}{PB_{Max}}$$

- In cochlear lesion: Rollover ratio <0.40
- In neural lesion: Rollover ratio >0.45.

Bekesy Audiometry

A self-recording audiometer in which the changes in frequency as well as intensity are done automatically by means of a motor while the patient controls the intensity through a button. The patient is instructed to press the button as soon as he just hears the sound and release it as he stops hearing the sound.

Pure tone are recorded under various conditions including—

- Sweep frequency (Continuously variable from low-to-high frequency or from high-to-low frequency)
- Discrete frequency (at selected fixed frequencies).

Two tracings, one with continuous tone and the other with pulsed tone are obtained for each ear.

There are five different Bekesy audiograms as follows (Fig. 5):

Type I

- Continuous and pulsed tracings overlap showing an interweaving pattern with a tracing width which is constant over frequency and average about 10 dB
- It is seen in normal hearing/middle ear lesion/presbyacusis.

Type II

- The tracings for continuous and pulsed tone are superimposed up to 1000 Hz and then continuous tracing falls slightly below that for the pulsed tone. Gap usually does not exceed 20 dB in high-frequencies

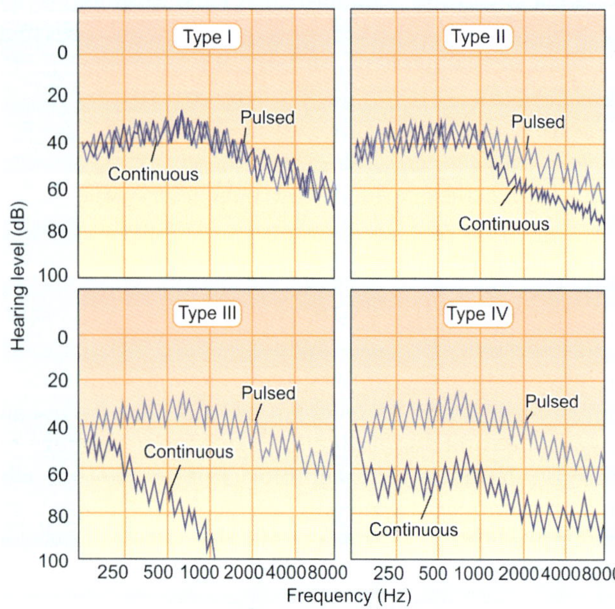

Fig. 5: Different types of Bekesy audiograms

- Width of continuous tracing is smaller than the pulse tone tracing at high-frequencies
- It is seen in cochlear lesions/presbyacusis.

Type III

- Continuous tracing drops sharply below the pulsed
- It usually diverges at low-frequencies (100–500 Hz)
- Width of the tracing remains normal
- It is seen in VIIIth CN lesions (retrocochlear lesion)/sudden loss of hearing.

Type IV

- Continuous tracing falls consistently below the pulsed at all frequencies but not sharply like type III. Tracing width may or may not become abnormally small
- It is seen in VIIIth CN lesions (neural lesions).

Type V

- Continuous tone is above that of the pulsed tone
- Associated with malingering (Functional).

SPECIAL TESTS FOR HEARING

Tone Decay Test

Tone decay test (TDT) is a measure of nerve fatigue. Normally, a person can hear a tone continuously for 60 seconds. In nerve fatigue, he stops hearing earlier.

Procedure (Carhart's Method)

- To determine threshold (at 1K/2K/4K)
- Tone is raised to 5 dB sensitivity level and to determine the time for which it is heard
- If patient stops hearing it before 60 seconds have elapsed, tone is raised by further 5 dB and it is continued until—
    - Patient can hear tone for full 60 seconds or
    - 30 dB SL is reached and patient fails to hear tone at that level for at least 60 seconds or
    - Maximum limit of audiometer is reached.

TDT is usually done at 500 Hz/1000 Hz/2000 Hz/4000 Hz. Rosenberg's criteria for interpreting tone decay tests:

I   Normal: 0–5 dB in 60 seconds.

II   Mild: 10–15 dB in 60 seconds.   } Indicating involvement of Organ of Corti

III   Moderate: 20–25 dB in 60 seconds.

IV   Marked: 30 dB or more in 60 seconds.   } Indicating Retro-cochlear pathology

SISI (Short Increment Sensitivity Index)

Short increment sensitivity index is designed specifically as a test of site of lesion in the auditory system.

The test is performed at 500 Hz/1000 Hz/2000 Hz/4000 Hz.

A continuous tone is presented at 20 dB above the threshold at the frequency being tested and sustained for about 2 minutes.

Every 5 seconds, the tone is increased by 1dB and 20 such blips are presented. Patient indicates the blips heard. Each correct response is counted as 5% and so all 20 correctly indentified makes for a 100% score at the test. Interpretation of SISI test:

- Score >70% suggests cochlear pathology
- Score <30% is of normal people/SNHL (Retrocochlear)
- Score of 30–70% has only limited diagnostic significance.

Modified SISI

Carrier tone is presented at 80 dB SPL (rather than at 20 dB above threshold for the test frequency).

- Score >90% is typical of cochlear pathology
- Score <90% suggest normal people
- Score <40% hints retrocochlear pathology.

Recruitment Test

Recruitment test is defined as an abnormally steep growth of loudness with increasing intensity and is usually associated with a sensorineural deafness due to a cochlear pathology. The ear which does not hear low intensity sound begins to hear greater intensity sound as loud sound or even louder than normal hearing ear.

- It is seen in lesions of cochlea, e.g. Meniere's disease, presbycusis
- In normal and CHL, the test is negative
- It is to differentiate a cochlear from a retrocochlear SNHL.

Derecruitment of loudness—It is abnormally slow growth of loudness, that is characteristic of retrocochlear disorder.

Loudness Discomfort Level

- Loudness discomfort level (LDL) is the minimum intensity that the listener designates as uncomfortably loud
- First the reception threshold of the patient is determined. Then the stimulus intensity is gradually increased until the patient reports that the level is uncomfortable and further increase would be painfully loud
- In normal ear people experiences—discomfort at the intensity of 90–105 dB HL.
  - Dynamic range ~ 90–105 dB
    (Intensity between auditory threshold to discomfort level is dynamic range)
  - Patients with conductive HL/retrocochlear lesion experience discomfort at the intensity greater than 110 dB HL (beyond the limit of the audiometer)

- Cochlear lesions (Meniere's disease/Noise-induced HL/etc.) are associated with increased reception threshold but the discomfort level is within the limits of the audiometer is said narrow dynamic range.
- Dynamic range (LDL-threshold) ≤60 dB
  - It indicates auditory recruitment that is characteristics of cochlear lesion.

Most Comfortable Listening Level

Most comfortable listening level (MCL) is the level that listener designates as most comfortable speech.

This is also obtained at reduced levels above hearing threshold when auditory recruitment is present.

MCL for Speech in

- Normal people is 55 dB> SRT
- Patients with Meniere's disease is 22 dB> SRT

In this test, speech is presented at varying intensities and the patient is asked to report when speech is at a level that is most comfortably loud.

Alternate Binaural Loudness Balance Test of Fowler

Alternate binaural loudness balance (ABLB) test of Fowler is used to detect recruitment in unilateral cases.

- In this test, a tone is played alternatively into normal and deaf ear, the intensity is gradually increased in the affected ear until the sound is heard equally in both ears.
- Test is usually done at 20 dB/40 dB/60 dB/80 dB above the threshold in the poorer ear and result plotted on a Laddergram (Fig. 6). In positive recruitment—Ladder pattern becomes horizontal at higher intensity.

In CHL and SNHL (Retrocochlear), initial difference is maintained throughout.

In cochlear lesion, partial, complete or over — recruitment is seen.

IMPEDANCE AUDIOMETRY [9]

It is an objective test, widely used in ENT practice. It consists of:

- Tympanometry
- Acoustic reflex measurements.

Tympanometry

Tympanometry is defined as the measurement of the change of impedance of the middle ear at the plane of the tympanic membrane as a result of change of air pressure in EAC.

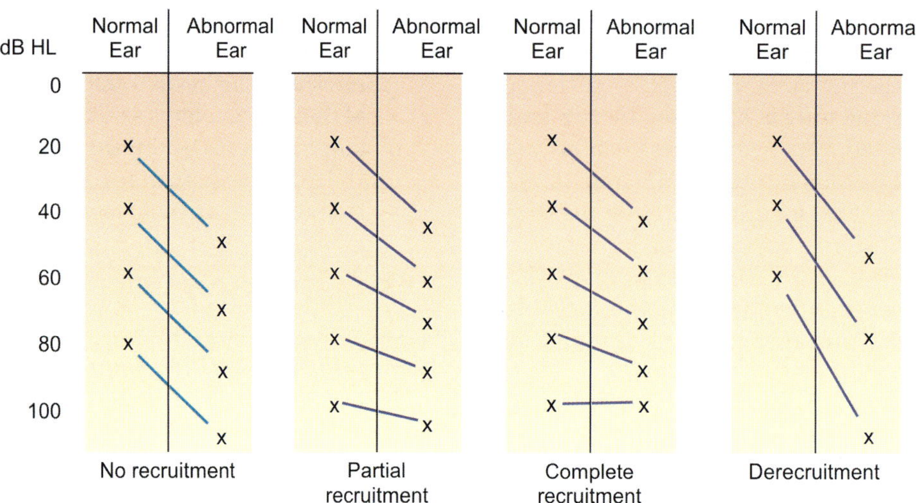

Fig. 6: Laddergrams in ABLB test

- It can be thought of as electronic pneumatic otoscopy that measures the mobility or compliance of TM and middle ear system.

Principle

When a sound strikes TM, some of the sound energy is absorbed while the rest is reflected. A stiffer TM reflects more of the sound energy than a compliant one. By changing the pressure in a sealed EAC and then measuring the reflected sound energy, the compliance or stiffness of tympano-ossicular system as well as healthy or diseased status of middle ear can be assessed. The compliance of TM is at its maximum when air pressure on both sides of TM is equal. It consists of a probe fitted into EAC and has three channels.

   i. An oscillator to deliver a tone of 226 Hz
  ii. An air pressure pump is used to alter the pressure in EAC from positive to normal to negative
 iii. A microphone to pick up the reflected sound.

- Tympanometry results are represented by air pressure/compliance graphs known as tympanograms
- The peak air pressure of tympanogram is equal to the patient's middle ear pressure
- Range of middle ear pressure from~ 0 to - 100 mm of H_2O generally indicates normal Eustachian tube function, Middle ear pressure more negative than -100 mm H_2O indicates poor Eustachian tube function.

Types of Tympanogram (Fig. 7)[10]

Type A—Normal middle ear function.
Type As—Tympanic membrane is stiffer than normal (lower compliance) in presence of normal middle ear pressure (e.g. otosclerosis).

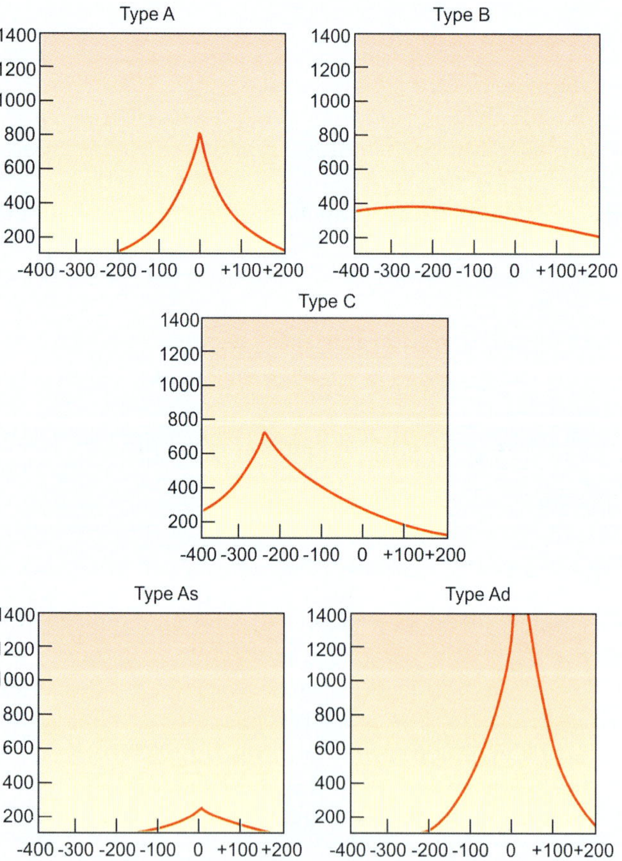

Fig. 7: Different types of tympanograms

Type Ad—Tympanic membrane is more flaccid than normal (High-compliance) in presence of normal middle ear pressure, e.g. ossicular discontinuity, lax or thin TM.

Type B—Known as a flat tympanogram, it shows no pressure peak and indicates nonmobility of TM, e.g. Middle ear effusion or perforated TM or thick TM.

Type C—Tympanic membrane shows a peak in the negative pressure range (< –100 mm H_2O), e.g. poor Eustachian tube function or retracted TM.

Static compliance—It is defined as the compliance of the auditory conductive apparatus as measured at the TM.

C1 reading = Compliance value at +200 mm of H_2O (when TM is stiffened) ~volume of EAC.

C2 reading = Maximum compliance value (TM maximum mobility) ~volume of whole system.

The static compliance (CX) is obtained by subtracting C1 from C2.

Cx = C2-C1 = Compliance of middle ear space.

It increases with discontinuity of ossicles and decreases with middle ear effusion. Increased C1 hints TM perforation. The range of normal static compliance is ~ 0.35–1.40 mL.

Pathologies with increased compliance:

- Ossicular chain discontinuity
- Scaring of the tympanic membrane
- Very large TM (rare)
- Poststapedectomy ear.

Pathologies with decreased compliance:

- Otosclerosis
- Adhesive or SOM
- Tumors in the middle ear, e.g. Glomus jugulare
- Ossicular fixations, e.g. fixed malleus syndrome
- Tympanic sclerosis or thickening of the TM.

Pathologies with normal compliance:

- Eustachian tube obstruction only without OME
- Some cases of otosclerosis.

Acoustic Reflex (or Stapedial Reflex) (Fig. 8)[11]

Acoustic reflex is the reflex contraction of stapedius muscle in response to sound stimulation when muscle contracts it pulls in the direction perpendicular to the main axis of the ossicular chain so as to stiffen the chain, thus increasing compliance of the middle ear system and the TM. The reflex is consensual in that sound stimulation of one side stimulates almost equal contraction of stapedius muscles on both sides. Testing the contraction of stapedius muscle by measuring the change of compliance of TM is known as the acoustic reflex.

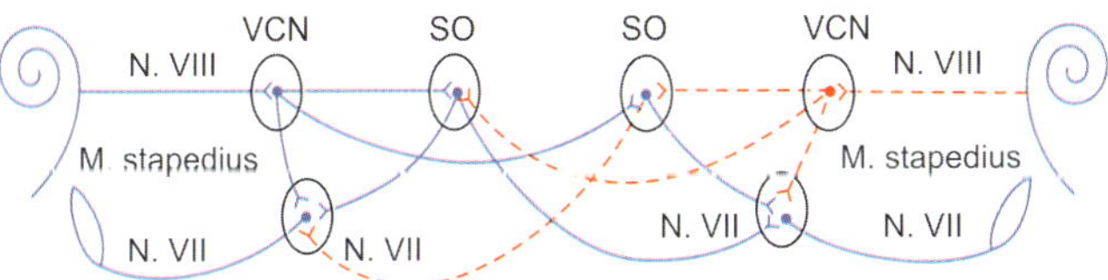

Fig. 8: Acoustic reflex pathway

Stapedius usually contracts at around 70–100 dB hearing level (85 dB). This causes a change in compliance which can be measured in both ears.

The acoustic stapedius reflex arc:

- When acoustic reflex is present at usual stimulus level indicates normal middle ear function
- When acoustic reflex is elevated indicates SNHL, VIIth CN/VIIIth CN disorder or absent indicates middle ear disorder.

Assessment of Eustachian Tube Function by Tympanometry in Intact or Perforated Tympanic Membrane

Toynbee test

The baseline tympanogram is obtained. The patient is then asked to swallow while pinching the nares, afterward the patient is to release the nares and not to swallow. Another tympanogram is recorded. If the Eustachian tube is patent, the tympanic membrane will retract medially. Ear canal pressure is increased until the pressure indicator deflects in the direction back to zero daPa indicating the forced opening of the Eustachian tube. If the pressure indicator does not return to zero daPa as in perforated TM, the patient is then asked to swallow repeatedly (usually 5 swallows in 20 seconds), the clinician then observes whether the pressure indicator returns to zero daPa. If the patient is unable to equilibrate the pressure completely, then it is assumed that the patient has Eustachian tube dysfunction in case of perforated eardrum.

Valsalva Maneuver (William Test)

This maneuver is used to assess the Eustachian tube function in intact tympanic membrane. The patient is instructed to pinch the nares and inflate the cheeks through forced expiration with the mouth closed until the air feels full. The patient is then asked to release the nose and to refrain from swallowing. A tympanogram is then obtained and the shift in tympanometric peak pressure during this maneuver is 47–79 daPa in adults with normal, Eustachian tube function. In case of patulous Eustachian tube the tympanometric peak pressure will be less than or equal to 45 daPa.

EVOKED RESPONSE AUDIOMETRY

Evoked response audiometry is an objective test that measures electrical activity in the auditory pathways in response to auditory stimuli. It has the following types:

- Auditory brainstem evoked response (ABR)
- Cortical evoked response audiometry (CERA)
- Electrocochleography (ECoG).

Auditory Brainstem Response (ABR) or Brainstem Evoked Response Audiometry (BERA)

Auditory brainstem response (ABR) is a far field recording of neuroelectric activity of the eight CN and brainstem auditory pathways that occurs over the first 10-15 milliseconds after a suitable sound stimulus delivered to the ear.

It is designated as a far field recording because of the relatively large distance between the recording electrodes on the scalp and the actual generators of the response in the brainstem.[12]

Stimulus Parameters

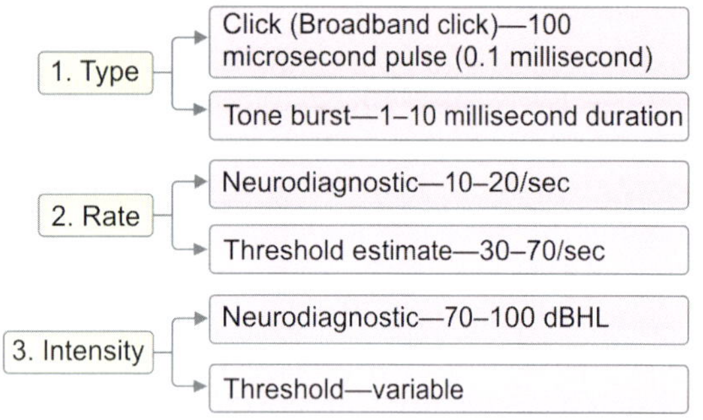

Electrode Sites

Active electrode (+) is placed on vertex. Reference electrode (–) on Ipsilateral lobule/mastoid. Ground electrode on forehead.

A series of clicks or tone bursts are delivered to the patient through inserted earphones, it elicits or evokes a series of small electrical events (Potentials) along the entire peripheral and central auditory pathway that is picked up the surface electrodes, amplified and averaged with a computer. This electrical activity is displayed as a waveform with latency specific wave peaks.

It measures hearing sensitivity in the range of 1000–4000 Hz.

In a normal person, 7 waves are produced in 1st 10 milliseconds (Fig. 9).

The 1st, 3rd and 5th waves are most stable and studied for
- Absolute latency
- Interwave latency (usually between wave I and V).
- Amplitude
- Morphology.

Remember pneumonic ECOLI for origin of waves:
Wave I—Eight nerve action potential.
Wave II—Cochlear nucleus.
Wave III—Olivary complex (superior).
Wave IV—Lateral lemniscus.
Wave V—Inferior colliculus.
Wave VI and VII—Not definitely known.

It is a noninvasive technique and is used—
- As a screening for infants
- To determine the threshold of hearing in infants, children and malingerers
- To diagnose CP angle tumors (Retrocochlear pathology)
- To diagnose brainstem pathology, e.g. multiple sclerosis or pontine tumors
- To monitor CNVIII intraoperatively in the surgery of acoustic neuromas.

Prolongation between:

Wave I and wave III is associated with—8th CN disorder and lower brainstem lesion.

Wave III and wave V is associated with—Upper brainstem disorder.

Wave V is the largest and most consistent.

Latency is dependent upon intensity of the stimulus.

Latency at threshold is ~ 8.5 milliseconds.

Latency at 50–60 dB HL is ~ 5.5 milliseconds.

Patient with middle ear pathology is associated with—
- Delayed response
- Normal morphology and
- Normal interwave intervals.

Cochlear lesions are associated with—
- Well-formed responses
- Normal absolute latencies and interwave intervals.

Retrocochlear disorders are associated with—
- Poor morphology
- Prolonged interwave intervals.

Auditory Steady State Responses[13]

Auditory steady state responses (ASSR) are auditory evoked neural potentials through steady state stimuli which have a frequency or amplitude modulation or both (Fig. 10). ASSR potentials are stimulated with a series of repeating stimuli. The potential difference originates in the VIII cranial nerve and the auditory brainstem, allowing acquisition of these

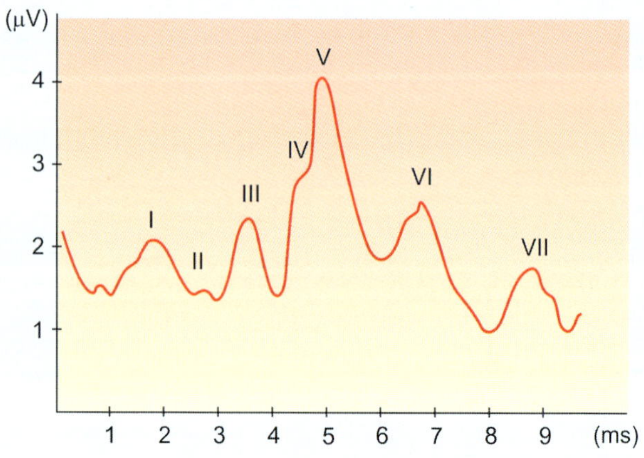

Fig. 9: Normal ABR waveform

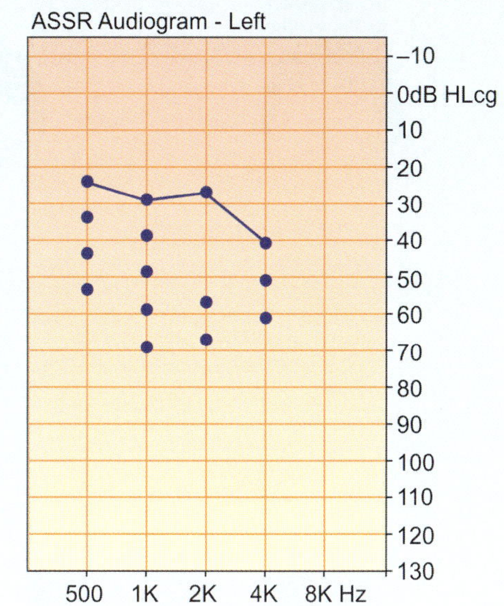

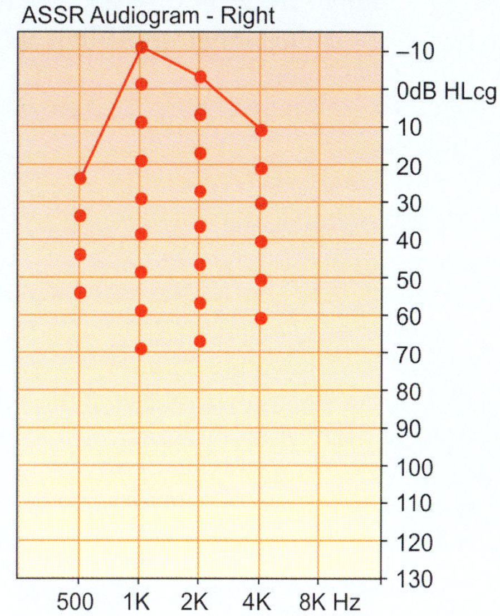

Fig. 10: ASSR response audiogram

differences by averaging the acquired signal over a specified period of time. ASSR and ABR have important differences, too. Rather than depending on amplitude and latency, ASSR uses amplitudes and phases in the spectral (frequency) domain. ASSR depends on peak detection across a frequency domain. ASSR is evoked using repeated sound stimuli presented at a high repetition rate. In ASSR, positive electrode is placed in nontest mastoid, negative electrode at test ear mastoid and ground electrode is placed at forehead. The ASSR is a far-field potential and extremely small compared to the background electroencephalographic (EEG) noise. In young infants, response amplitudes are largest when recorded from the ipsilateral mastoid (Table 3).

Recommended Test Settings

Table 3: Recommended settings for ASSR acquisition	
Parameter	**Suggestion**
Stimulus	500 Hz, 1 kHz, 2 kHz and 4 kHz tones, binaural stimulus at repetition rates of 70 Hz to 110 Hz
Transducers	Insert earphones
Intensity	70 dB SPL for starting point then up or down for threshold search
Filters and gain	These may not be modified
Notch filter	Off/On if there is excessive electrical line noise present
Analysis time window	1 sec
Sweeps	400 max
Electrode montage	Ipsilateral array

Advantages

- It can be used as a screening tool
- Identification of frequency specific air conduction threshold
- Identification of frequency specific bone conduction threshold
- Identification of frequency specific sound field threshold
- It can be used in pre- and post-hearing aid fitting tool
- To identify auditory neuropathy spectrum disorder.

Electrocochleography (ECoG)[14]

This is the measure of the electrical potentials arising within the cochlea and the auditory nerve in response to the auditory stimuli within first 5 milliseconds. Parameters measured by ECoG are:

- Cochlear microphonics (CM)
- Summating potential (SP)
- VIIIth CN action potential (AP).

The parameters are measured by transtympanic placement of electrode on promontory or on round window; reference electrode is placed on mastoid and ground electrode on forehead (Fig. 11).

Cochlear Microphonics (CM)

It is the electrical activity occurring in cochlea in response to sound stimulus.

- The source is hair bearing surface of the hair cells
- The onset is immediate and it mimics waveform of the acoustic stimulus

- The response obtained from promontory is diffuse and gives no definite information regarding specific population of the hair cells
- It is decreased in cochlear lesions and normal in retrocochlear lesions.

Summating Potential and VIIIth CN Action Potential

AP is the electrical activity obtained in VIIIth CN. SP is complex measurements of many electrophysiological parameters taken together.

Source: Hair cells.

- It represents asymmetry in movements of the basilar membrane during stimulation by sound
- It appears superimposed on the VIIIth CN action potential, seen as a direct current shift of baseline of the recording in a negative direction
- Normally SP is 30% of AP, the ratio is increased in Meniere's disease.

Application of electrocochleography:

- Testing for thresholds—Thresholds for clicks/Tone burst is equal to audiogram thresholds
- Study of Meniere's disease—Increase in negative summating potential is associated with increased periods of hearing loss in Meniere's disease
- Study of Acoustic Neuromas—Acoustic neuromas are associated with abnormal VIIIth CN action potentials
- Intraoperative monitoring of peripheral auditory system.

Advantages (Fig. 12)

- Totally objective test
- No masking of contralateral ear is required
- Accurate measurement of hearing threshold can be made between 1000 and 8000 Hz.

Disadvantages

These tests need for placement of transtympanic needle. It gives us information about cochlear integrity only. Recently, extratympanic electrodes are of clinician's choice. Wick electrodes, impregnated mesh with jelly, foam tip, and wings of flexible plastic are the most available extratympanic recording electrodes as per various manufacturers' specifications.

Middle-Latency Responses[15]

The middle-latency response (MLR) is derived from the medial geniculate body, inferior colliculus and the primary auditory cortex (Fig. 13). The MLR is used to assess auditory cortical functions, whether the person has function or does not have function. If there is an abnormality, it determines the side that is affected. The MLR produces waveforms that

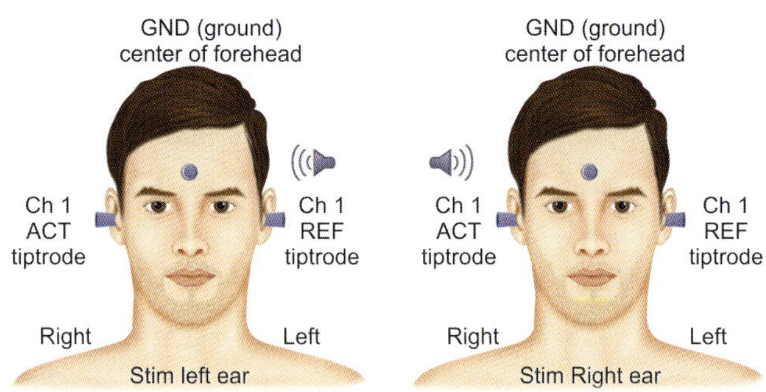

Fig. 11: Horizontal montages for ECoG

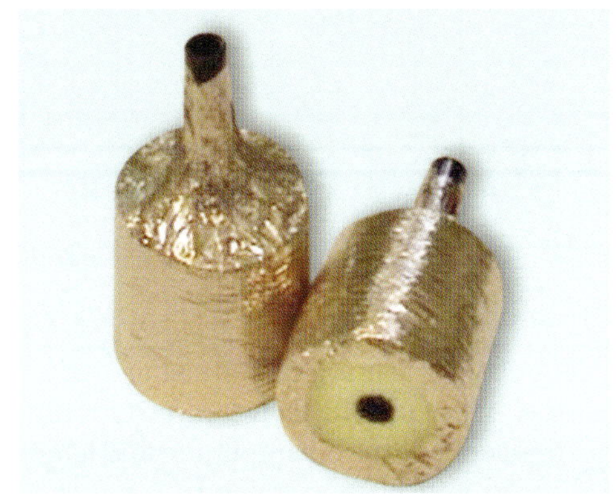

Fig. 12: Tiptrode

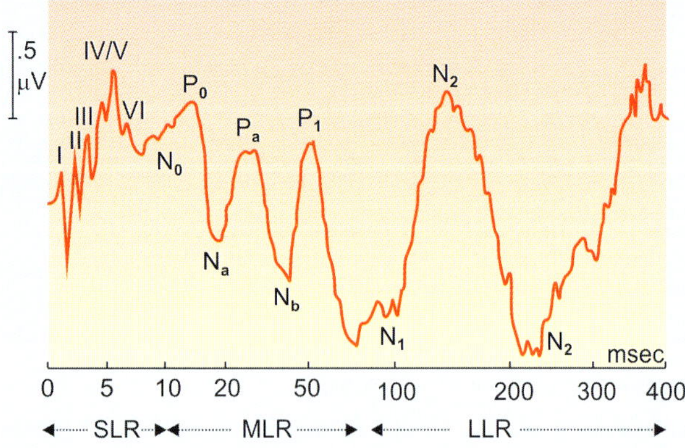

Fig. 13: Middle latency response

Abbreviations: SLR, short latency response; MLR, middle latency response; LLR, late latency response

are identifiable at or near threshold and may be useful in identifying low-frequency auditory sensitivity. However, the ABR latencies are more consistent between tests than with MLRs. MLR has larger amplitude than the ABR and is less dependent on neural synchrony. The latency of the response is unchanged whether the patient is asleep or awake, but the amplitude is highly affected. In single channel MLR, positive electrode is placed in nontest mastoid, negative electrode at test ear mastoid and ground electrode is placed at forehead. In dual channel MLR, positive electrode is placed at vertex, negative electrodes are placed at mastoids and ground electrode is placed at forehead. The response amplitude decreases with faster rates, so it is easier to record the MLR if a slower rate is used. The filters are 10–300 Hz, so they are much narrower than for ECoG or ABR. The MLR is a much later potential, so the sweep time is relatively as long as 80 milliseconds. It is a large response so not as many sweeps are needed to collect this response, about 1,000 sweeps will do, and it always stops the collection if a robust response appears. A 10 millisecond prestimulus delay is recommended.

P300[16]

P300 is considered a late-latency response (LLR) that generally occurs at approximately 300 milliseconds. P300 is dependent on internal thought process and is generated by the hippocampus where short-term memory functions are stored. The patient must be awake and alert to the stimuli. In single channel P300, positive electrode is placed in nontest ear mastoid, negative electrode at test ear mastoid and ground electrode is placed at forehead. In dual channel P300, positive electrode is placed at vertex, negative electrodes are placed at mastoids and ground electrode is placed at forehead. The P300 is generated from conscious discrimination of different stimuli. The purpose of the counting task is to ensure they are attending to the stimuli and that their brain is staying alert. That attention is what generates the P300 response. The P300 is a slow, broad response with a peak at 250–300 milliseconds. A decrease in amplitude and an increase in latency are indicative of dementia, Alzheimer's or other various neurological or psychiatric diseases. Therefore, if there is a disorder of cognitive functioning, the P300 typically will be abnormal. The parameters for the P300 vary from the other evoked potentials. The default intensity for both stimuli is 75 dBnHL (dB normalized hearing level). Insert earphones with an alternating polarity for the tone bursts is the default. The frequency can be selected for both tones, but the default is 1000 Hz and 2000 Hz. The gain is usually lower for later potentials because they are such large responses. The artifact rejection level for the P300 is just below the amplitude. That can help to ensure the eye-blink artifacts excluded in the P300 response (Fig. 14).

Cortical Responses[17]

The cortical response is derived from a slow-vertex response, is a form of sensory cortical responses (150–1000 ms). It produces waveforms that are identifiable near a threshold and may be useful in identifying hearing status

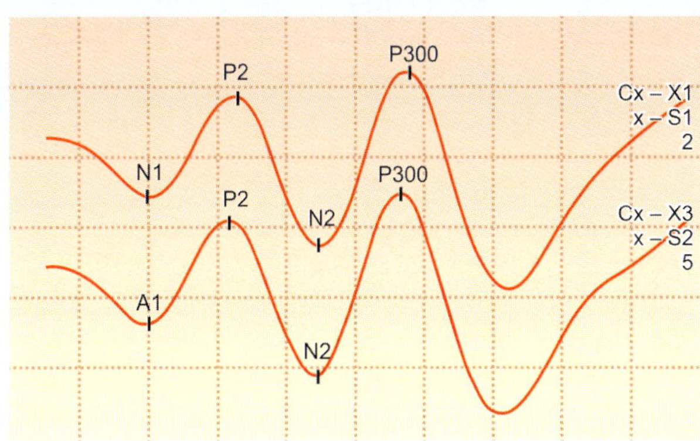

Fig. 14: P300

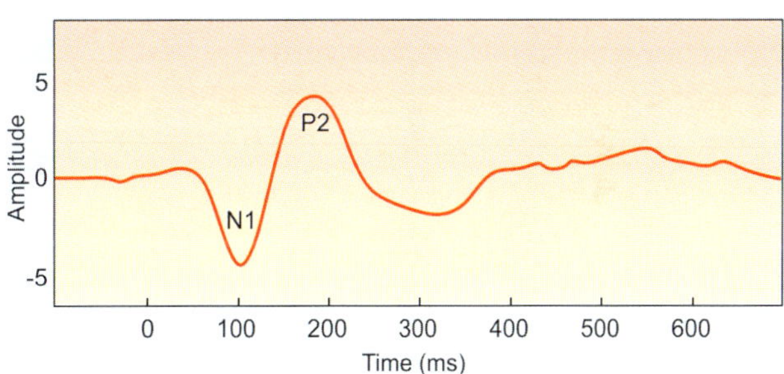

Fig. 15: Cortical response

using tone burst stimuli. It is used for medicolegal cases or for patients who are difficult to test with behavioral audiometry. The one disadvantage to cortical responses is that the response is not fully matured until the late teen years. In cortical response identification, positive electrode is placed in non-test mastoid, negative electrode at test ear mastoid and ground electrode is placed at forehead. The response is collected using a 2000 Hz tone burst presented at 70, 50 and 30 dB with N1 to P2 marked. The benefit is that a robust response appears with very few sweeps (Fig. 15).

Otoacoustic Emission (OAE)

Otoacoustic emissions are sounds that originate in the cochlea and propagate through middle ear and into the ear canal where they can be measured by using a sensitive microphone placed in the external auditory canal. OAE's are first described by David Kemp in 1978. OAE's are generated by the somatic motilities of OHC's and non-linear mechanics of the OHC stereocilia bundle. Prestin is assumed to be the molecular motor responsible protein for somatic OHC motility. These outer hair cells are stimulated in a manner that causes them to act on the signal. One byproduct of that action is the production of a sound, which travels back out of the cochlea, through the middle ear, and into the ear canal. This sound is referred to as an otoacoustic emission or OAE.[18] OAE's are classified majorly as two types:

- Spontaneous otoacoustic emissions (SOAE)
- Evoked otoacoustic emissions (EOAE)

EOAE is divided into three types:

- Transient otoacoustic emissions (TEOAE)
- Distortion product otoacoustic emissions (DPOAE)
- Stimulus frequency otoacoustic emissions (SFOAE).

SOAEs are measured in the absence of the external simultaneous and are measureable in approximately 50% of normal hearing children and adults. SOAE can be measured in ears having hearing loss no greater than 25–30 dBnHL in patients having normal middle ear function excluded by impedance audiometry.

TEOAE is the evoked OAE, measured after the presentation of a transient or brief stimulus. A click or tone burst is presented to the ear, and the response occurs after a brief time delay. TEOAE can be measured in ears having hearing loss no greater than 35–40 dBnHL (Fig. 16).

DPOAE's are measured simultaneous with the presentation of two pure tone stimuli called 'primaries' to the ear. The frequency of the primaries are conventionally designed as F_1 and F_2 ($F_1 < F_2$) and the corresponding levels of the primaries are named as 'L1' and 'L2'. The F_1 and F_2 are reasonably close in frequency, interaction of the two primaries on the Basilar membrane result in the output of energy by the cochlea at other discreet frequencies that are arithmetically related to the frequencies of primaries (e.g. $F_2 - F_1$, $2F_1 - F_2$, etc.). DPOAE can be measured in ears having hearing loss no greater than 55–60 dBnHL.

SFOAE occurs at the same frequency and at the same time as a continuous pure tone applied to the ear. The microphone in the ear canal records the combination of the pure tone being presented to the ear and the SFOAE is evoked by the pure tone. Averaged SFOAE levels generally

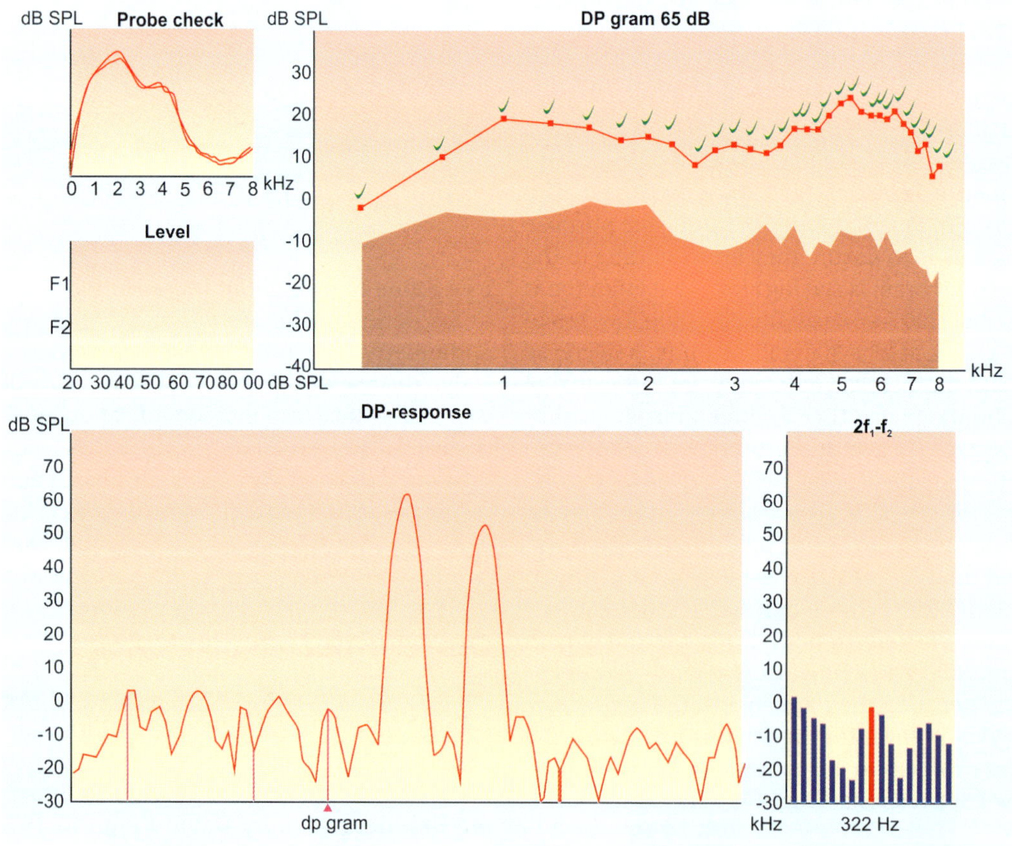

Fig. 16: Two dimension picture of DPOAE findings (DPGRM)

grow linearly for low stimulus levels and then saturate for high stimulus levels.

Applications

- Identification of hearing loss
- Prediction of hearing thresholds
- Diagnosing auditory neuropathy spectrum disorder in collaboration with ABR findings
- Globally accepted tool for newborn hearing screening
- Monitoring cochlear functions with reference to ototoxicity.

REFERENCES

1. American National Standards Institute. Specifications for audiometers (ANSI S3.6-2004). (2004). New York: Author.
2. American National Standards Institute. Maximum permissible ambient noise levels for audiometric test rooms (ANSI S3.1-1999;Rev. ed.). (2003). New York: Author.
3. Carhart R, Jerger JF. Preferred method for clinical determination of pure-tone thresholds. Journal of Speech and Hearing Disorders. 1959;24:330-45.
4. American Speech-Language-Hearing Association. Guidelines for manual pure-tone threshold audiometry. (2005). Rockville, MD: Author.
5. American Speech-Language-Hearing Association. Guidelines for audiometric symbols. (1990). Rockville, MD: Author.
6. Jerger J, Speaks C, Trammell J. A new approach to speech audiometry. Journal of Speech and Hearing Disorders. 1968;33:318-28.
7. Gelfand SA. Essentials of Audiology, (2009) 3rd ed. New York: Thieme Medical Publishers, Inc.
8. Jerger J, Jerger S. Diagnostic significance of PB word functions. Arch Otolaryng. 1971;93:573-80.
9. Measurement of acoustic impedance and rectance in the human ear canal. The Journal of the Acoustical Society of America. 1994;95:372-84.
10. Rosowski JJ, Nakajima HH, Hamade MA, Mahfoud L, Merchant GR, Halpin CF, Merchant SN. Ear-canal reectance, umbo velocity, and tympanometry in normal-hearing adults. Ear and Hearing. 2012;33(1):19-34.
11. Asai M, Roberson JB Jr, Goode RL. Acoustic effect of malleus head removal and tensor tympani muscle section on middle ear reconstruction. Laryngoscope. 1997;107:1217-22.
12. Roger A. Ruth and Paul R. Lambert. Auditory brainstem response, The Otolaryngologic clinics of North America, April. 1991;24(2):353-69.
13. Beck DL, Speidel DP, Petrak M. Auditory steady-state response (ASSR): a beginner's guide. Hearing Review. 2007;14(12): 34-7.
14. McPherson DL. (1996). Late Potentials of the Auditory System. San Diego: Singular.
15. Hall JW. (1992). Handbook of auditory evoked responses. Boston: Allyn and Bacon.
16. Näätänen R. (1992). Attention and Brain Function. Hillsdale. NJ: Lawrence Erlbaum Associates.
17. Davis H, Mast T, Yoshie N, Zerlin S. The slow response of the human cortex to auditory stimuli: Recovery process. Electroenceph Clin Neurophysiol. 1966;21:105-13.
18. Hall JW. HandBook of otoacoustic emissions. (2000). Clifton Park, NY: Singular Thomson Learning.

Hearing Loss

Asok K Saha

INTRODUCTION

- Conductive hearing loss
- Sensorineural hearing loss
- Sudden hearing loss
- Nonorganic hearing loss.

HEARING LOSS

Classification

Classification of hearing loss is an important and essential component for assessing hearing status of an individual. Hearing loss is classified as:

Organic

- Conductive hearing loss (CHL)—Sound transmission obstructed in external or middle ear or both
- Sensorineural hearing loss (SNHL)—Involvement of cochlea and/or the auditory nerve
- Mixed hearing loss—Combination of CHL and SNHL
- Central hearing loss—Dysfunction in the central nervous system
- Auditory neuropathy—Absence of neural function.

Nonorganic or Functional Hearing Loss

Hearing loss not substantiated with routine auditory tests.

Conductive Hearing Loss

Conductive hearing loss results from any condition that may obstruct to the flow of sound energy from external ear to the inner ear. Anatomically this pathway of obstruction includes external auditory canal, tympanic membrane and ossicles of middle ear (Fig. 1).

The flow of sound energy may be blocked by cerumen impaction, otitis media with effusion or any pathology that

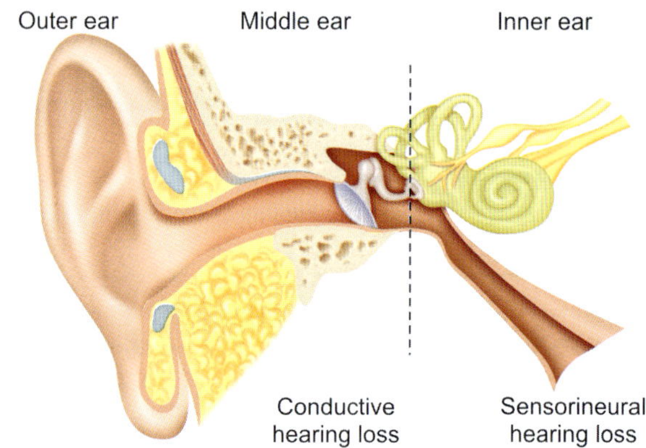

Fig. 1: Anatomical pathway of obstruction of sound energy from external ear to inner ear resulting in hearing loss

may cause ossicular discontinuity or fixation resulting in changes with sound conduction system of the middle ear.

Criteria for CHL

- Tuning fork test with 512 Hz (CPS) shows (Fig. 2):

Rinne Test is Negative

Heinrich Rinne first described the test in the year 1855. The test is performed by placing base of the vibrating tuning fork firmly on the mastoid bone and then placing the prongs of the vibrating tuning fork in the air closer to the ear. The patient is asked whether he or she hears louder when the fork is in the air or placed on the bone. In normal individual or patient with sensorineural hearing loss is heard louder when the fork is placed in the air compared with when it is placed on the bone. This response is called positive Rinne test. The person with CHL will hear the sound louder when the fork is placed on the bone than in the air. This response is said negative Rinne test. At least an air-bone gap of 18 dB is in need to get negative Rinne test.

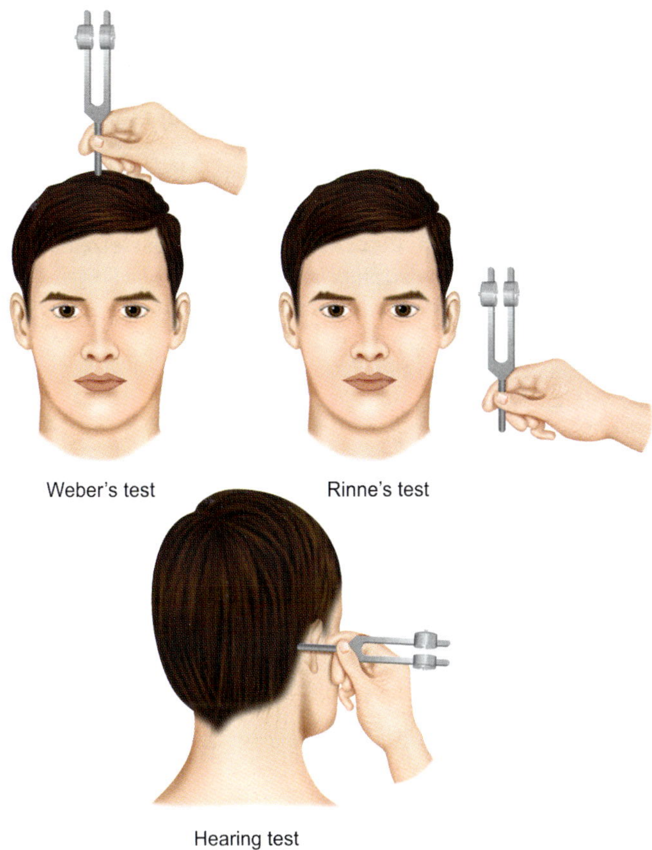

Fig. 4.2: Tuning fork test

- If tuning fork test with 256 Hz (CPS) is negative it hints mild conductive loss with 20–30 dB air-bone gap
- Tuning fork test with 512 Hz (CPS) is negative indicating moderate conductive loss of 30–45 dB air-bone gap
- If tuning fork with 1024 Hz (CPS) is negative it indicates a maximum conductive loss with air-bone gap of 45–60 dB.

Weber is Lateralized to the Diseased Ear

Wilhelm Weber first described the test in the year 1825. In Weber test base of vibrating tuning fork (512 Hz) is placed firmly on the top of the head or forehead and patient is asked whether he or she hears the sound louder in one ear. In patient with CHL, the sound is lateralized to the ear of disease side. In unilateral SNHL the sound is lateralized to the better ear. In normal individual, the sound is central. When a mixed hearing loss is present, sound is lateralized to the ear with conductive impairment. In CHL, lateralization of sound indicates a hearing loss of only 10–15 dB.

Reasons of Lateralization

- Ambient sound theory (Noise Theory)—Ambient sound is the sound that is always present in environment. In normal individual as ambient sound is heard, tuning fork sound is not heard. In CHL, ambient sound is not heard, so tuning fork sound is heard well.
- Theory of dispersion—Vibration of tuning fork is dispersed via bone in all directions-middle ear, external ear and inner ear after reaching the medial wall of middle ear. In CHL, all sounds from tuning fork is conducted to the inner ear and not to the exterior because of disease of the middle ear and/or external ear. Sound is, therefore, heard well in the ear with CHL.[1]

Some patient refuses to accept that the vibration of tuning fork is heard in the ear with conductive impairment. Bing test is done to clarify this.

- Bing Test—This is a bone conduction test, first described by Albert Bing in the year 1891. Vibrating tuning fork is applied to mastoid bone and then external auditory canal is occluded by pressing on the tragus. If hearing is louder, Bing test is positive seen in normal person or one with SNHL.

  If hearing remains same or less, Bing test is negative indicating CHL. This test is useful even in mixed hearing loss where conducting impairment is minimal and tympanic membrane is intact as in otosclerosis.
- Gelle's Test—It is also a bone conduction test where a vibrating tuning fork is placed on mastoid bone and air pressure in the ipsilateral external auditory canal is increased intermittently by Siegle's speculum or pneumatic otoscope or by pressing finger on tragus. Decrease in loudness of a bone conducted sound is present in people with normal conductive mechanism and with SNHL and no change in loudness of hearing is observed in ossicular fixation or discontinuity. This test is useful to detect conductive impairment in otosclerosis.
- Lewis Test—A vibrating tuning fork is placed on mastoid bone. When conducted sound is no longer heard, stem of the fork is placed on the tragus and gentle pressure is applied to occlude the ear canal. If tympanic membrane and ossicles are intact but ossicular fixity is present, sound is not heard when fork is placed on the tragus. In normal condition and SNHL vibration of tuning fork is heard well.

Absolute Bone Conduction (ABC) Test is Normal

ABC or Pomeroy's test—Bone conduction is a measure of cochlear function. In ABC test, bone conduction of the patient is compared to the bone conduction of the examiner. A vibrating tuning fork is placed on the mastoid and external ear canal is occluded by pressing on the tragus. When the patient stops hearing the vibration tuning fork is placed on the mastoid bone of the examiner to hear the vibration. If the examiner still hears the vibration of the sound, the bone conduction of the patient is diminished indicating SNHL.

In CHL, the patient and the examiner hear the vibration of Tuning fork for same duration of time and then ABC of the patient is normal.

Schwabach's Test — This is a crude comparison of bone conduction of the patient to that of examiner (normal hearing person) without occluding ear canal. The test is said to be diminished in SNHL and equal or lengthened in normal person or in CHL.

Low Frequencies are Usually Affected in CHL

Pure tone audiometry (PTA) which is the gold standard of assessing hearing threshold shows air-bone gap of about 10 dB or more while bone conduction level is normal (15 dB–20 dB). Air-bone gap represents quantitative measurement of CHL on audiogram. Greater the air-bone gap more is the conductive hearing loss (Fig. 3).

A CHL can produce maximum losses of 60 dB. Ossicular disruption is considered with hearing losses greater than 50 dB.[2] Speech discrimination score is good in CHL.

- Impedance audiometry represents the compliance of tympanic membrane to different pressure changes.
  - Low-compliance (type As) is seen in ossicular fixation
  - High-compliance (type Ad) is obtained with ossicular discontinuity
  - Decreased compliance (type B or C) hints fluid in middle ear

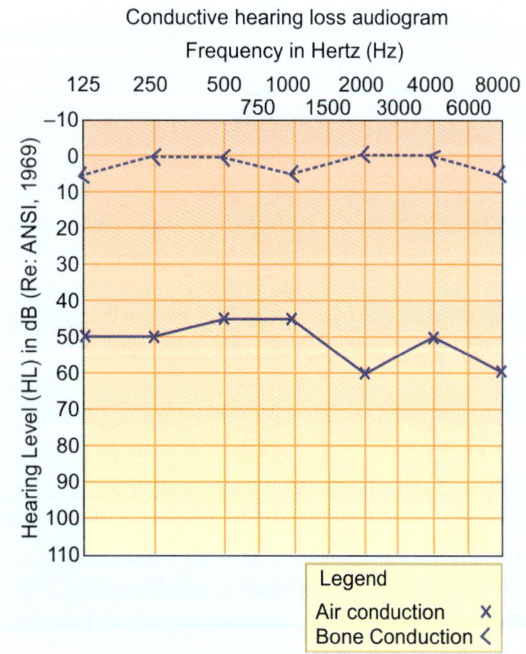

Fig. 3: Audiogram of left ear conductive hearing loss with A-B gap

- Flat tympanogram (type B) reveals perforation in tympanic membrane.
- Stapedial reflex is absent if CHL is greater than 40 dB. It is useful in evaluating quantitative measurement of hearing loss.
  - CT scan of temporal bone is helpful imaging in CHL. It reveals the status of middle ear and mastoid, ossicular discontinuity, otosclerosis and labyrinthine fistula.[3]

Causes of conductive hearing loss (CHL)
- Pathologies in external ear
  - Wax impaction
  - Foreign body in the ear
  - Otitis externa
  - Atresia of ear canal
  - Bony exostosis
  - Tumors
  - Cyst and canal cholesteatoma.
- Pathologies in middle ear
  - Perforation of tympanic membrane
  - Tympanosclerosis
  - Otitis media with effusion
  - Ossicular discontinuity
  - Ossicular fixity—fixation of malleus head or otosclerosis
  - Cholesteatoma
  - Tumors.
- Temporal bone fracture/hemotympanum
- In adults, most common cause of CHL is wax impaction followed by tympanic membrane perforation. 1% of population is affected by otosclerosis
- In children, the most common cause is otitis media with effusion.

Key points
- Complete obstruction of ear canal results in CHL of about 30–40 dB
- Perforation of tympanic membrane causes CHL ranging from negligible to 50 dB, depending on frequency, perforation size and position as well as middle ear air space volume[4,5]
- Otitis media with effusion (OME) causes conductive loss of up to 30–35 dB[6] because of reduction of ossicular coupling caused by fluid.
- Atelectasis of tympanic membrane results in CHL varying from negligible to 50 dB, because of reduction in ossicular coupling caused by atelectatic tympanic membrane
- Complete ossicular interruption with an intact tympanic membrane can cause CHL of about 60 dB[7] as ossicular coupling is lost, sound input to oval window results from acoustic coupling only and ossicular coupling is about 60 dB larger than acoustic coupling

- Loss of tympanic membrane, malleus and incus may cause CHL ranging from 40–50 dB. This is explained by loss of ossicular coupling as well as in enhancement of acoustic coupling by 10–20 dB in comparison to normal individual.[8]
- Ossicular fixity as is seen in otosclerosis or tympanosclerosis causes CHL of 5–60 dB depending on the degree of fixation. Footplate fixation results in reduction in ossicular coupling causing CHL. Stiffness of the annular ligament which is the primary effect of otosclerotic lesion affects hearing loss mainly in low-frequencies.[9] Malleus fixation is associated with CHL of 50–25 dB which is less compared to stapes fixation as complete fixation does not occur and some motion is present across the incudomalleolar joint resulting less reduction in ossicular coupling.[10]

SENSORINEURAL HEARING LOSS (SNHL)

Sensorineural hearing loss is the reduction in sensitivity of auditory threshold due to lesion in the cochlea and/or in the auditory nerve and central auditory pathways (retrocochlear) (Fig. 4).

Criteria of SNHL

- Weber test shows sound lateralizes to better ear
- Rinne test is positive, air conduction > bone conduction Both air and bone conductions are equally decreased but the difference between them remains unchanged
- Absolute bone conduction test or Schwabch test shows bone conduction is reduced
- Audiogram reveals both air and bone conduction lines are below the normal thresholds and air-bone gap is 10 dB or less
- Hearing loss usually involves high-frequencies and may exceed 60 dB. Speech discrimination score is poor
- Difficulty of hearing in noise
- Certain sounds seem too loud.

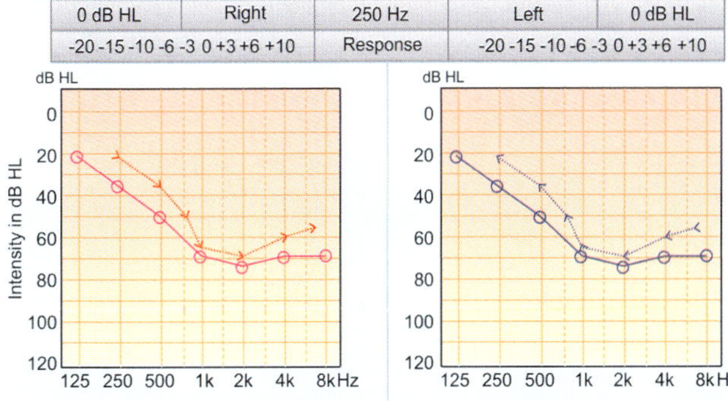

Fig. 4: Audiogram shows symmetrical sensorineural hearing loss of both ears

Causes of SNHL

Congenital

- Malformations of the cochlea
- Chromosomal syndromes
- Congenital infections—infection that passes from mother to baby (e.g. Rubella, CMV).

Acquired

- Presbyacusis—age-related sensorineural hearing impairment
- Noise-induced hearing loss
- Ototoxicity—aminoglycosides, loop diuretics, cytotoxic drug, antimalarials
- Acquired infections—measles, mumps, toxoplasmosis, meningitis, herpes type I and type II and syphilis
- Immune-related hearing loss
- Familial progressive SNHL
- Meniere's diseases
- Trauma to inner ear or VIII CN, e.g. temporal bone fracture, ear surgeries, etc.
- Tumors, such as acoustic neuroma
- Idiopathic SNHL.

Etiology, assessment and management of SNHL of infants and children are covered in Chapter 14.

Common Conditions of SNHL

Presbyacusis—Age-related sensorineural hearing impairment.

The term presbyacusis comes from Greek word Preys meaning 'elder' and akousis meaning 'hearing' or age-related SNHL. It is defined as bilateral, symmetrical and progressive SNHL presenting in people older than the age of 65 years where hearing loss caused by other primary conditions, such as noise-induced hearing loss, ototoxicity, atherosclerosis, hypothyroidism, head injury, etc. are excluded. As the loss of hearing is so gradual the people with presbyacusis does not realize this diminishing hearing loss. Environmental noises contribute significantly and half of the people with presbyacusis are genetically determined. The hearing loss is seen in high-frequency (>2000 Hz). Speech discrimination is significantly poor and difficulty in hearing is realized by people in noisy background. Men suffer more than women.

Pathological Changes

Inner Ear

Pathological changes of inner ear are evident; these are sensory, neural, vascular or strial and cochlear conduction.

- Sensory presbyacusis—There is loss of hair cells at the basal end of corti.[11,14] High-frequencies are affected with good speech discrimination (Fig. 5)

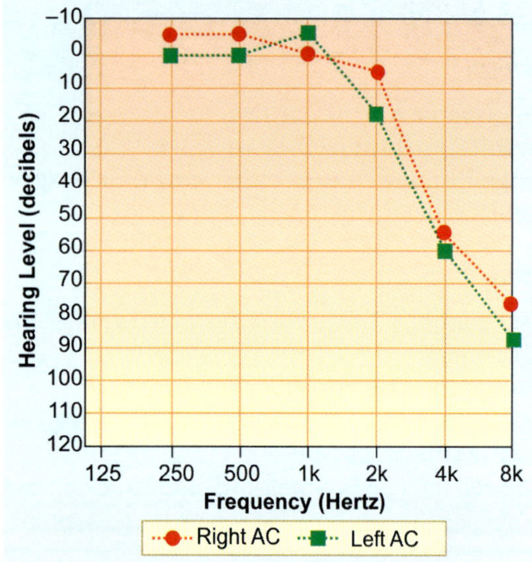

Fig. 5: Sensory presbyacusis with good speech discrimination

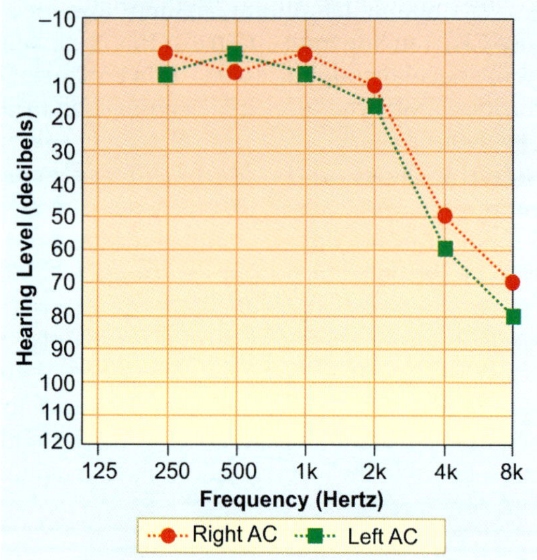

Fig. 6: Neural presbyacusis similar to sensory presbyacusis but poor speech discrimination

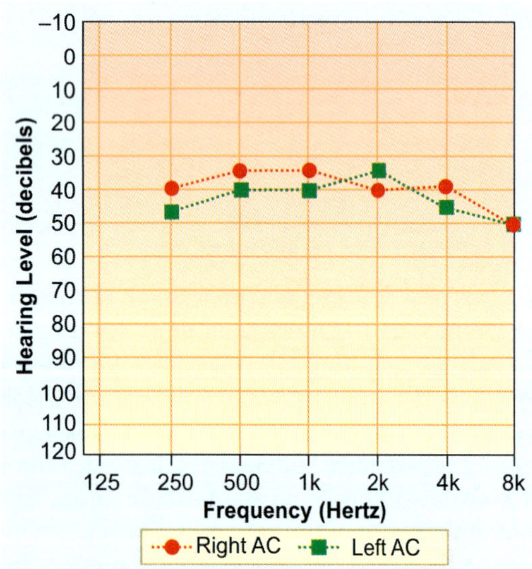

Fig. 7: Vascular or strial presbyacusis

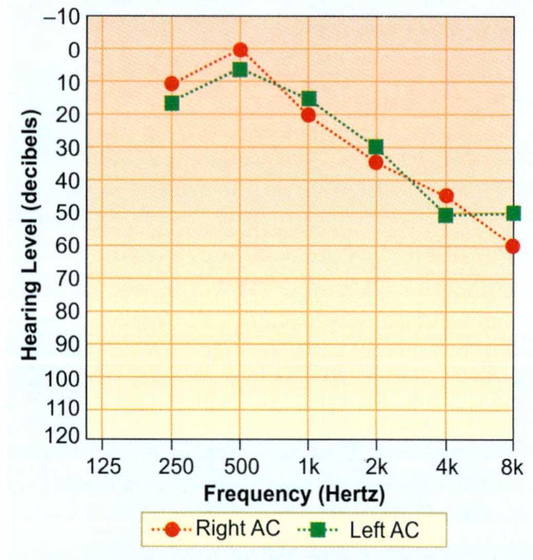

Fig. 8: Cochlear conductive presbyacusis

- Neural presbyacusis—There is degeneration of neurons of cochlear nerve resulting in loss of cochlear ganglion cell. A high tone loss with poor speech discrimination is indicative of neural presbyacusis (Fig. 6)
- Vascular or strial presbyacusis—There is atrophy of stria vascularis with loss of strial tissue in the apical and middle turns of the cochlea.[12,14] A flat threshold curve in audiogram is significant in strial presbyacusis (Fig. 7)
- Cochlear conductive presbyacusis—There is alterations in the physical characteristics of the cochlear duct associated with stiffness of the basilar membrane because of increase number of fibrillar layers of basilar membrane.[13,14] A sloping threshold pattern is present in audiogram (Fig. 8).

External Ear and Middle Ear

It is now known that the loss of some sensitivity sometimes is caused by changes in external ear and or middle ear. Such changes may include reduced epithelial migration, increased hair growth or potential collapse of external ear, reduced function of tympanic membrane or ossicular chain for carrying sound waves from tympanic membrane to the inner ear.

Genetic Factors are important in age-related hearing loss. A clear familial aggregation occurs in sensory presbyacusis phenotype and strial presbyacusis phenotype. The aggregations are stronger in women than in men and greater for the strial phenotype than for his sensory phenotype.[15,16]

Diagnostic evaluation is based on pure tone audiogram which shows a mild SNHL at higher frequencies in early condition. As the condition worsens the audiogram reveals hearing loss at mid frequencies (1–2 kHz) and at low-frequencies (250–500 kHz).[17] If significant asymmetry in hearing exists, MRI is required to rule out CP angle tumor.

Treatment

- Presbyacusis is not curable. Properly fitting hearing aid helps to improve hearing in people with presbyacusis
- There are no specific criteria where hearing aid is to be recommended. Usually, when high-frequency loss is greater than 40 dB on audiogram a trial of hearing aid is indicated. Lesser degree of hearing loss may need hearing aid trial if professional or social life requires fine hearing[18]
- Assistive listening devices are also beneficial role to amplify sound without disturbing other people with normal hearing
- Lip reading helps the people with poor speech discrimination and hearing aid user to hear well in background noise
- Cochlear implants are helpful in some people having bilateral cochlear changes with intact spiral ganglion and normal central auditory pathways where severe hearing loss is not improved with the help of hearing aid
- Trial for treatment of hearing loss by gene therapy, cellular or pharmacotherapy to regenerate hearing cells in the damage region of the cochlea is on progress. Endogenous stem cell study of inner ear may help to unlock the regenerative potential of such cells to improve the fundamental deficit in presbyacusis with stem cell therapy.[19]

NOISE-INDUCED HEARING LOSS (NIHL)

Noise-induced hearing loss is the impairment of hearing caused by one time exposure to high intense sound or repeated exposure to sounds at less intense levels for a period of time (Fig. 9).

The hearing loss may be temporary and it recovers after short interval of time (a few minutes to a few hours). This is described as temporary threshold shift (TTS).

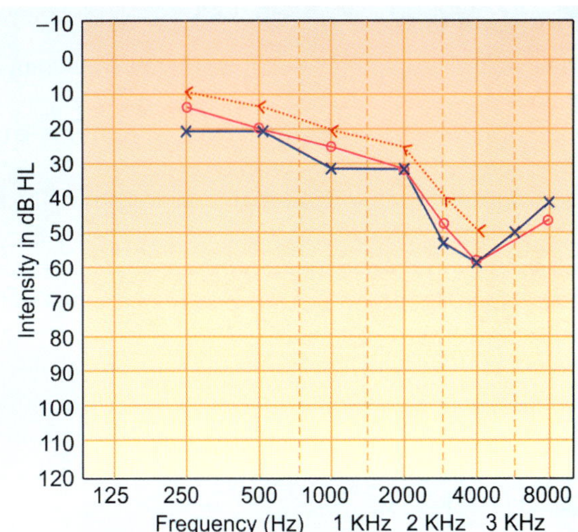

Fig. 9: Noised-induced hearing loss

The hearing loss may be permanent and it does not recover with time. This is described as permanent threshold shift (PTS). This may happen following TTS or following one time exposure to noise.

The term 'acoustic trauma' is used when hearing impairment is caused by single exposure to high-intense sound with immediate hearing loss, such as explosions, gun fire or fire crackers.

Pathophysiology

Noise trauma leads to over stimulation of the hair cells resulting in excessive production of reactive oxygen species (ROS) that damages phospholipids in membranes and DNA leading to oxidative cell death. It is evident from studies that cochlear dysfunction includes[20]—

- Metabolic exhaustion of hair cells and
- Structural changes within the hair cells.

Metabolic Changes

Recovery of hearing from TTS implies metabolic mechanism. Possible metabolic mechanisms are as follows:

- Cochlear over stimulation from acoustic trauma leads to excessive release of glutamate that may contribute to NIHL based on the evidence that administration of glutamate receptor antagonists reduces TTS[21]
- Sound of moderate intensity increases cochlear blood flow whereas sound of high-intensity decreases cochlear blood flow. Noise induces changes in cochlear blood flow resulting in cochlear hypoxia[22]
- High-intense sound effects in outer hair cell plasma membrane fluidity and induces oxidative stress.[23, 24]

Structural Changes

Persistence of PTS is thought to imply structural mechanism; these include—

- Micromechanism changes and degeneration of structures within the hair cells
- Depolymerization of actin filaments in stereocilia that may be the substrate of TTS
- Swelling of stria vascularis and rupture of cell membrane
- Complete degeneration with loss of hair cells, neural cells and supporting cells.[25]

Corelation of NIHL with hair cell dysfunction is complex and controversial. Progression of outer hair cell death following cessation of noise indicates necrotic mechanism being involved in addition to metabolic and structural changes in organ of corti.[26]

Risk Factors for NIHL

Potential changes for risk of NIHL are considered with Ahl gene, smoking, diabetes and cardiovascular diseases. Individuals with blue eye color, alcohol and recreational drug use may cause greater chances of NIHL and tinnitus. Combination of ototoxicity and noise has synergistic effect on NIHL. Individual variability is also noted in the susceptibility of NIHL. Male are more susceptible than female.

Symptoms

Common accompanying symptoms are otalgia, tinnitus, hyperacusis, headache and sleep disturbance.

Investigations

- PTA—NIHL is characterized by a specific pattern in pure tone audiogram. It shows a notch-shaped high-frequency sensorineural loss that is worst at 4 kHz, although the notch appears at 3 kHz or 6 kHz as well with recovery at 8 kHz. It is usually symmetrical in both ears. Asymmetry may exist in audiogram when source of the noise is lateralized as seen in riffle or gun fire. However, all audiological results will not match the above description but significant hearing loss at frequencies below 2 kHz is rare. Speech recognition scores (SRS) correlate well with the level of loss. Significant reduction in speech recognition scores starts if frequencies are less than 3 kHz are affected[8, 27]
- Impedance audiometry is also essential to confirm normal middle ear function
- BERA is required in suspected cases of nonorganic hearing loss
- MRI—In case of significant asymmetric hearing loss on both sides, MRI helps to exclude any vestibular shwannoma. MRI is also done if hearing loss is more than 10 dB at same frequency when it is compared from both sides.

According to Occupational Safety and Health Administration (OSHA), Department of Labor, Exposure to 85 dB (A) of noise, known as exposure action value, for more, than 8 hours per day may cause permanent hearing loss.[28] It is evident that even with prolonged exposure to sound levels below 80 dB is safe.[29] Exposure to impulsive or impact noise should not exceed 140 dB peak sound pressure level as is also stated by OSHA. It is evident that every increase of 3 dB sound pressure level (SPL) results in a doubling of intensity. It indicates hearing loss occurs at a faster rate. So NIHL due to chronic exposure to noise is related to combination of the sound intensity and duration of noise.

As per Government of India, Ministry of Labor, model rules under factories act, permissible limits of time for various intensities of noise level are given in Table 1.

Preventive Measures

Noise-induced hearing loss is an irreversible hearing impairment. Therefore, it is essential to take preventable measures that include:

- Avoiding the exposure to excessive noise
- Using the correct hearing protective devices (HPDS), i.e. ear plugs or ear muffs
- Performing routine hearing test to find out any professional hearing loss
- Developing a noise protective program by employer in the working place. Occupations susceptible to hearing loss are agriculture, mining, construction, transportation and music conduction, etc.

Ear plugs and ear muffs can provide the users with 10 to 15 dB of sound attenuation. Active noise reduction is an electronic device that provides sounds inside a set of ear muffs. It cancels out the background noise and is an effective form of sound attenuation, usually at lower frequencies (<1000). Other measures used for severe hearing loss are infrared headphones for use with television, volume

Table 1: Various intensities of noise level

Noise level (dBA)	Permitted daily exposure (hours)
90	8
95	4
100	2
105	1
110	½
115	¼

controllable telephones, louder door bells and lip reading classes. Binaural hearing aids are providing excellent rehabilitative support. Again some treatable conditions are alleged to exacerbate NIHL, e.g. smoking, cardiovascular disease, diabetes mellitus, hyperlipidemia and ototoxic drug. Appropriate treatment of these conditions might improve NIHL.

OTOTOXICITY

Literally, the term ototoxicity means ear poisoning (oto = ear, toxicity = poison). More exactly, it refers to toxic insult to inner ear resulting from medication of drugs or chemicals that may affect hearing or balance or both. The ototoxic effect may be reversible and temporary or irreversible and permanent as well as dose limiting.

Commonly used drugs causing ototoxicity as a side effect of medication are:
- Antibiotics of aminoglycoside, macrolide and polypeptide groups
- Antineoplastic agents—Cisplatin and related compounds
- Loop diuretics—Frusemide, ethacrynic acid and bumetanide
- Antimalarial drugs—Quinine and Chloroquine
- Analgesics—Salicylates and nonsteroidal antiinflammatory drugs (NSAIDs)
- Other agents—Heavy metals, e.g. arsenic, mercury and lead
    - Organic solvents, such as propylene glycol, styrene or benzene.

Ototoxic antibiotics, antineoplastics and organic solvents are found to cause irreversible and permanent hearing loss and or/vestibular injury.

Other drugs like loop diuretics, analgesics and antimalarial agents have primarily reversible effect causing temporary hearing loss and tinnitus.

Ototoxic Drugs

Antibiotics of aminoglycosides are gentamicin, tobramycin, amikacin, netilmicin, neomycin and streptomycin. These are widely used against gram negative bacteria and mycobacteria. They affect the sensory neuroepithelium of inner ear. In cochlea, outer hair cells are more susceptible than inner hair cells and in vestibule type I hair cells are more affected than type II hair cells.[30] Within the vestibule the cristae ampullaries are more sensitive to ototoxicity than the maculae of utricle and saccule.

Aminoglycosides bind to NMDA (N methyl D-Aspartate) receptors in the cochlea and aggravate excitation of the neurons.[31] Aminoglycoside-induced production of hydroxyl radical causes cellular injury under oxidative stress.[32] Coadministration of N acetyl cysteine may prevent aminoglycoside-induced ototoxicity.[33]

Ototoxicity of gentimicin, amikacin and tobramycin are similar but netilmicin is comparatively less toxic.[34] Streptomycin is predominantly vestibulotoxic. Transtympanic administration of gentamicin for treatment of Meniere's disease suggests that it is primarily vestibulotoxic but it appears to have similar vestibulotoxicity and cochleotoxicity during systemic administration.[35] Neomycin, amikacin and dihydrostreptomycin are primarily cochleotoxic. Systemic use of neomycin is prohibited because of severe ototoxicity. Amikacin is less cochleotoxic than neomycin. Oral dose containing aminoglycosides primarily causes vestibulotoxicity and rarely causes cochleotoxicity.[36]

Other antibiotics, such as macrolide group, e.g. erythromycin, azithromycin and clarithromycin are associated with reversible ototoxic effect. Polypeptide antibiotics, e.g. viomycin and vancomycin also have ototoxic effect (Fig. 10).

Patients at risk for ototoxicity are those:
- Having renal or liver failure
- Receiving aminoglycoside treatment for longer period of time or other ototoxic drugs
- Having genetic susceptibility to aminoglycosides caused by 1555A to G substitution on mitrochondrial 12S – rRNA[37]
- Elderly patients and especially who had an organ transplantation.

Antineoplastic Agents

Platinum containing antineoplastic agents that are effective against head and neck cancer include cisplatin,

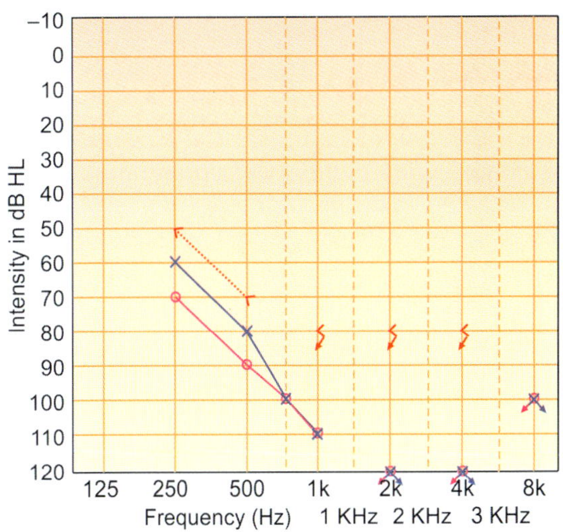

Fig. 10: Gentamicin-induced cochleotoxicity

carboplatin and oxaliplatin. They are associated with bilateral, symmetric and high-frequency sensorineural loss with tinnitus.

Cochleotoxicity results from loss of cochlear outer hair cells and to less extent inner hair cells through oxidative stress via increased intracellular production of reactive oxygen species and free radicals that bind with cell membrane phospholipids to generate aldehydic lipid peroxidation products accelerating programmed cell death.[38] Cisplatin-induced cochleotoxicity is dose dependent occurring with cumulative doses greater than 200 mg/m^2. Vestibulotoxicity is detected with cumulative doses greater than 400 mg/m^2. Cristae ampullaris are more susceptible than maculae of utricle and saccule.

Ototoxicity is less frequently detected with related compound oxaliplatin due to decreased uptake of the drug by cells of the cochlea.[39]

Risk factors for cisplatin ototoxicity are:
- Cumulative dose
- Previous noise exposure
- Renal or liver dysfunction
- Hypoalbuminemia or low RBC level.

Loop Diuretics

Loop diuretics block the transport of sodium and chloride ions in the ascending loop of Henle. They damage the striavascularis of cochlear duct with loss of endocochlear potential which is the driving force for hair cells. SNHL and its recovery are parallel to the loss of endocochlear potential. The hearing loss is usually reversible and flat SN type on audiogram. Hearing loss may be permanent also. Frusemide is associated with ototoxicity with doses greater than 240 mg/hr.[40] Ethacrynic acid has a higher risk of ototoxicity while Bumetanide has a lower risk of ototoxicity compared to frusemide.[41]

Antimalarial Drugs

Quinine which is used as antimalarial drug has ototoxicity characterized by reversible SNHL and tinnitus associated with nausea and vomiting. It primarily affects the motility of outer hair cells.[42] Use of quinine by mother during first trimester of pregnancy may result in congenital deafness and hyperplasia of cochlea in children.

Chloroquine a synthetic antimalarial drug may be used in the treatment of rheumatoid arthritis or systemic lupus erythematosus may result in permanent SNHL on prolonged use.[43]

Salicylates and NSAIDs—At high doses **salicylates** may cause high-pitch tinnitus and high-frequency bilateral sensorineural hearing loss, typically reversible on discontinuation of the drug. Ototoxic effect of salicylates is due to changes in ionic conductances through the outer hair cells. At doses when salicylate is used to treat pyrexia it protects the cochlea against gentamicin toxicity. Here it acts as a radical scavenger and metal chelator (Fig. 11).

Isolated cases of SNHL associated with transient tinnitus have been found with **NSAIDs** like indomethacin, phenylbutazone and ibuprofen.

NSAIDs impair the active process of outer hair cells and affect peripheral and central auditory neurons although recent studies show NSAIDs are potential therapeutic agent against cochlear insults.[45]

Other agents—Ototoxic effects are seen with some heavy metals such, as mercury and lead. Subclinical **mercury** toxicity may be detected by auditory brain stem recordings (ABR) that shows prolongations of wave I-V. **Lead** has ototoxic effect on both the peripheral and central auditory pathways.[46]

Desferoxamine, an iron chelating agent is mainly used for iron intoxication and iron overload in patient receiving multiple transfusions particularly in the treatment of thalasemia. Mechanism for toxicity is due to direct toxic effect on the cochlea and on the higher auditory pathways.

Solvents, such as propylene glycol used in many oral preparations have been shown to be ototoxic in animal models.[47]

Some disinfectants, such as chlorhexidine, alcohol, iodine and quaternary ammonium compounds used in external auditory canal prior to ear surgery to reduce bacterial load may damage the inner ear in presence of perforated tympanic membrane.[48]

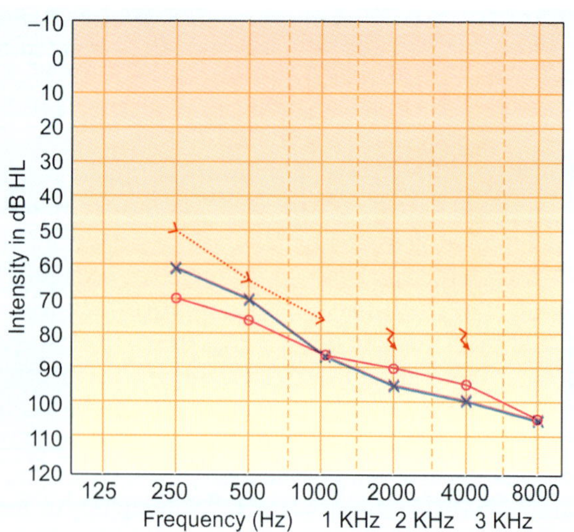

Fig. 11: Salicylate induced hearing loss

Monitoring Ototoxicity

Monitoring ototoxicity for drugs, such as aminoglycosides or cisplatin involves two elements—cochlear and vestibular.

Cochlear Monitoring

It Includes:
- Ultra high-frequency (up to 12 kHz) pure tone audiometry—Early ototoxicity is recognized by high-frequency SNHL which is gradually involving lower frequencies. Ultra high-frequency pure tone audiometry can detect early ototoxicity. Conventional audiometric testing confined to less than 8 kHz can detect around 80% of cases of hearing loss.[49] High-frequency audiometry testing up to 12 kHz can detect around 95% of cases of hearing loss. This testing cannot be technically possible at bed side and in nonambulant patients (Fig. 12)
- Otoacoustic emissions (OAEs)—It is more sensitive in monitoring auditory dysfunction than ultra high-frequency pure tone audiometry.[50] Transient OAEs and distortion product OAEs (DPOAEs) can be measured easily at bed side and even in comatozed patient for detection of ototoxicity. DPOAEs are more sensitive than transient OAEs.

Vestibular Monitoring

It Includes:
- Electronystagmography (ENG)—It is done to monitor early vestibular dysfunction and is the test only for lateral semicircular canal function. It has poor sensitivity in bilateral vestibular loss as is seen in early systemic ototoxicity
- Rotational chair—It is a test of high-frequency vestibular function and can differentiate between central and peripheral lesion
- Computerized dynamic posturography—It measures everyday activity and is useful in rehabilitation
- Head shake test—It is clinical bedside test and gives information about asymmetrical vestibular dysfunction.

Treatment

- Permanent hearing loss should be treated with a hearing aid or cochlear implant. Hope for the possibility for the recovery even in case of permanent hearing loss may require assessment of hearing on regular basis following ototoxicity
- Genetic counseling (1555 chromosome mutation)—Screening of hearing loss in other family members is essential and helpful for familial nonsyndromic SNHL
- Vestibular dysfunction is to be treated by vestibular rehabilitation exercises to compensate vestibular function
- Perinatal counseling and hearing screening of infant by behavioral audiometry and objective tests, such as OAEs, BERA or steady state evoked potential audiometry may be necessary to follow the child for several years after birth.

IMMUNE-MEDIATED SNHL

Immune-mediated SNHL plays an important role in the etiopathogenesis and natural course of various inner ear disorders.[51] The disorder is one of only a few forms of sensorineural hearing loss that can be treated. It is characteristically presented as an asymmetrical bilateral rapidly progressive SNHL with or without endolymphatic hydrops. The SNHL usually involves high-frequencies and is often represented by down-sloping audiogram.[52] The age of presentation is variable from 20–50 years of age group; the female suffers more than the male. The incidence is about less than 1% of all cases of hearing impairment with dizziness. It is either a separate disease entity or part of generalize disease process. It involves various causes ranging from vasculitis to type II collagen-related disorders. Immune-mediated disorders can cause SNHL include systemic lupus erythematosus, polyarteritis nodosa, Wegener granulomatosis, Behcet's disease, ankylosing spondylitis and Cogan syndrome.

All the cases of SNHL due to autoimmune disorders are not steroid responsive. Only those associated with aortitis syndrome (Takayasu disease) are steroid responsiveness.[53]

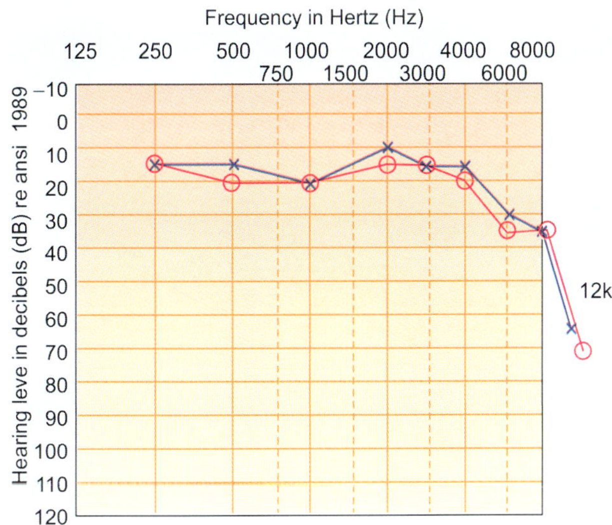

Fig. 12: High-frequency audiometery testing of gentamicin-induced cochleotoxicity detects hearing loss at higher frequencies

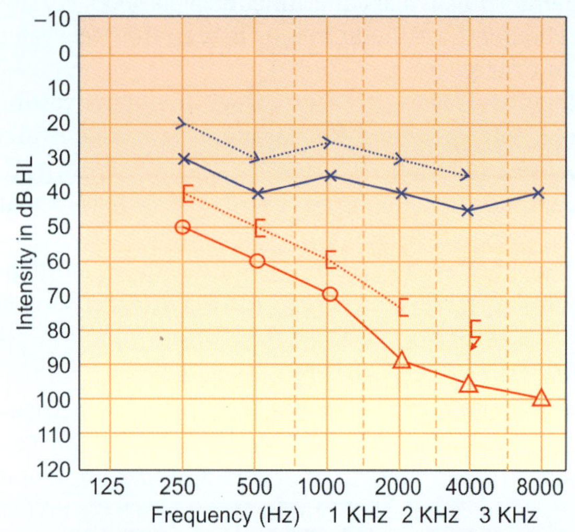

Fig. 13: Pure tone audiogram showing SNHL in systemic lupus erythematosus (SLE)

- Special tests of hearing, such as speech reception thresholds (SRT), speech discrimination score (SDS), tone decay (TD) and short increment sensitivity index (SISI) show hair cell lesion
- CT scan reveals no abnormal inner ear defect
- Serology reveals no abnormality in most cases
- More than 40 genes have been identified to cause hearing loss.[54]

Both autosomal dominant and recessive genes are involved to cause SNHL. In a family with dominant gene for deafness, direct transmission to offspring is inherited from only one parent. If genetic hearing loss is caused by recessive gene indirect transmission to offspring is inherited a few generations later from both parents.

Genetic hearing loss may be syndromic or nonsyndromic. Syndromic hearing loss comprises 20% of genetic hearing impairment. Nonsyndromic is implicated in 80% of cases (Fig. 15 and 16). Again among the nonsyndromic hearing

These patients have elevated level of IgE and type I immune reaction that respond to steroid therapy. The hallmark of diagnostic criteria is rapidly progressive SNHL and steroid responsiveness. The audiogram is variable and speech discrimination score is poor relative to hearing loss (Fig. 13).

Treatment

Aim of treatment is to control abnormal immune response to inner ear antigens.

Treatment Includes:
- Steroid therapy which is indication in most cases
- Cytotoxic drugs, such as cyclophosphamide, methotrexate, azothiopine are given when hearing loss does not improve with steroid alone
- Treatment with dexamethasone and cyclophosphamide remarkably improves hearing.

It is evident that hearing improves with initiation of treatment, worsens with cessation of medicine and recovers with repetition of therapy.

FAMILIAL HEREDITARY PROGRESSIVE SENSORINEURAL HEARING LOSS

Hearing loss may result from hereditary disorder. It is evident that tradition of consanguineous marriages results in an increased risk of having hearing impaired children. The hearing loss is characterized by bilateral sensorineural type starting at 1 kHz frequency and gradually pure tone audiogram shows sloping to mid frequency and high-frequency pattern.

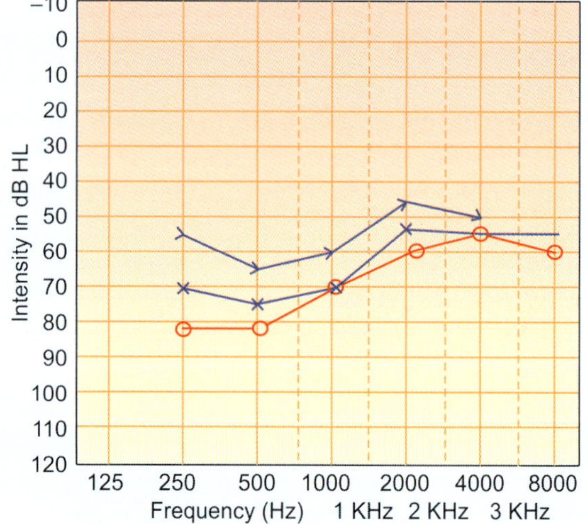

Fig. 14: Meniere's autoimmune hearing loss

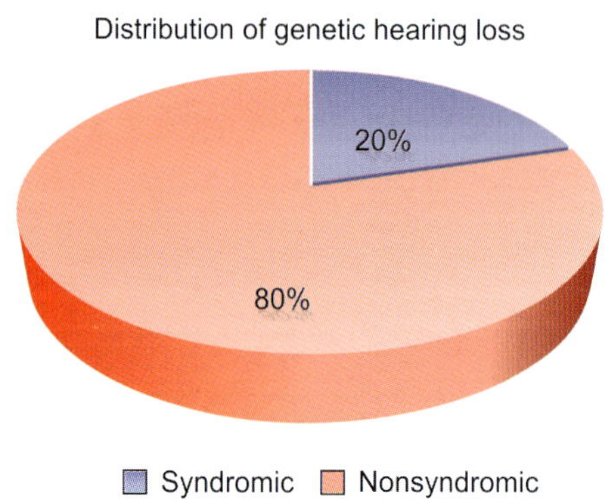

Fig. 15: Distribution of genetic nonsyndromic hearing loss

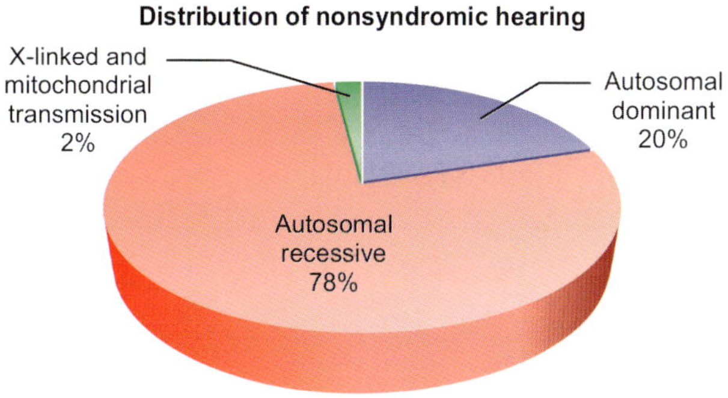

Distribution of nonsyndromic hearing

Fig. 16: Distribution of genetic hearing loss

loss cases 15–25% is autosomal dominant, 75–80% is autosomal recessive and less than 2% of cases X-linked and mitochondrial transmission.[55] Mitochondrial genes are unique group where inheritance is transmitted through female. The A1555G mutation in 12 Sr-RNA is most common in hereditary hearing loss with mitochondrial transmission.

In autosomal dominant inheritance, profound childhood hearing loss is rare; in most cases, child is presented with mild hearing loss that worsens significantly in later life. Gene mapping studies have identified both nonsyndromic dominant (DFNA #) and recessive (DFNB #) forms of hearing loss. DFN stands for deafness, A stands for autosomal dominant, B stands for autosomal recessive and suffix means X-linked.[56]

About 50% of genetic hearing loss is DFNB$_1$ also known as Conexin 26 deafness or GJB2 (Gap-Junction-Beta 2) related deafness.[57]

- Most common autosomal dominant syndromic forms of hearing loss are Stickler syndrome (high myopia, cataract, arthropathy, cleft palate and hearing loss) and Waadenburg syndrome (pigmentary abnormality and hearing loss)
- Most common autosomal recessive syndromic forms of hearing loss are pendred syndrome (thyroid organification defect and hearing loss), large vestibular aqueduct syndrome and Usher syndrome (retinitis pigmentosa and hearing loss)
- Hearing impairment in DFNA$_1$ is more severe as compare to DFNA$_6$. DFNA$_9$ is midlife on set progressive hearing loss resembling Meniere's disease.

In clinical practice, careful family history including syndromic and nonsyndromic patterns of hearing loss, annual pure tone audiometry along with vestibular function test and diagnostic DNA laboratories for genetic mapping should be considered in addition to usual workup for SNHL.

SUDDEN SENSORINEURAL HEARING LOSS (SSNHL)

Sudden sensorineural hearing loss is defined as the sudden hearing loss of 30 dB or more occurring at at least three contiguous audiometric frequencies over a period of 3 days or less. The hearing loss is sensorineural in origin, usually unilateral; and it may be bilateral in about 2% of cases. Highest incidence occurs in 50–60 years of age and the incidence is equal in male and female.

The classification of SSNHL is made as low-tone (type I), flat (type II) and high-tone or total (type III).

Etiology

In only 10% of cases definite diagnosis can be evaluated and most of the cases the etiology remains idiopathic.

Causes

Causes of idiopathic SSNHL include viral infection, vascular compromise, intracochlear membrane breaks and autoimmunity.

Viral Infection

Viral infection causing SNHL is favored by the clinical and pathological evidences.

Site of lesions are cochlea and components of the 8th cranial nerve. The cochlear lesion is said as viral endolymphatic labyrinthitis and neural component involvement is called as viral neuronitis and ganglionitis.[58] Common viruses are mumps, measles, influenza, adenoviruses and herpes zoster virus.

Temporal bone histopathological study from bone that was acquired shortly after the hearing has lost proposed a new hypothesis which states that ISSNHL is due to the activation of cochlear nuclear factor Kappa B by endogenous or exogenous stimuli. This hypothesis has no direct proof of its support.

Vascular Compromise

Vascular occlusion, thrombosis, hemorrhage and spasm may cause SSNHL. Vasospasm of cochlear artery may result from stress and emotional disturbance causing sudden hearing loss. Thrombosis due to arteriosclerosis and IHD may affect old age group. Thromboembolic changes due to congenital or rheumatic valvular disease may affect young age group.

Vascular changes may be precipitated by diabetes, hypertension, polycythemia or sickle-cell trait evidenced by temporal bone histopathologic study.[59]

Intracochlear Membrane Breaks

- Spontaneous rupture or break of Reissner's membrane resulting from pressure changes during sneezing, coughing, valsalva maneuver or sudden physical activities done by the patient may cause sudden deafness. Proof of membrane break is evident from study of temporal bone histology[60]
- Spontaneous rupture of round window membrane may result in perilymph fistula causing SSNHL. Improvement of hearing and vertigo is established by surgical sealing of round window.[61]

Autoimmunity

Autoimmune inner ear disease (AIED) was first described by McCabe in 1975.[62] In AIED patients, complain of rapidly progressive bilateral sensorineural hearing loss in absence of any other systemic manifestations that distinguishes it from other known autoimmune-related deafness. About 50% of patients have episodic vertigo with occasional tinnitus during active disease. Positive lymphocyte inhibition test and substantial improvement with steroid therapy hint autoimmune etiology.

Management

Primary goal of treatment is to exclude any treatable causes and to evaluate the patient as a medical emergency for which definite deafness treatment still remains obscure. Clinical examination and laboratory testing are essential. About 1/3rd of patients note their hearing loss first when these wake up in the morning and about half of patients have associated vertigo and tinnitus.

Pure tone audiogram and tympanogram including stapedial reflex are done in all patients with SSNHL. Audiogram helps for establishing diagnosis as well as provides prognostic information (Fig. 17).

Majority of patients will have hearing loss in the range of 41dB–70 dB with severe/profound loss in others and mild loss in a few patients (Fig. 18).

MRI of internal auditory meatus—cerebellopontine angle with contrasts is useful for patients with asymmetric hearing loss.

Other laboratory investigation include:
- Complete blood count and erythrocyte sedimentation rate
- Glucose, urea, creatinine
- T_3, T_4, TSH and lipid profile
- PTI, APTT
- VDRL, FTA-ABS, HIV (I and II), HBsAg, anti-HCV
- Heat-shock protein 70 antibody and lime titer.

Treatment

Treatment for sudden SNHL is still a subject of controversy. High-percentage of patients (50%) undergoes spontaneous recovery. Treatment is directed towards the known etiologies involved for hearing loss.

Following treatment modalities are empirically used where underlying cause for hearing loss remains obscured.
- Steroid therapy—High-doses of prednisolone 80 mg in a single morning dose for 5 days and then tapered in 2 weeks are given as anti-inflammatory agent to relieve edema
- Antiviral—Acyclovir (200 mg 5 times/day for 5–10 days) and valacyclovir (500 mg/day in 1–2 divided doses for 5–10 days) are used
- Vasodilators—Carbogen inhalation therapy—Inhalation of carbogen (5% CO_2 with 95% O_2) improves cochlear blood flow. It is considered in cases where underlying

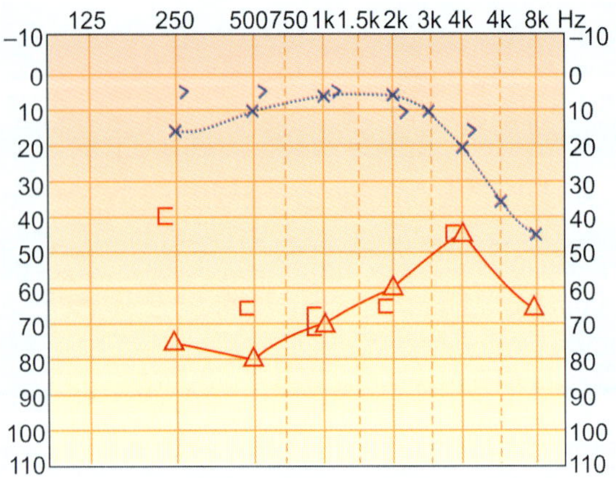

Fig. 17: Idiopathic sudden sensorineural hearing loss

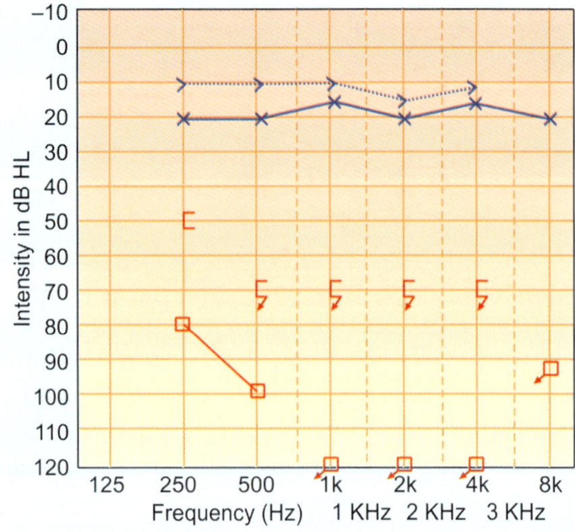

Fig. 18: Profound hearing loss in idiopathic sudden sensorineural hearing loss

causes are noise, vasospasm or thromboembolism[63] Other vasodilators used are papaverine, buphenine, prostacyclin, nicotinic acid and pentoxifylline.[64]

- Volume expander/hemodilators—Hydroxyethyl starch and low molecular weight dextran are effective in increasing cochlear blood flow by decreasing blood viscosity. They are contraindicated in cardiac failure and bleeding disorders
- Defibrinogenators, e.g. Batroxobin and calcium channel antagonists, e.g. nefedipine are also used
- Hyperbaric oxygen therapy given in the first month of onset of hearing loss is effective in some cases
- Diuretics, such as hydrochlorothiazide, triamterene and furosemide are useful in patient with autoimmune SNHL showing endolymphatic hydrops
- Other agents, such as vitamins, iron, intravenous histamine and procaine have also some benefits for this condition.

The current practice for sudden SNHL is to use short courses of oral steroid and antiviral agents in an otherwise healthy individual resulting in significantly higher rate of hearing recovery compared to either drug alone. No single treatment is unequivocally recommended to be effective till death.

Prognosis

It is evident from the study that following four variables are affecting the recovery of Idiopathic sudden sensorineural hearing loss (ISSNHL):[65]

- Time since onset—Earlier the patients' treatment is started better is the recovery. About 56% of the recovery is seen if patients are seen within 7 days of their treatment while 27% of recovery is noted if patients are presented on 30 days or later
- Age of the patients—Average age for better recovery is 42 years and below 15 years and over 60 years are poorer recovery rate
- Vertigo—In patients with severe vertigo recovering of hearing loss is worse than in patients with no vertigo
- Audiogram—In patients with profound hearing loss, recovering rate of hearing loss is decreased while patients with hearing loss between 40–90 dB are an excellent recovery rate.

Conclusion

Etiology for the majority of the patients with SSNHL remains undiagnosed. Minimal investigations, such as audiometry and MRI for those patients with asymmetric hearing loss should be undertaken. Steroid therapy provides significant improvement of hearing recovery in the treatment of idiopathic and autoimmune forms of SSNHL. Several other agents proposed for treatment required further study to prove their efficacy.

NONORGANIC HEARING LOSS (NOHL)

Hearing loss that lacks the evidences of any organic lesion and involves the psychological or malingering problem is called nonorganic hearing loss.[66] It is also known as functional hearing loss. The individual seems to have impairment of hearing, but actually he/she is normal hearing. Nonorganic hearing loss is of two types:

1. Psychogenic—Individual simulates hearing loss unconsciously due to emotional or psychological conditions which is also known as conversion deafness.
2. Malingering—Individual deliberately pretends deafness for claiming hearing handicapped certificate and compensations related to industrial noise, ototoxicity and head injury or for motive in avoiding work responsibility, although he/she is normal hearing.

Suspicions of Malingering

Quality of voice—Unlike deaf individual malingerer has normal voice.[67]

On exposure to loud sound, twitching of pinna or contraction of palpebral muscles is absent in deaf persons whereas these reflexes are present in malingering individuals.

In malingerers, hearing loss appears suddenly and disappears suddenly. When they pretend bilateral, individual remains mute.

Individual shows exacerbated efforts to hear placing cupped hand behind the pinna or asked for repetition of the words for hearing.

Lombard's Test

The test is based on Lombard's principle. The principle states that one raises his/her voice on speaking in noisy environment. While performing the test one is allowed to read a book. Noise is then introduced into the ear and gradually increases till the individual raises his/her voice or stops reading. No change in voice loudness level indicates the individual does not have any organic hearing loss.

Tuning Fork Test for NOHL

Stenger Test

This test is based on Stenger's phenomenon. The phenomenon states that, when an individual is presented with same type of sound in both ears, he/she will hear a single sound only in the ear which receives tone of louder intensity.

Procedure—Individual is blindfolded during the procedure. Two tuning forks with equal frequency (512 Hz) after vibrating are kept at an equal distance from both the ears, one should hear equally well in both sides. In malingerer, even if the tuning fork is moved too close to the feigned ear, the patient denies that he is having hearing in the said normal ear. This test can be done with a double channel audiometer using pure tone or speech signals.

Teal's Test

A vibrating tuning fork is placed over the mastoid process of so called deaf ear, the patient accepts to hear it. Patient is now blindfolded and with a nonvibrating tuning fork placed on the mastoid process, the malingerer claims to hear the sound.

Chimani-Moos's Test

This is a variation of Weber's test. Normally in Weber's test, the patient hears better in the occluded ear. Malingerer does not accept to hear better in the occluded ear.

Pure Tone Audiometry

During performing pure tone audiometry following characteristics are suggestive for NOHL.[68]
- Inconsistent response on repeat pure tone audiometry and speech audiometry. Normally, results of repeat tests are within ±5 dB. Gross discrepancy more than ±15 dB suggests NOHL
- Air conduction shadow test—Maximum interaural attenuation (IA) of air conduction tone for any frequency is about 80 dB, average attenuation across various frequencies would be 63 dB. Therefore, unmasked IA which exceeds 80 dB for any frequency or 70 dB over a range of frequencies indicates NOHL
- Bone conduction shadow test—Maximum bone conduction transcanal hearing loss is found to be less than 15 dB. A difference of unmasked bone conduction hearing threshold between both ears greater than 15 dB suggests NOHL
- Inconsistency in PTA (pure tone average in pitch frequencies) and SRT (speech reception thresold) Normally SRT is within ±7 dB of PTA. If the discrepancy is more than 10 dB between the two hints NOHL.

Objective Test for NOHL

Acoustic Reflex Threshold

In normal individual, stapedial reflex is elicited at 70–100 dB. If malingerer individual claims totally deaf but the reflex is elicited, it indicates NOHL.

Bekesy Audiometry

Two tracings, one with continuous tone and the other with pulsed tone are recorded. In normal hearing, continuous and pulsed tracings overlap showing an interweaving pattern with a tracing width of about 10 dB (type I). In patient with malingering, tracing of continuous tone is above that of the pulsed tone which is known as type V pattern.[69]

BERA Test

It is an objective test to elicit brain stem responses to auditory stimulation by clicks or tone bursts. It measures hearing sensitivity in the range of 1–4 kHz. It can establish hearing acuity of the person within 5–10 dB of the actual threshold, therefore, it is helpful in malingerer to determine the threshold of hearing.

Auditory Steady State Response (ASSR)

It is also evoked electrophysiologic response used to estimate hearing sensitivity as well as to detect the integrity of the auditory system like BERA test except it utilizes long duration stimuli (~1000 msec); short duration stimuli (<5 msec) is used in BERA. ASSR is helpful to cross check the hearing threshold of pure tone audiometry in malingerer.

Otoacoustic Emissions (OAEs)

Otoacoustic emissions may present in normal hearing person where hearing loss does not exceed 35 dB. It informs cochlear damage only providing middle ear function is normal as is determined by impedance audiometry. It is helpful for screening hearing loss in children and in malingerer.

Nowadays, the above screening tests are essential to weed out malingerers and to identify exact beneficiaries to ensure that the incentives should reach the deserving individual.

REFERENCES

1. Sasikumaran Nair, Zakir Hussain, Instrument in Otorhinolaryngology, second edition. Paras medical publisher. Hyderabad; India: 2006. p-50-8.
2. Yoshikawa N, Bruce W, Murrow and Stephen P. Cass-ENT Secrets, 3rd edition. 2005. p-32–8.
3. Alexander AE Jr, et al. Clinical and surgical application of reformatted high resolution CT of the temporal bone. Neuroimag clinic North America. 1998; 8:631-50.
4. Voss SE, Rosowski JJ, Merchant-SN, Peake WT. How do tympanic membrane perforations affect human middle ear sound transmission? Acta Otolaryngol (stockh). 2001;121:169-73.

5. Voss SE, Rosowski JJ, Merchant-SN, Peake WT. Middle ear function with tympanic membrane perforations II; a simple model, J. Acoust Soc Am. 2001;1445-52.

6. Fria T, Cantekin E, Eichler J, Hearing acuity of children with otitis media. Arch Otolaryngol. 1985;111-10-6.

7. Peake WT, Rosowski JJ, Lynch TJ III. Middle ear transmission: Acoustic versus Ossicular coupling in Cat and human. Hear Res. 1992;57:245-68.

8. Merchant SN, John J. Rosowski Auditory physiology, Glasscock-Shambaugh Surgery of the ear, 5th edition. 2003.p-69-73.

9. Schuknecht–HF, Stapedectomy, Boston: Little, Brown and Co; 1972. pp. 406-10.

10. Vincent Ri Lopez A, Sperling NM. Malleus-ankylosis: a clinical, audiometric, histologic and surgical study of 123 cases. Am. J. Otol. 1999;20:717-25.

11. Schuknecht H. Pathology of Presbycusis, In: Goldstein J, Kashima H, Koopman C (eds). Geriatric otolaryngology. Toronto: BC Decker; 1989. 40-4.

12. Weinstein BE. Geriatric audiology, New York: Thieme; 2000. 1993.

13. Schuknecht H. Pathology of the ear, 2nd edn. Pennsylvania: Lea and Fibiger; 1993.

14. http://www.ihsinfo.org/ Presbycusis—A Look into the Aging Inner Ear By Patricia E. Connelly, PhD, CCCA.

15. Baguley DM, Evan Reid and Andrew McCombe. Age-related Sensorineural hearing impairment, Scott-Brown's Otorhinolaryngology, head and neck Surgery. 2008;7(3): p 3540-2.

16. Gates GA, Couropmitree NN, Myers RH. Genetic associations in age-related hearing thresholds. Archives of otolaryngology-head neck Surgery. 1999;125:654-9.

17. Gates GA, Cooper JC. Incidence of hearing decline in the elderly, Acta Oto-laryngologica. 1991;III:240-8.

18. http:// www.uptodate, com/ contents/Presbycusis.

19. Martinez-Monedero R, Oshima K, Heller S. Edge As-The potential role of endogenous Stem cells in regeneration of the inner ear, Hear Res. 2007; 227-48.

20. Gelfand S. Auditory System and related disorders. Essentials of Audiology, 2nd ed. New York: Thieme; 2001.P.202.

21. Chen GD, Kong J, Reinhard K, Fechter LD. NMDA receptor blockage protects against permanent noise-induced hearing loss but not its potentiation by carbon monoxide. Hearing research. 2001;154:108-15.

22. Lamm K, Arnold W. Noise-induced cochlear hypoxia is intensity dependent, correlates with hearing loss and precedes reduction of cochlear blood flow. Audiology and Neuro-otology. 1996;1:148-60.

23. Chen GD, Zhao HB. Effects of intense sound exposure on the outer hair cell plasma membrane fluidity. Hearing research. 2007;226:14-21.

24. Henderson D, Bielefeld EC, Harris KC, Hu BH. The role of oxidative stress in noise-induced hearing loss. Ear and Hearing. 2006;27: 1-19.

25. Lim DJ. Effects of noise and ototoxic drugs at the cellular level in the cochlea: a review. American Journal of Otolaryngology. 1986,7.73-99.

26. Baguley DM, McCombe A. Noise-induced hearing loss, Scott – Brown's Otorhinolaryngology, head and neck surgery. 2008; 7(3):P 3548-57.

27. Agarwal SK, Schindler DN, Jackler RK, Robinson S. Occupational hearing loss, current diagnosis and treatment, Otolaryngology head and neck surgery, edited by Anil K Lalwani. Tata Mc Graw Hill; 2008.3:P 732-9.

28. ^ab "Hearing Conservation" Occupational Safety and health administration. 2002.

29. Mangiardi JR, Sperling NM. Noise-induced hearing loss, comprehensive text book of otology, In: Kirtane MV, Brackmann D, Borkar DM, Chris de sonza. 2010.P 372-75.

30. Garetz SL, Schacht J. Ototoxicity of Mice and Men. In van De Water TR, Popper AN and Fay RR (Eds). Clinical aspects of hearing, New York: Springer Verlag; 1996.P 116-54.

31. Basile AS, Huang Jm, Xie C, Webster D, Berlin C, SKolnick P. N-methyl – D- aspartate antagonists limit aminoglycoside antibiotic-induced hearing loss. Nature medicine. 1996;2(12):1338-43.

32. Wu WJ, Sha SH, Schacht J. Recent advances in understanding aminoglycoside ototoxicity and its prevention. Audiology and Neuro-otology. 2002;7(3):171-4.

33. Tepel M. N-acetylcysteine in the prevention of ototoxicity. Kidney International. 2007;72(3):231-2.

34. Aran JM, Erre JP, Guil haume A, Aurousseau C. The comparative ototoxicities of gentamicin, tobramycin, and dibeKacin in the guineapig. A functional and morphological cochlear and vestibular study, Acta Oto-Laryngologica. Supplementum. 1982;390:1-30.

35. WinKel O, Hansen MM, Kaaber K, Rozarth K. A Prospective study of gentamicin ototoxicity, Acta oto-laryngologica. 1978; 86:212-6.

36. Marais J, RutKa Ja. Ototoxicity and topical eardrops. clinical Otolaryngology. 1998;23:360-7.

37. Prezant TR, Agapian JV, Bohlman MC, BuX, Oztas S, Qiu WQ, et al. Mitrochondrial ribosomal RNA mutation associated with both antibiotic–induced and nonsyndromic deafness. Nature Genetics. 1993;4:289-94.

38. Stephen O'Leary. Ototoxicity Scott-Brown's otorhinolaryngology, head and neck Surgery, 7th edition. In: Gleeson M, et al. 2008;3:3567-73.

39. Hellberg V, Wallin I, Eriksson S, et al. Cisplatin and oxaliplatin toxicity: Importance of cochlear kinetics as a determinant for ototoxicity. Journal of the National Cancer Institute. 2009;101(1):37-47.

40. Roland, Peter S. Ototoxicity. Hamilton, Ont: B.C. Decker. 2004.

41. Voelker JR, Cartwright-Brown D, Anderson S, et al. Comparison of loop diuretics in patients with chronic renal insufficiency. Kidney International. 1987;32(4):572-8.

42. Puel JL, Bobbin RP, Fallon M. Salicylate, Nefenamate, meclofenamate and quinine on cochlear potentials. Otolaryngology–Head and neck surgery. 1990;102: 66-73.

43. SecKin U, Ozoran K, Ikinciogullari A, Borman P, Bostan EE. Hydroxychloroquine ototoxicity in a patient with rheumatoid arthritis. Rheumatology International. 2000;19:203-4.

44. Dinis TC, Maderia VM, Almeida LM. Action of Phenolic derivatives (acetaminophen, salicylate and 5-amino salicylate) as inhibitors of membrane lipid peroxidation and as peroxyl radical scavengers. Archives of Biochemistry and Biophysics. 1994;315:161-9.

45. Tauchi K, Nishimura B, NaKamagoe M, Hayashi K, Nakayama M, Hara A. Ototoxicity: Mechanisms of Cochlear impairment and its prevention. Department of Otolaryngology, graduate school of comprehensive human sciences university of TsuKuba, 1-1-7 Tennedai, TsuKuba, 305-8575, Japan.

46. Alamadi AM, Rutka JA. Ototoxicity, PS Roland and JA Rutka (eds): BC Decker Inc; 2004. section II, Chapter 3, http://otologytextbook.com/webtext/ototoxicity.pdf.

47. Tom LWC, Elden LM, Marsh RR. Topical Antifungals in Ototoxicity, edited by PS Roland and JA Rutka. BC Decker Inc; 2004. Section III, chapter 15.

48. Scott AR, Prepagern N, Rutka JA. Surgical Disinfectants and Antiseptics. In: antiseptics in ototoxity, edited by PS Roland and JA Rutka (eds). BC Decker Inc; 2004. Section III, Chapter 16.

49. Fausti SA, Henry JA, Schaffer HI, Olson DJ, Frey RH, McDonald WJ. High-frequency Audiometric monitoring for early detection of aminoglycoside ototoxicity. Journal of infectious diseases. 1992;165:1026-32.

50. Stavroulaki P, Apostolopoulos N, Dino-Poulou D, Vossinakis I, TsaKaniKos M, Douniadakis D. Otoacoustic emissions—an approach for monitoring aminoglycoside induced toxicity in children. International Journal of pediatric otorhinolaryngology. 1999;50:177-84.

51. Veldman J. Department of otorhinolaryngology, Utrecht university hospital, The Netherlands. Immune-mediated sensorineural hearing loss.

52. http://www.medilink.com/medlinkcontent.asp

53. Kanzaki J. Immune-mediated sensorineural hearing loss, Acta — Otolaryngol suppl. 1994; 514:70-2.

54. Matsunaga T. "Value of genetic testing in the otological approach for sensorineural hearing loss". The Keio Journal of Medicine. 2009;58(4):216-22.

55. Nicolas Gurtler. Hereditary hearing impairment, current diagnosis and treatment. Otolaryngology head neck surgery, 2nd edition. Lalwani AK (ed). Tata Mcgraw-Hill; 2008.697-704.

56. Cremers C. Otosomal dominant nonsyndromic sensorineural hearing impairment, Scott – Brown's otorhinolaryngology, head and neck surgery. 2008;7(3):3558-65.

57. Sabag AD, Dagan, Avraham KB. Connexins in hearing loss: A comprehensive overview. Journal of Basic and clinical physiology and pharmacology. 2005;16:101-16

58. Deka RC. Sudden sensorineural hearing loss: Recent concept of etiology and AIIMS experience with steroid therapy – otolaryngology review. Shah VH, Karnik PP (eds). 2000;P130-2.

59. Gussen R. Sudden deafness of vascular origin. A temporal bone study. Ann Otol Rhinol Laryngol. 1976;86:55-60.

60. Gussen R. Sudden deafness associated with bilateral Resissner's membrane rupture. Am J Otolaryngol. 1983;69:27-32.

61. Goodhill V Harris I, et al. Sudden deafness and labyrinthine window rupture. Ann Otol Rhinol laryngol. 1973;82:2-12.

62. Mc Cabe, Brian F. Autoimmune inner ear disease: results and study. Adv Otorhinolaryngol. 1991;46:78-81.

63. Witter HL, Deka RC, et al. Effects of prestimulatory Carbogen inhalation on noise-induced temporary threshold shift in human and chinchilla. Am J Otol. 1980;1:227-32.

64. Snow JB, Suga F. Labyrinthine Vasodilators. Arch. Otolaryngol. 1973;97:365-70.

65. Byl FM. Sudden hearing loss: Eight years experience and suggested prognostic table. Laryngoscope. 1984;94:647-61.

66. Hinchcliffe J. clinical tests of auditory function in the adult, Audiology. 1974;3:439-51.

67. Mc Dermott BE, Feldman MD. Malingering in the medical setting Psychiar. Clin North Am. 2007;30(4):645-62.

68. Lt Col. Metha AK. Screening test for nonorganic hearing loss MJAF. 2000; 56:79-81.

69. Drtbalu's Site, Nonorganic Hearing Loss, drtbalu's otolaryngology. https://sites.google.com/site/drtbalusotolaryngology/otology/non-organic-hearing-loss-by-drtbalu.

Physiology of Balance and its Disorders

Asok K Saha

INTRODUCTION

Inner ear has two components—cochlea and vestibule.

Cochlea is the sense organ of hearing whereas vestibule is the sense organ of balance.

Parts of Vestibule

Vestibule has following parts (Figs 1A and B)

- Saccule and utricle — they are known as otolith structure and concerned with linear movements of the body along all the axis.
    - Saccule plays a role in postural control and senses linear movement along vertical axis, such as sensation experienced while moving in a lift
    - Utricle is concerned with linear movement along horizontal axis, such as moving forwards in a car. It also senses orientation of head relative to the pool of gravity.
- Semicircular canals are responsible for angular or rotational head movements in all planes. Lateral semicircular canal responds to side to side head movement on vertical axis—yaw plane (shaking head 'no'). Posterior and superior semicircular canals are concerned for anterior-posterior head movements on transverse axis—pitch plane (shaking head 'yes'). The semicircular canals are also responsible for detecting head movement in roll plane (tilting head to the side).[1]
- Endolymphatic sac—terminal part of endolymphatic duct is dilated to form endolymphatic sac between two

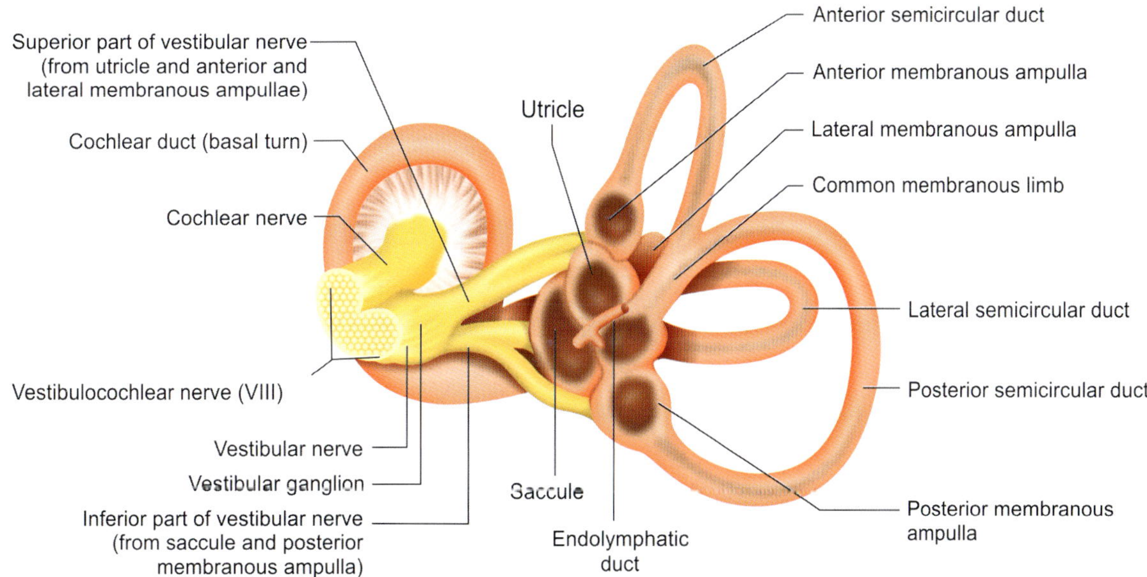

Fig. 1A: Membranous labyrinth with nerve: Posteromedial view

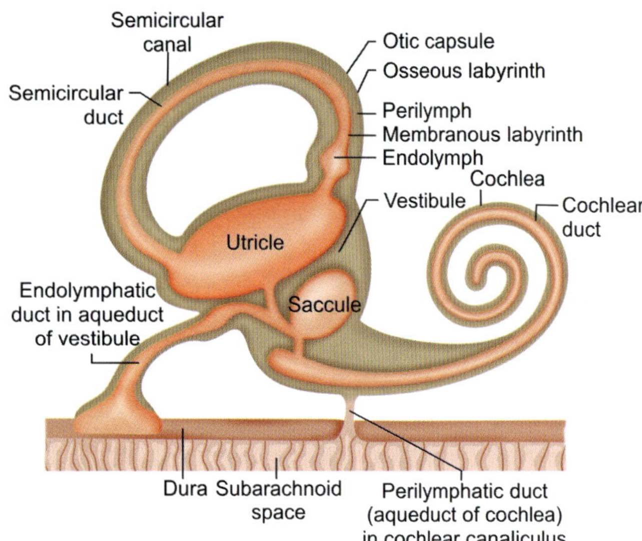

Fig. 1B: Bony and membranous labyrinth

layers of dura on petrous temporal bone. It is functioning for absorption of endolymph.

Inside bony labyrinth membranous labyrinth lies in between two, there is perilymph. Membranous labyrinth contains endolymph which has a high ratio of potassium to sodium in contrast with the perilymph where ratio of sodium is more than that of potassium in chemical composition. Five sensory organs are housed within the membranous labyrinth (Fig. 2A).

Macule is the sensory neuroepithelium present in otolith organ—utricle and saccule. Macule of the utricle lies in the floor of utricle in horizontal plane. Macule of saccule lies on the medial wall of saccule in the vertical plane. Both the saccule and utricle sense linear movements as well as static tilts of the head. This is possible by means of an otolithic membrane which is a gelatinous membrane stacked with calcium carbonate crystals known as otoconia. Hair cells are projected at the base of the gelatinous membrane. Any movement of the membrane results in the stimulation of the hair cells. The density of the otolithic membrane is higher than that of endolymph. This difference in density allows utricle to respond to linear acceleration caused by translational movement of the head as well as static head tilt (Figs 2B and C).

Cristae ampullaris is the sensory neuroepithelium present in the ampullated ends of three semicircular canals. A gelatinous membrane called cupula extends from the surface of crista to the ceiling of the ampulla forming partition or diaphragm that is intensely sensitive to motion. It displaces to one or the other side like a swing door with movements of endolymph. Cupula has a density similar to the density of the endolymph. It is therefore, insensitive to prolonged static tilt.[1]

Deflection of otoconial mass results in hair cell depolarization. Backward deflection is seen when head is tilted backwards or when accelerating forwards. Similarly, forward deflection happens when head is tilted forwards or when accelerating backwards (deceleration) (Fig. 3).

As per Einstein's equivalence principle—no single physical device can distinguish gravity from linear acceleration. This is same for otoliths also. Otoliths cannot differentiate between linear acceleration and tilt. Interplay of visual, proprioceptive and vestibular senses enables central nervous system to distinguish tilt from linear

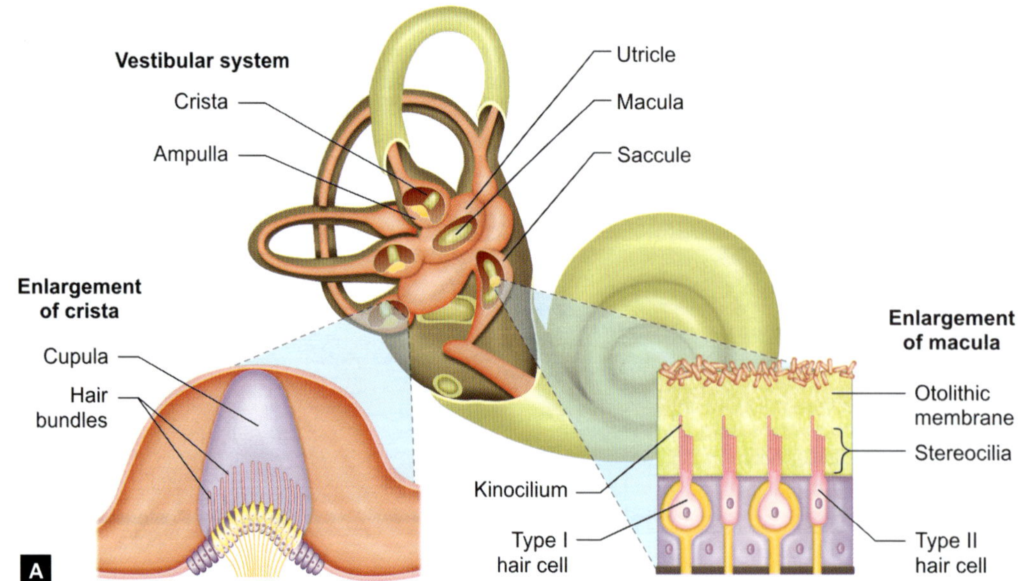

Fig. 2A: Cut section of bony labyrinth, crista ampullaris and structure of macula of utricle and saccule

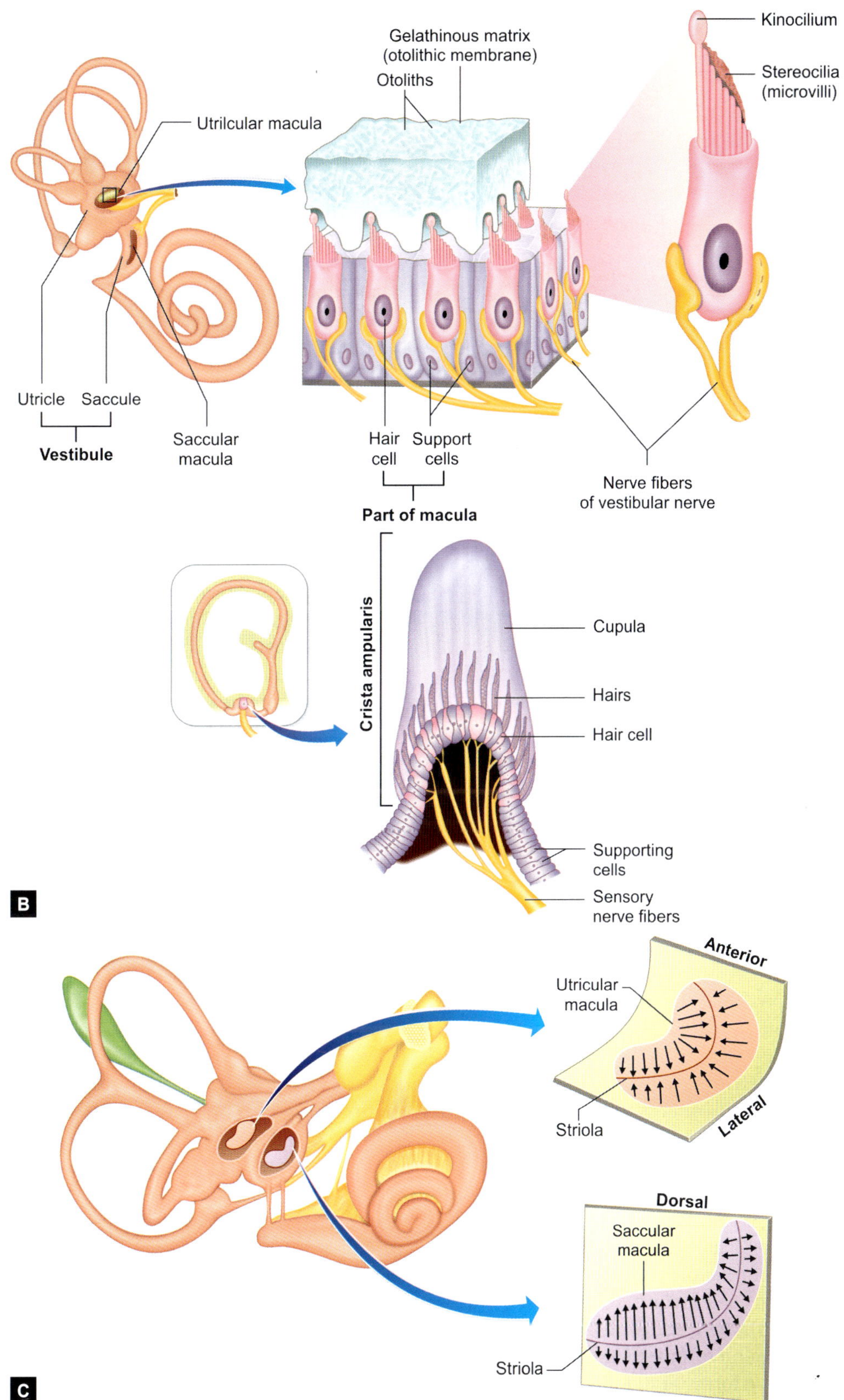

Figs 2B and C: Structure of macula and crista[2]; (C) Shows maculae of utricle and saccule

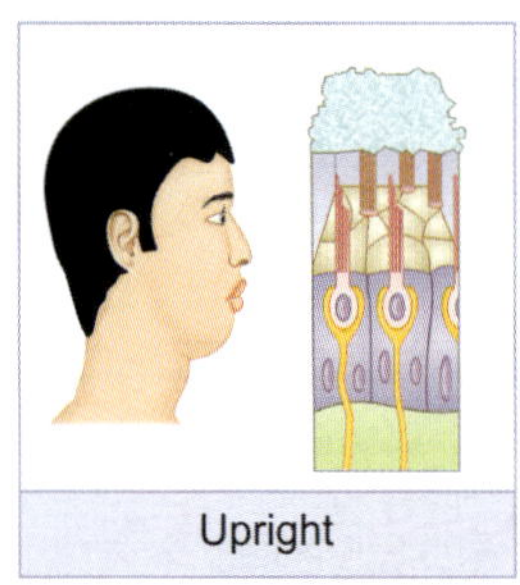

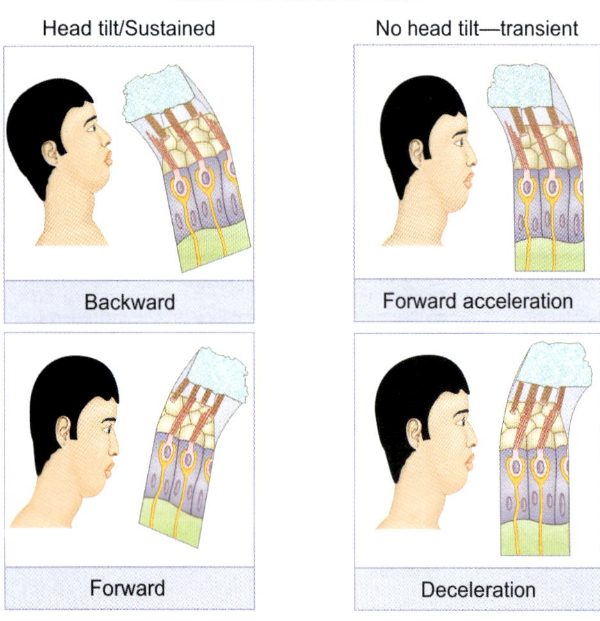

Fig. 3: Force acting on the head and resulting displacement of the otolithic membrane of utricular macula

translation under normal condition. In movements (active or passive), the otoliths sense sum of the acceleration acting on the head, called gravitoinertial acceleration (GIA). In static (no movement) otoliths sense only the direction of gravity.[3]

As per Newton's law—object in motion stays in motion until acted upon by a force and force acting on an object equals mass times acceleration (F = m.a). Movements of body and head are related to force or acceleration. Moving endolymph in semicircular canal is the prime trigger for detection of movement of head. For rotational movement Torque equals mass of inertia times angular acceleration (T = i.a), i.e. Torque = force × perpendicular distance to the axis of rotation. During constant rotation, no force triggers the sensory epithelium of semicircular canal to move the cupula. Only changes of rotation are detected by the canal system. The semicircular canal system is entirely adapted for transient rotations, such as back and forth movements of the head or during walking and running. Vestibular apparatus is not adapted to passive forms of motion as generated by aeroplane, merry-go-round or cars resulting in motion sickness.

Biomechanics of response of semicircular canal — Three forces act upon the endolymph and cupula in the canal.
- The inertial force which is proportional to the mass of the endolymph and cupula
- Elastic restoring force of the cupula that forces the cupula back to the central position after stimulation
- Viscous force that acts upon the fluid when flows through the tube. Viscous force is dependent on the speed of endolymph movement in the canals.

The behavior of the semicircular canal is referred to as the pendulum model summarized as:

Inertia of the endolymph + Endolymph viscous behavior + cupular spring response = head angular acceleration.

Therefore, head angular acceleration induces a number of reaction within the canal responded by endolymph–cupular system. This includes movements of fluid determined by its inertial mass with its viscous drag along the wall and restoring force of cupula pulling the cupula back to the central position after stimulation. Cupular deflection triggers hair cell depolarization or hyperpolarization and it is proportional to the head angular velocity. For high head rotation of 500°/second, cupular deflection is only 1.5°. Again dynamic systems are frequency dependent. Typical frequencies of natural head movements in man during walking and running for yaw, pitch and roll are between 0.5 and 5 Hz. Human resonant frequency for locomotion is 2.00 ± 0.03 Hz, for vertical head movement regardless of activity (walking, ridings a bike up hill, cleaning).[2]

Coplanar pairing of the semicircular canals—Spatial arrangement of six semicircular canals causes three coplanar pairings:
- Right anterior (superior) canal lies in the plane of left posterior canal (RALP)
- Left anterior and right posterior (LARP) lies in same plane
- Right and left horizontal canals are in same lateral plane.

The horizontal canal makes an angle of 30° with the horizontal axis of upright head. Angles of vertical canals are 45° with the saggital plane of the head.

This allows a push-pull arrangement of two sides. As head turns, right semicircular canal will increase firing rate and left semicircular canal will decrease firing rate (Fig. 4).

Physiology of balance—It is a multiaxonal complex reflex that has afferent sensory system and efferent motor system.

Afferent sensory system includes:
- Vestibular part
- Visual system
- Proprioceptive part
- Superficial sensory system.

Information from these four sources is integrated in the brainstem and cerebral cortex.

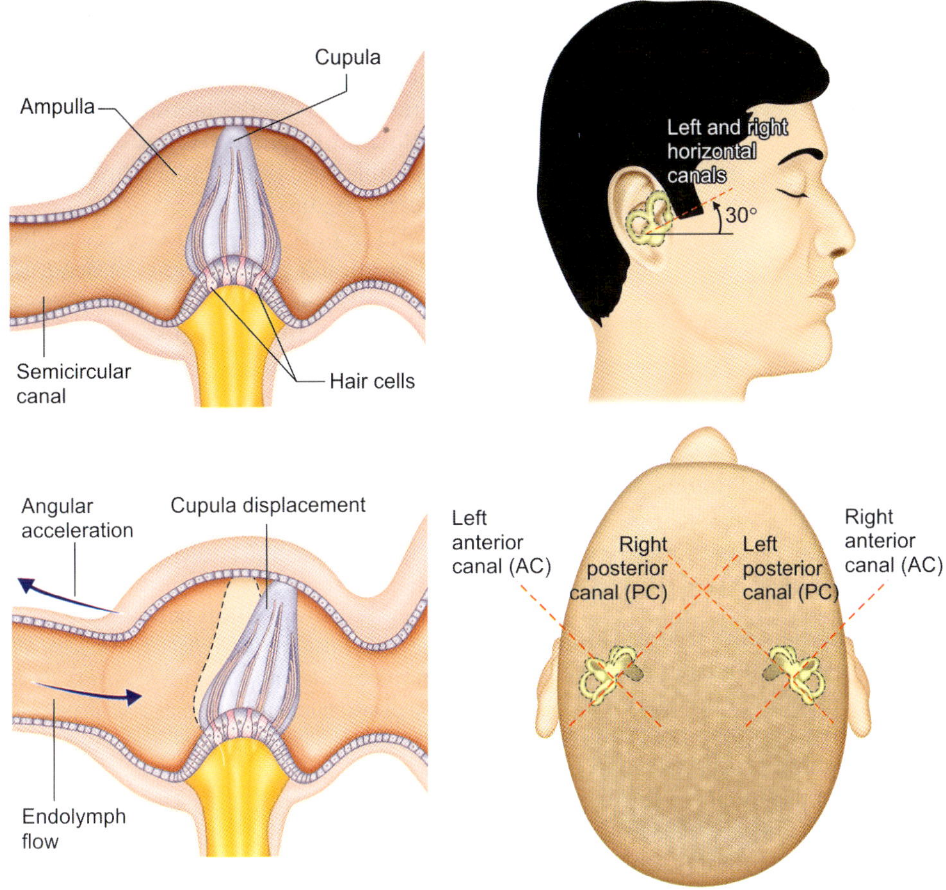

Fig. 4: Cristae ampularis of the semicircular canal

Efferent motor system is directed to:

- Muscles of limbs/trunk/neck (vestibulospinal reflex)
- Muscles of eyeball (vestibulo-ocular reflex)
- Cerebellum (vestibulocerebellar fibers) controlling fine tunes of motor output.

Ewald's law (Fig. 5)—Over a century ago (1892), Ewald made observations relating to vestibular physiology. Ewald attached a cannula to the lateral semicircular canal of the pigeon, there upon producing head and eye movements in response to mechanical stimulation of the membranous canal.

- Head and eye movements always occur in the plane of the canal being stimulated/and in the direction of the endolymph flow
- In the horizontal canal, ampullopetal endolymph flow causes a greater response than the ampullofugal flow
- In the vertical canals ampullofugal flow of endolymph causes a greater response than the ampullopetal flow.

The physiology of balance involves:

- Central processing system—
  It processes information in conjunction with other sensory inputs for position and movement of head in space

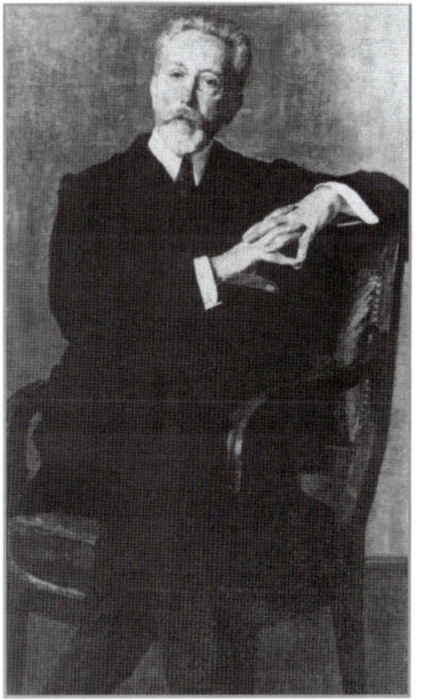

Fig. 5: J. Richard Ewald, 1855–1921

- Peripheral sensory apparatus—
  It detects and relays information about angular and linear velocity of head to central processing system. It orients the head with respect to gravity
- Motor output system—
  It generates compensatory eye movements and compensatory body movements during head and postural adjustments.

Vestibular Control System

It controls movements of head, body, limbs and eyes. The control of eye movements is a vital function of the vestibular system. The control signals sent by the vestibular system to the premotor system generate compensatory eye movements helping to keep visual targets on the foveae during head movements.

Central Vestibular Connections (Fig. 6)

Afferent nerve fibers from the semicircular canals and otolith organ enter CNS via the vestibular portion of the 8th nerve. These nerve fibers are bipolar and their cell bodies lie in scarpa's ganglion. Their peripheral process synapse on the hair cells and their central processes synapse on the cells of the ipsilateral vestibular nuclei. A few bypass the nuclei and proceed directly to the cerebellum.

The vestibular nuclei lie on the floor of 4th ventricle. At least ten distinct nuclei can be distinguished on each side, but four of these are prominent: the superior nucleus, the lateral nucleus (or Dieter's), the medial nucleus (schwalbe) and the descending (spinal nucleus).

These nuclei receive afferent fibers from the labyrinth as well as input from spinal cord, reticular formation, contralateral vestibular nuclei and especially from

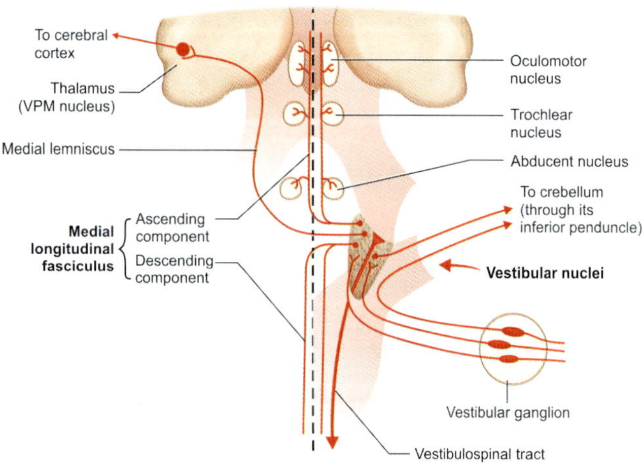

Fig. 6: Central vestibular connections

cerebellum. The influence of cerebellum on the vestibular nuclei is primarily inhibitory. Vestibular nuclei sent efferent fibers to the same part of the brain from which they receive afferent fibers. Vestibular nuclei sent efferents to:

- Nuclei of CN III, IV, and VI via medial longitudinal bundle (vestibulo-ocular reflexes) concerned for genesis of nystagmus
- Motor part of spinal cord (vestibulospinal fibers) coordinating movements of head, neck and body for maintaining balance
- Cerebellum (vestibulocerebellar fiber) for input information for body balance
- Autonomic nervous system
- Vestibular nuclei of opposite side
- Cerebral cortex (temporal lobe) for subjective awareness of motion.

Function of Vestibular System

It supplies information concerning gravity, rotation and acceleration. It performs function as a reference for somatosensory and visual systems. It helps to integrate arousal and conscious awareness of the body via connections with vestibular cortex, thalamus and reticular formation. It provides:

- Gaze and postural stability
- Sense of orientation
- Information about linear and angular movement.

Vestibular Hair Cells

These are the sensory structure for the vestibule and stimulated by movement and position relative to gravity. Approximately 10,000 sensory cells are packed side by side in each sensory area. Hair cells are of two types in mammalian labyrinth (Fig. 7).

Type I — Flask-shaped with a single cup-like nerve terminal surrounding the base.

Type II — Cylindrical with multiple nerve terminals at the base.

On the upper surface each vestibular hair cell has two types of cilia — one kinocilium and several stereocilia arranged in 'stair–step' pattern (Fig. 8A).

Kinocilium is the largest of the cilia and stereocilia are progressively shorter across the hair cell.

- In resting state, each hair cell has a resting electrical potential. With any motion this potential changes from base line. The potential will increase or decrease depending on relative position of hair cells. Any movement that causes flow of stereocilia towards the kinocilium results in depolarization of the hair cell and an increase in electrical potential described as excitatory. Any movement that causes flow of stereocilia

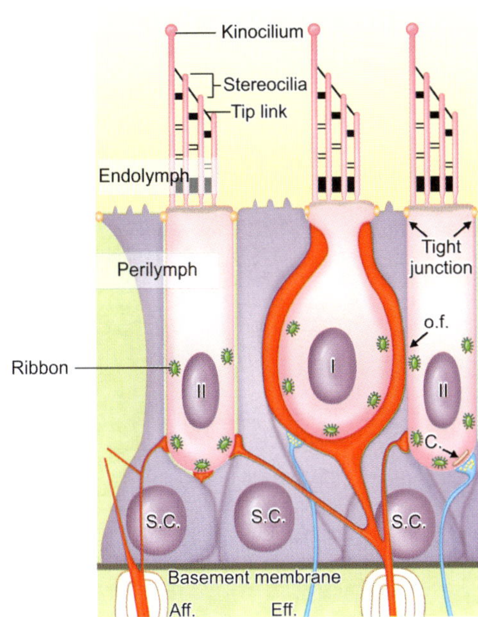

Fig. 7: Vestibular hair cells: Type (I) and type (II)
Abbreviations: SC, supporting cells; Aff, afferent; Eff, efferent; of, outer face; C, synapse and subsynaptic cistern

away from kinocilium results in hyperpolarization and a decrease in electrical potential described as inhibitory. If hairs are bent in direction perpendicular to the plane of polarization no change in the firing rate occurs

- The orientation of the hair cells in semicircular canal is such that rightward horizontal head movements result in an excitatory response from right horizontal canal and a corresponding inhibitory response on left horizontal canal. The hair cell orientation in the anterior and posterior canals is just reversed. Posterior canal is matched to the opposite anterior canal. Hair cell orientation in otolith organ (utricle and saccule) is more than one direction. Some hair cells are oriented to provide an excitatory response to forward movement. Whereas others are oppositely oriented resulting inhibitory response. The otoliths work as matched pairs, any movement causing a primarily excitatory response on one side is paired against a primarily inhibitory response on opposite side
- Hair cells affect the firing rate of the primary vestibular afferents to the brainstem.

Three groups of vestibular afferents are present in mammalian labyrinth based on their responses to motion and innervation patterns in the sensory epithelia of the labyrinth — the calyx only the afferents, Bouton only afferents and dimorphic afferents.[4] The neuroepithelium of cristae has three zones (Fig. 8B).

- Central (c), intermediate (I) and peripheral (p) zones.

Calyx group of afferents has fibers endings on to type I hair cells in the central zone. These afferents are irregularly discharging and have low rotational sensitivities.

Bouton only afferents have fibers ending on to type II hair cells in peripheral zone. These afferents are discharging regularly and have low rotational sensitivities.

Dimorphic afferents have both calyx fibers ending on to type I hair cells and bouton fibers ending on to type II hair cells. Dimorphic fibers are found throughout. Dimorphic afferents ending in peripheral zone are regularly discharging while dimorphic fibers terminating near the central zone are irregularly discharging with higher rotational sensitivities.

KEY POINTS

- Depolarization of the ipsilateral hair cells occurs during angular head movements
- Hyperpolarization of contralateral hair cells occurs at the same time
- At rest hair cells are able to hyperpolarize. Inhibitory influences from movement going to opposite direction are cut off, even if the ipsilateral hair cells continue to spike higher firing rates
- Vestibular nerve and vestibular nuclei have a normal resting firing rate of 70–100 cycles/second
- Baseline firing rate is present without head movement
- Tonic firing is equal in both sides; if it is unequal a sense of disequilibrium is felt, e.g. Vertigo, tilt, impulsion and spinning
- Excitation and inhibition of vestibular system may occur from stimulation of the hair cells.

Pathways of Vestibular Impulses (Flowchart 1 and Fig. 8C)

Vestibular impulses arise from the three cristae of semicircular canals and two maculae of sacule and utricle. They are carried by the dendrites of the nerve cells in scarpa's ganglion (first order neurons which is the peripheral neurons). Axons of these cells form the vestibular division of 8th cranial nerve. The nerve enters the central nervous system in the lower border of pons and ends in the following ways:

- Some fibers directly enter the cerebellum through the inferior peduncle, relay in the cerebellar nuclei and end in the cerebellar cortex
- The remaining fibers terminate in the vestibular nuclei. The vestibular nuclei (VN) are divided into four — superior vestibular nucleus of Bechterew (SVN), lateral vestibular nucleus of Deiters (LVN), medial vestibular nucleus (largest and situated in 4th ventricle — MVN) and inferior or descending vestibular nucleus (DVN).

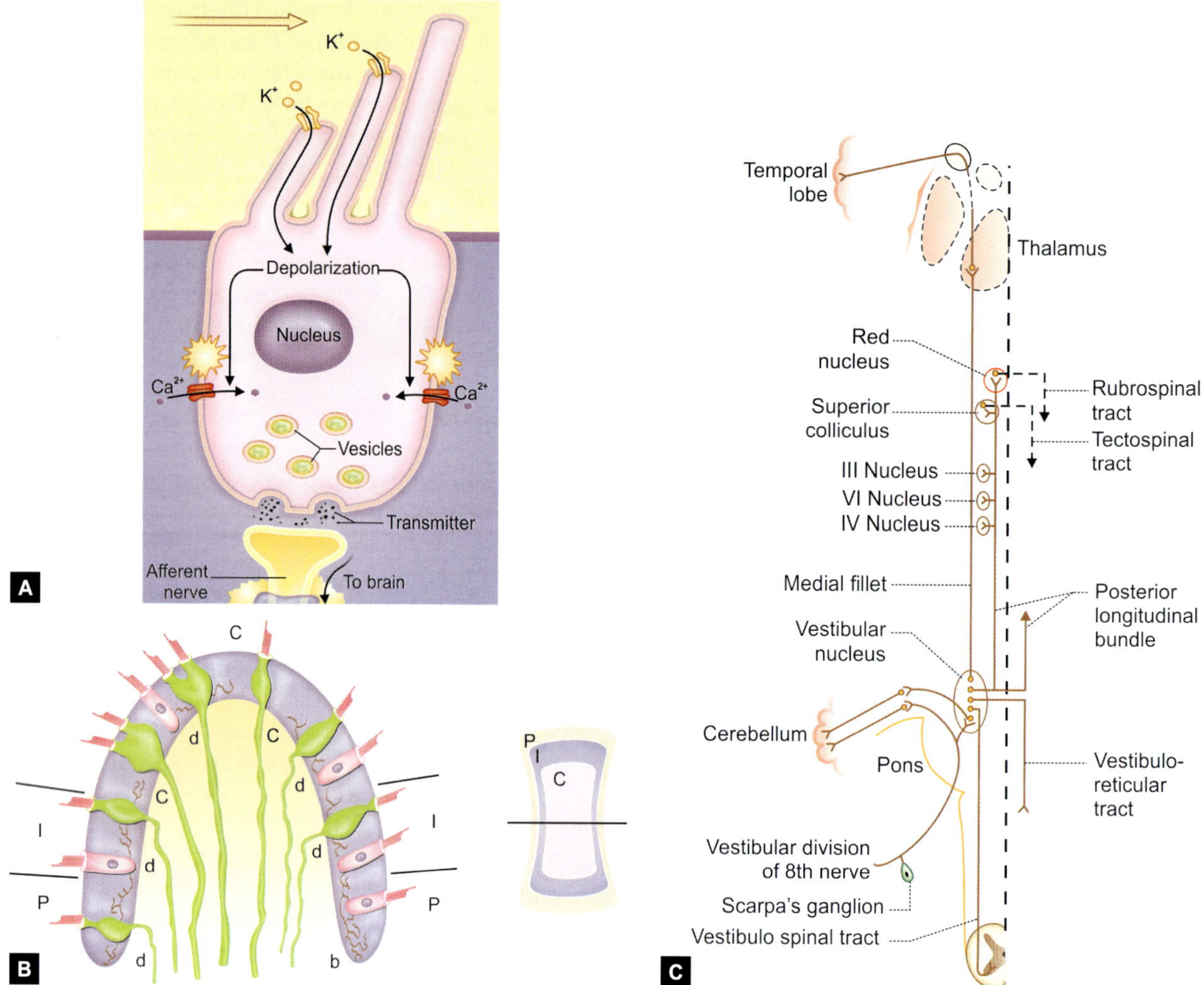

Figs 8A to C: (A) Vestibular hair cells; (B) Innervation of chinchilla crista, which is divided into central (*C*), intermediate (*I*), and peripheral (*P*) zones. Type I and type II hair cells are found throughout the neuroepithelium. Calyx (*c*) fibers are confined to the central zone; bouton (*b*) fibers, to the peripheral zone. Dimorphic (*d*) fibers innervate all three zones; (C) Pathway of vestibular impulse

The cell bodies of second neurons are situated in the vestibular nuclei. From here, second order neurons goes as follows—

- Vestibulo-ocular tract—It connects the vestibular nuclei (chiefly Deitor's nucleus) to the 3rd, 4th and 6th nerve nuclei through medial longitudinal fasciculi of both sides. The tract is concerned with reflex eye movements in response to vestibular stimuli. A few fibers of the tract end in the red nucleus and also in the superior colliculus of the same side
- Vestibulocerebellar tract—It enters the cerebellum through the inferior cerebellar peduncle and ends in flocculonodular lobe and fastigial nucleus of same side in cerebellum

- Vestibuloreticular tract—It ends in the bulbar nuclei in the reticular formation of brain stem
- Vestibulocortical fibers—The fibers enter the medial fillet and end in thalamus where 3rd order neurons arise. The fibers then pass with auditory fibers through posterior limb of internal capsule to end in temporal lobe of brain. The fibers are concerned with conscious vestibular sensation
- Vestibulospinal tract—Lateral vestibular tract originates from lateral vestibular nucleus (Deiter's nucleus) and descends the entire length of the spinal cord and ends in the medial part of the anterior horn cells of the gray matter. It exerts facilitatory influences on reflex spinal activities and also spinal mechanism underlying the muscle tone.

Flowchart 1: Vestibular impulse

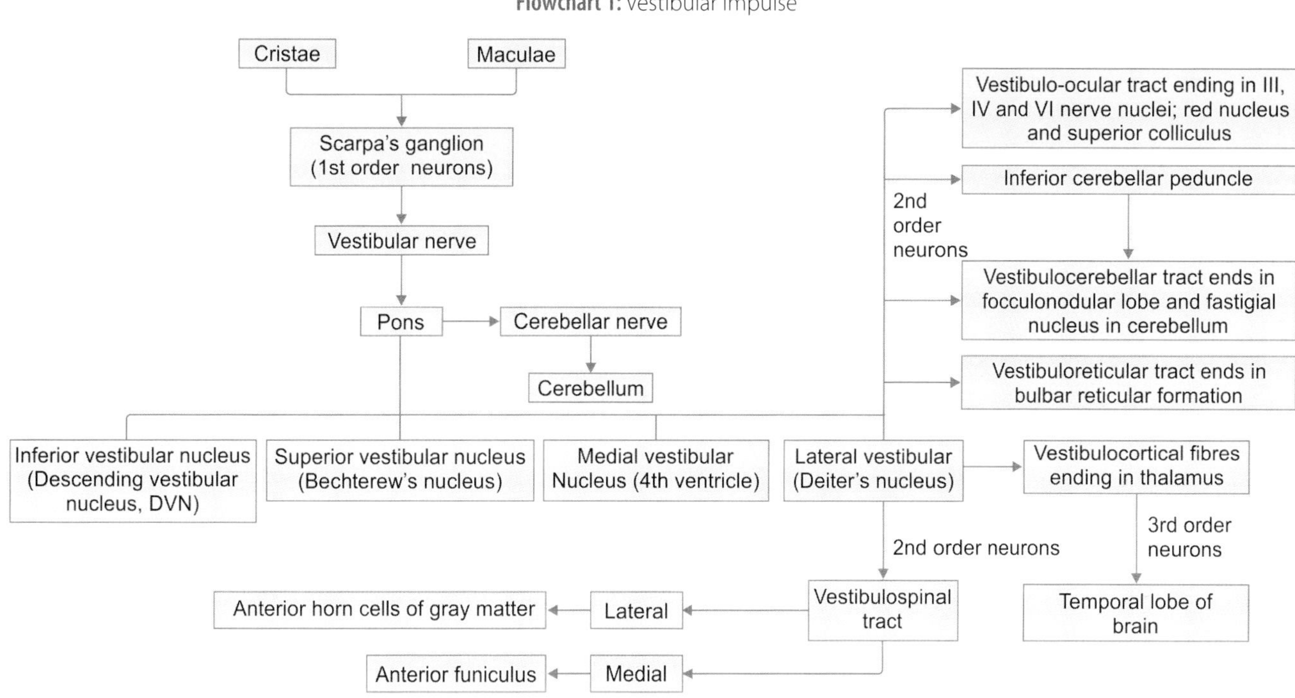

The medial vestibular tract originates from medial and inferior vestibular nuclei, descends in medial longitudinal fasciculus up to upper thoracic spinal segment and enters the area of anterior fasciculus.

Besides some fibers to the reticular formation of brain stem, this tract gives fibers to the visceral motor nuclei, such as dorsal motor nucleus of vagus, autonomic cell groups and secretory nuclei. It is responsible for nausea, vomiting, palpitation, perspiration, pallor, eye and neck movements.

Vestibular Ocular Reflex (VOR)

Vestibular ocular reflex is actually a reflex eye movement in response to head movement. When head rotates, the eyes move in a direction opposite to the direction of head rotation, maintaining visual fixation on stationary points. This is a short latency response resulting directly from changes in labyrinthine electrical potentials. During horizontal head movement to right or left, the difference of polarization happens resulting in asymmetric activity at the level of vestibular nuclei with increase activity on ipsilateral side and corresponding decrease activity on contralateral side; projections of the vestibular nucleus pass to the nuclei of cranial nerve III (oculomotor) and VI (abducens). Connections to the oculomotor nucleus and to the contralateral abducens nucleus are excitatory whereas connections to ipsilateral abducens nucleus are inhibitory. Oculomotor nucleus is connected to the medial rectus of left eye and abducens nucleus is connected to the lateral

rectus of the right eye. This circuit causes contraction of medial rectus of left eye and lateral rectus of right eye. Thus, the eye moves to the right that is in the direction away from the left when head rotates to the left. Again head movement to the right causes increased activity in right horizontal canal and has opposite effect on eye movement. The rectus muscles work in an antagonistic way as per law of reciprocal innervations. Contraction of the lateral rectus muscle is accompanied by relaxation of the opposing medial rectus muscle. All this response results in eye movement that is equal and opposite to the head movement with minimal latency. The latency of response for the VOR is less than 16 milliseconds (ms) whereas the latency for a voluntary eye movement is approximately 70 ms under ideal predictable conditions (Fig. 9).

The VOR represents one mechanism by means of which humans stabilize gaze while head is moving. The clinical measurement of the oculomotor response to precise vestibular stimuli, mediated through the semicircular canal — ocular reflex enables quantification of labyrinthine function to be made.[5] VOR is compromised with damage to one or both peripheral vestibular apparatus.

It is noted that the vestibulo-ocular reflex arc bypasses the horizontal gaze center and proceeds directly to the oculomotor nuclei. However, horizontal gaze center lesions abolish vestibular eye movements. It should be unlikely. Most probably the reason is that the signals in the vestibulo-ocular reflex arc by themselves are insufficient to produce

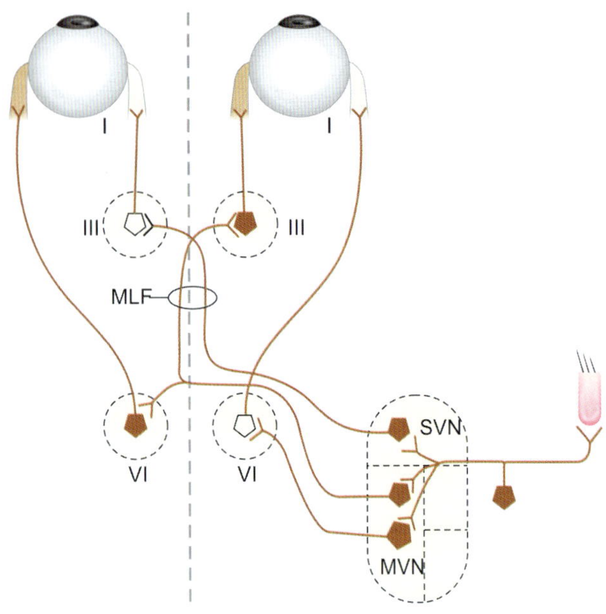

Fig. 9: Schematic diagram of the vestibulo–ocular reflex arc
Abbreviations: SVN, Super vestibular nucleus; MVN, Medial Vestibular Nucleus; MLF, Medial Longitudinal Fasciculus; III, 3rd nucleus; VI, 6th nucleus (Barber and stock well, manual of electronystagmorgraph[6])

eye movements. Vestibular signals also reach oculomotor neurons via the multisynaptic neural integrators in the premotor system that may depend on the horizontal gaze centers.[7]

VOR Dysfunction

- Direction of gaze will shift with the head movement
- It causes degradation of the visual image
- In severe cases, visual world will move with each head movement.

Modular View of Vestibular System (Flowchart 2)

Dizziness and disequilibrium: The sensation of dizziness and disequilibrium is caused by defects in one or more of the followings:

- Vestibule
- Vestibular nerve
- Brainstem (vestibular nucleus)
- Vestibular cortex
- Cerebellum
- Spinal cord
- Eyes, limbs, trunk and neck muscles and or nerves
- Each of these anatomical structures may get affected by various disease and condition resulting imbalance—dizziness or vertigo.

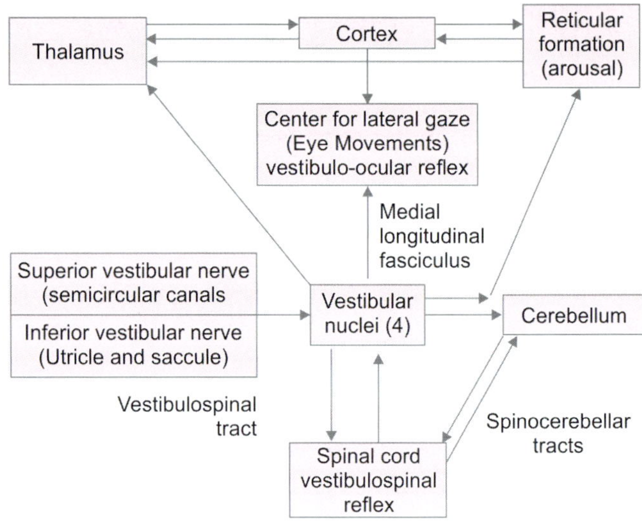

Therefore, various diseases and conditions may result sense of vertigo or imbalance, if there is—

- Mismatch between the information obtained from the afferents—vestibules, eyes or proprioception or mismatch between both the vestibules
- CNS (Brainstem and cerebral cortex) fails to integrate the afferent information
- Cerebellum fails to generate the motor output
- Defect in motor output system, i.e. in the nerves and muscles of the eyes/limbs/trunk/neck.

REFERENCES

1. Desmond A. Function and dysfunction of the vestibular system, vestibular system: Evaluation and treatment. Published by Thieme Medical and Scientific Publishers' Private Limited Ltd; 2009. 21-43.
2. Hole's Human Anatomy and physiology, 7th edition, by Shier, et al. TM Higher Education group, Inc; 1996.
3. Wuyts FL, An Boudewyns. Physiology of equilibrium, Scott Brown's otolaryngology, head and neck surgery, 7th edition. Vol-3: chapter 230; p 3210-3.
4. Baird RA, Desmadryl G, Fernandez C, Goldberg JM. The Vestibular nerve of the chinchilla. II. Relation between afferent response properties and peripheral innervation patterns in the semicircular canals. J Neurophysiol. 1988;182-203.
5. Kerr AG, Groves J. (eds). Scott-Brown's otolaryngology vol. I Butterworth and con. Ltd; I987. p116.
6. Barber HO, Stockwell CW. Manual of electronystagmography. 2nd edition. Saint Louis: The Cv Mosby co; 1980.
7. Shavenski AA, Robinson DA. Role of the abducens neurons in vestibulo-ocular reflex. J. Neurophysiol. 1973;36:724.

Vestibular Function Tests

Asok K Saha

A patient with balance disorder for evaluating the vestibular function, two groups of testing are done:

- Clinical testing
- Laboratory testing.

CLINICAL TESTING

Nystagmus

The control of eye movements is the vital function of the vestibular system. Nystagmus is a disturbance of ocular posture characterized by a more or less rhythmical oscillation of the eye.[1] There are two basic types of Nystagmus:

Pendular Nystagmus: Here ocular oscillations are almost equal in velocity in both directions. The nystagmus is usually horizontal.

Phasic or jerk Nystagmus: It is characterized by rhythmic oscillations in which movement in one direction is significantly faster than in other direction. The slow movement is pathological. But the fast or corrective movement is used to denote the direction of Nystagmus (Figs 1 and 2).

Null point is the position in which nystagmus is least marked.

To see the Nystagmus, patient is seated in front of clinician or lies supine in bed. Patient is asked to gaze at the tip of the clinician's index finger. The clinician keeps his or her finger 30 cm away from the patient's eye and then move it laterally and vertically not more than 30° to avoid gaze nystagmus, which is the tracking function.

Classification

Nystagmus is Classified as

Spontaneous Nystagmus

It is associated with rhythmic eye movements on forward gaze. It represents a tonic imbalance in the vestibular system. It may be horizontal, vertical or rotatory (Fig. 3).

- Purely vertical or purely torsional nystagmus is the sign of central lesion (vestibular nuclei, mid brain,

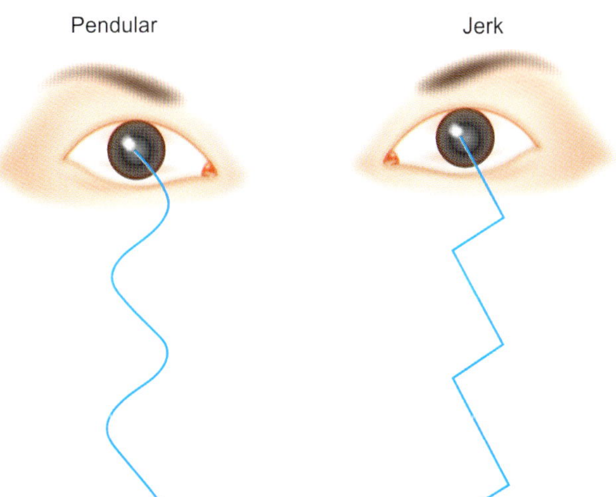

Fig. 1: Pendular and Jerk Nystagmus

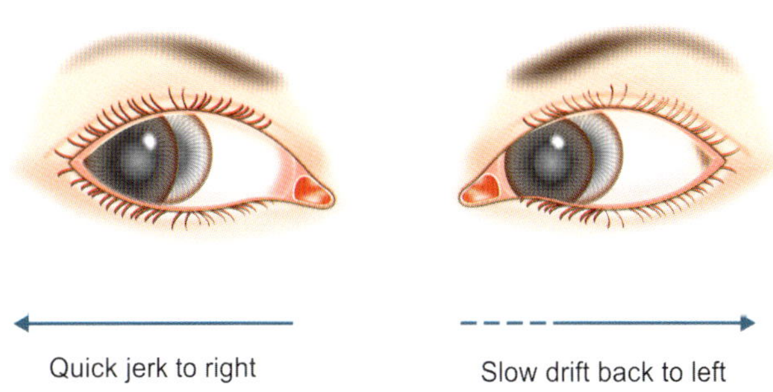

Fig. 2: Eyes looking to right associated with jerky involuntary eye movements of slow and fast components

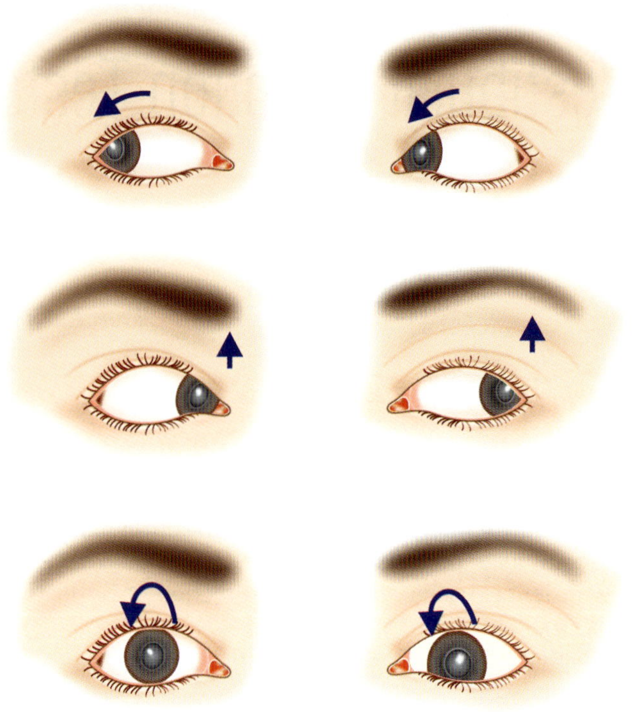

Fig. 3: Horizontal, Vertical and Torsional Nystagmus

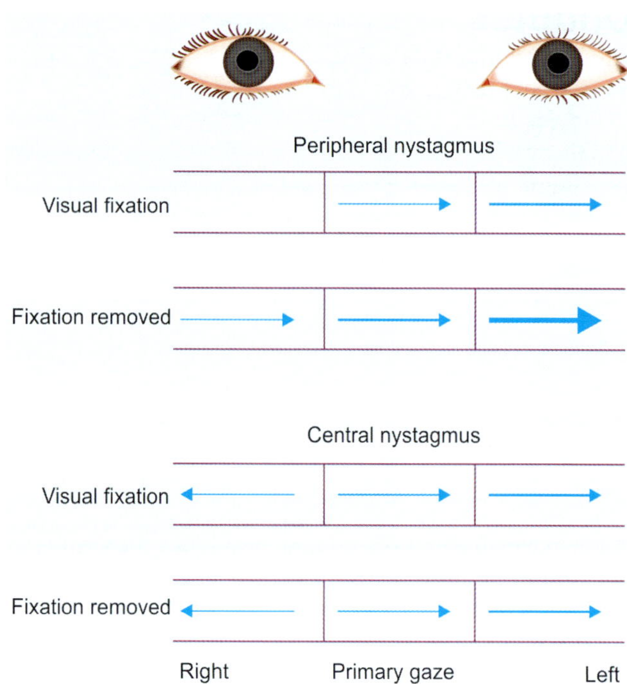

Fig. 4: The direction of the fast phase of the nystagmus is indicated by the direction of the arrows and the intensity of the nystagmus is represented by the thickness of the arrows

cerebellum) whereas horizontal rotatory nystagmus is considered the peripheral vestibular lesion (labyrinth or VIIIth nerve)

- The vestibular nystagmus that is peripheral in origin is rarely oblique and it diminishes with visual fixation, on the other hand, the central nystagmus is not affected by visual fixation rather the nystagmus may increase. Frenzel glasses (magnifying lenses 20 diopter) are used to see the nystagmus by preventing visual fixation which may cause suppression of nystagmus in peripheral lesion
- Peripheral vestibular nystagmus is usually conjugate whereas central nystagmus is disconjugate (more intense in one eye)
- Down beating nystagmus is seen in patient with diffuse cerebellar atrophy
- True vertical nystagmus is rarely seen in peripheral vestibular disease.

Gaze Nystagmus

It is demonstrated by altering the gaze to the right or left or up or down.

- The central origin nystagmus changes its direction with different gaze positions. The peripheral origin nystagmus has fixed direction in all gaze positions
- Again it is noted that in peripheral origin the intensity of nystagmus increases when visual fixation is removed

while in central origin the intensity of nystagmus is relatively unaffected by visual fixation (Fig. 4).

Spontaneous nystagmus or gaze nystagmus is the test for static vestibular function.

Causes of spontaneous nystagmus—

- Labyrinthine lesions
- CNS lesions
- Toxic drugs (alcohol/barbiturates/tranquillizers/anticonvulsants)
- Ocular (e.g. Amblyopia)
- Congenital.

Labyrinthine Nystagmus

It is phasic nystagmus with following characteristics:

- Associated with sense of vertigo
- Always unidirectional
- Increased on looking in the direction of the fast phase
- Enhanced on removal of occular fixation.

Following labyrinthine destruction, it decreases with time and disappears clinically in 4 weeks.

Irritative lesions of labyrinth as in serous labyrinthitis result in nystagmus to the side of lesion. Paralytic lesions as in purulent labyrinthitis result in nystagmus to the healthy side.

Alexander's law states that the intensity of nystagmus seen during the acute phase (first 1 to 3 days) of peripheral vestibular asymmetry can be increased by moving the eyes in the direction of fast phase and decreased by moving the eyes in the direction away from the fast phase.

Ocular tilt reaction (OTR) indicates tonic imbalance of activity of VOR consisting of skew deviation (vertical misalignment), ocular counter rolling (fixed torsion) of the eyes and head tilt towards the side of lesion.

Key Points

- Nystagmus is therefore, described under following headings—
  - Direction—right beating or left beating
  - Plane—horizontal, rotator or vertical
  - Intensity—1°, 2° and 3°
- 1st degree nystagmus—It is weak nystagmus and is present when phasic eye movements are detected when patient is looking in the direction of the quick phase
- 2nd degree nystagmus—It is more intense than 1st degree and is present when phasic eye movements are seen on looking straight ahead
- 3rd degree nystagmus—It is strongest nystagmus and is present when phasic eye movements are seen when patient is looking in the direction away from the direction of quick phase.

CNS Lesions Nystagmus

CNS lesions produce nystagmus associated with following characteristics:

- Bidirectional nystagmus (direction changing)
- Vertical nystagmus, although labyrinthine lesion may cause an upbeat nystagmus as seen in excitation of the posterior canal crista (as in BPPV) or transection of the posterior ampullary nerve may cause a down beat nystagmus
- Unidirectional nystagmus whose intensity is decreased by removal of fixation or intensity does not vary in amplitude or velocity in different directions of gaze
- Mono-ocular nystagmus—Nystagmus involving only one eye
- See-saw nystagmus where one eye presents upbeat nystagmus and the other down beat nystagmus.

Toxic Drugs

Drugs are the most common cause of vertical nystagmus. Toxic drugs are alcohol, barbiturates, tranquilizers and anticonvulsants. Effect of most drugs is on the central nervous system (CNS).

- Ocular lesions—Any lesion involving the macula, especially where the peripheral vision is still maintained, e.g. amblyopia, may result in nystagmus which is usually pendular. The nystagmus has velocity equal in either direction.

Congenital Nystagmus

Congenital nystagmus is often familial with following characteristics:

- Nystagmus has very long duration
- Usually horizontal and pendular, although it may be phasic (jerk)
- The null point is close to the position of forward gaze
- Nystagmus continues even when eyes are turned upwards
- Closure of the eyes results in decreased intensity in the nystagmus but the effect of darkness with eyes open is variable, some situation nystagmus increases.

Head-Shake Nystagmus (HSN)

Head-shake nystagmus is a procedure to detect an imbalance in dynamic vestibular function. Patient with Frenzel glasses or close eyes is advised to shake head back and forth in horizontal plane about 30 times with chin kept about 30° downward.

Head shake is stopped abruptly, examiner looks for any nystagmus. Normal persons usually have no nystagmus or just one or two beats of nystagmus. In persons with unilateral labyrinthine lesion, a brief period of horizontal nystagmus with slow phase component initially directed towards the lesion side is noted. This is due to dynamic asymmetry within the vestibular ocular reflex (VOR) (Fig. 5).

Three patterns of post-HSN is noted—

- Within the first several seconds a brief horizontal nystagmus beating towards the intact labyrinth occurs

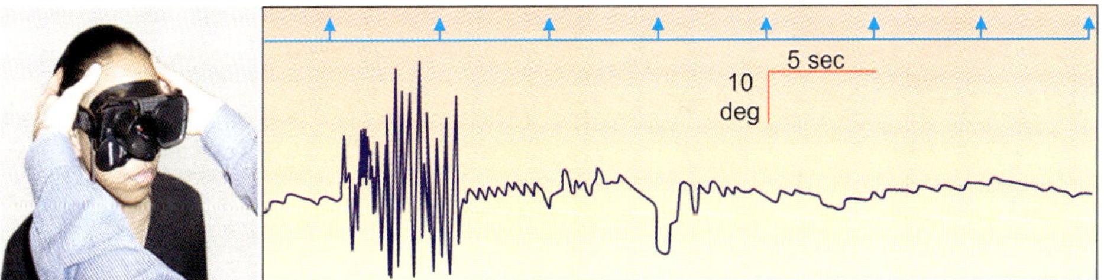

Fig. 5: Inducing head-shaking Nystagmus—position trace. The head is shaken after which a nystagmus ensues, typically for about 15 seconds, with a peak velocity of about 15°/sec (Wei et al. 1989)

- About 20 seconds after the head shake, a horizontal nystagmus beating towards the lesion side develops. This is due to central compensatory response (Recovery Nystagmus)
- A 3rd pattern involves an initial burst of nystagmus towards intact labyrinth, then a reversal in the direction towards the lesion side. This is due to compensatory response to the peripheral vestibular asymmetry.

Key Points

- Presence of HSN correlates with peripheral vestibular function
- HSN is also noted in patient with cerebellar dysfunction where a vertical component following horizontal head shake is identified
- HSN test has a low sensitivity (27%) but good specificity (85%) for assessment of vestibular dysfunction.

Head Thrust Test

Head thrust test is dynamic evaluation of vestibular dysfunction involving VOR in response to head movement. Patient's head is rotated in the YAW plane (as in shaking the head 'no'), first at slower speed then applying brief, high acceleration head thrust about 15°–30° lateral to central.

The patient's eye is kept focused on a centered target (usually on the examiner's nose). The examiner should monitor the patient's eye movements. A lack of visual fixation and subsequent catch up corrective saccade eye movements to regain fixation indicate dysfunction in the corresponding ipsilateral semicircular canal. If patient maintains visual fixation, it is suggestive of normal vestibular function.

Lateral semicircular canal is tested by moving head in horizontal direction whereas the anterior (superior) and posterior semicircular canals are tested by moving head in a diagonal direction[2] (Fig. 6).

Dynamic Visual Acuity (Fig. 7)

It is also dynamic evaluation of vestibular function test involving VOR where patient is asked to read a snellen eye chart to establish visual acuity. Then patient moves his head back and forth at a speed of 1–2 Hz while reading the chart. Missing of one line seems to be normal. Missing of three lines indicate VOR deficit. Scoring of visual acuity is done by viewing the lowest line on which patient cannot correctly recognize at least 50% of the optotypes (characters).[3]

Fistula Test

Nystagmus is induced by increasing pressure in the external auditory canal which is then transmitted to the labyrinth, if fistulous connection is present between middle ear and inner ear. The test is done by applying intermittent pressure on the tragus or by using pneumatic otoscope, Siegle's speculum or the air pump of a tympanometer. In normal condition, the test is negative as pressure change in the external auditory canal cannot reach to the labyrinth. A negative fistula test is possible in presence of fistula also, if there is dead labyrinth due to disease process.

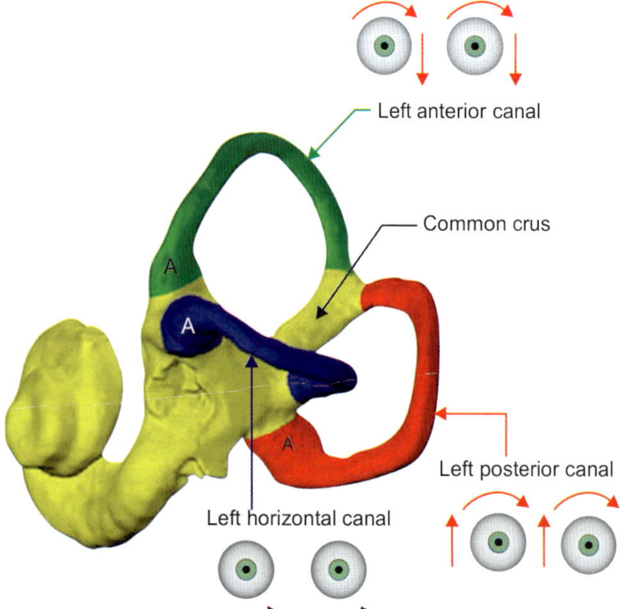

Fig. 6: Left Horizontal canal is tested by moving head in horizontal direction while left anterior and posterior canals are tested by moving head in diagonal direction

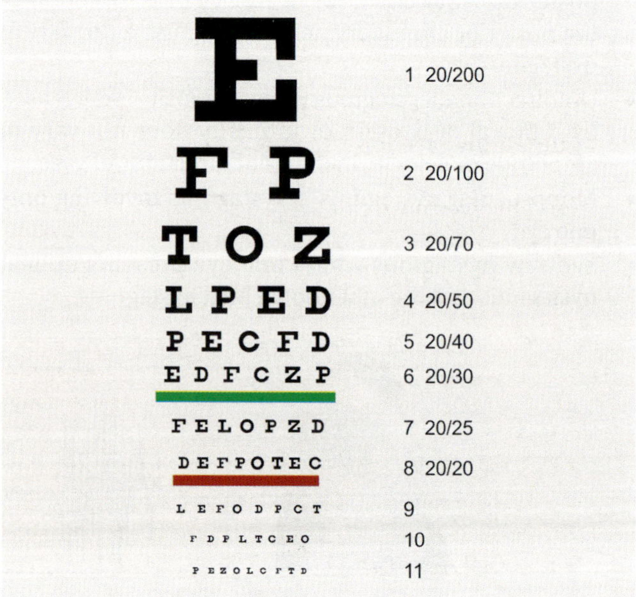

Fig. 7: Snellen Eye chart

A Positive Fistula Test Hints

- Erosion of lateral semicircular canal by cholesteatoma in CSOM creating third window into the perilymphatic space that enables movement of endolymph and stimulation of the vestibular end organs. Palpation of fistula while probing the ear results in severe vertigo
- Poststapedectomy fistula in oval window
- Rupture of round window membrane
- The labyrinth is still functioning.

A false positive fistula test (Hannebert's sign)—It occurs when there is a positive fistula test with an intact tympanic membrane and no evidence of middle ear disease. It is seen commonly in congenital or late tertiary syphilis, in condition causing endolymphatic hydrops, such as Meniere's disease.

Hannebert's sign is seen using slow and sustained negative pressure change of tympanometer. The pathophysiology of this sign is still obscure but it is thought to be due to adhesions in the vestibules or pressure of third window in labyrinth caused by osteitis.[4]

A false negative fistula test—It is seen when cholesteatoma seats the site of fistula thereby pressure change is not transmitted to the labyrinth.

Dix Hallpike Maneuver (Positioning Test)

- This test is designed to elicit nystagmus and vertigo related to benign paroxysmal positional vertigo (BPPV)
- Patient is seated on the table, the patient's head is then turned 45° to the right. The examiner standing behind the patient holds the patient's head and pulls him/her rapidly backwards without rotating the neck into supine position with the head hanging over the end of the table 30° below the horizontal. Patient is asked to look straight forward and his/her eyes are observed for at least 20 seconds for nystagmus. Then patient is turn to the sitting position. The maneuver is repeated with patient's head turned 45° to the left side. In most cases, BPPV involves posterior semicircular canal. A burst of intense nystagmus that is rotatory and beats upwards and towards the undermost ear is the hallmark of BPPV (Fig. 8).

In BPPV nystagmus has four characteristic features:[5]

- First, nystagmus has short latency (2–15 seconds) that is nystagmus appears after an interval of 2–15 seconds after the patient reaches the head hanging position
- Second, nystagmus is short duration (15–45 sec) that is nystagmus rapidly builds up in intensity, reaches a crescendo, slowly abates and finally disappears while head is held in position
- Third, the nystagmus is accompanied by vertigo that follows the same course as nystagmus

- Fourth, the nystagmus is fatigable that is on subsequent repetitions of Hallpike maneuver it becomes weaker, finally disappears altogether.

Suchuknecht (1969) proposed that otoconia are dislodged from utricular macula and become settle on cupula of posterior semicircular canal making cupula heavier than the surrounding endolymph. Therefore, it becomes sensitive to gravity. Any head movement that reorients the posterior canal relative to gravity causes deflection of the cupula resulting vertigo and nystagmus.

As per Suchuknecht latency or delay in onset of nystagmus is due to time taken to get the mass of otoconia into motion, short duration or transience of nystagmus is caused by return of the cupula to normal position after the otoconia have left the cupula and fatigability of nystagmus is caused by the dispersal of otoconia after repeated maneuver.

Sometimes patient with disorders other than BPPV develops nystagmus following Hallpike maneuver where nystagmus is purely vertical or persistent because of

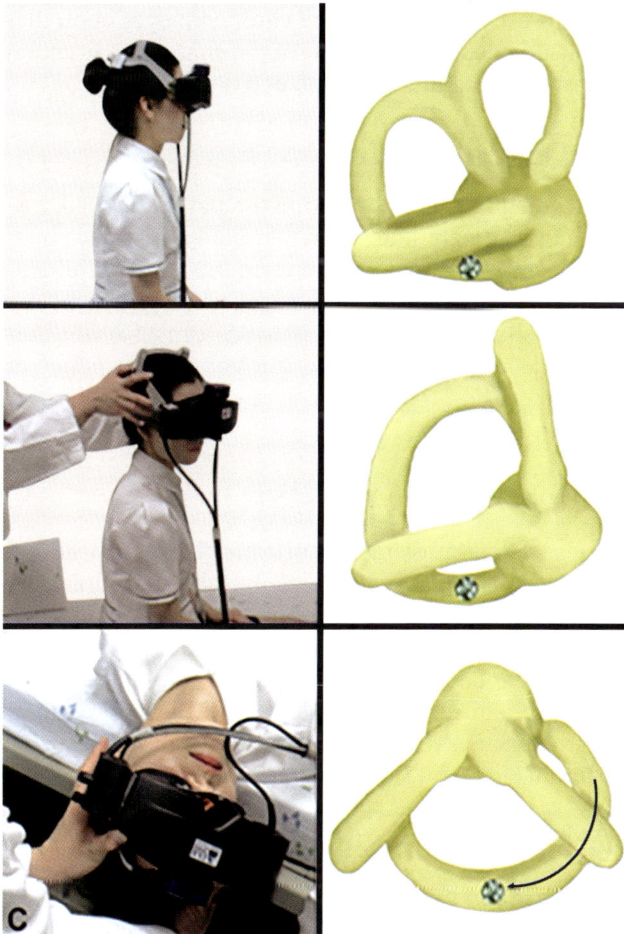

Fig. 8: Maneuver for the diagnosis of BPPV involving right posterior semicircular canal

possibility of central lesion. BPPV may occur in horizontal or anterior (superior) semicircular canal but duration and direction of nystagmus may vary accordingly.

Romberg Test (Fig. 9)

The test was originally devised by Romberg for evaluating postural instability characteristic of leutic posterior column disease. It is later refined and designed for screening test of postural stability. The test is performed by asking patient to stand with feet together and arms by the side with eyes first open and then closed (Fig. 10A).

- Excessive sway with eye closed relative to open indicate vestibular lesion. The side to which patient sways most indicates the side of the lesion.
- Equal but excessive sway with eye open and eye closed indicates proprioceptive weakness.
- Patient with compensated vestibular dysfunction is stable on the Romberg test. In this case a tandem or sharpened Romberg test is performed to evaluate the postural stability where patients stand heel to toe and arms are folded across the chest with eyes open then closed. Instability to perform the sharpened Romberg test hints vestibular dysfunction (Fig. 10B).

Tandem Walking Test

The test is performed by asking the patient to walk heel to toe in a straight line or circular pattern with eye open and closed. If patient can perform this test, it indicates intact cerebellar function. An ataxic gait is common sign of cerebellar dysfunction. There are causes other than cerebellar dysfunction that result poor performance on tandem walking tasks. The specificity of the test is therefore low (Fig. 11).

Fukuda Stepping Test (FST)

The test is done by asking patient to march in place with eyes closed for 100 steps. Normal patient is able to complete the test without moving more than 1m or without rotating more than 45°. Patient with vestibular dysfunction deviates from centre and rotates in the direction of the affected labyrinth. The simple observation can provide information about patient's balance when visual and somatosensory feedback is eliminated (Fig. 12).[6,7]

Dysdiadochokinesis Test

It is the inability to make finely coordinated rapid alternating movements seen in patients with cerebellar disorder. The test is done by asking patient to perform rapid supination and pronation of the hands against knee. Poor performance

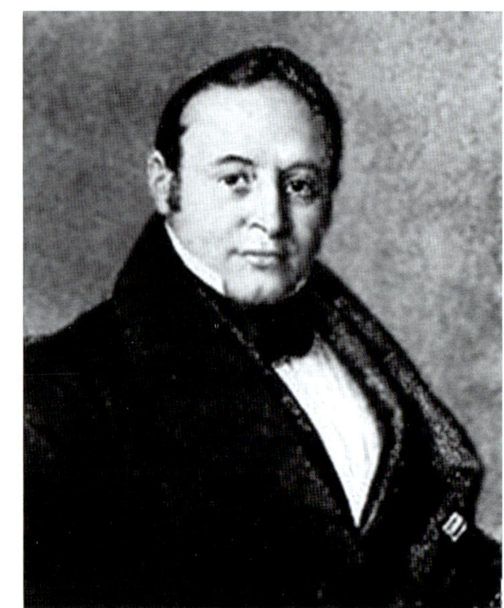

Fig. 9: Moritz Heinrich Romberg (1795–1873)

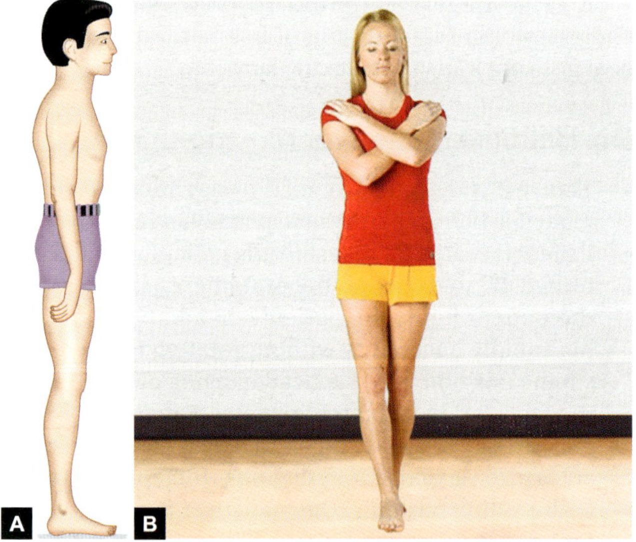

Figs 10A and B: (A) Romberg test; (B) Sharpened Romberg test

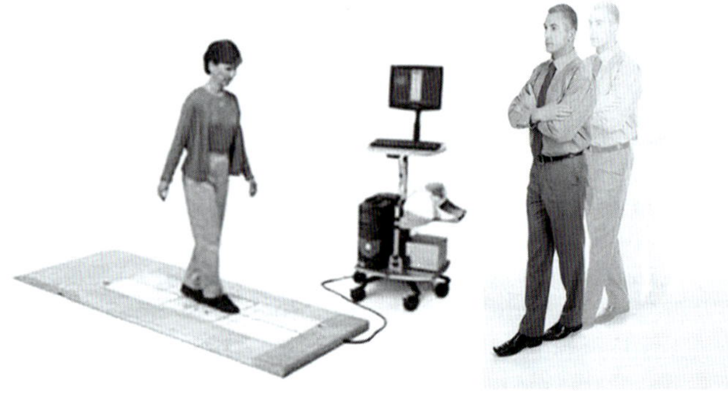

Fig. 11: Tandem Walking

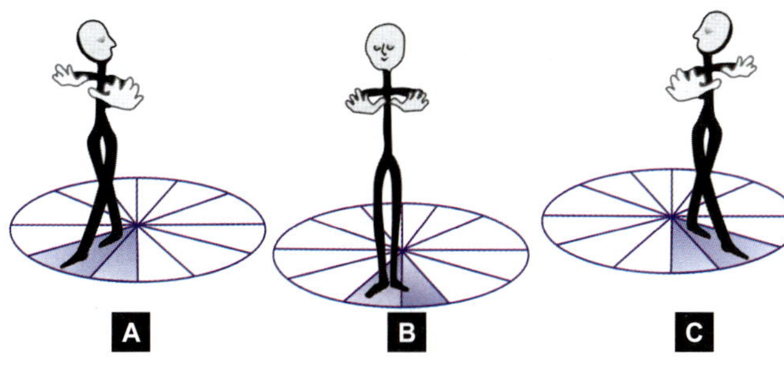

Figs 12A to C: The subject stands upright in the center of Fukuda ring with eye closed and arms stretched outward horizontally in front of him and he is asked to step on the spot hundred times raising his knee high. The maneuver is repeated with head straight ahead, then turns to right and then to left. (B) A normal subject does not go out of the hatched area. (C) With head turns right he deviates to the left. (A) With head turns to left he deviates to the right

of the test indicates inappropriate timing of muscle activity preventing the patient from quick stopping movement. The coordinated antagonistic movement requires efficient initiation and cessation of movements that can be poorly performed by patient with cerebellar dysfunction.[8]

Testing for orthostatic (postural) hypotension—Postural dizziness is usually correlated to postural or orthostatic hypotension where patient complain of dizziness or light headedness on rising from sitting or supine position to standing position.

Orthostatic hypotension (OH) is defined as a reduction of systolic BP of at least 20 mm of Hg or diastolic BP of at least 10 mm of Hg within 3 minutes of standing from sitting or supine position.

Orthostatic hypotension may be symptomatic or asymptomatic. The symptoms include light headedness, dizziness, blurred vision, weakness, fatigue, cognitive impairment, nausea, palpitation, headache and neckache. The symptoms resolve on resuming the lying position from erect position. It is commonly seen in patients taking antihypertensive drug or in patient with autonomic nervous system neuropathy or in older population.

Orthostatic hypotension is evaluated by measuring BP in recumbent position following 5–10 minutes patient having in lie down position. The patient is then ask to stand up quickly and BP is measured immediately and again after about 1 minute.[9]

LABORATORY TESTS (FOR VESTIBULAR FUNCTION)

Caloric nystagmus is one of the forms of induced nystagmus. It can be produced by stimulation of semicircular canals by thermal stimuli. It was known in later part of 19th century (Brown-Sequard)[10]. Hot and cold water are commonly used.

Warm irrigation excites the horizontal canal of the irrigated ear and provokes nystagmus beating towards that ear. Cold irrigation inhibits the horizontal canal of the irrigated ear and provokes nystagmus beating to the opposite side. Vestibular nystagmus can be strongly suppressed by a number of extravestibular sources, e.g. visual fixation, lack of mental alteration,[11] CNS depressant drugs.[12]

Electronystagmography (ENG)

This method utilizes the potential difference between electropositive cornea and electronegative retina where eye is a battery, cornea is positive pole and retina is negative pole. The potential difference between two poles (that is a corneoretinal potential) is 1mV. This potential difference (PD) is picked up by the circumorbital electrode and fed into electronic amplifying and recording system.

ENG is of specific value in the following ways:
- It makes it possible to discover nystagmus that is otherwise suppressed by ocular fixation
- It makes it infinitely easier to decide that the patient has a normal vestibular mechanism, disease of one or other labyrinthine end organs or retrolabyrinthine or CNS disease
- Various parameters of nystagmus can be studied, e.g. latent period, total number of beats, total duration, total amplitude and maximum speed of slow component
- The study of nystagmus can be carried out in certain odd position, e.g. lying down and during rotation
- It provides the kind of objective record that will be of significant advantage in medicolegal problems involving the vestibular sytem.[13]

The limitation of ENG is the rotatory nystagmus that cannot be recorded.

Schott (1922)[14] and Meyers[15] were the first to devise a method to utilize the corneoretinal potential for recording nystagmus. They thought that the action potential was due to contraction of extraocular muscles.

Mowrer et al. (1936)[16] confirm the presence of action potential and thought that it is not due to muscular contraction. A persistent corneoretinal potential difference presumably arises from high metabolism of retina and relatively low metabolism of cornea. According to them, this potential difference is 0.50–0.75 mV for the movements of eye from the median position to an extreme lateral and vertical position.

Fenn and Hursh[17] noted that corneoretinal potential varied from 0.2–0.8 mV and it remained constant for an individual. Retina was the site of origin of corneoretinal potential as stated by Marg.[18]

Neoll[19] studied the effect of medication on corneoretinal potential. He postulated that the site of origin of potential difference was the sensory element.

The free end of visual cell was thought to be negative with respect to its base in the cephaloid retina. Chemical destruction reduced or abolished the potential.

ENG usually consists of six tests.[12]

1. **Gaze test:** Nystagmus is recorded when patient looks forward, looks to right, looks to left, looks up and looks down. The test is done to detect inappropriate vestibular nystagmus induced by various eye movements.

2. **Saccade test:** Saccades are rapid eye movements performed to take an object of interest into the center of the line of sight (foveal vision). Two pairs of dots are placed on the wall. One pair is placed so that its members are separated by 20° visual angle and imaginary line between them is horizontal. The second pair is placed so that its members are separated by same distance and imaginary line between them is vertical. Patient is asked to look back and forth between the two members of the horizontal pair and then back and forth between the two members of the vertical pair, keeping the head still. The patient's eye movements are recorded. The procedure is performed to calibrate the recording system and to evaluate the saccade eye movements control system.

3. **Tracking test:** It is the recording of the nystagmus while the patient follows a slowly moving visual target. The test is done to evaluate the pursuit eye movement control system.

4. **Optokinetic test:** It is the recording of nystagmus while patient looks vertical stripes moving at several different speeds to the right and then to the left. Tracing of nystagmus helps to determine whether the nystagmus generated by stimulus becomes stronger if the stimulus strength increases and whether the nystagmus is stronger in one direction than in the other direction.

5. **Positional test:** It is the recording of nystagmus induced by placing the patient in various positions (usually sitting, supine, right lateral, left lateral and head hanging) with the patient's eyes both open and closed.

6. **Caloric test:** It is designed to determine whether appropriate nystagmus response is generated by thermal stimulation of labyrinth.

ENG and caloric stimulation: Jongkees et al.[20] 1964 mentioned that caloric testing is an essential part of ENG examination.

Brown-Sequard[10] was the first to observe the response of the vestibular organ to the syringing of cold water into the outer auditory canal.

Barany[21] (1906) was the first to see the clinical importance of this reaction and also the first to give a theory as to the origin of the reaction. During syringing with water, temperature is transmitted towards the semicircular canals and its surrounding endolymph. It causes lowering specific gravity by heating and raising specific gravity by cooling resulting flow of endolymph. The first canal reached is the lateral one in its most lateral part. Maximum effect of the caloric test is produced in the semicircular canal when it is in a vertical position. This in turn means that the maximum vestibular response is elicited when the patient is examined lying in the supine position with the head elevated on a cushion about 30°. He used larger quantities of water which produced unpleasant sensation of nausea and vomiting. This method is known as mass irrigation.

Kobark[22] stressed the importance of employing small quantities of water in executing the test. Initially, only 5 cc of ice water for 60 seconds was employed to build the threshold level of nystagmus; if there is no response ear is irrigated with 10 mL, 20 mL and 40 mL of ice water. Normally nystagmus beating towards the opposite ear is seen with 5cc of water. If response is seen with increase amount of water (i.e. 5–40 mL of ice water) the labyrinth is said hypoactive. If no response even with 40 mL of ice water the labyrinth is considered dead.

Fitzgerald and Hallpike[23] recorded nystagmus using alternate hot (44°C) and cold (30°C) water, i.e. 7°C above and below the body temperature. The stimulus was just strong enough to evoke a vestibular reaction and avoid unnecessary disturbance to patients causing nasuea and vomiting. They irrigated the ear with 250 cc of water at 44°C and 30°C for 40 seconds. The position of the patient was supine with head flexed 30° forward (Fig. 13).

Use of 50cc of water at 30°C and 40°C was recommended by Jonkee.[24] The interval between the tests need not be longer than six months. He studied the influence of quantity of water irrigated in the caloric response using 5 cc, 10 cc, 25 cc, 50 cc and 500 cc of water and found little correlation between the volume of water irrigated and duration of caloric nystagmus. Again the velocity of irrigation has little influence.

Temperature of water is more important than the volume. Cold water produces nystagmus of longer duration than that produced by hot water. Cold water produces nystagmus to opposite side and warm water to the same side (mnemonic cows→cold—opposite, warm—same).

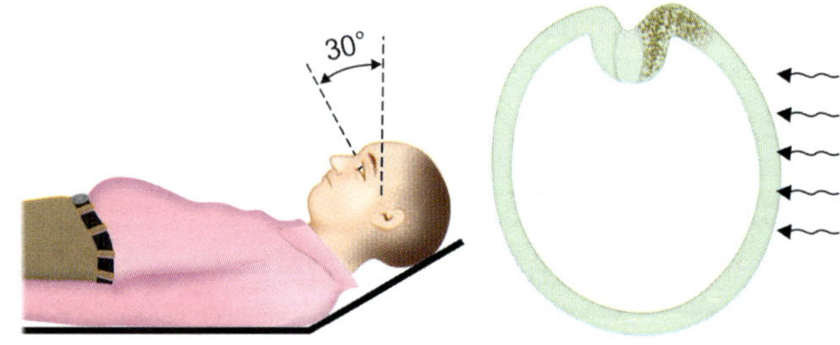

Fig. 13: Caloric test position and effect of warm water irrigation on right lateral canal

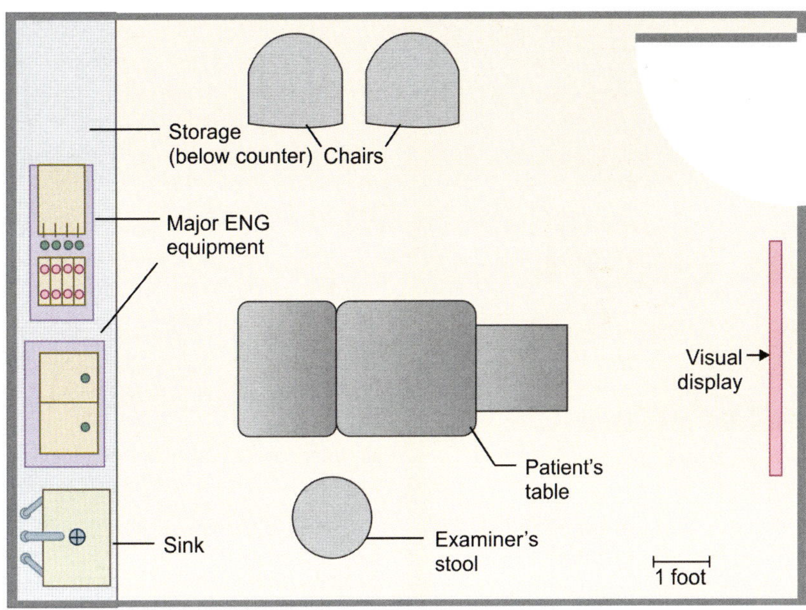

Fig. 14: Layout of an ENG laboratory (*Source:* Barbar HO, Stockwell CW. Manual of electronystagmography. 2nd edition, 1980.)

Methodology

Assessment of vestibular functions is performed according to Fitzgerald and Hallpike's Bithermal caloric test (1942) to induce nystagmus. The test is conducted in a dimmy light, sound treated and air conditioned vestibular laboratory with special shielded walls and ceiling to cut extraneous electronic disturbances (Fig. 14).

Equipment (Figs 15 to 17)

- Nystagmus is recorded electrically with the help of dual channel AC electronystagmography machine. The machine is properly earthed and operated on stabilized voltage. The preamplifiers are of AC type with long time constant of 4.5 seconds

- The machine has a knob to control the heat of stylus, another to control the gain or amplification of recording and a third to control the position of stylus on the recording paper. By a separate control the speed of recording paper is preset at 10 mm/second
- A 4 inch wide curved wooden plank painted white is hung from the ceiling to face towards the patients
- Distance between the plank and the eyes of the patient is 132 cm. The midpoint of the plank is in straight alignment with the glabella of the patient
- At an equidistant of 11.5 cm from the midpoint of the plank two small bulbs are fixed on either side. These

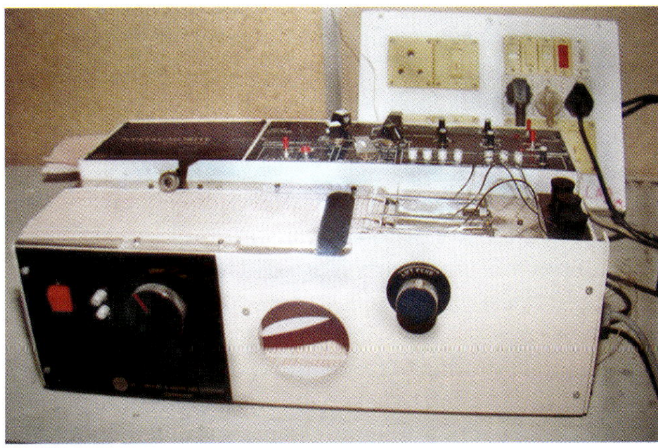

Fig. 15: Nystagmograph (front view)

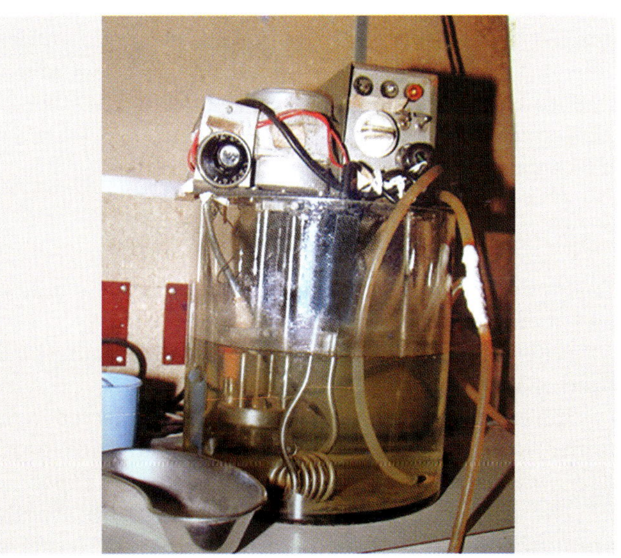

Fig. 16: Thermostatic water bath

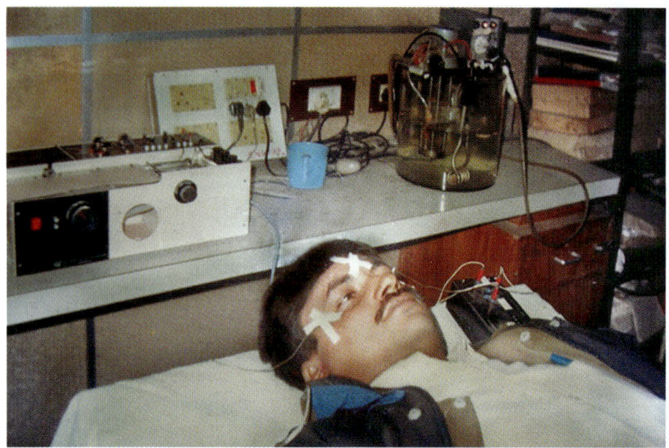

Fig. 17: Set up for recording of nystagmus

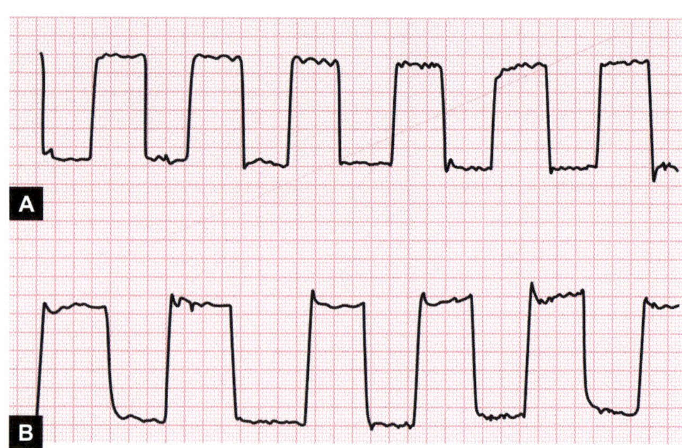

Figs 18A and B: (A) Horizontal calibration with bitemporal leads and DC recording system; (B) Vertical calibration with vertical leads (left eye) and DC recording system

bulbs are connected to an AC coupler which when switched on, lighted those bulbs alternately
- The distance between the two bulbs is so adjusted as to give rise of 10° of eye movement, on the patient being made to follow the alternately lighting bulbs.

Procedure

The procedure is at first explained to the patients. They are told not to move the head or to feel apprehensive. At the same time patients' mental alertness and cooperation are sought.

Patients are asked to lie supine quietly and comfortably on an examination table with head end elevated at an angle of 30° from horizontal.

An area of skin 1cm lateral to external canthi on either side and in between the eyebrows is cleaned with solvent ether for better contact between electrode and skin.

A saucer-shaped metal electrodes of 8 mm diameter are applied to the above sites, the positive electrode on right side and negative electrode on left side and neutral over forehead that are held in place by application of adhesive plaster on top. This arrangement of electrode is known as bitemporal arrangement.

Calibration (Figs 18A and B)

Calibration is carried out prior to recording of nystagmus and at the completion of procedure in each case.

Patients are asked to look alternately at the lighting bulbs fixed on wooden plank.

The eye movement towards the right is reflected in the form of upward deflection of the stylus and towards the left as downward deflection on the recording graph paper.

The gain control is manipulated to obtain the amplification of recorded graph as near to 10 mm as possible for 10° eye movements. A mean average of 10

readings before and 10 after the recording is calculated. This is used for the calculations of various parameters in degree.

Caloric Stimulation

The technique of Fitzerald and Hallpike (1942) is employed to induce nystagmus. The temperature of water used for cold stimulation is maintained at 30°C and for hot stimulation at 44°C. 250 cc of water is irrigated in each ear for 40 seconds. 10 minutes time is allowed in between the test.

The caloric irrigation is done through metal nozzle of 44 mm diameter fixed to the end of rubber tubes connected to electrically operated water pumps. This machine pumps out water from water reservoirs at a constant rate of 7 mL/second. The water in the reservoir is kept at constant temperature of 30°C and 40°C with the help of thermostat controlled water heaters.

The subject's eye is kept closed during the procedure. The recorder is switched on immediately on commencement of irrigation. The end point of nystagmus is determined by appearance of a square wave[25] or first beat in opposite direction[26] or absence of two consecutive waves within a time span of 5 second.[27]

Caloric stimulation are done in the following orders in all cases—right cold, left cold, right hot followed by left hot (Fig. 19).

The electronystagmographs are studied, analysed and compared under following parameters:
1. Latency of nystagmus (LP): This is computed from beginning of the stimulus to the onset of first nystagmus beat.
2. The total duration of nystagmus (TD): This is estimated as the time period between the onset of caloric irrigation and last beat of nystagmus in the same direction. Any after nystagmus in the reverse direction is not included.

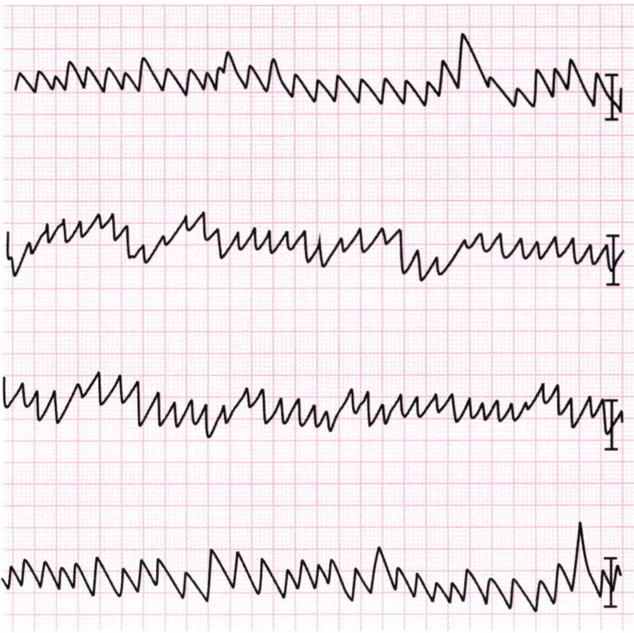

Fig. 19: Right hot, Right cold, Left hot and Left cold Caloric stimulation resulting nystagmus as recorded by ENG. Right hot and Left cold producing right beating nystagmus and Right cold and Left hot producing left beating Nystagmus.

3. **Total amplitude of the first component (TA):** It is calculated by summing the amplitude of first component of all beats from the graphic record with the help of a map measured by tracing over the individual beat. The total distance indicated on the map measure is converted in degree of rotation by the use of calibration.
4. **Total number of beats (TB):** It is established by counting the well-formed nystagmus beats from the onset of induced nystagmus to the end. All the beats with slow and quick components are included.
5. **Maximum speed of slow component (MSS):** It is calculated by dividing the amplitude by the duration. It is obtained by taking the average of slow phases of nystagmic beats within 10 seconds during the culmination period, i.e. when the nystagmus is most intense (Barber and Stockwell).[12] MSS is generally accepted to be a most sensitive parameter.[26]

A comparison between the responses obtained from right and left irrigation from same individual giving the difference between the excitability of each right and left side is considered as unilateral weakness (canal paresis).

Correspondingly, the difference between right beating and left beating nystagmus is considered as a relative value of directional preponderance. These relative values are generally calculated by using the formulae originally introduced by Jongkess, Mass and Philipzoon (1962).[28]

Unilateral weakness (%)

$$= \frac{(L_{30°C} + L_{44°C}) - (R_{30°C} + R_{44°C})}{(L_{30°C} + L_{44°C} + R_{30°C} + R_{44°C})} \times 100$$

Where, L= left; R= right

Positive values give right unilateral weakness in percentage and negative values give left unilateral weakness in percentage. It is indicative of depressed function of the ipsilateral labyrinth, vestibular nerve or vestibular nuclei as seen in Meniere's disease, acoustic neuroma, post-labyrinthectomy or vestibular nerve section.

Directional Preponderance (%):

$$DP = \frac{(L_{30°C} + R_{44°C}) - (R_{30°C} + L_{44°C})}{(L_{30°C} + L_{44°C} + R_{30°C} + R_{44°C})} \times 100$$

Positive values give right and negative values give left directional preponderance in percentage. Directional preponderance occurs towards the side of central lesion, away from the side of peripheral lesion.

Summation of mean and 2SD (95% limit of normal) is calculated from control group for both unilateral weakness and directional preponderance and this serves as a parameter to decide whether the results of study group are normal or pathological. The 95% limit of normal variation is 25% for unilateral weakness (UW) and 29% for directional preponderance.

Posturography

Posturography is used to mention any test described for postural stability or standing balance.

Body sway is recorded and measured by means of force platforms that register the position of the centre of pressure and the vertical, horizontal and transverse ground forces during standing. The standard Romberg's position is commonly used with eye open and closed for 15 seconds to 1 minute.

Statokinesiometry is the recording and measurement of radial displacement or total length in millimeters of the line or the locus of the body's center of gravity traced for a given period. The area of the locus displacement is obtained from an x-y recorder in which 'x' represents lateral and 'y' represents anteroposterior displacements (Fig. 20).

- **Stabilometry** is the recording of 'x' and 'y' displacements separately. AC and DC recordings of the oscillations of the locus are made. The frequency analysis determined by power spectra is applied.

Two basic coefficients are—

- **Romberg coefficient =**
  Value obtained with eyes closed/value obtained with eyes open
- Ratio of anteroposterior/lateral sway which is greater than 1.

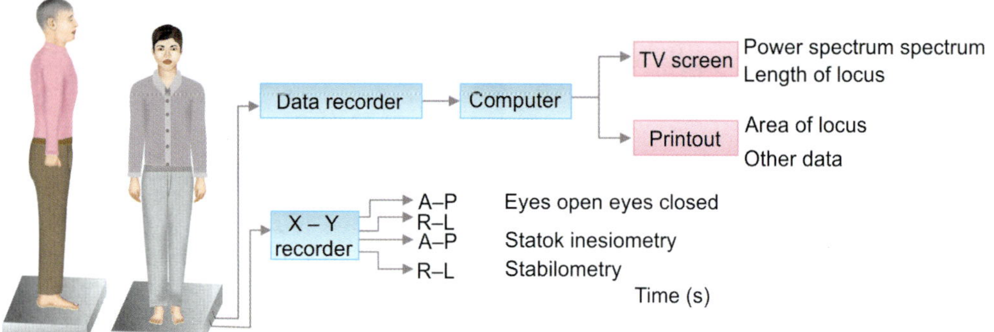

Fig. 20: Schematic representation of posturography. A-P: anteroposterior body sway; R-L: Lateral body sway.
(*Source:* Scott-Brown`s Otolaryngology 5th edition Vol 2)

In vestibular disorders the lateral sway is more marked than anteroposterior sway. The ratio of anteroposterior (AP) and lateral sway (R-L) is less than unity.

In patient with bilateral vestibular lesion, the main posturographic feature is an increase in anteroposterior sway at 0.4 Hz.

Posturography is not a test of the VOR as standard tests of VOR evaluate the response of horizontal semicircular canal only without providing any information about the otolith structures or the vestibular spinal reflex (VSR). Posturography is a test of VSR function. To evaluate the vestibular function the most useful form of posturography is the **sensory organization test** (SOT). SOT measures the patient's response to a variety of visual and somatosensory altered conditions. Patient is able to properly utilize the three main sensory inputs—the visual, somatosensory and vestibular to the central nervous system (CNS) for maintaining posture and equilibrium. SOT involves six sensory conditions (Fig. 21).

Condition 1: Stable platform with eye open in a stable visual environment. Patient can utilize full use of sensory inputs—visual, vestibular and somato sensory information.

Condition 2: Stable platform with eye closed. Patient is able to use of vestibular and somatosensory inputs.

Condition 3: Stable platform with moving visual environment. Patient is able to suppress a false sense of visually induced movement and utilizes vestibular and somatosensory information.

Condition 4: Unstable platform with eyes open in a stable visual environment. Patient utilizes vestibular and visual information.

Condition 5: Unstable platform with eyes closed. Patient is primarily dependent on vestibular information as visual and somatosensory inputs are eliminated.

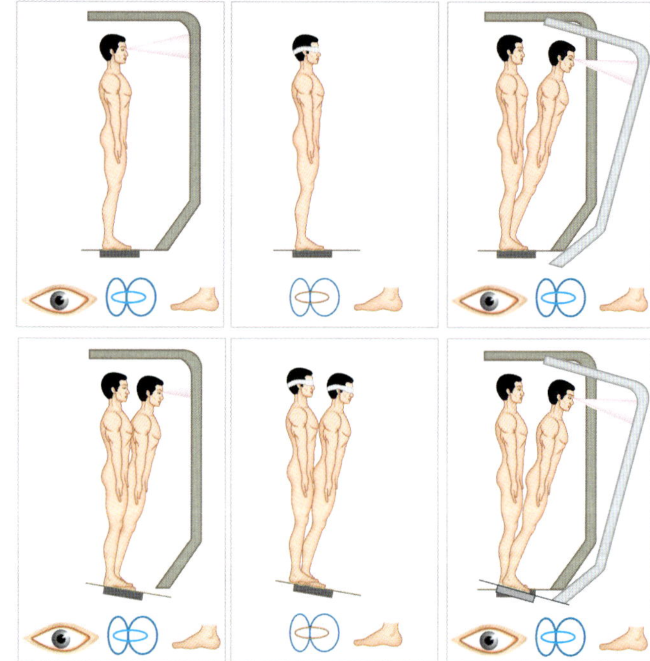

Fig. 21: Six conditions for SOT as performed on Eqitest by Neurocom International

Condition 6: Unstable platform and unstable visual surround. Patient is primarily dependent on vestibular input and is able to suppress a false sense of visually induced movement.

The 'gold standard' of posturography is computerized dynamic posturography (CDP) (Fig. 22). CDP is developed as a means to evaluate relative contribution of each of peripheral senses related to postural stability. It is marked in the name of uquitest system produced by Neurocom International (www.onbalance.com)

The equitest produces an unstable visual environment by providing wall in front of the patient to move in response

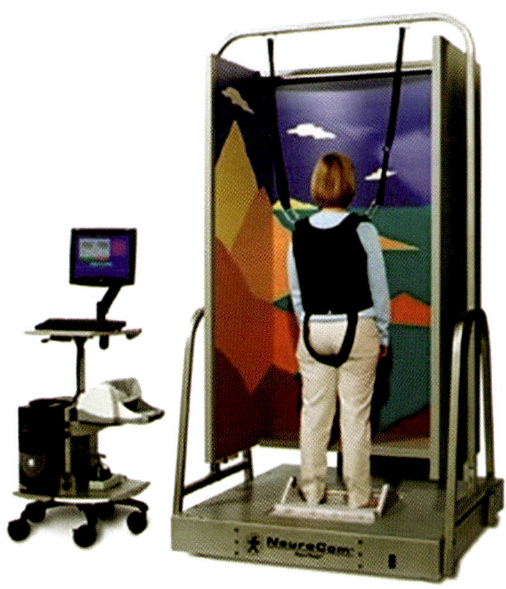

Fig. 22: Computerized Dynamic Posturography

to patient's sway as measured on the base platform. When patient leans forward, the wall synchronously moves forward, thereby disturbing visual feedback of the movement. The reduced somatosensory feedback is done successfully by movement of the base platform in response to patient's sway. When the patient leans forward the platform moves also, thereby reducing or distorting proprioceptive input received from the stretch receptors of the lower legs.

Key Points

- CDP is not a diagnostic site of lesion test. It provides an assessment of functional balance under a variety of conditions
- Two tests are performed in CDP—
  - The sensory organization test (SOT)—It involves measurement of postural stability or sway while systematically removing or distorting visual and somatosensory information used for balance
  - The motor control test (MCT)—It helps to assess disorders of motor coordination to maintain posture and equilibrium. The force platform is allowed to undergo sudden translations forwards and backwards. The patient's way is monitored and analyzed by the computer. A somatosensory input is sent in by changing the ankle angle. This input from muscle stretch receptor in ankle passes through spinal tract to brain stem –cerebellar complex - then to motor cortex. From motor cortex the input goes

down through descending spinal tract to appropriate muscles of the body to contract ensuring postural stability. Any disorder in motor coordination is assessed by MCT.

Galvanic Test

When galvanic stimulation is applied to the mastoid, the subject tends to fall towards the anode current. Falling tendency begins with a current of as low as 1–1.5 mA.

The test is carried out by asking patient to stand in the tandem position (Mann's Standing Test) with application of binaural galvanic current of 1–1.5mA near the ear or mastoid. The site of stimulation is considered to be scarpa's ganglion. The normal subjects tend to fall towards anode.

The body sway is a measure of response to galvanic stimulation. Body sway can be studied by special platform. The test is done to differentiate an end organ lesion from that of vestibular nerve (Fig. 23).

Rotatory Test (Barany's Technique)

Rotatory test is first carried by Barany (Fig. 24). Patient is seated in Barany's revolving chair (Fig. 25) with his head tilted 30° forwards and then rotated for about 20 seconds. The rotation is abruptly stopped. The nystagmus induced by sudden stop is 10–30 seconds in duration in normal subject that is fairly symmetrical in clockwise and counter clockwise in rotation. Gross asymmetries in duration between the response to clockwise and counter clockwise rotation are taken as a vestibular pathology. In this test, actually the postrotatory nystagmus is assessed. Nowadays with the advent of more precise device like torsion swing chair for rotating and ENG for recording nystagmus, both prerotatory and as well as postrotatory nystagmus is evaluated.

Cranio-Corpo-Graphy (CCG)

Cranio-corpo-graphy is the photographic recording of patient's head and body movements. It provides the functional measurement of balance that reflexes vestibulospinal function.

The patient is made to wear a helmet fitted with two small bulbs in sagittal axis, one on the forehead and other on the occiput. Another two small bulbs are fitted to each shoulder of the patient. The examination room is darkened and has a convex mirror fitted on the roof. A polaroid camera with an adjustable stand is kept between head of the patient and convex mirror on the roof. The lens of the camera is directed towards the convex mirror. An eye mask is used for blind folding the patient. The patient is then asked to perform Fukuda Stepping test and Romberg's test.

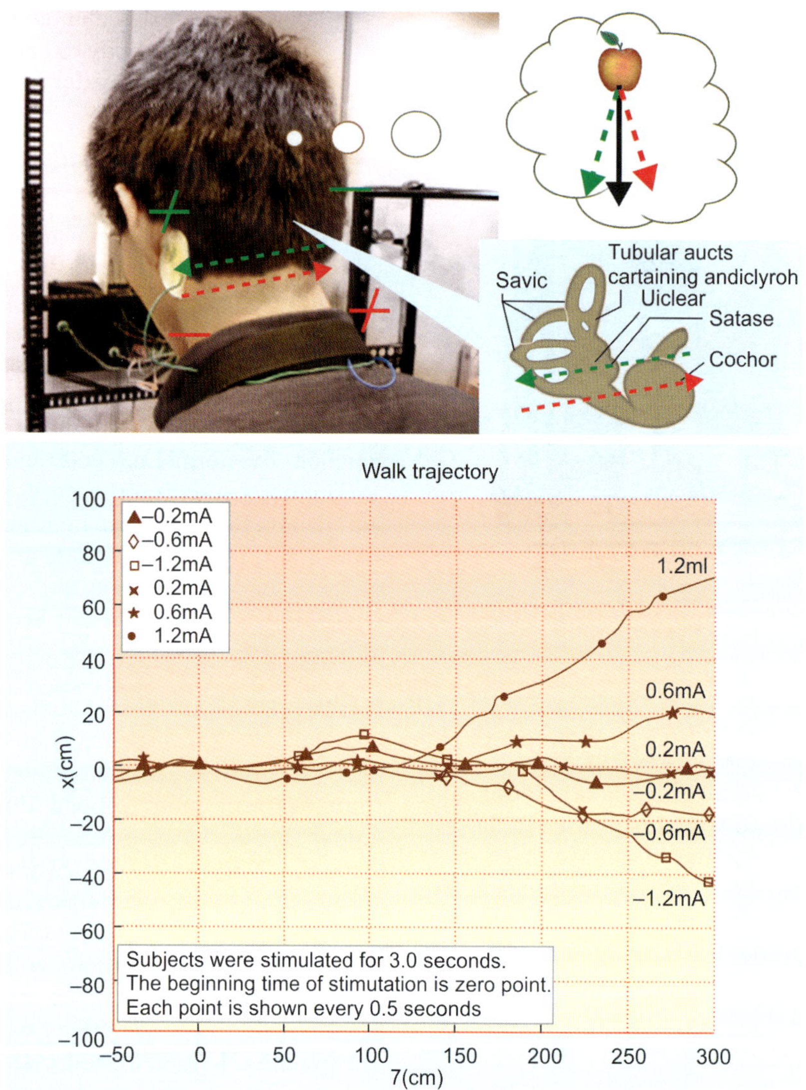

Fig. 23: Galvanic Vestibular stimulation causing a person to sway while he is standing in Tandem Position

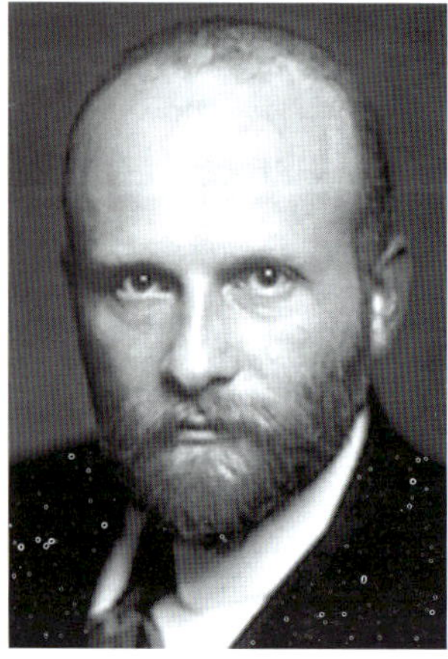

Fig. 24: Robert Barany. (April 22, 1876-April 8, 1936)
Noble Prize in medicine 191

The movements of the patient during the stepping test and Romberg test are monitored by the lights that are reflected onto the convex mirror and from there to the film in the camera. The camera kept in constant exposure records the movements of the patient on the film during the stepping test and Romberg's test.[29]

Parameters, such as longitudinal sway, lateral sway, forehead covering area, torticollis angle (Romberg's test), longitudinal deviation, lateral sway width, angular deviation and self-spin and Unterberger Fukudas test are automatically measured.

Indications

- To recognize a normal or abnormal pattern of body balance

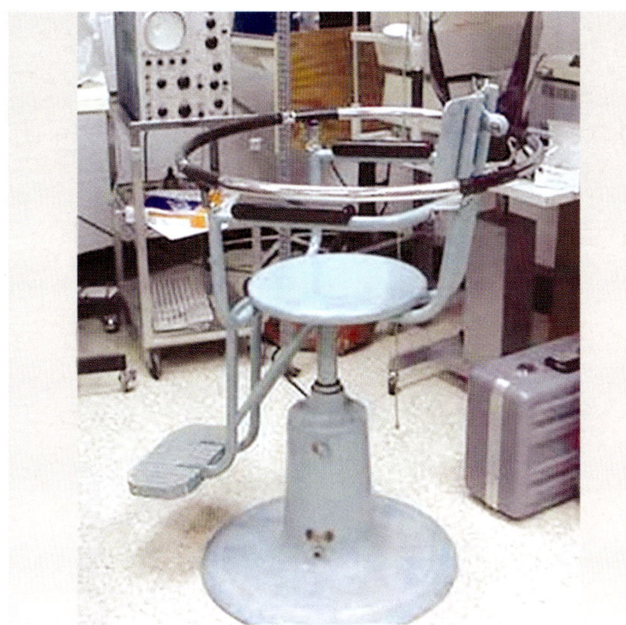

Fig. 25: Barany's chair

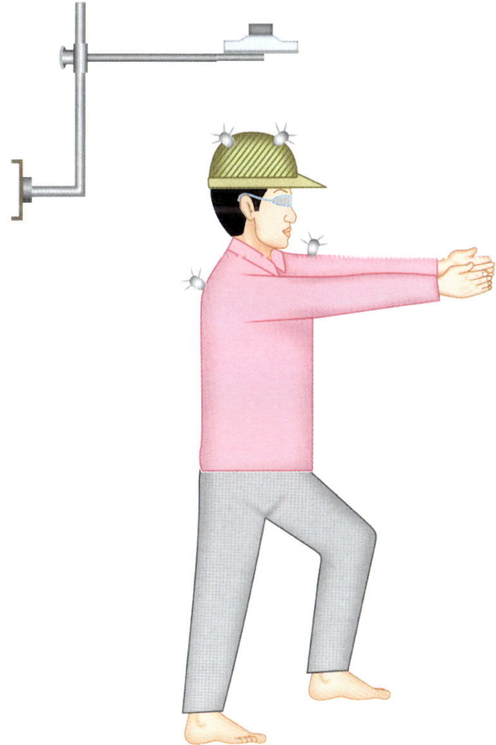

Fig. 26: CCG set up as devised by Claussen

- To monitor the evolution of vertiginous patients on treatment
- To identify sensorimotor lesions in patient with tinnitus.

REFERENCES

1. Kerr AG, Vertigo. Scott Brown's otolaryngology, 5th edition. 1994. 437.
2. Harvey's, Wood.D, and Feroah T. Relationship of the head impulse test and head shake nystagmus in reference to caloric testing. Am J Otol. 1997;18(2):207-13.
3. Longridge NS, Mallinson AI. The dynamic illegible E (DIE) test: a simple technique for assessing the ability of the vestibule-ocular reflex to overcome vestibular pathology. J Otolaryngol. 1987;16(2):97-103.
4. Schuknecht H (Editor). Pathophysiology. In pathology of the ear. Cambridge, mass: Harvard University Press. 1974;97-163.
5. Charles W Cummings (Editor). Otolaryngology-head and neck surgery. 1990;4:2750-52.
6. Fukuda T. The stepping test: two phases of the labyrinthine reflex. Acta Otolaryngol. 1959;50:95.
7. Allison L. Balance disorders, In: D .Umpherd (Ed.), Neurologic rehabilitation. 3rd Edition, St Louis: Mosby Year Book. 1995;802-37.
8. Urbscheit NL, Oremland BS. Cerebellar dysfunction. In: DA Umphered (Ed), Neurologic rehabilitation. St Louis: Mosby Year Book; 1995. 657-80.
9. Puisieux F, Boumbar Y, Bulckaen H, Bonnin E, Houssain F Dewailly. Intraindividual variability in orthostatic blood pressure changes among older adults: The influence of meals. J Am Geriartr soc. 1999;47:1332-6.
10. Brown Sequard C. Course of lectures on the physiology and pathology of the central nervous system. Philadelphia: Collins; 1860. P187.
11. Collins WE. Arousal and vestibular habituation in kornhuber HH (editor). Hard book of sensory physiology. Vol.6, No:2, New York: Springer Publishing Co. Inc. 1974. pp.361-8.
12. Barber HO, Stockwell CW. Manual of electronystagmography, 2nd edition. Saint Louis: The CV Mosby Co; 1980.
13. Rubin W, Norris c. Specifications for electronystagmographs (emdash) clinical and research. J. Assn Advance Med Instr. 1967.
14. Duke-Elder, Sir WS. The textbook of ophthalmology: Development, ff and function of visual approaches. Vol. 1. Henry Kimpton: London; 1842.
15. Meyers L. Electronystagmography–A graphic study of the action currents in nystagmus. Arch n Psychiat. 1929;21:901-18.
16. Mowrer OH, Ruch TC, Miller NE. Corneo repotential difference as the basis of the galvanometric method of recording of eye movements. Amo J Physiol. 1936;114:423-8.
17. FennWo, Hursh JB. Movements of the eye when the lids are closed. Am J Physiol. 1937;118:8-14.
18. Marg E. Development of electro-oculography. AMA Arch Opthal. 1951;45:169-85.
19. Neollwk. Azide sensitive positive difference across the eye ball. Am J Physiol. 1952;170:217-38.
20. Jongkees, Philipzoon AJ. Electronystagmography. Acta otolaryngol suppl. 1964;189:1-111.
21. Balany R. untersuchungem uber den Vom. Vestibul arapparat des ohres refl ektorischansgel osten Nystagmus and seine begleit Mschr. Oh. 1906;40:193-7.
22. Kobrak F. Beitrage zum experimental nystagmus, Beitrz physiol path. 1918;10:214.

23. Fitzgerald G, Hallpike CS. Studies in human vestibular function. Observation on the directional preponderance(Nystagmus bere) of caloric nystagmus resulting from cerebellar lesions. Brain 1942;65:115-37.

24. Jongkees JBW. Which is the preferable method of performing caloric test. Arch Otolaryngol. 1949;49:594-608.

25. Stable J, Bergman B. The caloric reaction in Meniere's disease. An electronystagmographical study in 200 patients. The laryngoscope. 1967;77:1629-43.

26. Jongkees JBW, Mass JPM, Philipzooh AJ. Clinical nystagmography. Practice otolaryngologia. 1962;24:65-93.

27. Gordon MA. The genetics of oto. A review. Am J Otal. 1969;10:426-38.

28. Morrison AW. Genetic factors in otosclerosis. Annals of the Royal college of S og England.1967;41:202-37.

29. A Bis was vestibulo spinal tests, clinical audio-vestibulometry for otologists and Neumologists, 3rd edition. 2002. 148-9.

Diseases of the External Ear

Asok K Saha

External ear comprises Pinna, External Auditory Canal (EAC) and Tympanic membrane (TM).

Morphology of these structures is bilaterally symmetrical that helps in sound transmission to middle ear in frequencies of 2–4 kHz. Diseases of external ear are common entities in clinical practice resulting in hearing loss with poor communication as well as psychological trauma for aesthetic sense. Diagnosis and management of these diseases need precise knowledge of embryology, anatomy and physiology of ear that has been discussed in Chapter 1 and 2.

Diseases of the external ear are caused by—

- Congenital anomalies
- Inflammatory conditions
- Trauma and tumors.

Congenital Anomalies

Congenital anomalies include:

- Congenital anomalies of pinna
- Atresia and stenosis of the EAC
- Preauricular sinus or pit
- Collaural fistula
- Congenital swellings of pinna.

Congenital Anomalies of Pinna

Pinna begins to form by fusion of six hillocks or tubercles. Three of these hillocks are derived from first branchial arch (Mechel) and three from the second branchial arch (Reichert) during 5th and 6th weeks of intrauterine life. By the 20th week pinna takes adult shape (Fig. 1).

External auditory canal is formed from an invagination of surface epithelium from the first branchial cleft in the 5th week of gestation. As the cells grow inward, they meet the similar evagination of entodermal tissue of developing tubotympanum trapping a layer of mesoderm in between. Fusion of these cells results in formation of tympanic membrane having three germinal layers. The solid core of tissue then recanalizes forming the epithelial lining of bony meatus in about 16th embryonic week. EAC is completely developed at about 28 weeks of gestation (Fig. 2).[1]

First three hillocks form the tragus, helical crus and the helix and second three hillocks form anti helix, scapha and the lobule. Circumference of the pinna is formed by helix, lobule and tragus. Inner fold of pinna comprises antihelix and antitragus. Antihelix divides external ear superiorly into superior and inferior crus. Between the crura is triangular fossa. Between helical rim and antihelical fold is scapha or scaphoid fossa. Between antihelix and tragus is conchal bowl which is divided by root of the helix into cymba concha above and cavum concha below. Tragus overlies the opening of ear canal. Height of a normal pinna is 55–65 mm width is 30–45 mm and pinna is rotated so that top is 15°–30° more posterior than the ear lobule. Angle between pinna and head is <21° in female and <25° in male. The angle

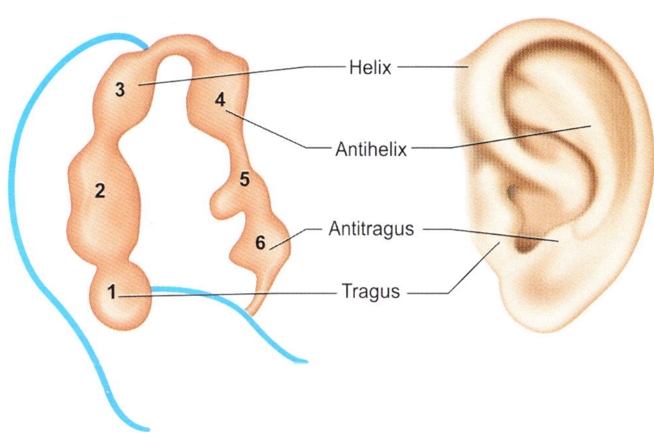

Fig. 1: Development of Pinna

of the ear is parallel to the dorsum of the nose. Root of the ear is 60–70 mm posterior to lateral canthus.[2]

Anomalies of pinna may occur in isolation or may be associated with anomalies of EAC, middle ear and inner ear. These may be the part of syndromic diseases.

Anotia

Anotia—is the complete absence of pinna. One or two small rudimentary tubercles may be present. EAC is usually absent or replaced by a blind-ended pit. It is a rare congenital disorder caused by thalidomide-induced embryotoxicity in 50% of cases (Fig. 3).[3]

Microtia

Microtia—pinna is smaller than normal and is deformed. The deformities may vary from mild to severe distortion of anatomic landmarks. Atresia or stenosis of EAC is also associated with certain degree of microtia. Association of inner ear deformities is rare in patients having microtia with atresia of EAC. 50% of microtia is associated with other anomalies of face (Figs 4 and 5).

Incidence

Its incidence is rare, about 0.03% of live births. These deformities commonly occur unilaterally, more on the right side. Males are predominant (Male: Female= 3:1). Multigravida with 4 or more pregnancies has high-risk of bearing baby with microtia. Japanese are affected more than other populations.

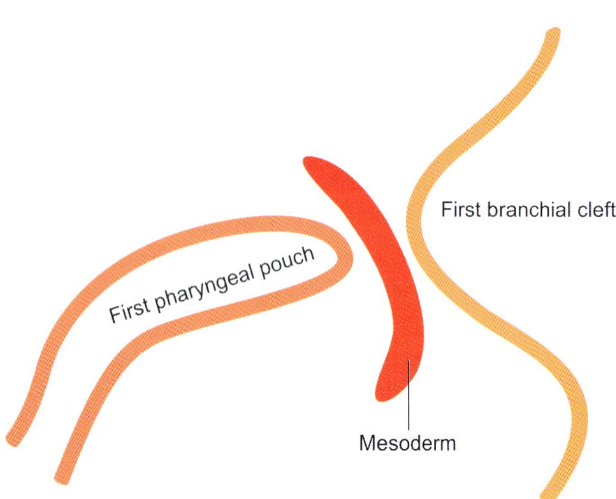

Fig. 2: Development of EAC and tympanic membrane

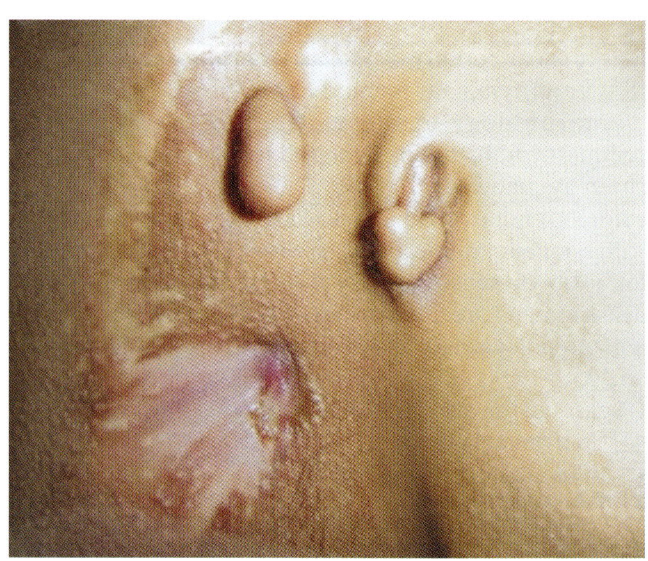

Fig. 4: Microtia of right ear

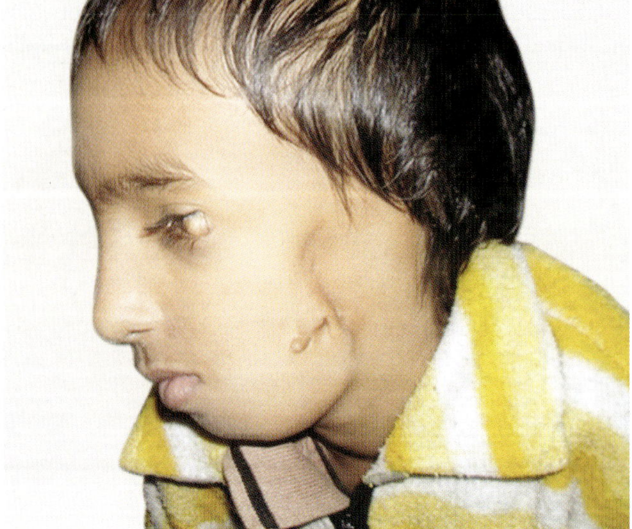

Fig. 3: Anotia—Absence of pinna and EAC

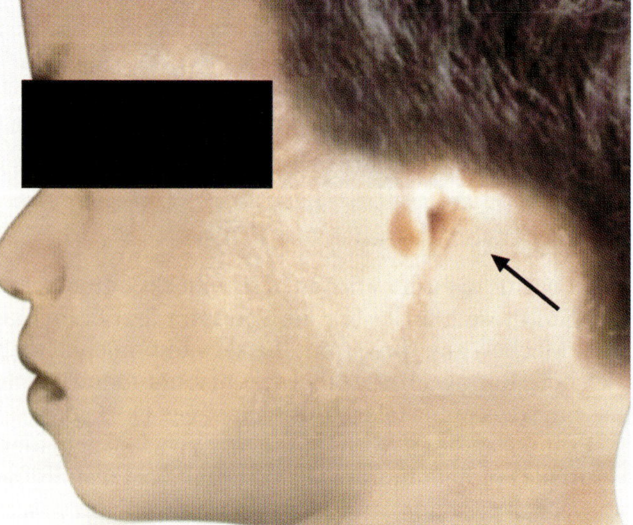

Fig. 5: Microtia of left ear

Etiology

The cause of microtia is unknown but it may be due to—

- Genetic aberrations or a single gene deletion, e.g. Goldenhar syndrome
- Mother's use of teratogens like thalidomide, accutane, vitamine A, etc.
- Vascular insult to the ear of the growing fetus
- Fetal exposure to environmental toxins.

Types of microtia are graded according to severity of malformed pinna by Marx (1926).

Grade 1 microtia—The pinna is malformed and small but retains most of the component of a normal pinna. EAC may or may not be present.

Grade 2 microtia—The pinna is abnormal; parts of the pinna are not recognizable.

Grade 3 microtia—Only very small auricular tag is present. EAC is absent.

Grade 4 microtia—Complete absence of pinna (anotia).

Microtia accompanied by atresia is difficult to put into simple grades.

Two other classification systems proposed by Jahrsdoerfer and De La Cruz are commonly used now a days. Jahrsdoerfer[4] proposed a scoring system for selection of patients with congenital aural atresia (CAA) based on CT scan findings and appearance of external ear using 10 points scale.

Patients with scoring 8–10 surgical outcomes are good to excellent; scoring 7–6 fair to marginal. Patients with score 5 or less surgical outcomes are poor (Table 1).

De la Cruz classification divides the malformation into major and minor categories that correlate to surgical outcome. Minor deformities are better group for surgical reconstruction and major deformities are treated with hearing aids.[5]

Management

Before surgical management following points are essential.

- Attention is to be given to rule out other associated cervico facial congenital anomalies
- Skin quality over the deformed pinna is to be noted as well as facial nerve examination to be done and documented
- Hearing status of the affected side is to be assessed
- CT scan helps to know the middle ear and inner ear anatomy. Congenital cholesteatoma may be present in these patients should be ruled out from CT imaging.

Surgery for unilateral microtia is performed as a staged procedure with an interval of 3 months between these stages using autogenous rib cartilage by Tanzer procedure (1959) (Later modified by Brent, 1974). Operation is performed when the child reaches 6 years of age for sufficient growth of the rib cartilage at the donor site (Figs 6 to 10).

Table 1: Jahrsdoerfer scoring system of conenital aural atresia

	Score
Stapes Present	2
Oval window open	1
Middle ear space	1
Facial nerve	1
Malleus incus complex	1
Mastoid pneumatization	1
Incus stapes connection	1
Round window	1
Appearance of external ear	1
Total available points	10

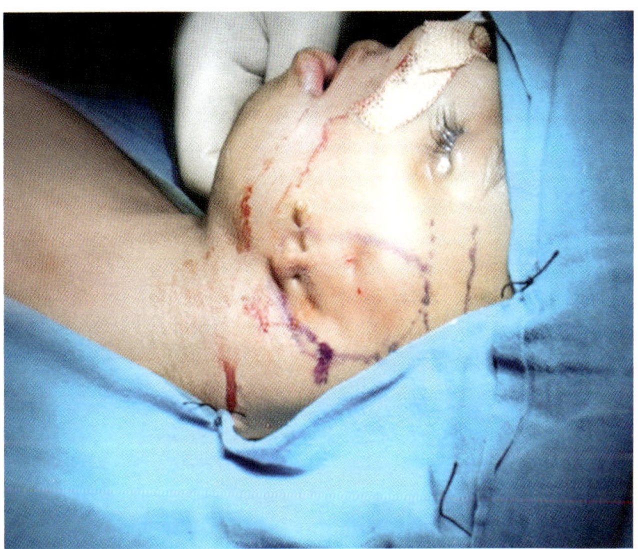

Fig. 6: Incision mark being made

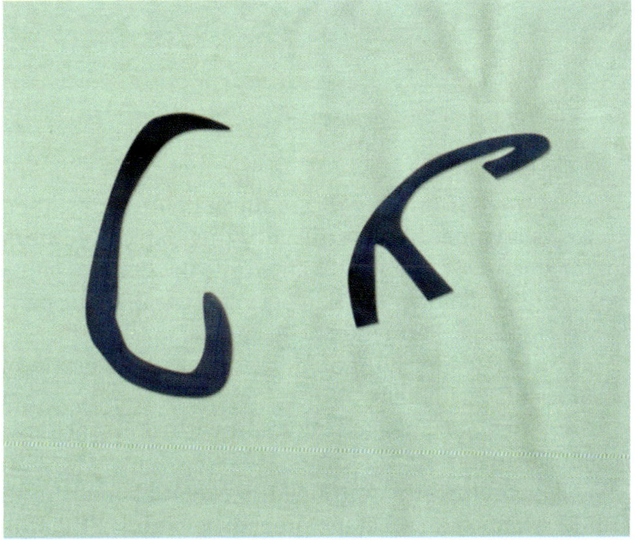

Fig. 7: Template of normal ear is designed with X-ray plate

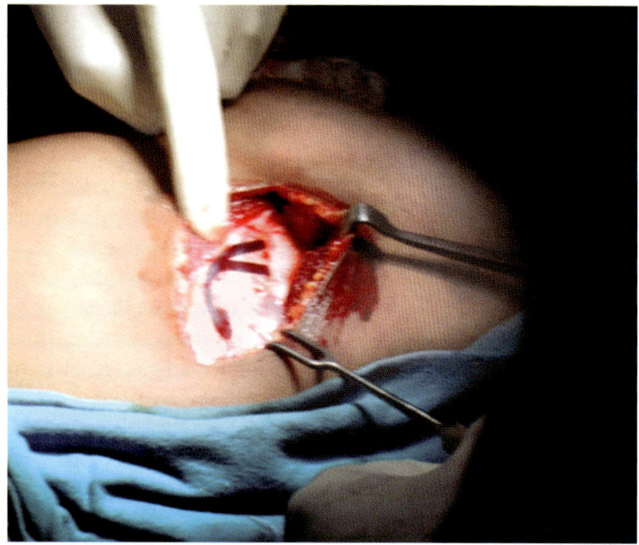

Fig. 8: Rib cartilage harvested from 6th to 8th ribs

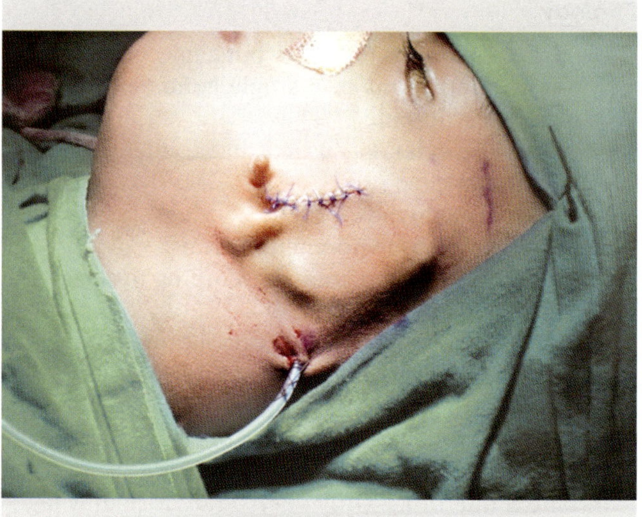

Fig. 10: Cartilage placed under skin pocket

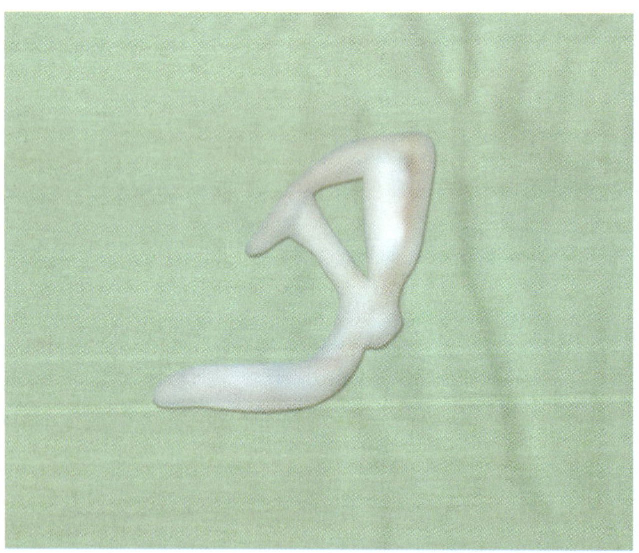

Fig. 9: Rib cartilage framework made into shape of pinna

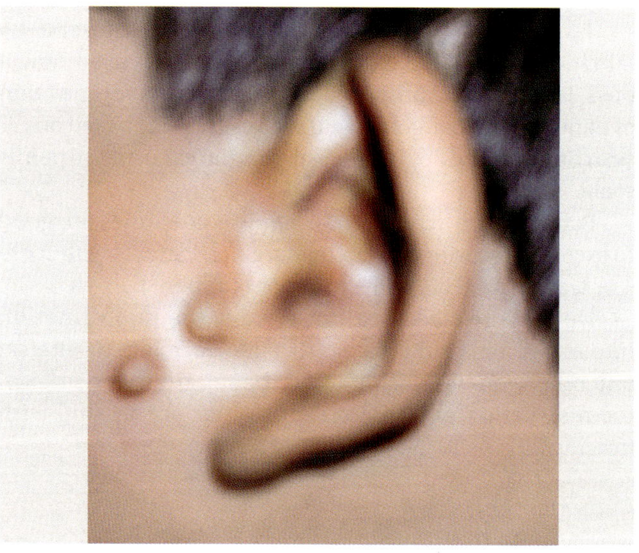

Fig. 11: Melotia of left ear with atresia of EAC

First stage: Template of the normal ear is designed to use as a guide. A rib cartilage is then harvested from contralateral 6–8 ribs and sculptured into the shape of pinna which is placed under the skin pocket of the microtic ear.

Second stage: Formation of the lobule.

Third stage: Elevation of framework with insertion of postauricular skin graft.

Fourth stage: Tragus is created with skin/cartilage composite graft from contralateral ear.

Other technique employed is Nagata's technique (1985) which is a two stage procedure with six months interval and usually performed at 10 years of age with chest circumference of at least 60 cm.

Stage I: Fabrication of auricular framework from ipsilateral costal cartilage, creation of tragus and transposition of lobule.

Stage II: Elevation of framework. A split-thickness skin graft is harvested to cover posterior aspect of the graft.

Melotia is the caudo-ventral displacement of ears (Fig. 11).

Polyotia is the presence of an extra-auricle on one or both sides of the head (Fig. 12).

Complications of auricular reconstruction are mainly of two types:

Complication at the cartilage donor site—

- Immediate complication like pneumothorax and atelectasis

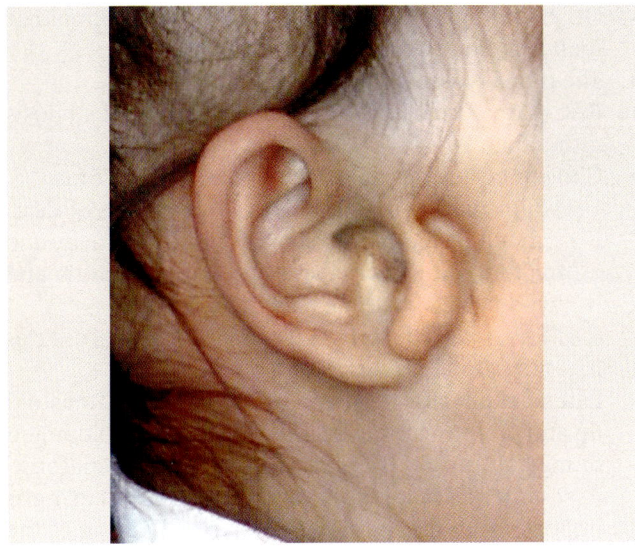

Fig. 12: Polyotia of right ear

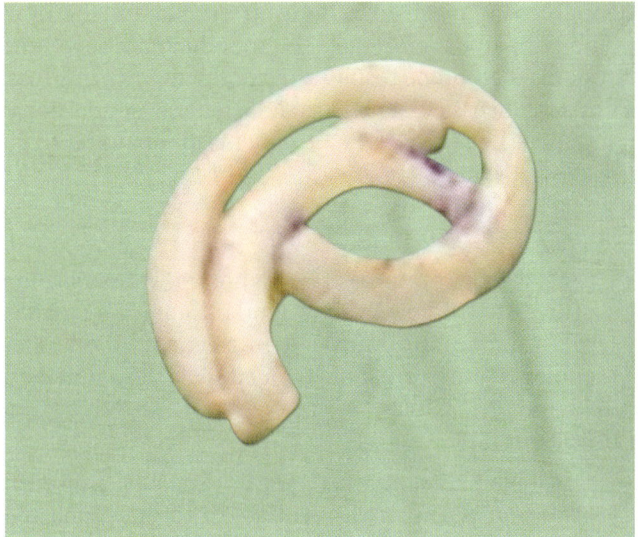

Fig. 13: Alloplastic material for auricular reconstruction

- Delayed complications include anterior chest wall deformity and scarring. Posterior perichondrium, if kept intact helps to prevent this complication.

Complications at ear reconstruction site include—

- Extrusion of the framework due to skin flap necrosis
- Resorption of the frame work due to tightly placed suture or placement of framework in scarred ischemic bed.

Alloplastic Material for Auricular Reconstruction

The auricular reconstruction can be done by alloplastic materials. It provides a more consistent aesthetic value and avoids harvesting costal cartilage (Fig. 13).

Various alloplastic materials used are made of silastic framework for auricular reconstruction which has excellent result, but long-term follow-up shows high rate of implant exposure. Minor trauma or abrasion results in implant exposure and failure for which silicon implant has been abandoned.

Nowadays use of porous polyethylene like Porex, Porex surgical and Newman provides good short-term results. Temporoparietal fascia flap that completely surrounds the implant results in significantly reduced failure rate.[6]

Prosthetic Reconstruction

The osseo-integrated anchoring devices approved by the FDA for use extra-aurally are practised recently by providing direct structural connection between living bone and a load carrying implant.

Indications for prosthetic microtia reconstruction are as follows:

- Failed autogenous reconstruction

- Significant soft tissue/skeleton hypoplasia
- Low or unfavorable hair line
- Acquired total or subtotal auricular defect in adult.

However, autogenous auricular reconstruction is still the choice of treatment for children with congenital auricular deformity.

Tissue Engineering

The technology of the tissue engineering provides potential to grow autogenous cartilage in predetermined shape. The study of transplantation of bovine chondrocytes onto a scaffold in the shape of human ear and its implantation for twelve weeks in mice result in new cartilage formation with gross morphology of human ear. Human chondrocytes can multiply well in vitro and have the ability to multiply new cartilage.[7] This idea can offer the advantage of autogenous reconstruction without morbidity associated with rib harvest.

Atresia and Stenosis of External Auditory Canal

It is a rare congenital disorder (1 in every 10,000 live births). Unilateral atresia is seven times more common than bilateral atresia.[8] The right ear is more often involved than left ear. About 15% of the patients have positive family history. Males are affected more often than females. It occurs with associated deformity of pinna. Average age of diagnosis is 3.5 years. Kisselback in 1882, first performed operation for correction of atresia of EAC. Unfortunately, the operation left with complication like facial nerve paralysis. Failure of canalization of the epithelial plug causes congenital atresia of EAC. Persistence of the tympanic ring results in a bony atresia plate at the level of the tympanic membrane. The sound cannot reach the tympanic membrane resulting in conductive hearing loss. Concomitant ossicular malformation may cause additional conductive hearing loss. Some patients may have SNHL in the affected ear.

Etiology

- Exact etiology of atresia of EAC is not known, association of atresia with low birth weight, intrauterine trauma, toxin or infection have been advocated. Genetic etiologies are being studied for craniofacial anomalies.

Presentation

- Congenital aural atresia (CAA) is usually diagnosed at birth. Some cases, such as child with normal pinna and partially patent are not noticed at birth and are detected during screening being done in nursery school
- Bilateral atresia may affect speech and language development of the children and may need earlier correction. Children with unilateral aural atresia usually have normal speech and language development
- Otitis media (OM) is a common disease in children. Congenital aural atresia complicates the diagnosis of OM. Symptoms of pain, fever, hearing loss or disequilibrium together with HRCT temporal bone may prompt earliest correction of CAA and oral antibiotics may be started on presumption. Cholesteastoma may be present medial to atretic ear canal and may need surgical treatment along with antibiotics
- Along with otologic assessment complete head neck examination is essential to find out any anomalies

- Other anomalies like cardiac, renal or ophthalmologic malformation should be ruled out
- The pinna is assessed for microtia
- EAC—Meatus of EAC if pinpoint hints canal stenosis rather than atresia
- Congenital atresia can be of major or minor forms
    - Major malformations include—absence of EAC, tympanic membrane, a small middle ear cavity and malformations of malleus and incus. Microtia and hypoplastic mandible may be associated
    - Minor malformations comprise of abnormal ossicles with patent EAC and small but intact TM.
- Lateral skull—Relationship of TM joint with mastoid tip and middle ear is to be assessed. Poor development of mastoid tip hints abnormal facial nerve anatomy. Assessment of facial nerve function and hearing is important before surgical repair. The grading of the facial nerve is based on the House and Brackman system
- Clinical photography of anomalies should be taken for reference and the objective analysis of the surgical output
- Children with CAA are associated with other syndromes in 10% of the cases. These are discussed below:

Goldenhar Syndrome

It is a rare congenital defect involving mandibular hypoplasia resulting in facial asymmetry, ear or eye malformation and vertebral anomalies with deafness (Fig. 15). It is also known as hemifacial microsomia, oculo-auriculo-vertebral dysplasia. Facial asymmetry involves one side of the face. It affects other organs, such as heart, kidney, lungs and nervous system. This disorder was first documented by Maurice Goldenhar in 1952. It is sporadic,

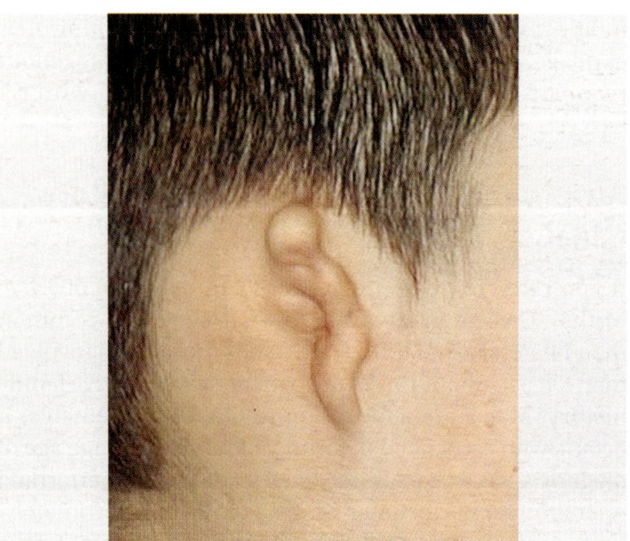

Fig. 14: Atresia of EAC with microtia of right ear

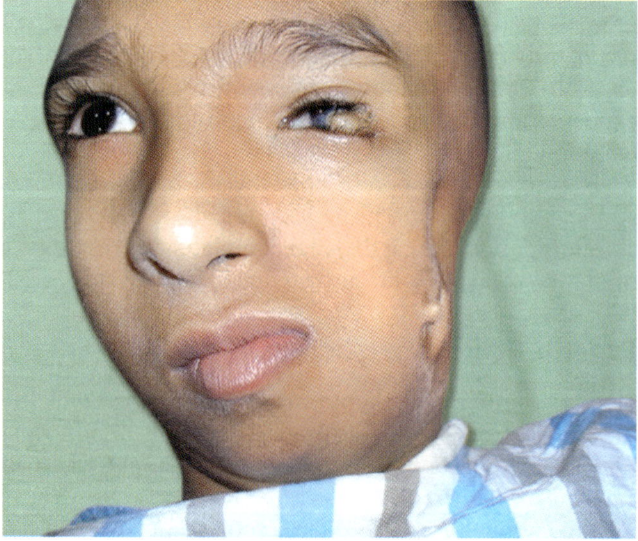

Fig. 15: Goldenhar syndrome

rarely an autosomal dominant pattern. Diagnostic tests include X-rays, MRI, CT scan, ultrasonography and genetic testing of child saliva to identify DNA. Additional test of hearing and cardiac evaluation may be needed.

Treacher Collins Syndrome (TCS)

It is a rare autosomal dominant congenital disorder involving craniofacial deformities characterized by downward slanting eyes, micrognathia, conductive hearing loss, hypoplastic zygoma, drooping of lateral lower eyelids and absent or malformed ear (Fig. 16). The condition was first described by the English surgeon and ophthalmologist Edward Treacher Collins in 1900. $TCOF_1$ gene mutations are the most common cause of the disorder.[9] Mutation of $TCOF_1$ gene reduces the production of rRNA, which triggers apoptosis of certain cells involved in development of facial bone and soft tissue.

Crouzon Syndrome

It is an uncommon genetic disorder involving features of early closure of skin suture (craniosynostosis) and abnormal development of orbit and midface, affecting shape of head, appearance of face and alignment of teeth (Fig. 17). The syndrome was first described by French neurosurgeon Dr Crouzon in 1912. It is caused by mutation in one of the fibroblast growth factor receptor genes—$FGFR_2$ on chromosome 10 and $FGFR_3$ on chromosome 4.

Fifty five percent of patients with Crouzon syndrome have conductive hearing loss and some are born with absence of EAC. Neurological manifestations include hydrocephalus or Chiari malformation. Cleft palate is a rare presentation. Some patients develop skin abnormalities called acanthosis nigricans.

Diagnostic Tests

Diagnostic tests are CT scan head and PNS, X-ray spine and head, genetic testing to confirm the diagnosis.

Children with all these syndromes are not candidates for surgical repair of atresia. Auditory rehabilitation with bone anchored hearing aid (BAHA) should be considered as early aiding is of utmost importance for language development. Compared to surgical reconstruction BAHA provides better outcome and superior audiological results.

Radiology

- HRCT temporal bone (noncontrast) of axial and coronal sections is required
- It helps to determine the relationship of TM joint with mastoid tip and middle ear structures
- Presence of congenital cholesteatoma. Congenital cholesteatoma is rarely seen in children with CAA
- Extent of external ear, middle ear, inner ear and mastoid development and facial nerve localization.

Audiology

- Audiogram shows conductive hearing loss in children at 5 years of age
- Behavioral testing is done when the child is able to sit and turns to stimuli around 6 months of age
- Brain stem evoked response audiometry (BERA) is done if children fail to undergo behavioral testing
- Bone conduction BERA is very useful to identify the sensorineural component in CAA.
- Vestibular evoked myogenic potentials (VEMPs)—A promising vestibular function test in children with bilateral CAA

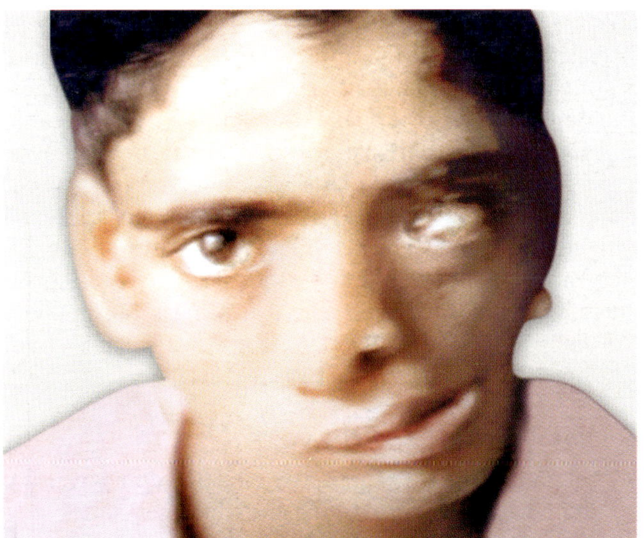

Fig. 16: Treacher Collin syndrome

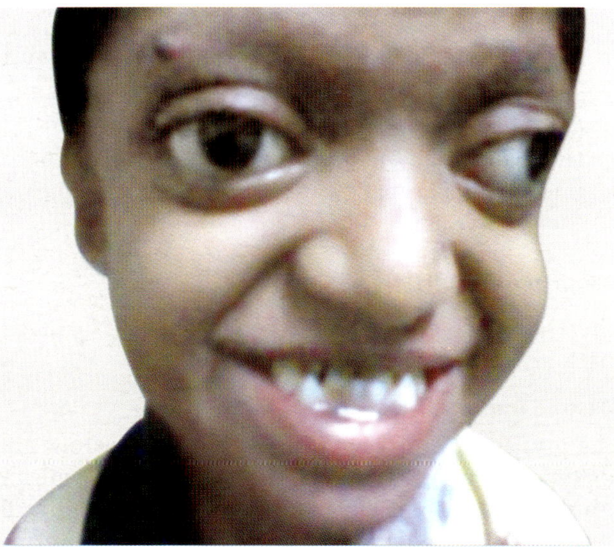

Fig. 17: Crouzon syndrome

- Electroneuronography (ENog)/Electromyography (EMG) is indicated for facial nerve dysfunc before and after surgery.

  Following rules to be remembered before surgical planning for CAA:
- Detailed audiological assessment, radiological evaluation and facial nerve function test should be done
- Early ABR testing and subsequent early placement of hearing aids greatly helps the language development
- HRCT temporal bone should be taken to assess the status of inner ear, temporal bone pneumatization, course of facial nerve, presence of oval window and footplate or any cholesteatoma
- Even with normal inner ear anatomy, SNHL is contraindication of surgery
- Atresia repair follows microtia repair by 2 months to preserve the vascular supply of skin and subcutaneous tissue
- For patient with binaural microtia and CAA surgery is done at 6 years of age
- For patient with unilateral atresia, CAA repair may be delayed or unwise
- Presence of internal auditory meatus and inner ear anatomy is essential for planning of surgery
- Severe hypoplasia of tympanum with little middle ear space is contraindication of surgery. Poorly formed ossicles or absent stapes results in poor outcome of surgery.

Many classification systems have been advocated for the staging of the degree of atresia of EAC. The commonly used classification system is De La Cruz's classification.

Minor
- Mastoid pneumatization normal
- Normal oval window
- Normal inner ear
- Facial nerve and oval window relationship acceptable.

Major
- Mastoid poorly pneumatized
- Oval window absent or abnormal
- Inner ear malformation
- Facial nerve aberration.

Surgical Approaches

There are two approaches for repair of atresia of EAC- mastoid approach and anterior approach.

Mastoid Approach

The procedure starts with the drilling of mastoid and identifying sinodural angle. It leaves a large cavity which is prone to postoperative infection. Again it is often difficult in case of distorted anatomy because of risk of injury of aberrant facial nerve, vestibular system and other structures.

Anterior Approach

This approach is often used. A postauricular incision is made. Soft tissue and periosteum are elevated anteriorly to the glenoid fossa. A tympanic bone remnant is searched for as it points the way of middle ear. If any tympanic bone is present, drilling is made at the cribriform area of the mastoid process. If no tympanic membrane is present drilling is done at the temporal line just posterior to the glenoid fossa. About 1.5 cm in diameter of bone opening is recommended. Drilling is continued to follow the dense atretic bone medially. The most common anomaly of middle ear space is fused incus-malleus complex, whereas stapes remains normal. In extreme malformation, attachment of incus to stapes may be absent. Fixation of stapes footplate is found only in 4% of cases. Conversely in minor ear malformation confined to middle ear only stapes fixation is common. The atretic bone overlying the middle ear is thin and removed carefully, uncovering the ossicles. The ossicular chain is then assessed. The first landmark seen by surgeon is body of the incus which is confirmed by the gentle palpation to note the mild movement of the ossicles. Facial nerve is always medial to the ossicular chain and must be avoided while bone is drilling away in posterior-inferior middle ear space. Facial nerve monitoring is used routinely. Drilling is continued until new canal is about 1 cm of size. Ossiculoplasty is done with either the patient's native ossicles or prosthesis as situation needs. The tympanic membrane is then created by using temporalis facia graft (1.5 cm in diameter) placed directly on the ossicular mass.

A split thickness skin graft measuring 0.006–0.008 inches is harvested. The skin graft is cut to the size of 3–6 cm and notched. The skin graft is used to line the new EAC; notched edges of skin graft are reflected onto the temporalis fascia graft tympanic membrane. Finally, the meatoplasty is done by using 'U-shaped' pedicle flap-hinged at tragus. The pedicle flap is then positioned in the new ear canal and sutured to the periosteum at the level of glenoid fossa. It gives excellent skin coverage of soft tissue of the new ear canal at the anterior part. External ear is then stabilized with subcutaneous sutures. Interrupted sutures with 5-0 vicryl attach the skin graft to the meatus. A merocel is then put into the ear canal. The mastoid dressing is then applied. Normally reduction in diameter of new ear canal is about 30% postoperatively.[10]

Complications of CAA Repair

- Lateralization of TM graft. It can be prevented by using gelfoam pack to support the graft during healing.
- Stenosis of new ear canal can be avoided by regularly cleaning and treating of infection, if any.

- Facial nerve damage can be avoided by drilling of bone away posteriorly and inferiorly and using of facial nerve monitoring
- High-frequency SNHL, it can happen from acoustic drill trauma.

Preauricular Sinus or Pit (Fig. 18)

This was first described by Heusinger in 1864. It is a common congenital developmental defect resulting from incomplete fusion of hillocks of first and second branchial arches during formation of pinna and is characterized by a small opening or dimple located in front of the crus of helix. It is inherited through an autosomal dominant gene with incomplete penetrance and in rare cases associated with bronchio- oto-renal (BOR) syndrome that includes external ear deformity, preauricular sinus and renal disorder.[11]

The sinus is bilateral in 25–50% of cases. The bilateral sinuses are more likely to be hereditary. When unilateral, left side is more affected.

Anatomically, it is lateral and superior to the facial nerve and parotid gland. The sinus tract may vary in length. It may be short or may extent to the cartilage. It may arborize and follows a tortuous course adjacent to the external ear. It may extend in the parotid gland. The sinus tract is lined with squamous epithelium. When it is blocked it results in recurrent infection at the site, ulceration and scarring.

If the sinus is free of infection it may be left alone. Once infected the sinus become infected with recurrent acute exacerbations.

Differential diagnosis—Basal cell carcinoma/epidermal inclusion cysts.

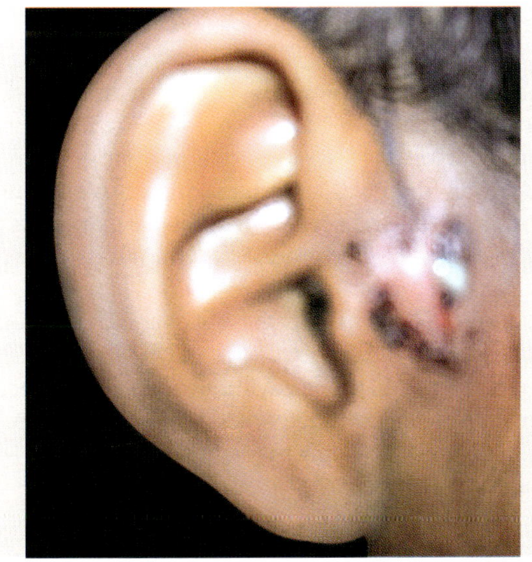

Fig. 18: Infected preauricular sinus

Laboratory Test

- If discharge from sinus is present, swab soaked with discharge is sent for culture and sensitivity study for appropriate antibiotic therapy
- Ultrasonography—USG depicts preauricular sinus and its relation to superficial temporal artery, anterior crus of helix and tragus. When there is high suspicion of Bronchio-oto-renal (BOR) syndrome, USG abdomen helps to rule out kidney anomalies.

Treatment

If sinus is infected, systemic antibiotics are given. If an abscess is formed, it must be incised and drained and pus is sent for Gram stain and culture sensitivity study for covering proper antibiotics. If sinus tract is once infected, recurrent acute exacerbation is the rule; it may need surgical excision of the tract. To prevent recurrence following surgery (about 20% on large study) due to incomplete removal, proper delineation of tract by probing or injection of methylene blue dye into the tract during surgery is essential for successful surgery.

The standard technique for excision of sinus tract is—

- An incision is made around the sinus and then the tract is dissected up to the cyst near the helix
- A portion of the auricular cartilage attached to the tract is also excised
- For treatment of recurring preauricular sinus, supra-auricular approach that extends the incision postauricularly provides best surgical outcome by wide local excision of the sinus[12]
- Use of operating microscope can improve the effectiveness of surgery to remove remnants and can help to prevent recurrence[13]
- Radiofrequency thermal ablation versus cold steel excision for excision of preauricular sinus is reported. It is concluded that radiofrequency associated local wide excision appears to be superior to cold steel excision as former provides better visualization, minimal bleeding and easier dissection.[14]

Factors contributing to recurrence after surgery are as follows:

- Incomplete removal of sinus tract
- Active infection at the time of surgery
- Surgery under local anesthesia
- Failing to remove auricular cartilage at the base of the sinus
- Poor delineation of the entire sinus tract during surgery.

Prognosis

Prognosis is good following excision of entire sinus tract.

Collaural Fistula (Fig. 19)

It is a rare congenital anomaly resulting from developmental defect of the first branchial cleft, characterized by a fistulous tract between external auditory canal and the skin of the neck just below and behind the angle of mandible. Internal opening of the fistula is mainly present in the cartilaginous part of the ear canal and rarely in the bony part. Outer opening of the fistula is in the neck at a point between the angle of the mandible and the sternomastoid muscle. The fistulous tract traverses through the parotid gland and may run medial to, lateral to or through the facial nerve.

Clinical Features

It accounts less than 8% of all anomalies.[15] Initially patient presents with neck swelling which later bursts out resulting in formation of discharging skin sinus. It is associated with ear discharge which is refractory to any medical treatment. Onset of symptoms goes since birth. On examination, skin is excoriated around the sinus opening. The skin opening is pulled in upward direction because of fibrosis resulting from recurrent infection. Ear examination shows opening in the floor of external auditory canal (EAC). Tympanic membrane (TM) looks normal.

Fistulogram shows the entire tract with no branching patterns.
CECT scan of neck shows complete tract starting from skin sinus to bony or cartilaginous EAC and traversing through parotid gland.

Treatment

Surgery is the main treatment modality for this disorder.[16]

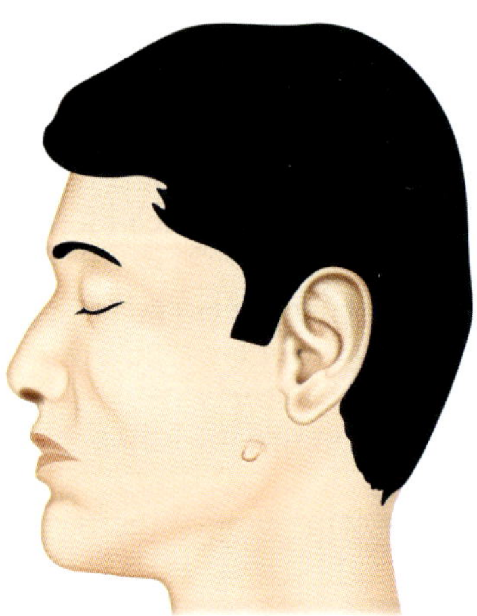

Fig. 19: Collaural fistula

- Preoperative methylene blue dye is injected through the skin opening to delineate the fistulous tract during operation
- Modified parotidectomy incision is made including ear opening at the upper end and neck opening at the lower end
- Superficial parotidectomy is done for better visualization of the tract
- Elliptical incision is made on the skin opening
- The fistulous tract is then traced in upward direction
- A cord like structure is seen on dissection and it is dissected entirely from skin opening up to the opening in EAC. The tract is found in close relation to the facial nerve
- Bony or cartilaginous defect in EAC is repaired with muscle and fat support
- The skin incision is closed following placing a drain.

Essential points to be remembered
- Fistulogram and CECT scan neck are essential to know the entire extent of the tract
- Adhesion of the tract to parotid tissue and its close relation to facial nerve make the dissection difficult
- Inattentive pulling of facial nerve intraoperatively may lead to facial nerve injury. Superficial parotidectomy provides clear exposure of the tract with decreased chances of facial nerve injury
- Patient should be informed regarding the possibility of facial nerve injury.

Congenital swellings of pinna include—
- Dermoid cysts
- Hemangiomas
- Lymphangiomas.

Dermoid Cysts (Fig. 20)

They are rare tumor, often present at birth. They occur anywhere in the body. About 7% of them are found in the head and neck region.[17] They are cystic teratomas composed of fibrous wall lined with stratified squamous epithelium. They consist of skin, hair follicles and sweat glands. As they contain mature tissue and grow slowly, dermoids are usually benign cysts.

The dermoid cysts usually present as smooth, spherical, spongy growth on the medial surface of the pinna, over the upper part of mastoid process without any punctum or scar. They are nontender, nonfluctuant, skin over them is mobile. Differential diagnosis being made include:[18]
- First branchial arch cyst
- Preauricular sinus
- Acquired cyst following ear pricking
- Keloid

- Lipoma
- Sebaceous cyst.

Gardner's syndrome is if cysts are multiple and appear before puberty.[19]

Diagnosis is done by USG, CT Scan and MRI imaging. FNAC shows presence of epithelial remnants, desquamated squamous cells and cellular debris.

Treatment—Surgical excision is the treatment of choice. An elliptical incision is made over the cyst using ellipse with width of 1/3rd to 1/2 circumference of swelling to allow primary closure without much redundant skin.[20] The cyst is found to be attached to the underlying perichondrium.

Prognosis—5% of the cysts may develop malignant transformation.

Hemangioma of Pinna (Fig. 21)

It is a congenital benign vascular tumor arising from arterioles, venules and capillaries. It affects female more than male. It is deep red or deep purple compressible mass which is increased in size when patient strains. It usually occurs in association with hemangiomas involving other parts—parotid gland, face and neck. If the lesion involves both superficial and deep elements it is called mixed hemangioma. Usually, the lesion undergoes involution over time. Persistent lesion may need treatment by cryosurgery or laser excision or if by large ligation or embolization of feeding vessels.

Auricular hemangiomas associated with extensive and multiple skin ulcerations have been documented.[21]

Arteriovenous malformations (AVMs) are rarely involving the pinna but are commonly found intracranially. They are usually present at birth but they manifest later in life necessitating treatment. AVM differs from hemangioma which is a neoplasm involving endothelial proliferation histologically while AVM is the developmental vascular defect producing blood flow malformations.[22]

Patient presents with pain, ulceration, hemorrhage, persistant warm sensation and deformity of pinna. Physical examination reveals a soft ill-defined pulsatile mass with discoloration and sometimes ulceration of overlying skin or mucosa. On auscultation, a continuous bruit synchronous with pulse of patient is heard. EAC and TM look normal. Pure tone audiometry shows normal hearing sensitivity.

- Plain X-ray and CT scan have little role in diagnosis
- Color Doppler ultrasonograpy confirms the diagnosis
- MRI is the investigation of choice to know the extent and multiplanar imagings helps to differentiate between high- and low-flow lesions[23]
- MR angiography shows tortuosity of the feeding vessels having corkscrew appearance.[24]

Treatment

Surgical total resection is the treatment of choice. It requires a wide field resection of all the involved tissue to prevent recurrence. Partial resection that may lead to rapid recurrence needs intravascular embolization of the remaining AVM tissue.[25] Reconstruction using split thickness skin graft and pedicle or free flap is done during same sitting.

Lymphangiomas of Pinna

They are benign lesions arising from malformation of lymphatic system. It may be congenital associated with

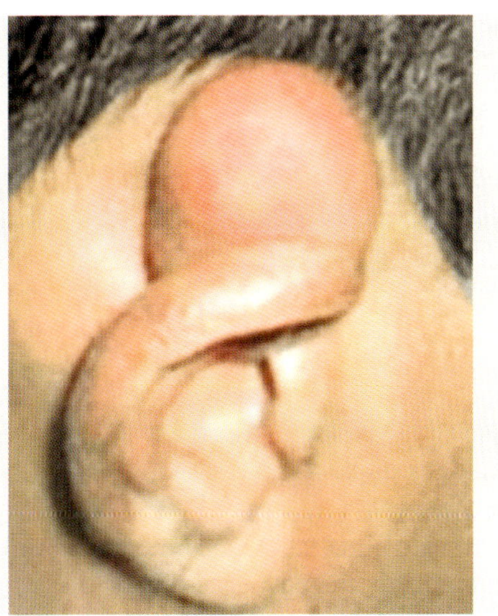

Fig. 20: Dermoid cyst of pinna

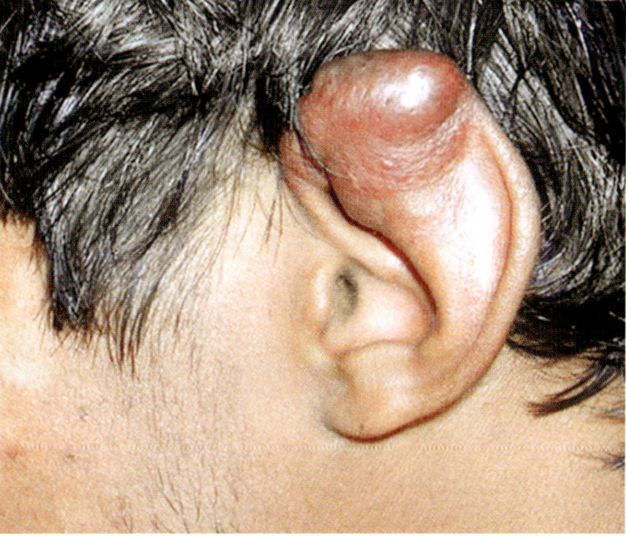

Fig. 21: Hemangioma of auricle

chromosomal abnormalities, such as Turner syndrome or acquired resulting from trauma, infection or obstruction of lymphatic system.

Classification of Lymphangiomas

Based on microscopic features includes:
- Capillary lymphangiomas involving capillary-sized lymphatic vessels located in epidermis
- Cavernous lymphangiomas comprising dilated lymphatic vessels invading surrounding tissues
- Hemangiolymphangioma—Lymphangioma with vascular component and irregular dilated space are seen in dermis (Fig. 22).

Based on size of their cysts—
- Microscopic—Each cyst size measures less than 2cm³ in volume
- Macroscopic—The cyst size more than 2cm³ in volume
- Mixed lymphangiomas containing both microscopic and macroscopic component.

Based on location and extent of lesion[26]—
- Stage I—Unilateral infrahyoid
- Stage II—Unilateral suprahyoid
- Stage III—Unilateral infra- and suprahyoid
- Stage IV—Bilateral suprahyoid
- Stage V—Bilateral suprahyoid and infrahyoid.

90% of the disorder occurs in children below 2 years of age involving head and neck region.

Lymphangioma of pinna is extremely rare. It originates from posterior aspect of pinna extending to anterior parotid region.[27] It is soft cystic slow growing doughy mass.

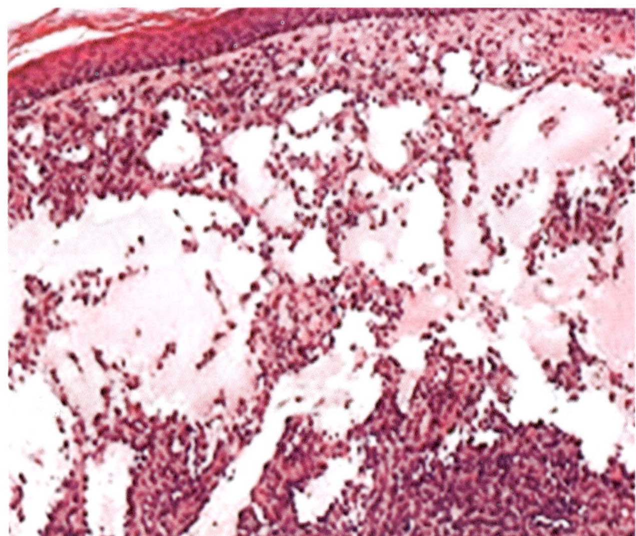

Fig. 22: Microscopic histologic feature of lymphangioma showing irregular dilated space in dermis

Prenatal hemangioma is diagnosed by fetal ultrasonography. Amniocentesis is recommended for diagnosis of associated genetic disorder. Diagnosis of lymphangioma is made commonly by ultrasonography and is confirmed by histologic findings.

Treatment

- Aspiration—It provides temporary relief and helps to confirm diagnosis by cytological study
- Surgical excision provides excellent result, but idea of additional procedure should be kept in mind as it regrows
- Laser excision—Microcystic lymphangioma can be treated with laser but it may cause port wine stain or vascular lesion[28]
- Sclerotherapy—Sclerosing agents, such as 1% or 3% sodium tetradecyl sulfate/doxycycline or ethanol is directly injected in the lesion by interventional radiologist resulting in ablation of endothelial cells of feeding lymphatic channels to lymphocel[29]
- Radiotherapy: It is not effective for treatment of lymphangioma as it is with hemangioma.[30]

Prognosis

It is reported that lymphangioma is rarely transferred into lymphosarcoma, if the preexisting lesion is exposed to radiotherapy.

Inflammatory Conditions of External Ear

Inflammatory conditions affecting external ear are divided into infective and noninfective groups based on etiological factors.

Infective Group Includes

- Bacterial, viral, fungal, and other rare organisms, such as rickettsia or parasites.

Noninfective Group

- Noninfective group may be immune-mediated inflammation or radiation exposure or environmental insult.

Inflammatory Conditions of Pinna

Erysipelas of Pinna (Fig. 23)

It is superficial infection of skin involving lymphatic system, usually caused by group A *streptococcus* secondary to abrasion or laceration. It is also known as St Anthony's fire (1095) named after the Egyptian saint of middle age who is said to have been able to cure it.[31]

It may affect infant children and adult. Pinna is bright red, hot and tender. It is diffusely oedematous because of lymphatic vessel involvement. Unlike localized infection, systemic symptoms of fever and chill (flu like symptoms) are common. Infection may spread to face and adjacent periorbital region. Streptococci produce toxins, such as streptokinase and DNAase B which results in marked reaction visible in skin. In 80% of the cases erysiplelas affect the leg. Erysiplelas is contagious disease. It is purely diagnosed on clinical basis and treated with antibiotics. Penicillin is the first line of therapy administered orally or parentally for 10 days. If patient is allergic to penicillin first generation cephalosporin or macrolide, such as erythromycin or azithromycin may be considered. In severe infection of infant, elderly and immune-compromised patients, hospitalization for close monitoring and intravenous antibiotics is recommended. Topical use of aluminium acetate solution 8% as mild astringent helps the skin to dry up. Uncomplicated erysipelas has excellent prognosis and complete recovery.

Cellulitis of Pinna (Fig. 24)

It is the bacterial infection involving skin and subcutaneous tissue of pinna, usually caused by gram positive cocci, sometimes *Pseudomonas aeruginosa* or other organisms.

The affected ear is warm, red, swollen and tender; suppuration may intervene. Regional neck node may be palpable. Fever or malaise is uncommon. Cellulitis is usually localized to ear following trauma, laceration, burns or insect bite. The condition usually affects patients having diabetes, immune deficiency or vascular disease or history of previous cellulitis.

Community acquired methicillin resistant *Staphylococcus aureus* (CA-MRSA) may cause life threatening infection with rapidly developing necrosis and hemorrhage because of panton–valentine leucocidin (PVL) toxin. PVL is produced from genetic material of bacteriophage that infects *Staphylococcus aureus* making it more virulent.[32]

Treatment Includes

High dose of oral antibiotics effective against gram positive, such as amoxicillin and clavulanic acid, amoxicillin and sulbactum, clindamycin or ciprofloxacin.

In severe infection, intravenous antibiotics are administered.

Perichondritis of Pinna (Fig. 25)

It is the infection or inflammation involving perichondrium of external ear—Pinna and EAC. It is commonly described as continuation of diseased conditions of external ear ranging from erysipelas (infection of overlying skin), cellulitis (infection of soft tissue) and true perichondritis (infection of perichondrium) to chondritis (infection of cartilage).[33]

Etiology: It results from infection secondary to laceration, hematoma, surgery to external ear, high piercing of ear lobe to insert ear rings. It may also be due to spread of infection from diffuse otitis externa or a furuncle of the meatus.

Microorganisms most commonly isolated are *Pseudomonas aeruginosa* (75-90%) and S*taphylococcus aureus* (50%).[34] Other organisms include Proteus, *Escherichia coli* and streptococci.

Clinical features: The pinna is red, warm, painful and stiff. The ear lobule, devoid of cartilage is spared. Pain

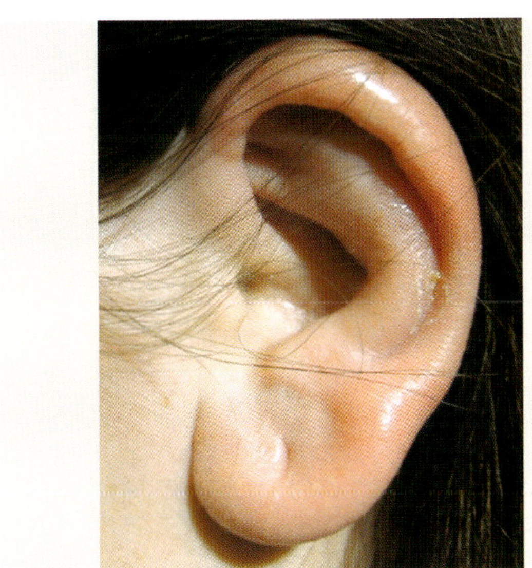

Fig. 23: Erysipelas of pinna

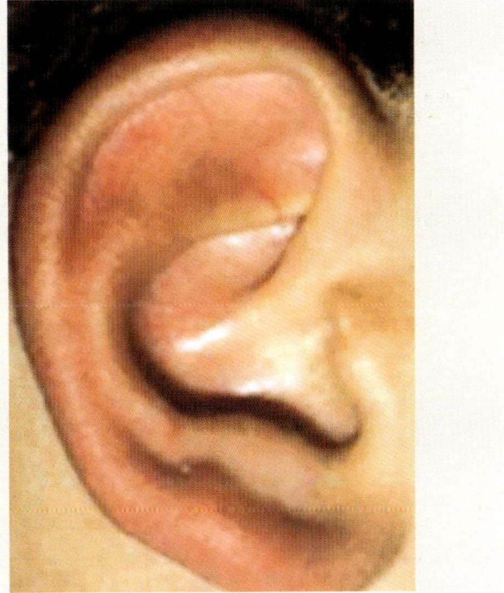

Fig. 24: Cellulitis of pinna

and tenderness are more in perichondritis compared to erysipelas or cellulitis of pinna. The condition is differentiated from relapsing polychondritis which is associated with systemic illness and is an autoimmune disease. Perichondritis if left untreated causes necrosis of cartilage and results in deformity of pinna (cauliflower ear).

Treatment: In mild form, perichondritis is managed by high dose of oral antibiotics to cover both gram-positive and gram-negative organisms. Subperichondrial abscess needs incision and drainage. Pus is sent for gram stain and culture/sensitivity study for administering appropriate antibiotics.

In resistant and relapsing cases necrosed cartilage and devitalized skin and soft tissue should be resected. Intravenous antibiotics should be started. Continuous drainage and irrigation of subperichondrial abscess with antibiotic and steroid solution by placing fenestrated polythene tube twice daily provides good result and minimum deformity.[35]

In highly resistant cases, low dose radiotherapy 3 to 4 sittings of 0.8 Gy over a period of 2 days is used to kill the microorganism.[36]

Relapsing Polychondritis (Fig. 26)

It is an autoimmune rare disease presented as episodic inflammation and degeneration involving multiple cartilaginous tissue of the body, usually of pinna as well as connective tissue at various sites. Nasal, laryngeal, tracheal and costal cartilages are less frequently involved. When repiratory tract, heart valve or blood vessels are affected it becomes life-threatening. It was first described by Jacksh-Wartenhorst (1923) as polychondropathies.[37] The term relapsing polychondritis was coined by Pearson et al (1960).[38]

The disease manifests commonly in 45–55 years of age, however, children and young adults are also affected. Only one pinna is involved. The pinna is red, hot, swollen and tender. It is described as hot red ears. The lobule is spared. EAC becomes stenotic. Recurrent attacks lead to auricular deformity resulting in floppy or cauliflower ear. Saddle nose deformity is due to degeneration of septal cartilage.

Histopathology

It shows initial neutrophilic infiltration with loss of normal basophilia of cartilage and subsequent infiltration of histiocytes, plasma cells and lymphocytes resulting in atrophic cartilage with cystic space filled with gelatinous material.

Similar inflammatory and degenerative changes are also seen in other tissues rich in proteoglycan, such as eyes and cardiovascular system.

Etiology

It is an autoimmune response to type II collagen as evidence by immune fluorescent deposits of immunoglobulins and serum antibodies to type II collagen in acute phase.[39]

Diagnosis

No specific test is available for relapsing polychondritis. Patient with acute phase have high-level of inflammatory markers, such as ESR or CRP. Biopsy of cartilage of pinna shows inflammation, distraction and atrophic changes with

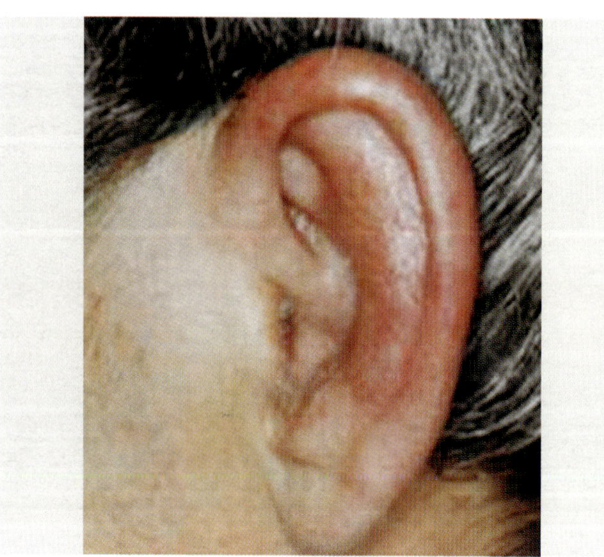

Fig. 25: Perichondritis of pinna

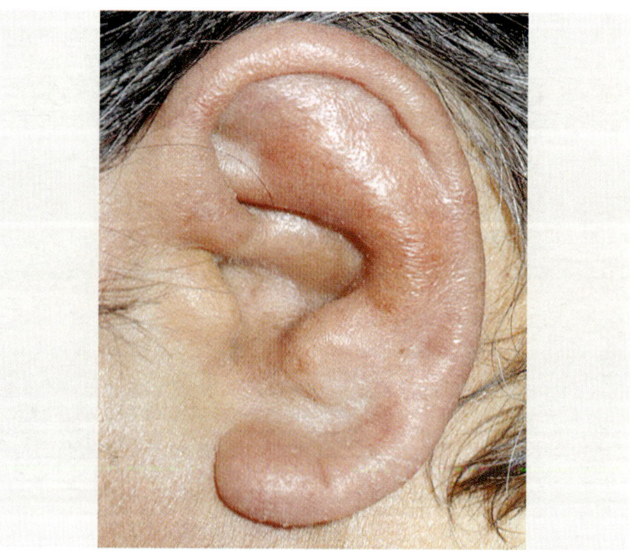

Fig. 26: Relapsing polychondritis

cystic spaces filled with gelatinous material. McAdam's criteria for diagnostic sign together with biopsy findings help to establish the final diagnosis.

Six signs as per McAdam's criteria[40] are as follows:

- Recurrent chondritis of both pinnae, deformed pinnae after acute inflammation
- Nonerosive inflammation of multiple joints
- Inflammation and deformity of septal cartilage resulting in saddle nose deformity
- Inflammation of eye including conjunctivitis, keratitis, scleritis and episclerites or uveitis
- Inflammation and deformity of cartilage including laryngeal/or tracheal cartilage resulting in hoarseness and airway compromise
- Recurrent inflammation and damage to the cartilage of inner ear resulting in SNHL, tinnitus/or vertigo.

If three or more of the above signs are present together with the support of histology, the diagnosis is confirmed.

Differential diagnosis includes systemic granulomatosis diseases, such as—

- Wegner's granulomatosis
- T-cell lymphoma
- Tuberculosis and sarcoidosis.

Treatment

Treatment of relapsing polychondritis involves suppression of immune system with systemic steroids. High dose of prednisolone orally or medroxy prednisolone intravenously is required for acute episodes. Steroid-induced osteoporosis can be prevented by supplementation of calcium, vitamin D and bisphosphonate. Immunosuppressant, such as azathioprine or methotrexate is often administered to reduce steroid dose. Use of dapsone has been reported.

NSAIDS and colchicine are effective in mild episodes. Use of anti-CD$_4$ monoclonal antibody and minocycline has been studied.[41]

Surgical management includes tracheostomy or stent insertion in case of airway compromise.

Inflammatory Conditions of External Auditory Canal

Infective group

Bacterial

- Furunculosis (localized acute otitis external)
- Diffuse otitis externa
- Malignant otitis extrnal.

Fungal

- Otomycosis.

Viral

- Ramsay Hunt syndrome.

Noninfective or reactive group

- Eczematous otitis externa
- Seborrhoeic otitis externa
- Neuro dermatitis.

Furunculosis of EAC (Fig. 27)

It is a localized acute infection of hair follicle present in cartilaginous part of the ear canal. The infection is usually caused by *Staphylococcus aureus* with swelling of the canal. Furuncle is usually single but it may be multiple. Source of infection is usually the patient's nasal vestibule harboring staphylococci from where they are transferred by patient's finger.

Patient may present with excruciating pain and tenderness with positive tragal sign. Tympanic membrane looks normal. A furuncle of posterior canal wall may cause edema of mastoid with obliteration of postauricular sulcus. Periauricular lymph nodes may also be enlarged and tender.

Treatment includes systemic antibiotics, analgesics and anti-inflammatory drugs. Ear pack of 10% ichthammol with glycerin provides splintage action and relives pain. Ichthammol has an antiseptic function and glycerin having hygroscopic action reduces edema. In case of recurrent infection, diabetes should be ruled out.

Diffuse Otitis Externa

It is diffuse acute bacterial infection of the ear canal, usually caused by *Pseudomonas aeruginosa*. It is also known as swimmer's ear as history of prolonged water exposure is present. History or trauma to ear canal by hair pins or paper

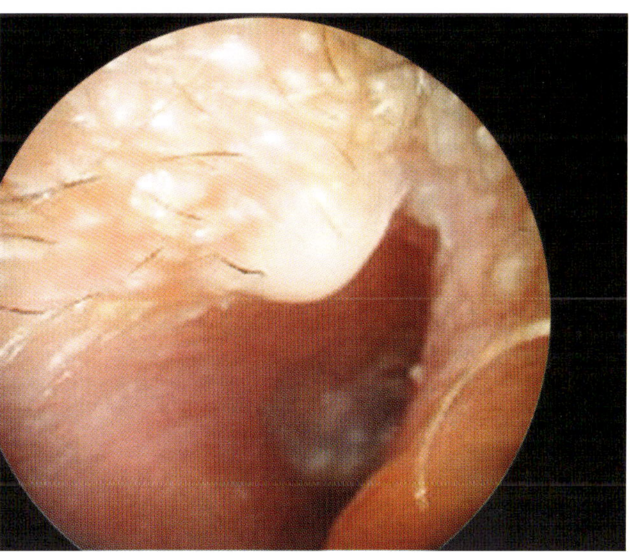

Fig. 27: Furunculosis of EAC

clips is also another initiative factor. A cardinal sign is the pain elicited by pulling the pinna upward and backward. On examination of skin EAC is red and edematous. Canal is narrowed obliterating the lumen with sticky yellow colored exudates. The infection is confined to EAC. Regional lymphadenopathy may be present.

Prolonged water exposure may change the bacterial flora of EAC from gram positive to gram negative bacteria, such as pseudomonas and enterobacter.[42]

Treatment for diffuse otitis externa in acute phase is mainly topical. All debris and exudates are removed, especially from anteroinferior meatal recess where discharge is accumulated by suction clearance or irrigating the canal with sterile normal saline. After thorough ear toilet a gauze wick smeared with antibiotic—steroid medication is inserted in the ear canal with alligator forceps and kept in place for 3 days. It is kept in moist with instilling 3 or 4 times of ear drops. A wick saturated with aluminium acetate solution (8%) can be used as astringent to dry up the canal. Ear should be kept away from water exposure for at least 3 weeks. A mixture of vinegar and honey as ear drop is effective in ear ache as it is acidic and hyperosmotic helping in killing bacteria and reducing edema. Most commonly used oral antipseudomonal antibiotic is ciprofloxacin. In severe cases, systemic antibiotics are used.

Prevention—The recurrent infection can be prevented by advising swimmers to use swim plugs and to instill boric acid drops into ear canal after swimming.[43]

Malignant Otitis Externa (MOE) (Fig. 28)

It is an invasive and life-threatening infection of external ear which may lead to osteomyelitis of temporal bone

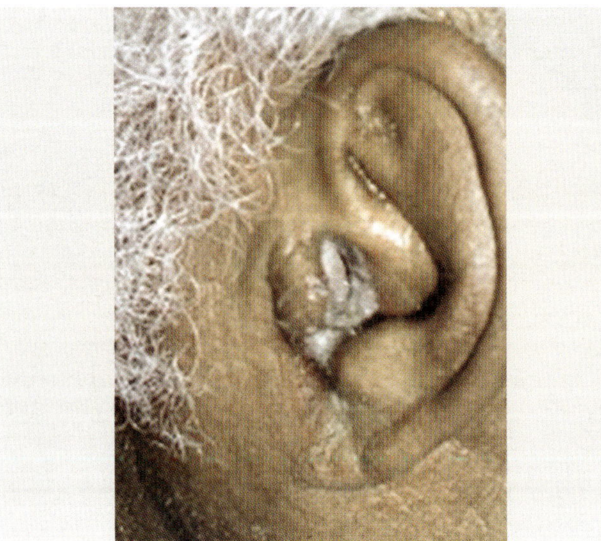

Fig. 28: Malignant otitis externa

and multiple cranial nerve palsies usually caused by pseudomonas infection in diabetic or immuno compromise patients. MOE was first reported by the physician, Tolmouche in 1838.[44] Chandlear coined the term malignant otitis externa in 1968.[45] He described it as malignant because of its aggressive clinical behavior, poor treatment outcome and high mortality rate. The term malignant otitis externa is misnomer as it is not a neoplastic disease. It is also known as skull base osteomyelitis and necrotizing external otitis.

Clinicoradiological Staging System of MOE

Stage 1   Clinical evidence of malignant Otitis Externa with infection of soft tissue beyond EAC but negative TC-99 bone scan

Stage 2   Soft tissue infection beyond EAC with positive TC-99 bone scan

Stage 3a   Soft tissue infection beyond EAC with positive TC-99 bone scan together with single cranial nerve paralysis

Stage 3b   Soft tissue infection beyond EAC with positive TC-99 bone scan together with multiple cranial nerve paralysis

Stage 4   Meningitis, empyema, sinus thrombosis or brain abscess

Pathophysiology

Malignant otitis externa (MOE) is an infection that starts from EAC and extends to the surrounding structure. It subsequently involves the periosteum and bone of the skull base resulting in cellulitis, chondritis, periosteitis, osteitis and osteomyelitis. Later on facial nerve and other cranial nerves are affected. Spread of infection outside of EAC occurs through fissures of Santorini and osseo-cartilaginous junction. Involvements of Haversian system of compact bone and pneumatized part of temporal bone are late findings. Multiple microabscesses that are formed are found during surgery. In most of the cases, *Pseudomonas aeroginosa* is the positive organism (95% of cases). Rarely aspergillus may cause MOE.

Predisposing Factors

MOE is more common in males than in females. It commonly affects elderly diabetic (90%) both type I and type II and immunocompromised patients. Predisposing factors that impair host defence to pseudomonas include:
- Microangiopathy associated with diabetic
- Vasculitic properties of pseudomonas
- High pH of cerumen in diabetic patients that reduces bactericidal properties
- Decreased cell-mediated immunity associated with AIDS. In AIDS, patients are generally younger,

granulation tissue in EAC is absent, positive organism is other than pseudomonas and poorer outcome than diabetic.

Clinical Presentation

Patient presents with history of diabetes (90%) or immune suppression and develops—
- Severe deep-seated otalgia and temporal headache
- Purulent ear discharge
- Dysphagia hoarseness and/or facial paralysis.

On Examination

Marked tenderness is present between tip of mastoid and angle of mandible. Granulation tissue is present on the floor of EAC just lateral to the osseo cartilaginous junction. This is the pathognomic of MOE. Otoscopy reveals exposed bone, tympanic membrane looks intact. Fever usually is absent. Deterioration of mental status hints intracranial complications.

Spread of the Disease and Complications

Presence of cranial nerve palsy indicates advanced disease with increase mortality rate (up to 80%). Facial nerve is affected most commonly (60% of cases with palsies), usually at stylomastoid foramen. Recovery of facial nerve paralysis is poor and unpredictable. Infection spreads to skull base and jugular foramen resulting in paralysis of cranial nerves IX, X, and XI followed by paralysis of cranial nerve XII at hypoglossal canal. Cranial nerve V and VI may be affected if infections spread to the petrous apex. Anterior spread of infection involves temporomandibular fossa, Posterior spread to mastoid and medial spread to middle ear and petrous bone. Disease may spread to the central venous sinuses, extradural space and meninges. Infective thrombophlebitis or thrombosis of internal carotid artery is the final outcome.[47]

Diagnosis and investigation of MOE: Diagnostic criteria for MOE are based on clinical features of pain, granulation, otorrhea and resistance to local therapy for 10 days in a diabetic or immunocompromised patient supported by positive bone scan and presence of *Pseudomonas aeroginosa* on culture together with cranial nerve paralysis.
- Culture sensitivity from EAC—It detects positive organism and should performed before antimicrobial therapy is started
- Biopsy is obtained from EAC to rule out carcinoma or other diseases. Otic capsule is resistant to disease process
- Nonspecific measures of inflammation include ESR and CRP, these are elevated in untreated patient; these parameters are helpful to measure the response of treatment. Leucocyte count is usually normal or mildly elevated
- High-resolution computed tomography (HRCT) looking at bone window can reveal bone erosion which becomes evident until 7 days or more after the onset of disease
- Technetium (TC-99) radio nucleide bone scan may show hotspot (positive) within 1–2 days after the onset of bone erosion. Isotope is absorbed by osteoclasts and osteoblasts and scan remains positive for up to 9 months. It is useful for detecting bone erosion at an earliest time
- Gallium (Ga-67)—The isotope is absorbed by leucocyte and is sensitive monitor of infection. This scanning can be used to ascertain the resolution of infection, watching for fading of residual hotspot
- MRI is useful to ascertain the extent of soft tissue inflammation beneath the skull base and helps to differentiate between malignant process and inflammation.

Treatment of MOE

Treatment includes aural toilet, topical and systemic antibiotic therapy, Control of diabetes, hyperbaric oxygen therapy and surgery.

Aural toilet—is essential to control granulation and to relieve local pain. Topical preparations include acetic acid solution and gentamicin drop are used. Use of topical antibiotics is controversial as it may alter the micro biological flora of EAC and misguide culture sensitivity report.

Systemic antibiotics—antipseudomonal antibiotic fluroquinolones that attain high-level in serum and soft tissue with oral doses are effective alone. Subsequently, oral ciprofloxacin monotherapy has been recommended at least for 6 weeks.

Till now, no established antibiotic treatment guideline is available.

Parental antibiotics—ciprofloxacin with or without aminoglicoside and first or third generation cephalosporin (ceftazidime) given initially, with transition to oral antibiotics once the CRP and ESR stars to fall are advocated by many experts.[48]

Monotherapy with ceftazidime—Ciprofloxacin resistant to P. aeroginosa appears to be increasing; mono therapy with ceftazidime may be used. Tobramycin is also effective with minimal toxicity. Gallium citrate (Ga-67) scanning is helpful in determining duration of treatment. Treatment should be ended one week after Ga-67 scan finding returns to normal.

Implantable gentamicin beads are recently applied with success when oral therapy is contraindicated. It may cause sensorineural hearing loss.[49]

Hyperbaric oxygen therapy is used as an adjunct to antibiotics and is indicated in patient with poor response to therapy or recurrence cases.

Surgery—Chandler reported surgery when appropriate antibiotics were not available with 50% mortality rate.

Surgery is indicated if patients are deteriorating clinically even with medical treatment. Surgery includes—

- Removal of sequestra
- Drainage of pus
- Debridement of necrotized tissue and granulation
- Mastoidectomy with facial nerve decompression and partial temporal bone resection

Control of diabetes—Cure of MOE needs meticulous control of diabetes. Patient may require shifting from oral hypoglycemics to insulin. Insulin must be continued for at least 6 weeks alone with antibiotic

Otomycosis

Otomycosis or fungal infection of ear is an inflammation of primarily outer ear and EAC caused by fungi, such as *Aspergillus fumigatus*, *Aspergillus niger*, *Candida albicans* and *Candida tropicalis* (Fig. 29). Other rare fungi are Rhizopus, Phycomycetes, Actinomyces and Penicillium. It comprises 20% of all cases of otitis externa.

Factors precipitating otomycosis are as follows:

- Moisture in EAC due to swimming, sweating and high humidity
- High environmental temperature
- Use of topical antibiotics or steroids in otitis externa or middle ear suppuration
- Diabetes or immunocompromised patients.

It is a superficial mycotic infection characterized by superficial epithelial exfoliation, mass of fungal debris containing hyphae, suppuration and earache with intense itching.

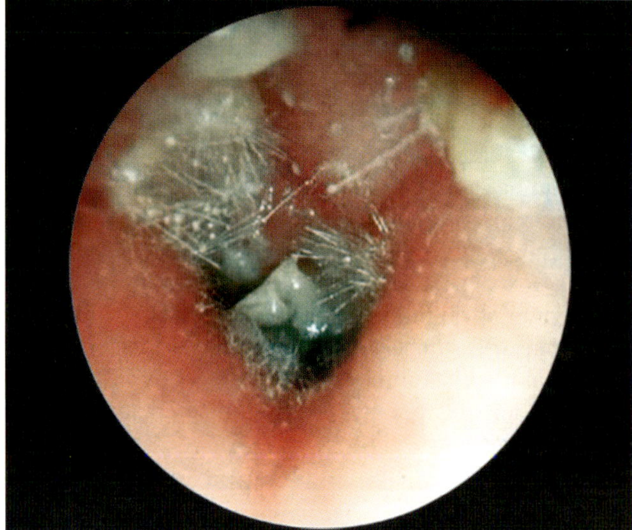

Fig. 29: Otomycosis

Clinical Features

Clinical features of otomycosis include watery discharge, blockage of ear, pain, itching and hearing loss. Hearing loss is due to accumulation of fungal debris. Otoscopy shows white, gray or black debris like a piece of wet blotting paper.

Clinical features of infection by Aspergillus species differs from that of Candida species. The organisms are airborne in spore form and belong usually to moist surface.

Aspergillosis is characterized by mild inflammation of the deeper ear canal filled with sheets of keratin. Under microscope, hyphae and candidiospores (fruiting head) of mature fungus can be made out. *Aspergillus niger* appears as black head filamentous growth; *Aspergillus fumigatus* look as green- or blue-colored mycelia.

Candidiasis is characterized by marked oedema and epithelial exfoliation of deeper ear canal, lumen is filled with curd like material. Candida is dimorphic fungus existing as budding yeast or pseudo-hyphaenated form. Diagnosis is confirmed by fungal smear showing fungal elements on KOH preparation and positive fungal culture.

Chronic or recurrent otomycosis hints to investigate underlying causes such as diabetes or immunocompromised diseases.

Treatment

Treatment of otomycosis includes aural toilet, debridement of EAC and instillation of topical antifungal drops. Deep canal may be smeared with antifungal cream. For candidiasis, tolnaftate is useful and it may be used as cream, powder or drop. 2% salicylic acid is also used as keratolytic agent. Other antifungal agents are cotrimazole, nystatin and ketoconazole. Itraconazole is used as long-term systemic oral therapy and effective for aspergillosis.[51] Application of 1% gentian violet to the affected ear is effective before starting long-term systemic therapy. Treatment of mycotic infection elsewhere in the body including athlete's foot needs attention in case of resistant otomycosis. Immunotherapy with dermatophyte (trichophyton, epidermophyton and oidiomycetes) extract is effective to treat dermatophytid reaction resulting from mycotic infection in a remote location.

Otomycosis may be associated with bacterial infection with intense itching; antibiotics and steroid preparation along with oral antihistamines are helpful.

Herpes Zoster Oticus

It is characterized by intense ear pain and erythematous vesicular rash on external auditory canal and pinna caused by Herpes zoster virus (VZV) with lower motor neuron type of ipsilateral facial palsy. This is commonly known as

Ramsay Hunt syndrome when the VIIIth nerve is involved to a varying degree resulting in hearing loss, tinnitus and/or vertigo.[52] It may also involve Vth nerve resulting in anesthesia of ipsilateral face. This was first described by John Ramsay Hunt (1907).[53] It is discussed in Chapter 9 Facial Nerve and Its Disorders.

Eczematous Otitis Externa

It is a chronic relapsing, inflammatory condition involving pinna or EAC characterized by itchy red rash followed by vesiculation, oozing, crusting and scaling. It results from hypersensitivity to environmental irritants and allergens. Triggering factors are:
- *Staphylococcus aureus* infection of skin
- Topical ear drops
- Extreme temperature and humidity
- Dietary factors (food allergy) and its association with gut dysmotility
- Stress and hormonal change in women.
  Atopic eczema affects 15–20% of school children and 2–10% of adults.[54]

Diagnostic Criteria

- History of intense itching that may cause scratching. It results in lichenification, thickening or pigmentary changes of the skin
- History of asthma or hay fever
- Estimation of Immunoglobulin E (IgE) and specific radioallergosorbent test (RASTs) may confirm the atopic nature of the individual.

Treatment

- Emolients are used 3–4 times daily to ensure rehydration of the skin
- Tropical corticosteroids are recommended once or twice daily. Mild to moderate preparations of corticosteroids are used according to the severity of atopic eczema. High-potent preparations should not be used in children.[55]
  Complications include impetigo, herpes simplex infection and superficial mycotic infection.

Seborrheic Otitis Externa (Fig. 30)

Seborrheic dermatitis of ear is a chronic inflammatory skin disorder characterized by fine scaling and erythema associated with oily skin. It involves EAC, lobule and postauricular area. It is associated with scalp lesions. In infants seborrheic dermatitis presents as thick glossy scales occurring in scalp. In adolescents and adults, it presents as mild greasy scales occurring in postauricular skin, nasolabial folds and scalp. It is evident that the susceptibility of this disease is more in patients with Human immunodeficiency disease (HIV). Incidence is higher among males than females. Etiology is still unknown. Risk factors include mycotic infection, maternal androgen level during puberty, trace oily skin, inflammatory response involving elevated CD16+ and NK1 cell count, depressed T-cell function and activation of complement system. The disease is associated with Parkinson's disease, Alzheimer's disease, Schizophrenia and mood disorders.

Treatment

Seborrhea cannot be cured but it can be controlled by good hygiene. Topical steroids are used. Oil-based preparations of corticosteroids are avoided. Coal tar, salicylic acid and selenium sulfide are effective.

Neurodermatitis

It is also known as lichen simplex chronicus which is an itchy skin disease similar to atopic dermatitis. The disease is characterized by localized, symmetrical patches of itchy dermatitis with lichenification. The condition improves when the scratch-itch cycle is stopped. Exact cause is not known. It is associated with other skin disorders, such as dry skin, eczema or psoriasis. The stress and anxiety trigger the itching. Chronic itching and scratching may result an

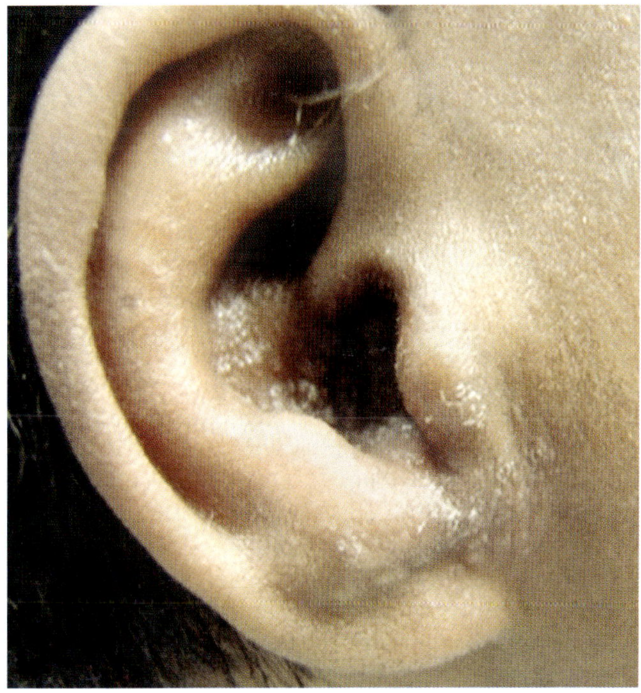

Fig. 30: Seborrheic otitis externa

affected skin to become thick and leathery. Treatment includes sympathetic psychotherapy. Antibiotics are given for any secondary infection, if present. Ear pack and mastoid bandage are helpful to prevent scratching. Topical corticosteroids and antihistamines are given to relieve itching. Anxietolytic drugs help to prevent itching associated with the disorder. Complications are persistant scratching that may result in bacterial infection of skin, permanent scars and sleep disturbance.

Traumatic Conditions of External Ear

Hematoma of Pinna (Hematoma auris)

It is caused by blunt trauma to the pinna during wrestling, boxing or rugby. When trauma occurs the blood accumulates between the perichondrium and cartilage. Perichondrium supplies nutrition to the auricular cartilage. Collection of blood following trauma results in mechanical barrier formation between perichondrium and cartilage, thereby jeopardizing nutrition of the cartilage. This results in necrosis of underlying cartilage followed by fibrosis and neocartilage formation.[56] It results in typical deformity of the pinna called cauliflower ear or wrestler's ear. If hematoma gets infected, perichondritis may develop.

Treatment Includes

- Needle aspiration of the hematoma under strict aseptic conditions from the most fluctuant or full area using 18 or 20 gauge needle. Local anesthesia is given with 1% lidocaine. This procedure has not been accepted by many surgeons because of chances of reaccumulation of hematoma.[57] If reaccumulation occurs, primary needle aspiration followed by incision and drainage, is recommended
- Incision and drainage—A small incision is given along the natural skin folds using a no. 15 scalpel. Skin and perichondrium are separated from the hematoma and cartilage. Hematoma is completely expressed or suctioned out. Care is taken to avoid damage to perichondrium. Normal saline irrigation of the portion with 18 gauge catheter is done. A drain is left at the incision site; it should be kept for 24 hours if no significant bleeding occurs. Reapproximation of the perichondrium to the cartilage is done
- Compression dressing—It is applied noninvasively by simple compression dressing or silicon splint to the medial and lateral surfaces of the pinna. Invasive surgical dressing with cotton bolsters or buttons using through-and-through sutures to the medial and lateral aspects of the pinna is done in some cases.

All patients should receive antibiotics that cover common skin flora for 7–10 days. Nonsteroidal antiinflammatory drugs (NSAIDs) or aspirin should be avoided for 10 days.

Hematoma less than 7 days old should not be left undrained. After 7–10 days aspiration is ineffective. Removal of organizing hematoma and new cartilage and perichondrium is necessary.

Complications are reaccumulation of hematoma, infection, chondritis and cauliflower ear.

Frost Bite of Pinna

It is a localized damage to the skin and soft tissues caused by freezing. It happens in the body parts furthest from the heart and usually involves extremities and face.

When the body is exposed to cold for long periods of time, blood vessels close to the skin undergo vasoconstriction which results in cold-mediated dehydration, endothelial injury, thrombosis and ischemia of auricular tissues. At the initial stage, the process is reversible but over time it leads to tissue necrosis.

There are four degrees of frost bite:
- First degree—only affects the surface of skin but deep tissues are not affected, this is called frost nip
- Second degree—skin may freeze and become harder; deep tissues are not affected
- Third degree—muscles, tendons, blood vessels and nerves are affected resulting in deep frost bite
- Fourth degree—this extreme degree of frost bite results in areas of purplish blisters turning to black areas due to gangrene. If it remains untreated, it may fall off.

Exposure to liquid nitrogen or other such cryogenic substances may cause frost bite.

Initially ear looks pale and cyanotic. Subsequently, as the ear thaws, pain, erythema and subcutaneous bullae secondary to extravasated extracellular fluid or blood may develop.[58] Risk factors for frost bite are diabetes, peripheral neuropathy and drugs, such as beta-blockers.

Treatment for Frost Bite Includes
- Rapid rewarming of the ear to 40°–42°C
- Debridement and/or amputation of the necrotic tissue is done. This should be delayed until demarcation of gangrene is complete. 'Frozen in January, amputate in July' with an exception in gas gangrene or signs of infection[59]
- Hyperbaric oxygen therapy as an adjunctive therapy can help in tissue salvage
- Analgesics for pain as rapid rewarming of frost bitten ear may cause pain
- Systemic antibiotics and vasodilators (plus doxycycline) for deep frost bite
- Antioxidants and thromboxane inhibitors in the form of Brufen are added

- An ointment of 10% aloe vera and Vitamin E are applied topically.

Pseudocyst of Pinna

It is an uncommon condition that results from a defect in auricular embryogenesis causing formation of residual tissue planes in auricular cartilage and these tissue planes may reopen due to repeated minor trauma or mechanical stress forming pseudocyst. It is also known as endochondral cyst, intracartilaginous cyst and idiopathic cystic chondromalacia. This condition was first described by Engel in 1966.

Presentation

Patient presents with painless cystic swelling in the anterior surface of pinna in scaphoid or triangular fossa seen predominantly in adult males before 20 and after 60 years of age. Right ear is affected more than the left ear. This is due to unusual sleeping habit on right side. Chinese population is involved more as they are using firm pillows while sleeping.

Etiology

- Etiology is unknown. Engel postulated that lysosomal enzymes released from chondrocytes cause damage to the auricular cartilage. But analysis of pseudocyst contents indicates lack of lysosomal enzymes with increase in the level of interleukins (IL-6) which stimulate chondrocyte proliferation. IL-1, a mediator of inflammation and cartilage damage induces IL-6 stimulating chondrocytes to synthesize protease and prostaglandin E2 and inhibits extracellular matrix formation
- Studies have shown that testosterone increases production of interleukin by monocytes which accounts for male predominance
- Traumatic etiology explains that repeated minor trauma results in elevated serum lactic dehydrogenase (LDH) and coenzymes LDH-4 and LDH-5 in pseudocyst fluid. These enzymes are released from degenerated auricular cartilage
- Autoimmunity—Antinuclear antibodies have been detected in the fluid of pseudocyst indicating autoimmunity.

Histopathology

Histopathological examination (HPE) in early stage shows intercartilaginous cavity without epithelial lining. In late stage, there is evidence of intercartilaginous fibrosis and granulation tissue formation with perivascular infiltration of lymphocytes.

Differential Diagnosis

Relapsing polychondritis, chondrodermitis nodular helicis, cauliflower ear, subperichondral hematoma.

Above conditions occur in subperichondral plane whereas pseudocyst pinna develops in intercartilaginous plane.

Imaging Study

MRI showing serous fluid collection within the auricular cartilage helps to establish the diagnosis.

Treatment

Aim of treatment of pseudocyst pinna is the restoration of anatomical architecture and prevention of recurrence. Treatment options include—

- Medical treatment with high dose of oral corticosteroids and intralesional corticosteroids has been advocated. Intralesional steroid injection may cause permanent deformity of the pinna for which this treatment option has not been widely accepted[60]
- Wide bore needle aspiration and pressure bandage along with systemic antibiotics. The success rate is about 60% with minimal complications[61]
- Incision and drainage—A helical incision is made and skin flap is elevated. Anterior wall of the cyst is excised along with the margin. Sterile buttons are sutured on anterior and posterior surfaces of pinna producing compression known as button surgery and kept for 7 days along with oral antibiotics and anti-inflammatory drugs (Fig. 31).

Complications

Complications involve perichondritis following excision with resultant cauliflower ear especially in patients with diabetes mellitus. Compression technique may cause necrosis that needs proper pressure application.

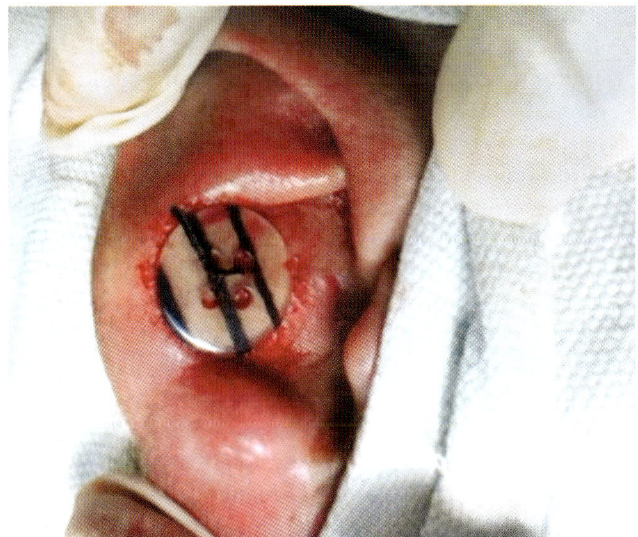

Fig. 31: Pseudocyst of pinna

Tumors of External Auditory Canal

Benign tumors are

- **Osteoma**—It is a benign slow growing bone tumor arising from cancellous bone at the tympanosquamous suture or tympanomastoid suture line. Patient may present with conductive hearing loss, otorrhea, otalgia, otitis externa and canal cholesteatoma if the lesion is obliterating the lumen or asymptomatic when the lesion is small and found incidentally during examination of the ear. On examination, the swelling is found to arise from posterior wall of the external auditory canal near its outer end as a single discrete pedunculated mass which is bony, nontender and fixed to the underlying bone. CT scan reveals a well-demarcated hyperdense attenuating outgrowth arising from the posterior wall of EAC obliterating the lumen.

  Histopathology—Osteoma is characterized by a dense squamous epithelium with an underlying periosteum, great abundance of fibrovascular channels surrounded by lamellated bone of increased density that is oriented in different directions.

  Treatment—Small lesions require frequent cleaning of the debris from EAC. Large lesion causing obstruction and hearing loss require surgical excision under general anesthesia

- **Exostosis**—Exostoses of EAC is characterized by benign growths of bone originating from periosteum presenting as multiple, bilateral often with anterior and posterior smooth sessile swelling in the deeper part of the meatus near tympanic membrane. These are accepted as a reactive condition secondary to repeated cold water exposure or recurrent otitis externa. A prevalence rate of 73.5% of exostoses is reported in surfing population;[62] hence ear with exostoses is called surfer's ear (Fig. 32).

  Exostoses and osteomas are separate clinical entities. Osteoma is generally a unilateral solitary discrete pedunculated bony growth arising from outer part of EAC.

  Exostoses are asymptomatic, if these are small and are incidental finding. When exostoses are large resulting in stenosis of greater than 80% of EAC common symptoms are conductive hearing loss that are fluctuant in early stage. Water and debris retained medial to it can cause otitis externa, otorrhea, otalgia and canal cholesteatoma that may extend medially in the middle ear, superiorly through tegmen into middle cranial fossa or posteriorly in the mastoid air cells. CT scan shows a broad-based lesion with no deep extension. It also helps to demonstrate extent of canal cholesteatoma, if present.

  Histopathology—Exostoses are covered by squamous epithelium with underlying periosteum. Internal structure is characterized by parallel concentric dense layers of subperiosteal bone abundant in osteocytes and lack of fibrovascular channels and their contents, so characteristic of osteoma.[63]

  Treatment—When patient is asymptomatic care includes—

  - Avoidance of cold water
  - Recommendation to use ear plugs for water sports
  - Aural toilet using suction clearance under microscope if collection of debris or otitis externa exists. Topical use of steroids, antibiotic and antifungal combination of ear drops is needed
  - Large lesion causing obstruction and hearing loss requires surgical excision. Surgery is done via postaural approach with careful elevation and preservation of skin overlying the exostosis. Care is also taken to avoid the injury of tympanic membrane and facial nerve. Bone of exostosis is removed by high-speed drill using both cutting and diamond burr. Outside lesion is removed first as its removal is less likely to injure facial nerve and thus enables the surgeon for better visualization of posterior region of EAC. Permeatal approach results in high incidence of complications and recurrence of the lesions. Complications include canal stenosis, tympanic membrane perforation, facial nerve palsy, sensorineural hearing loss and exposure of temporomandibular joint with chronic pain and joint subluxation.

- **Ceruminous gland tumors of EAC**—These are the tumors that arise from cerumen secreting modified apocrine glands in cartilaginous portion of EAC. Benign tumors that arise from ceruminous glands are:
  - Ceruminous adenoma
  - Ceruminous pleomorphic adenoma
  - Syringo cystadenoma papilliferum.

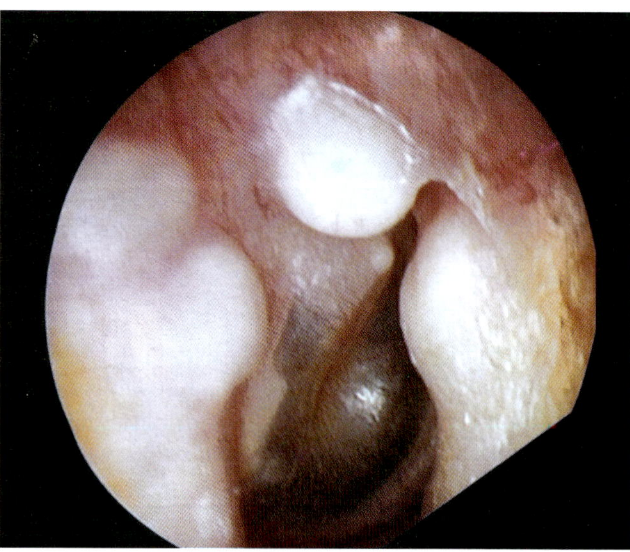

Fig. 32: Exostosis of EAC

Malignant tumors include ceruminous adenocarcinoma, adenoid cystic carcinoma and mucoepidermoid carcinoma. Histogenesis for most of these tumors is ceruminous gland or its embryonic anlage.

Ectopic salivary gland tissue is another possible origin for malignant tumors.[64] Primary adenocarcinoma, adenoid cystic carcinoma and mucoepidermoid carcinoma are rare and they may in fact arise from salivary tissue in adjacent parotid gland. Each has its unique histological pattern and clinical behavior with invasion or metastatic tendency.

Ceruminous gland tumors are rare neoplasms. It comprises 5% of neoplasms of EAC. Ceruminous pleomorphic adenomas are less common than ceruminous adenomas. Exact cause of these tumors is unknown. Otitis media is a risk factor for developing these tumors.

Mean age of these tumors is the 6th decade. Sex distribution is nearly equal for ceruminous adenoma whereas male predominance is seen for ceruminous pleomorphic adenoma. Syringocystadenoma papilliferum is an uncommon benign tumor usually found on scalp or face but rarely found in EAC and found in both men and women. Patients present with symptoms of unilateral hearing loss, pain, otorrhea and paralysis.

Histopathology of ceruminous adenoma is composed of two types of cells—first type consists of luminally placed cuboidal to low columnar epithelium with eosinophilic cytoplasm and apical caps (decapitation secretion). Second type comprises epithelial cells surrounded by a layer of myoepithelial cells with less apparent cytoplasm and a smaller hyperchromatic nucleus. Immunohistochemistry differentiates these two cell types.

Ceruminous pleomorphic adenomas are complex structures comprising chondroid to myxoid stromal components mixed with epithelial and myoepithelial components.

Syringocystadenoma papilliferum has a bilayered epithelial lining composed of inner cells with prominent eosinophilic cytoplasm and apical caps (decapitation secretion) and outer cells with less apparent myoepithelial cells.

Treatment—Extent of lesion is defined by CT scan or MRI of EAC.

Complete surgical excision is considered. Recurrences are due to incomplete removal. Pleomorphic adenoma is well known for recurrence. If histopathological examination shows malignancy, postoperative radiotherapy is given.

Malignant Tumors

Malignant tumors include basal cell carcinoma of pinna (BCC) and Ehrlich's ascites carcinoma (EAC).

Basal Cell Carcinoma of Pinna and EAC (BCC)

Basal cell carcinoma is the most common malignant neoplasm that rarely metastasizes, but invades the surrounding tissue and is considered malignant. It is known as rodent ulcer and arises from pleuripotent cells within the epidermis or hair follicles. Most of the lesion involves the head and neck region and it represents 45% of auricular malignancy (Fig. 33).

Risk factors for BCC include

Genetic Factors

Fair-skinned individuals with family history of BCC are more susceptible to skin damage to develop BCC. 3 out of 10 caucasians may develop a BCC in their life.[65] Syndromes, such as Xeroderma pigmentosum (autosomal recessive inheritance), Gorlin's syndrome (autosomal dominant inheritance) and Epidermodysplasia verruciformis have features of multiple BCC. In Xeroderma, pigmentosum resistance to ultraviolet ray-induced skin damage is lost. In Gorlin's syndrome, the disease is located at the tumor suppressor gene on long arm of chromosome 9.[66] Epidermodysplasia verruciformis is a disorder related to inability to resist human papilloma virus to develop BCC

Environmental Causes

- Sun exposure—BCC occurs commonly in sun-exposed areas of the body. UV radiation induces skin damage and initiates the pathogenesis of skin cancer. UVB is a major carcinogen affecting skin cells. UVC although a potent carcinogen, is filtered by ozone and have least effect on skin

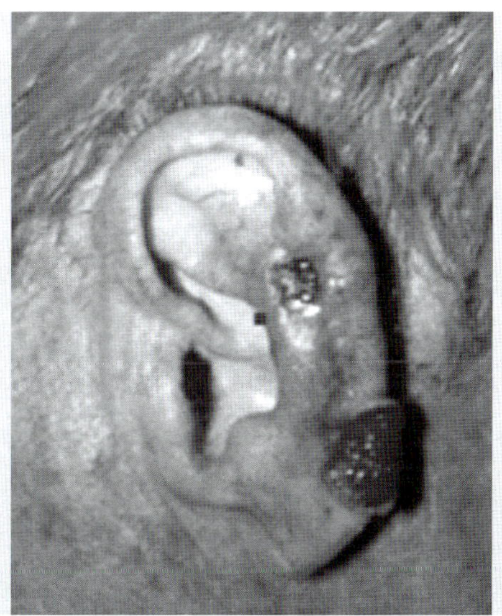

Fig. 33: Basal cell carcinoma of pinna

- Radiation factor—People working in radiology departments, mining, airlines and patients treated with radiotherapy are at higher risk of developing BCC. Radiation induced carcinogenesis depends on the total accumulation dose of radiation rather than the duration of exposure
- Chemical exposure—Chemicals, such as polycyclic aromatic hydrocarbons, psoralens and arsenic compounds are carcinogens and potentiates UV carcinogenesis induced by UV rays
- Immunosuppression—It predisposes to 30% of skin cancers which are highly aggressive.

Premalignant lesion—Sebaceous naevus of Jadassohn is a premalignant lesion presenting at birth as yellowish plaque. It may undergo malignant change in 10% cases.

Subtypes of BCC

Nodular

It is the most common and least aggressive subtype commonly arising in head and neck region. It is slow growing and appears as fleshy or pearly nodule.

Ulcerative

It presents with a central ulceration and pearly border.

Superficial

This lesion usually develops on the trunk as multiple erythematous scaly patches limited within the epidermis without any invasion in dermis. It may mimic the dermal lesions, such as eczema and psoriasis.

Pigmented

This lesion is similar to the gross appearance of nodular type but with brown pigmentation as it contains melanin and simulates melanoma.

Morpheaform

It usually develops on the face as yellowish indurated plaque with irregular border.

Basaloid

It is highly invasive keratinized lesion comprising 1% of BCC.

Clinical Examination

Patients may present with skin lesion of nodules, ulceration, pigmentation and/or bleeding. Auricular BCC predominantly develops on the posterior surface of pinna and preauricular region.

Diagnosis is confirmed by histopathological examination. CT scan and MRI may help to know the extent of the lesion to adjacent temporal bone and soft tissues of head and neck region. Metastasis may occur in less than 0.1% cases. Both lymphatic and blood borne metastasis have been reported.[67]

Differential diagnosis includes benign naevi, melanomas, cutaneous squamous cell carcinoma, eczema and psoriasis.

Treatment

Surgical excision with cancer free margin is the treatment of choice for BCC. Radiotherapy is indicated for unresectable lesions or surgically unfit patients. Chemotherapy, such as 5-Fluorouracil is not recommended for BCC, except for premalignant lesions like actinic keratosis. Intralesional injections of interferons into BCC are tried but its efficacy of cure is still not satisfactory with respect to others. Other treatment methods include:

Surgical Measure

Local excision provides excellent cure rate.
- If tumor is less than 2 cm, surgical excision with 4 mm margin gives about 95% cure rate
- If tumor is more than 2 cm with aggressive histological subtype, such as morpheaform BCC, wide excision with a staged reconstruction of the resultant defect is perforated.

Moh's Micrographic Surgery (MMS)

In 1932, Moh developed the procedure which involves surgical excision of lesion using repeated tissue sampling along lateral and deep margin to assess intraoperative histopathology under frozen section control for tumor evidence. Excision of free margin with 1.3–1.5 cm provides more than 95% cure rate. It is indicated in recurrent BCC larger than 2 cm or aggressive histopathology.

Electrodissection and Curettage (EDC)

This technique is used to excise the lesion and to dessicate the base done in some well-circumscribed superficial BCC resulting in about 97% cure rate.[68] Histopathological confirmation is not possible using this technique.

Cryosurgery

This is indicated in small (<1 cm) superficial lesions with less aggressive histopathology resulting in 97% cure rate. No histopathological confirmation is obtained.

CO_2 Laserization

CO_2 laser is used in patients with superficial BCC confined to epidermis. Hypopigmentation and scarring may result following use of CO_2 laser. Histopathological confirmation is difficult to obtain using this technique.

Conclusion

BCC can be prevented by minimizing sun exposure from 10 AM to 3 PM by wearing protective clothes and using UVB

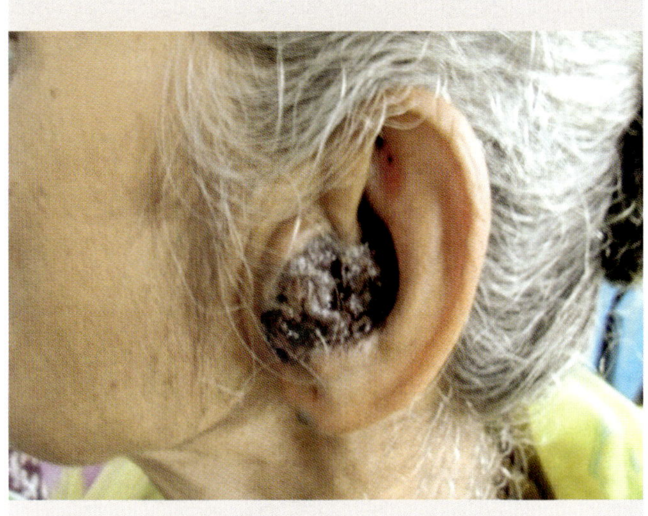

Fig. 34: Squamous cell carcinoma of pinna and EAC

protective sunscreens. Recurrence can be minimized by wide excision and frozen section control (MMS).

Squamous Cell Carcinoma (SCC) (Fig. 34)

Squamous cell carcinoma is a common form of cutaneous malignancy arising from basal layer of epidermis of skin. It accounts for 20% of skin cancer and has poorer prognosis than basal cell carcinoma. It invades the local tissue and metastasizes via lymphatics. Squamous cell carcinoma of EAC is about four times more common than basal cell carcinoma. The ratio is reversed in auricle. Auricular squamous cell carcinoma results from prolonged exposure of ultraviolet (UV) radiation usually from sunlight or UV lamps.

Risk Factors for SCC

Genetic factors: Syndromes, such as albinism (autosomal recessive inheritance), epidermolysis bullosa (variable genetic penetrance characterized by recurrent skin lesion) and porokeratosis (autosomal dominant inheritance characterized by abnormal keratinization) are susceptible to SCC.

Environmental factors: Environmental causes, such as sun exposure, radiation factors, chemicals and immune suppression are responsible for carcinogenesis as stated in BCC.

Premalignant lesion—Actinic keratosis which is the damage of skin caused by sunlight is a premalignant lesion resulting in SCC in 12% cases.

Subtypes of SCC based on microscopic appearance are as follows[69]

- Adenoid squamous cell carcinoma is characterized by a tubular microscopic pattern and keratinocyte acantholysis

- Basaloid squamous cell carcinoma is characterized by a predilection for tongue base
- Clear cell squamous cell carcinoma is characterized by keratinocytes appearing clear due to hydropic swelling
- Signet ring cell squamous cell carcinoma is characterized by concentric rings composed of keratin and large vacuoles
- Spindle cell squamous cell carcinoma is characterized by spindle-shaped atypical cells.

Clinical features—SCC of skin presents with variable appearances, such as small nodules, ulcerated lesion with raised edges or reddish skin plaques.

They are friable and have tendency to bleed. Tumors grow slowly and have substantial risk of metastasis. Auricular tumor occurs on helix or preauricular region but the lesion may usually present on sun-exposed areas. Clinically, positive lymph node is not uncommon and if present, indicates transformation of localised disease into regional or distant metastatic disease. During earliest stage, the lesion is said to be Bowen's disease. CT scan or MRI helps to detect adjacent temporal bone lesion or soft tissue invasion. Biopsy from lesion confirms the diagnosis.

Immunohistochemistry and specific dermal antibodies are helpful in differentiating poorly differentiated SCC from melanoma.

Staging—TNM staging system is used for squamous cell carcinoma of EAC (discussed in Chapter 16).

Differential diagnosis includes—
- Basal cell carcinoma
- Actinic keratosis
- Keratoacanthoma—It is a low-grade skin tumor which is unlikely to invade or metastasize and is considered as a variant of well-differentiated squamous cell carcinoma, commonly found on sun-exposed areas of the skin
- Melanomas and sarcomas.

Treatment—Surgical techniques include:
- For well-differentiated SCC less than 2 cm, local excision with surgical margin of 4 mm provides cure rate of 955
- For lesion more than 2 cm, excision with surgical margin of 10 mm is recommended
- For aggressive histopathology or irregular and indistinct borders involving eye lids, ears and lips and lesion more than 2 cm, Moh's micrographic surgery (MMS) is useful
- Electrodessication and curettage—It is used for well-differentiated small and superficial lesion. Histopathological study is difficult in this technique.

Nonsurgical options are as follows:
- Radiotherapy given as external beam radiotherapy or brachytherapy is indicated for unresectable lesions with cure rate of 90% or elderly patients surgically unfit with cure rate of 90% or an adjuvant therapy for metastatic or high risk cutaneous SCC. Systemic chemotherapy

is used for patients with metastatic lesion along with radiotherapy

- Topical chemotherapy, such as imiquimod cream and photodynamic therapy (PDT) are generally used in premalignant lesions or in-situ carcinoma lesions.

Prevention: Use of UVB-protective sunscreens and avoiding sun exposure between 10 AM and 3 PM help to reduce the risk of skin cancer.

Prognostic factors:[70] If the lesion is more than 2 cm local recurrence rate is 15.2% and metastasis rate is 30.3%. If lesion is more than 4 mm in depth local recurrence rate is 17.2% and metastasis is 45.7% Prognosis of the disease depends on histological subtype, size and local invasion of lesion.

For well-differentiated SCC, 5-year disease free survival rate is 75%–92%.

Melanoma of the External Ear (Fig. 35)

Melanoma originates from the Greek word 'melas' meaning 'dark' and is a cancer of melanocytes. Melanocytes produce dark pigment melanin and are predominantly present in skin but are also seen in other parts of the body, such as eye and GI tract. Melanoma of ear accounts for 1% of all cases of melanoma and 14.5% of all head and neck melanomas. It is less common than BCC or SCC but more aggressive if it is not detected in early stage. It is responsible for 75% of deaths related to skin malignancy.[71]

Types of Melanoma

- Lentigo malignant melanoma—It is characterized by hypopigmented macules occurring in sun exposed areas with better prognosis
- Nodular melanoma—The lesion invades dermis with risk of metastasis, predominantly seen on the trunk and less often in the head and neck region
- Superficial spreading melanoma—It is the most commom type (about 45%) and commonly localized to the anterior helix (about 49%).[72] The lesion is irregular and hypopigmented. It may have central nodularity, ulceration and bleeding indicating dermal invasion. There are two phases of growth, radial growth phase confined to epidermis (tumor thickness less than 1 mm) and vertical growth phase resulting in dermal invasion with risk of metastasis (tumor thickness more than 1 mm)
- Mucosal melanoma—Arising from mucosal surface of head and neck are rare lesions and are far more aggressive than cutaneous melanomas with poorer outcome.

Risk Factors for Melanomas

- Genetic factor
  - White individuals are mainly affected. Different genes have been identified as increasing risk for

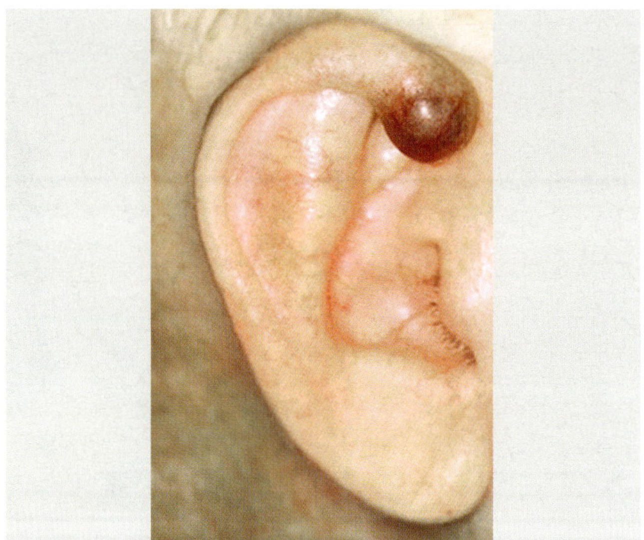

Fig. 35: Melanoma of pinna

developing melanoma. Loci for familial melanoma have been identified on the chromosome arms 1p, 9p and 12q
  - Atypical mole syndrome—An autosomal dominant disorder characterized by multiple naevi into one or more having dysplastic changes and 10% having chances of melanoma
  - Giant hairy naevus—Single naevus more than 20 cm has 18% chance of developing melanoma.
- Environmental causes—Sunlight exposure may induce melanoma by direct DNA damage.

  Dysplastic naevus is a premalignant lesion. It has 40% chance of transforming into melanomas.

Clinical Features

When an existing mole changes its shape, size or color, it hints towards early signs of developing melanoma. Subsequently, the mole may itch, ulcerate or bleed. A new swelling anywhere on the skin in case of nodular melanoma needs attention. Neck examination to note any enlarged lymph nodes, if any, indicates regional spread of disease. Paraneoplastic syndromes, such as loss of appetite, nausea, vomiting and fatigue are present in metastatic melanoma. Metastasis to brain, bones, liver and distant lymph nodes are common.

Prognostic Factors

Poorer outcomes are associated with—
- Male gender
- Head and neck primaries
- Thicker Breslow's depth (usually depth of lesion is less than 1 mm)
- Level of invasion (Clerk's level is usually 2)—Inverse relation to survival
- Increasing age and ulceration of primary lesion.[73]

Diagnosis

- Clinical diagnosis is still the mainstay of establishing the disease (mole changes in shape, size, color, itching or bleeding)
- Histopathology of skin biopsy and lymph node biopsy confirms the clinical diagnosis
- Liver function test helps to know the liver metastasis
- CXR is taken to rule out the lung metastasis
- CT, MRI and PET and/or PET/CT scanning are important to detect metastatic disease
- Radionucleide bone scan is used to know bony metastasis
- Diagnosis is further supported by presence of S-100 protein and HMB-45 markers that are specific for the evidence of melanogenesis.

Staging

As per American Joint Committee on Cancer (AJCC) the disease is broadly divided into four stages—

- Thin melanoma (<1 mm) with or without ulceration- 89-95% survival
- Thicker melanoma (1–4 mm) with or without ulceration- 45-79% survival
- Any thickness with regional nodal disease—24–70% survival
- Distant metastasis—7–19% survival

Treatment

- Surgery—Wide local excision (WLE) with 1–2 cm margins depleting on histological type and depth of tumor is the standard care for the disease
  - For tumor <1 mm thick, surgical excision with 10 mm margin is safe and effective[74]
  - For tumor 1–4 mm thickness, surgical excision of 2 cm margin is recommended[75]
  - For tumor thicker than 4 mm, no universally accepted excision or re-excision of margin is recommended despite their recurrence rate being high
  - For management of regional lymphatics and lymph nodes, a radical neck dissection and parotidectomy are the procedures to be done
  - Technique of sentinel lymph node biopsy (SLNB) is widely used procedure in the management of N_0 neck for tumor less than 1 mm thickness.
- Radiotherapy has little role in the treatment of melanoma. Various chemotherapy agents, such as dacarbazine and immunotherapy with interleukin-2 (IL-2) or interferon (IFN) are used in metastatic melanoma; these are still under evaluation.
- B-Raf gene—About 60% of melanoma contains mutation in B-raf gene. B-Raf inhibitor Dabraferib may lead to tumor suppression in the majority of patients[76]
- Other therapies, such as gene therapy using TILs (Tumor infiltration lymphocytes) and TCRs (T-cell receptors) or virotherapy where oncogenic viruses used to treat the diseases are under trial.

Miscellaneous

Keratosis Obturans

It is a condition characterized by accumulation of desquamated keratin debris in the external ear canal. It usually affects the young adults with a greater predilection for males.[77]

Etiology

Though the exact etiology for keratosis obturans is not known, yet it is postulated that the condition results from the abnormal migration of epithelial cells lining the skin of external auditory canal.[78] Risk factors for keratosis obturans include sinusitis and bronchiectasis.[79]

Pathology

Plugs of keratin and shedded epithelia get deposited in the lumen of EAC causing widening of its lumen. The keratin debris is deposited in lamina, thus appearing like onion peels. The deposited keratin plug may progress medially to involve the tympanic membrane as well.[77]

There are two types of keratosis obturans based on the etiology:[78]

- Inflammatory type—This type of keratosis obturans is caused by viral infection of the external ear canal. It is extremely benign and can be cured by simple removal of the keratotic plugs
- Silent type—This type is not associated with any preceding infection of the ear canal. It is believed to be caused by abnormal separation of keratin material from the epithelial cells of EAC.

Clinical Features

The usual clinical manifestations include severe otalgia, otorrhea, conductive hearing loss and widened EAC. However, some atypical cases of keratosis obturans may present with metallic taste. On examination, these patients are found to possess a widened hypotympanum with facial nerve and tympanic annulus exposed.[80]

CT scan of temporal bone shows an eroded external ear canal.[81]

Complications

These include sensorineural hearing loss, semicircular canal fistula, dehiscence of tegmen tympani and facial nerve palsy.[82]

Differential Diagnosis

External auditory canal cholesteatoma (EACC), squamous cell carcinoma of EAC.

Previously, EACC was considered to be a type of keratosis obturans.

But this theory has been discarded owing to the considerable differences in the pathology and clinical features of these two conditions. In keratosis obturans, the epithelial migration occurs circumferentially. Otalgia rather than otorrhea is the chief complaint of patients with this disease. It is mostly bilateral and leaves the canal skin intact.[83]

EACC, on the other hand, is characterized by formation of keratin pearls deposited on the floor of EAC. The condition presents unilaterally and causes ulceration of the canal skin and focal bony lesions. Since the keratin pearls do not block the external ear canal significantly, hearing is not compromised within these patients.

Otorrhea along with chronic dull earache are the chief complaints in this condition.[83]

Treatment

- Surgical removal of the keratotic mass is the treatment of choice
- Canal plasty may be helpful in cases of recurrent cholesteatoma
- Mastoidectomy is advised in case of EACC.

Cerumen Impaction

Cerumen or ear wax is a mixture of shedded epithelia, keratin debris and secretions from sebaceous and modified apocrine sweat glands located in the outer third of the cartilaginous part of external ear canal. The glandular secretions are rich in lipid materials like squalene, cholesterol esters, triacylglycerols, fatty acids, cholesterol and ceramides.[84] Ear wax lubricates the ear canal and provides antibacterial action. It gets removed from the ear canal time to time by jaw movements as in chewing.

Two types of cerumen are present, dry and wet type. This is determined by a specific genetic alteration, called single nucleotide polymorphism (SNP) in the ATP-binding cassette C11 gene. Individuals with dry type of ear wax possess two adenine bases while those having wet type ear wax require at least one guanine base in the gene. People with wet type cerumen produce sweat in profuse amounts and have armpit odor.[85]

Clinical Presentations

Patients with impacted cerumen present with
- Foreign body sensation in the ear
- Difficulty in hearing
- Otalgia
- Tinnitus
- Itching.

Supervening infection of impacted cerumen may result in otorrhea.

Prolonged impaction may also lead to ulceration of the canal skin and hence, severe earache.

Treatment

Conditions warranting removal of cerumen are:[86]
- Request of the patient
- Otitis externa
- Prior to fitting hearing aids
- Suspected external ear canal pathology
- During grommet insertion for management of Otitis media with effusion (OME).

Treatment options include—
- Manual removal—This technique is carried out with the help of a Jobson-Horne ear probe. Simultaneous use of an otoscope or a binocular microscope enhances visualization of and minimizes trauma to ear canal
- Irrigation—Irrigation of ear canal may be done alone or in combination with a ceruminolytic agent. Most commonly distilled water at room temperature is used for this purpose to avoid a caloric-reflex response. The nozzle of the aural syringe should be inserted gently inside the external ear canal and the water is pushed slowly in lateral to medial direction along the antero-superior wall of the EAC. Possible complication includes perforation of tympanic membrane
- Before performing irrigation, a complete history must be taken from the patient as to the presence of any middle ear disease, vertigo or radiation exposure of the ear. Presence of such condition is a contraindication to aural irrigation[87]
- Microsuction—Operating microscope and suction device capable of creating a pressure of 300 mm Hg are needed for microsuction[86]
- Application of ceruminolytics—Water-based, oil-based and nonwater/nonoil-based chemicals are commercially available as ceruminolytics. Water-based ceruminolytics include tri-ethanolamine polypeptide oleate condensate, 10% sodium bicarbonate and 2.5% acetic acid. They increase the miscibility of the cerumen and thus help in its removal from the ear. Oil-based ceruminolytics are arachis oil, olive oil, almond oil which lubricate the EAC. Choline salicylate and glycerol are examples of nonwater/nonoil-based preparations. Ceruminolytics should be avoided in cases of tympanic membrane perforation.[86]

Myringitis Bullosa

Myringitis bullosa or myringitis bullosa hemorrhagica is a clinical condition characterized by eruption of vesicles on the outer layer of tympanic membrane. The vesicles are present between the epithelial layer and the lamina propria of the tympanic membrane.

The exact etiology of this condition is not known, though Influenza virus or *Mycoplasma pneumoniae* has been suggested as the etiological agent. It predominantly occurs among children, adolescents and young adults. The condition is usually unilateral, but in 5% cases it occurs bilaterally. The patient presents with throbbing earache, blood-stained discharge and impairment of hearing associated with upper respiratory tract infections. On examination, bullae are found on intact tympanic membrane with serosanguinous secretion in the EAC.

Hearing impairment in myringitis may be conductive, mixed or pure sensorineural type as evident in audiometry. Impedance audiometry may hint towards presence of fluid in the middle ear. Assessment of facial nerve function is important to rule out herpes zoster infection. Examination under microscope is essential for establishing diagnosis. Fluid of bullae should be sent for PCR study in some patients with SNHL to exclude herpes zoster oticus or Ramsay Hunt syndrome.

Treatment: For uncomplicated cases without middle ear effusion and SN hearing loss, analgesics are given. In younger children, the condition should be treated as acute otitis media and antibiotics should be prescribed. Spontaneous resolution of the hemorrhagic blisters on TM may happen in most cases and complete recovery from sensorineural hearing loss, if any, occurs within 3 months.

REFERENCES

1. Donaldson JA, Ansm BJ. Surgical anatomy of the temporal bone, 4th ed. Donaldson JA, et al (Eds). New York: Raven Press; 1992. P.19.
2. Peggy Kelly, MD otoplasty. ENT Secrets Jafek & Murrow 2005, 3rd edition. P.203-307.
3. Pijush Jani and Tony Wright. Congenital abnormalities of the external and middle ear, diseases of the ear edited by Harold Ludman and Tony Wright, 1st Indian edition. Jaypee Brothers; 2006. P.279-81.
4. Gault D and Rothera M. Management of congenital deformities of the external and middle ear, Scott-Brown's Otorhinolaryngology, head and neck surgery, 7th edition. 2008;1:976-80.
5. Peggy E. Kelly, Melissa A. Scholes. Microtia and congenital aural Atresia. Otolayringol Clin N Am. 2007;40:61-80.
6. Zim SA. Mricrotia reconstruction an update current opinion in otolaryngology and head and neck surgery. 2003;11(4):275-81.
7. Walton RI, Bealm EK. Auricular reconstruction for microtia: Part II surgical technique. Plast Reconstr Surg. 2002;110(1):234-51.
8. Robert A. Jahrsdoerfer. Surgery for congenital aural atresia. Glasscock – shambaugh sufgery of the ear, 5th edition. 5th Indian reprint. 2007. P.389-99.
9. Dixon, Jill; Edwards, Sara J; Gladwin, Amanda J; Dixon, Michael J; StacieK; Bonner, Cynthia A; KoprivniKar, Kathryn; Wasmuth, John J. Positional cloning of a gene involved in the pathogenesis of Treacher collins Syndrome. Nature genetics. 1996;12(2):130-6.
10. Dela cruz A, Hansen MR. Reconstruction surgery of the ear: auditory canal and tympanum. In: Cummings CW, Feint PW, HarKer LA, et al (ed): Otolaryngology head and neck surgery, 4th edition. Philadelphia: Mosby; 2004. P. 4439-44.
11. Kemperman MH, StincKens C, Kumar S, Joosten FB, Huygen PL, Cremers CW. The bronchio-oto-renal syndrome. Advance in oto-rhino- laryngology. 2002;61:192-200.
12. Leopardi G, Chiarella G, Contis, Cassandro E. Surgical treatment of recurring preauricular sinus supra-auricular approach. Acta Otorhinolaryngol. Dec 2008;28(6):302-5.
13. Chang PH, Wu CM. An infidious Preauricular sinus. Presenting as an infected preauricular cyst. Int J Clin Pract. 2005;59(3):370-2.
14. Bajwa H, Kumar S. Radiofrequency thermal ablation versus cold steel for supra-auricular excision of preauricular sinus. Comparative study. J Laryngol Otol. Jun 11 2010;1-4.
15. D'souza AR, Uppal HS, De R and Zeitoun H. Updating concepts of first branchial cleft-defect: a literature review. Int. Journal of Pediatr Otolaryngology. 2002;62:103-9.
16. Lalit Kiran Saini, Deepchand and Gaurav Gupta. Complete fistulous tract with opening in Bony auditory canal: A rare presentation of collaural fistula. Indian Journal of medical case reports ISSN: 2319-3832. (Online) an online int. Journal available at http://www.cibtech.org/jcr.htm 2012 vol I(1) April- June, PP 15-17/Saini et al.
17. Singh AK. Multiple epidermoid systs of pinna: An uncommon presentation. Scholars Journal of applied medical sciences (SJAMS) Sch. J App Med Sci. 2013;1(5):378-9.
18. Prasad KC, Karthik S, Prasad SC. A comprehensive study on lesions of the pinna. Am J Otolaryngol. 2005;26(1):1-6.
19. Gardner EJ. Follow-up study of family group exhibiting dominant inheritance for a syndrome including intestinal polyps, osteoma, fibromas and epidermal cysts. Am J Hum Genet. 1962;14(4):376-90.
20. Ranganathan B, Douglas S, Mirza S. Skin incisions for the excision of spherical cutaneous and subcutaneous lesions. J Laryngol Otol. 2009;123(11):1250-1.
21. SM Gotam Rabbani, M Alamgir Chowdhury, Naseem Yasmeen, Mousumi Malakar. Hemangioma left pinna with extensive, multiple skin ulcerations. Bangladesh J. Otorhinolaryngology. 2010;16(1):70-2.
22. Anuj Goel. Arteriovenous malformation pinna: Review of literature otorhinolayingology clinics: An Int Journal. 2011;3(2):75-8.
23. Nussel F, Wegmuller H, Huber P. Comparison of magnetic resonance angiography, magnetic resonance imaging and conventional angiography in cerebral arteriovenous malformation. Neuroradiology. 199:33:56-61.
24. Burrows PE, MuliKen JB, Fellows KE, Strand RD. Childhood hemangiomas and vascular malformations: Angiographic differentiation and vascular malformations: Angiographic differentiation. AJR Am J Roentgenol. 1983;14:483-8.
25. PersKy MS. Congenital vascular lesions of the head and neck. Am J Surg. 1986;152:424-9.
26. Giguere CM, Bauman NM, Smith RJ. New treatment options for lymphangioma in infants and children. The annals of otology, rhinology and laryngology. 2002;111(12 Pt 1):1066-75.
27. Jee-nam song, So- Lyung Jung, Sung- Hak Lee, shinac Park. A case of large auricular lymphangioma. Int. Journal of Pediatric Otorhinolaryngology extra. 2012;vol 7(3):100-2.
28. Weigold DH, White PF, Burton CS. 'Treatment of lymphangioma circumscriptum with tunable dye lazer' Cutiz: cutaneous medicine for the practitioner. 1990;45(5):365-6.
29. Handbook of interventional radiologic procedures, 3rd edition. Kandarpa K and Aurny J. Lippincott 2002.

30. Goldberg, Kennedy (1997). Lymphangioma, Retrieved 2008. P. 11-10.
31. Loretta Davis MD. William D jams, MD. Eryspelos emedicine. medscape.com/article/1052445_overview.
32. Lina G, Piemonty, Godail-Gamot F, BeSM. Peter M, Gauduchon V, Vandenesch F, Etienne J. Involvement of Panton – Valentine Leucocidin-producing, staphylococcus aureus in primary skin infections and pneumonia. Clin infect Dis. 1999;29(5):1128-32.
33. James W Loock. Perichondritis of the external ear. Scott – brown's otorhinolaryngology, head and neck surgery, 7th edition. 2008;3:3358-61.
34. Martin R, YonKers AJ, Yarington CT. Perichondritis of the ear. Laryngoscope. 1976;86:664-73.
35. David B, Appelberg MD, Burton A, Waisbren MD, Frank W, Masters MD, et al. Treatment of chondritis in the burned ear by the local instillation of antibiotics. Plastic and reconstruction surgery. 1974;53:179-83.
36. Govrin- yehrdain J, Moscona AR, Hirshowits B. Treatment of acute suppurative perichondritis of the external ear by low dose X-ray irradiation. Burns, including thermal injury. 1983;10:140-4.
37. Loock JW. Relapsing polychondritis Scott- Brown's otorhinolaryngology, head and neck surgery, 7th edition. Vol 3. 2008. pp 3362-5.
38. Pearson CM, Kline HM, New comer VD. Relapsing polychodritis. New England Journal of medicine. 1960;263:51-8.
39. Foidart JM, abe S, Martin GR, Zizi CTM, Barnett EV, Lawley TJ, et al. Antibodies to type II collagen in relapsing polychondritis. New England Journal of medicine. 1978;299:1203-7.
40. Mc Adam LP, O'Hanlan MA, Bluestone R, Pearson CM. Relapsing polychondritis: Prospective study of 23 patients and a review of literature medicine (Baltimore). 1976;55:193-215.
41. Trentham DE, Le CH. Relapsing polychondritis. Annals of internal medicine. 1998;129:114-22.
42. Wright DN, Alexander JM. Effect of water in the bacterial flora in swimmer's ear. Archives of otolaryngology. 1974;99:15-8.
43. Jahn AF. Infection and inflammation of the external ear. Disease of ear, 6th edition. Harold Ludman and Tony Wright. Jaypee Brothers; 2006.pp 306-18.
44. Toulmouche MA. Observations of otorrhae cerebale suivis des reflexions. Gazette medicale de paris. 1838;6:422.
45. Chandler JR. Malignant external otitis laryngoscope. 1968;78:1257-94.
46. Carney AS. Malignant otitis externa, Scott-Brown's otorhinolaryngology head and neck surgery, 7th edition. 2008;3:3336-41.
47. Corey JP, Levendowski RA, Panwalker AP. Prognostic implications of therapy for necrotising external otitis. American Journal of Otology. 1985;6:353-8.
48. Holten KB, Gick J. Management of the patient with otitis externa. Journal of family Practice. 2001;50:353-60.
49. Ostfeld EJ, Kupferberg A. Biocompatible implantable antmicrobial release for fecrotizing external otitis. Journal of laryngology and otology. 1991;105-6.
50. Shupak A. Greanberg E. Hardoft R. Gordon C. Melamedy. Meyer WS. Hyperbaric oxygenation for necrotizing (Malignant) otitis externa. Archives of otolaryngology—head and neck surgery. 1989;115:1470-5.
51. Grunstein E, Santos F, Samuel H. Selesnick MD. Diseases of the external ear. Current diagnosis and treatment in otolaryngology – head and neck srgery. Edited by Lalwani AK. Vol 3. Tata McGraw-Hill. 2008. pp 625-40.
52. Sweeney CJ, Gilden DH. Ramsay-Hunt syndrome journal of neurology. New surgery and psychiatry. 2001;71:149-54.
53. Hunt JR. On hapetic inflammations of the geniculate ganglion. A new syndrome and it complications. Journal of nervous and mental disease. 1907;43:73-96.
54. Guidelines for management of atopic eczema, primary care dermatology socity and British Association of dermatologists (2006 updated October 2009).
55. Atopic dermatitis 9Eczema0- topical steroids; NICE technology appraisal (2004).
56. Giles WC, Lverson KC, King JD, Hill FC, Woody EA, BouKnight AL. Incision and drainage followed by mattress suture repair of auricular hematoma laryngoscope. 2007;117(12):2097-9.
57. Ghanem T, Rasamry JK, Park SS. Rethinking auricular trauma. Laryngoscope. 2005;115(7):1251-5.
58. Grunstein E, Santos F, Samuel H. Selesnick MD. Diseases of the external ear, carriear diagnosis and treatment in otolaryngology-head and neck surgery. Edited by Anil K Lalwani, Tata McGraw-Hill. 2008. pp 634-5.
59. Golant A, Nord RM, Paksima N, Posner MA. (Dec 2008) Cold exposure injures to the extremities. J Am Acad Orthop Surg. 2008;16(12):704-15.
60. Kim TY, Kim DH, Yoon Ms. Treatment of a recurrent auricular pseudocyst with intralesional steroid injection and clip compression dressing. Dermatol surg. 2009;35(2):245-7.
61. Patigaroo SA, Mahfooz N, Patigaroo FA, Kimani MH, Waheeda, Bhat S. Clinical characteristics and comparative study of different modalities of tritment of pseudocyst pinna. Ear Arch Otorhinolaryngol. 2012;269(7):1747-54.
62. Wong BJ. Cervantes W, Doyle KJ, Karamzadeh AM, Boys P, Brauel G, et al. Prevalence of external auditory canal exostoses in surfers. Archives of otolaryngology, head and neck surgery. 1999;125:969-72.
63. Graham MD. Osteoma and exostoses of the external auditory canal. A clinical histopathological and scanning electron microscopic study. Annals of otology, Rhinology, Laryngology. 1979;8:566-72.
64. Dehner LP, Chen KT. Primary tumors of the external and middle ear. Benign and malignant glandular neoplasm. Arch Otolaryngol. 1980;106(1):13-9.
65. Wong CS, Strange RC, Lear JT. Basal cell carcinoma. BMJ. 2003;327(7418):794-8.
66. Garrick AG, Michael G. Skin cancer of head and neck. Scott Brown's otorhinolaryngology , head and neck surgery, 7th edition. Edited by Michael Gleeson, at al. 2008;2:2394-98.
67. Motley R, Kersey P, Lawrence C. Multiprofessional guidelines for the management of the patient with primary cutaneous squamous cell carcinoma. British Journal of Dermatology. 2002;146:18-25. UK management guidlines. Zbar RIS. Cottel WI. Skin tumors: nonmelanoma skin tumors selected readings in plastic surgery. 2000;9:1-33. General overview.
68. Dubin N, Kopf AW. Multivariate risk scores for recurrence of cutaneous basal cell carcinomas. Archives of Dermatology. 1983;119:373-7.
69. Freedberg, et al. Fitz Patrick's Dermatology in general medicine, 6th ed. McGraw-Hill; 2003.

70. Rowe DE, Carroll RJ, Day Jr CL. Prognistic factors for local recurrence metastasis and survival rates in squamous cell carcinoma of the skin, ear and lip. Journal of the American Academy of Dermatology. 1992;26:976-90.
71. Jerant AF, Johnson JT, Sheridan CD, Caffrey TJ. Early detection and treatment of skin cancer. Am Fam Physician. 2000;62(2):357-68, 375-6, 381-2.
72. Ravin AG, Pickett N, Johnson JL. Fisher SR, Levin LS, Seigler HF. Melanoma of the ear: treatment and survival probabilities base on 199 patients. Ann Plast Surg. 2006;57(1):70-6.
73. Dong XD, Tyler D, Johnson L. Demato SP, Seigler HF. Analysis of prognosis and disease progression after local recurrence of melanoma, cancer. 2000;88(5):1063-71.
74. Veronesi U, Caseinelli N, Adamus J, Balch C, Bandiera D, BarchuK A, et al. Thin stage 1. Primary cutaneous malignant melanoma. New England Journal of Medicine. 1988;318:1159-62.
75. Balch LB, Urist MM, Keratousis CP, Smith TJ, Temgle WJ, Drzewiecki K, et al. Efficacy of 2cm surgical margins for intermediate thickness melanomas (1-4 mm). Annals of Surgery. 1993;218-7.
76. Christian Nordquist (4th June 2012). Darbraferib and Trametinib for metastatic melanoma meet primary and points in phase III studies medical news today.
77. McCoul ED, Hanson MB. External auditory canal cholesteatoma and keratosis obturans: the role of imaging in preventing facial nerve injury. Ear Nose & Throat Journal 2011. Available online at: http://www.entjournal.com/article/external-auditory-canal-cholesteatoma-and-keratosis-obturans-role-imaging-preventing-facial-
78. Gibson CM, Guddeti R. Keratosis obturans. Available online at: http://www.wikidoc.org/index.php/Keratosis_obturans
79. Piepergerdes MC, Kramer BM, Behnke EE. Keratosis obturans and external auditory canal cholesteatoma. Laryngoscope. 1980;90(3):383-91.
80. Persaud R, Chatrath P, Cheesman A. Atypical keratosis obturans. The Journal of Laryngology and Otology. 2003;117(9): 725-7.
81. Heilbrun ME, Salzman KL, Glastonbury CM, Harnsberger HR, Kennedy RJ, Shelton C. External auditory canal cholesteatoma: clinical and imaging spectrum. American Journal of Neuroradiology. 2003;24:751-6.
82. Saunders NC, Malhotra R, Biggs N, Fagan PA. Complications of keratosis obturans. The Journal of Laryngology and Otology. 2006;120(9):740-4.
83. Raz Y. Keratosis obturans and canal cholesteatoma. Myers EN, Eibling DE (eds) Operative otolaryngology: Head and neck surgery, 2nd edition. Saunders Elsevier; 2008. Chapter 110.
84. Bortz JT, Wertz PW, Downing DT. Composition of cerumen lipids. Journal of the American Academy of Dermatology. 1990;23(5):845-9.
85. Wikipedia. Earwax 2014. Available online at: http://en.wikipedia.org/wiki/Earwax
86. McCarter DF, Courtney AU, Pollart SM. Cerumen impaction. American Family Physician. 2007;75(10):1523-8.
87. van Wyk FC, Meyers AD. Cerumen impaction removal. Medscape 2012. Available online at: http://emedicine.medscape.com/article/1413546- overview#a01

Otitis Media

Asok K Saha

DEFINITION AND CLASSIFICATION OF OTITIS MEDIA

Otitis media (OM) is an inflammation of middle ear, Eustachian tube and mastoid (middle ear cleft). It can be acute, subacute or chronic. There is no absolute time period but in general—

- Acute—When the disease lasts for less than 3 weeks
- Subacute—When the disease lasts between 3 weeks and 3 months
- Chronic—When the disease persists for more than three months.

Histopathologically

Acute otitis media is accompanied with infiltration by polymorph nuclear cells associated with classical signs of acute inflammation.

Chronic otitis media is associated with infiltration of mucoperiosteum by round cells or cells of chronic inflammation.

Clinical Definition

- Myringitis is the inflammation of tympanic membrane (TM) alone or in association with otitis externa or otitis media
- Acute suppurative otitis media (ASOM) is clinically identified infection of middle ear with sudden onset and short duration
- Serous otitis media (SOM) is the presence of middle ear effusion behind an intact TM without acute signs and symptoms
- Chronic suppurative otits media (CSOM) is the chronic discharge from the middle ear through a perforation of the TM.

Suppurative refers to active clinical infection. Types of effusion associated with OM are:

- Serous
- Mucoid
- Purulent
- Hemorrhagic
- Combination of these

Complication is said to occur when the inflammatory process extends beyond the mucoperiosteum.

Sequelae refer to processes that remain within the mucoperiosteum and that have the capacity or potential for developing a complication.

Classification of Otitis Media[1]

1. Acute otitis media
   - Suppurative
   - Nonsuppurative
   - Recurrent.
2. Chronic otitis media
   - Suppurative
     - Tubotympanic
     - Cholesteatoma
   - Nonsuppurative
     - Otitis media with effusion.

Eustachian tube (E.tube) dysfunction is the major etiological contributing factor for pathogenesis of all forms of OM. The Eustachian tube is considered as a valve that connects the middle ear cleft to the nasopharynx. Normal physiologic functions of Eustachian tube are as follows:

- To ventilate the middle ear, it keeps the pressure of the both sides of TM equal
- To protect the middle ear from nasopharyngeal secretions

- To drain the secretion from the middle ear into the nasopharynx by mucociliary transport and a pump action of the Eustachian tube (E. tube).

Any condition that alters the normal functions of Eustachian tube may cause negative pressure in the middle ear that leads to accumulation of fluid in middle ear and mastoid. Ascending infection via Eustachian tube subsequently leads to infection in the accumulated fluid resulting in OM and possible mastoiditis.

Anatomic obstruction of Eustachian tube may come from

- Inflammation of Eustachian tube mucosa
- Extrinsic compression by tumor or large adenoids

Functional obstruction of Eustachian tube may occur from

- Failure of normal muscular mechanism of Eustachian tube as seen in cleft palate
- Insufficient stiffness of cartilaginous part of Eustachian tube as seen in infants and young children.

Younger children are predisposed to OM as Eustachian tube is in horizontal plane and has relatively short length and small lumen resulting in loss of protective function against the reflux of nasopharyngeal contents into the middle ear. In Down syndrome, the Eustachian tube is abnormally patent or short that may account for high incidence of OM. Again ciliary function of Eustachian tube may affect in viral infection, bacterial toxin or inherited increase rate of abnormalities of ciliary structure, results in OM.

Lillie's Classification[2]—

Type I—Permanent perforation Syndrome

- A persistent perforation of TM invades pars tensa. The margins are well-epithelialized
- Ear may remain dry for long period or it may discharge intermittently
- Degree of hearing loss varies considerably depending on size and site of perforation, maximum loss with large perforation.

Type II—Chronic tubotympanic mucositis

- It is long standing infection associated with odorless mucoid/mucopurulent discharge that becomes profuse and is associated with URTI
- A large total/near total perforation of TM
- Handle of Malleus may be necrosed
- Mucosa over promontory may be thickened and red. The exposed ossicles are buried in this thick, exuberant and oedematous mucosa.

Type III—Tympanic membrane perforation is associated with secondary cholesteatoma and necrosis of bone.

ACUTE OTITIS MEDIA (AOM) (FIG. 1)

Diagnostic Criteria (Table 1)

- Otalgia associated with ear tugging or irritability in children
- Pyrexia indicating an acute infection
- Tympanic membrane has a cart wheel appearance (Leash of blood vessel along the HOM and at the periphery of TM) or appears red and bulging with loss of landmarks. Yellow spot may be seen on TM when rupture is imminent
- Deafness, Tuning fork tests showing conductive hearing loss
- Otorrhea indicating perforation.

Pneumatic otoscopy is the gold standard for diagnosis of OM.

Table 1: Classification of Acute Otitis Media (AOM)

Acute Suppurative OM	*Nonsuppurative AOM*	*Recurrent AOM*
It is acute inflammation of middle ear by pyogenic organisms	It is the inflammation of middle ear cleft mucosa with or without formation of sterile effusion. It is often seen prior to or in resolution stage of acute suppurative otitis media	It is said as more or equal to three episodes of acute suppurative otitis media in a 3 months period or more or equal to four episodes in a 12 months period with complete resolution of symptoms and signs in between episodes

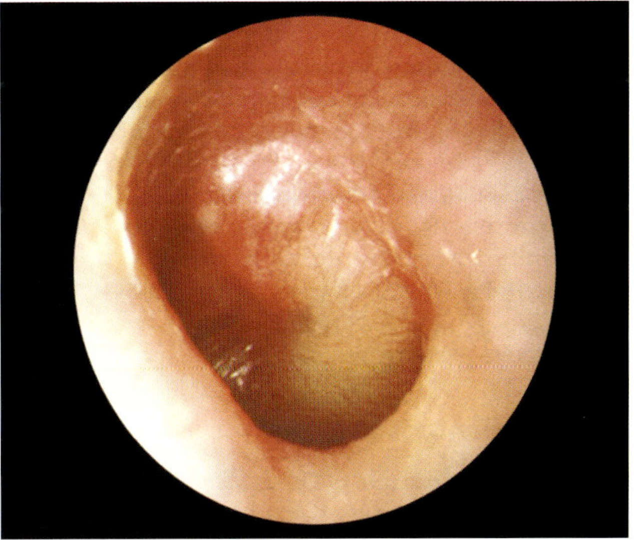

Fig. 1: Acute Otitis media (Stage of exudation)

Epidemiology

- It is a common childhood disease especially less than 2 years of age
- Greater risk is in first year of life.
- Children with an early OM onset are at high-risk for recurrent OM and Chronic OME
- Host factors:
  - Boys suffer more than girls
  - White suffers more than black. Genetic variation is related to anatomic and physiologic variations in Eustachian Tube
  - Children with congenital malformation like cleft palate and Down's syndrome suffer more than the normal
  - Patients with immunodeficiency, e.g. malignancy, immune suppressive therapy and AIDS suffer from OM because of abnormal host defense.
- Environmental factors:
  - Poor socioeconomic status suffers more than rich
  - Passive smoking impairs mucociliary clearance of Eustachian tube. It leads to increase chance of OM
  - Breastfeeding leads to decrease chance of OM. Breast milk provides antibacterial and immunologic benefits to infants
  - In colder seasons, high incidence of URTIs leads to increase susceptibility of OM.

Pathogenesis of Acute Otitis Media

Acute otitis media is considered a predominantly bacterial infection. Antecedent respiratory viruses play an important role in pathogenesis of AOM. Viral infection of URT induces release of inflammatory mediators in nasopharynx, increase bacterial colonization and has suppressive effect on host's immune defence. Most common organisms in infants and children are *Streptococcus pneumoniae* (40%), *Hemophilus influenzae* (30%) and *Moraxella catarrhalis* (20%). Less frequent organisms include *Streptopyogens, Staphylococcus aureus* and gram negative organism, such as *Pseudomonas aeroginosa*. Recently, PCR (Polymerase Chain reaction) method give positive result in patients in whom bacterial culture shows negative result.

Role of Adenoids in AOM

- Anatomic obstruction of Eustachian tube occurs when adenoids are enlarged
- A reservoir of bacteria is present in adenoids
- Tonsillitis is not considered a contributing factor in OM. Therefore, tonsillectomy is not recommended for treatment of OM.

Prevention of AOM

- Prophylactic antibiotics. Oral amoxicillin at the dose of 20 mg/Kg/day is recommended
- Vaccines—Pneumococcal vaccine is used for infants and children below 2 years of age and children above 2 years of age who are at high-risk of recurrent AOM
- Surgery—Prophylactic tympanostomy tube is inserted to reduce the episodes of AOM. Children undergoing a second tympanostomy tube insertion are recommended for adenoidectomy.

Clinical Course

The disease usually runs through four stages (Flowchart 1):

1. Hyperemia—It causes otalgia, ear fullness and fever with or without deafness. Pathogenic change comprises hyperemic edema beginning in Eustachian tube and tympanic cavity involving mucoperiosteum of mastoid antrum and air cells. Injection of blood vessels appears along the handle of malleus and at the periphery of the pars tensa and the pars flaccida giving it a cart wheel appearance.
2. Exudation—In absence of antibiotic therapy, stage of hyperemia is followed by stage of exudation. Tympanomastoid compartment gets filled with exudates under pressure, resulting otalgia, high fever accompanied by deafness. Tympanic membrane looks red, thick and bulging with loss of landmarks. X-ray reveals opacification of tympanomastoid compartment.
3. Suppuration—This is the formation of pus in the middle ear and mastoid air cells. Tympanic membrane bulges and finally ruptures resulting in otorrhea accompanied by otalgia and fever.
4. Resolution—Inflammatory process begins to resolve even without rupture of tympanic membrane. Otalgia is relieved and hearing returns to normal. When infection is severe and remains for 2 weeks, thickening of mucoperiosteum of epitympanum and periantral cells obstructs the drainage of mucopurulent discharge. It results in venous stasis, local acidosis and dissolution of calcium from adjacent bone walls. Osteoclast destroys the decalcifying septa resulting in stage of coalescence of mastoid air cells and surgical mastoiditis. Extension of infection beyond tympanomastoid compartment to

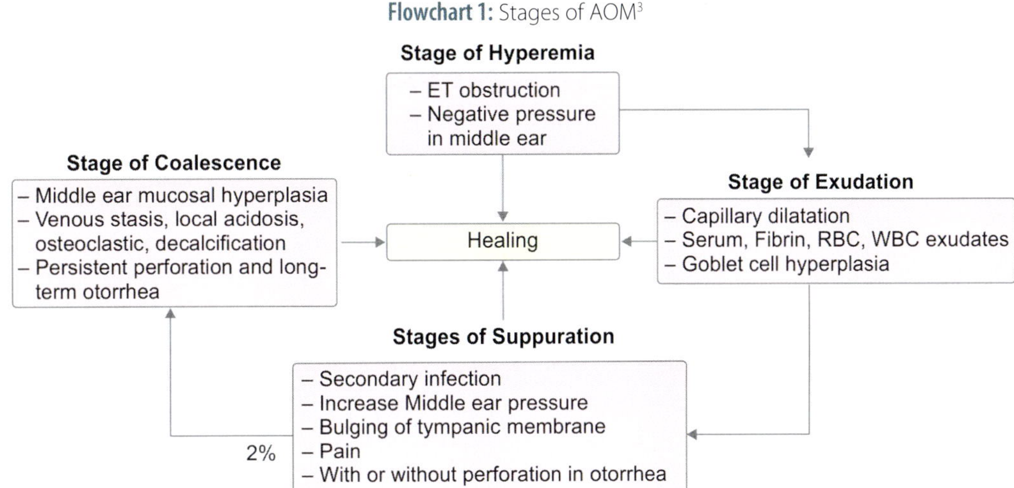

Flowchart 1: Stages of AOM[3]

adjacent structures results in the stage of complication. Acute otitis media (AOM) rarely progresses to this stage.

Medical Management of AOM

- Watchful waiting
- Control of environmental risk factors
- Antimicrobial administration
- Adjunctive therapy.

Watchful waiting: The current treatment protocol is the initial watchful waiting without antibiotic therapy for healthy 2 years old or older children with mild otalgia and fever less than 39°C. AOM symptoms improve in most cases within 3 days. For children less than 2 years old, watchful waiting is not recommended.

Control of environmental risk factor: Breastfeeding is to be given instead of bottle feeding to infants. Proping a bottle in a supine infant's mouth results reflux of milk in the middle ear through Eustachian tube. Other risk factors like passive smoking and attendance in a child care facility should be avoided.

Antimicrobial administration: If AOM does not improve after watchful waiting, antibiotic therapy should be started and continued for 10–14 days. A shorter course of five days may be curative. Amoxicillin (80 mg/kg/day in 3 divided doses) is considered the first line treatment; although many effective agents are available against *Streptococcus pneumonia, Hemophilius influenzae* and *Morexillae catarrhalis.* Antibiotics must have a convenient dose schedule, minimal side effect, cost-effective and good taste. In resistant case, amoxicillin is given in combination with clavulanic acid. Children with clinically defined treatment failure after three days of therapy needs second line treatment with oral cefuroxime, cefpodoxime proxetil and intramascular ceftriaxone. For selection of third line antibiotics, tympanocentesis is recommended for identification of pathogens and selection of appropriate antibiotics.[4]

Adjunctive Therapy

It Includes—

- Analgesic and antipyretics. Paracetamol relieves from pain and temperature
- Decongestant nasal drops (Oxymetazoline or Xylometazoline, 1% in adult and 0.5% in children) are used to relieve Eustachian tube edema to promote middle ear ventilation
- Oral decongestants or antihistamines have no role in treatment of AOM.[5]

Surgical Management of AOM

Most of the patients respond to medical treatment. Only a few patients, who fail to improve from medical treatment, need surgical management.

Myringotomy is indicated to allow the drainage of pus from the middle ear cleft. Indications are:

- Tympanic membrane bulges with otalgia
- Incomplete resolution with antibiotics with persistent conductive deafness
- Persistent effusion for more than 12 weeks.

Drug Resistant Pathogens

Drug resistant strains of Pneumococcus pyogens are found from 20–50% of cases of untreated AOM and from 45 to 90% of refractory AOM. Beta lactamase producing strains of Hemophilus influenzae are isolated in 40–50% of cases of OM. Therefore, clinician should be aware of the drug resistant pathogens.

Sequelae of OM

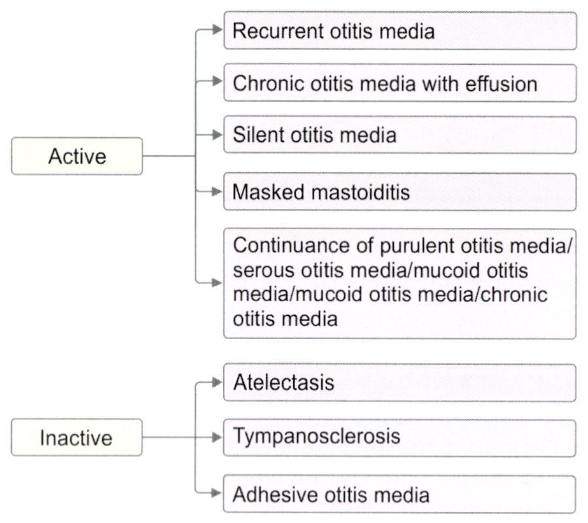

Silent OM

Silent OM is defined as clinically undetected or undetectable middle ear pathology. Here middle ear pathology exists but with an absence of perforation and otorrhea. It may be associated with—cholesteatoma behind the intact tympanic membrane

- Conductive/sensorineural hearing loss
- Pain
- Acute exacerbations of otitis media
- Labyrinthine fistulae
- Endolymphatic hydrops
- Temporal bone/intracranial complications.

Sequelae of silent OM are:
- Tympanosclerosis
- Atelectasis or adhesive otitis media
- Conductive hearing loss because of ossicular fixation or disruption
- Sensorineural hearing loss.

The concept of silent OM is especially significant in children below the age of 2 years because they often fail to communicate minor symptoms. In children having *Hemophilus influenzae* meningitis is likely to coexist with silent OM.

Treatment Includes

- First recognize the disease
- Second flexible surgical approach to remove the disease.

OTITIS MEDIA WITH EFFUSION

Otitis media with effusion (OME) is defined as fluid in the middle ear behind intact drum in absence of signs or symptoms of acute infection for 3 months or more. Various names have been given to this condition—chronic secretory otitis media, chronic serous otitis media, nonsuppurative otitis media and glue ear, etc. After several discussions at international symposia, the most acceptable nomenclature is otitis media with effusion[6]. The fluid in the middle ear cleft decreases tympanic membrane mobility that results in conductive hearing loss with type B tympanogram and normal external auditory canal volume. It is the most common cause of deafness in children and has increased incidence in preschool children. 50–60% is less than 1 year of age, 70% is more than 3 years of age. Predisposing factors for OME is closely related with those associated with AOM, e.g. poor general health, lower socioeconomic status, overcrowding, habit of smoking in parents, male more than female, winters more than summers. Breastfeeding offers protection.

Pathogenesis

Any condition that affects the function of mucociliary system of upper respiratory tract may cause to develop middle ear effusion (Flowchart 2).[7]

- Eustachian tube factor: The Eustachian tube opening dysfunction or muscular opening hypofunction in children is the primary endogenous etiological factor. Change in structure of Eustachian tube to adult type occurs at the age of 7 years
- Role of surfactant: The Eustachian tube epithelium is coated by a mixture of phospholipids identical to pulmonary surfactant. Eustachian tube surfactant is synthesized by Eustachian tube epithelium and secreted in the form of osmiophilic multilaminar bodies into the tubal lumen
- Immunological factors: In OME, an activated local immune system is present in middle ear and effusion is due to a local reaction. Various kinds of cytokines are detected in the middle ear fluid. Many of the cytokine are produced by T-lymphocytes
- Infection: The role of infective organisms in naso pharynx as a cause of inflammatory changes in middle ear is studied. Positive culture for *Hemophilus*

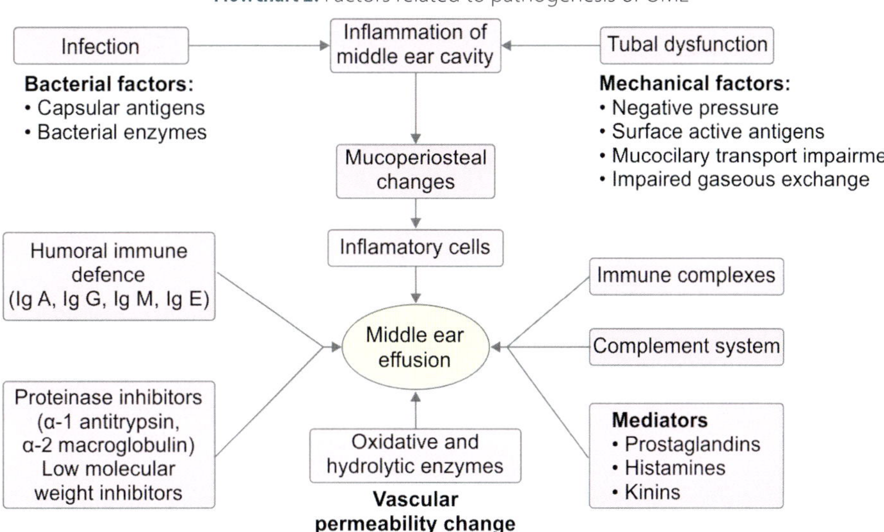

Flowchart 2: Factors related to pathogenesis of OME[8]

influenzae, Streptococcus pneumonia and *Moraxella catarrhalis* is seen in 30% of cases. A close relationship in incidence of respiratory syncitial viral infection and otitis media with effusion is studied

- Allergy: Higher prevalence rate of allergic condition is seen in children with OME
- Middle ear gas diffusion: The exchange of gas or air from middle ear via the Eustachian tube is an established fact. Middle ear gas content is controlled by Eustachian tube as well as by diffusion in the blood. Negative pressure created in the middle ear is due to increased diffusion in the blood due to increase vascularity from inflammation. A chemoreceptor mechanism is suggested within the middle ear under neural control
- Role of mastoid pneumatization: A well-pneumatized mastoid serves as a good middle ear pressure buffer system. Patients with mastoid pneumatization have a better long-term prognosis.

Etiology

In Children

- Adenoids—It may cause destruction and displacement of Eustachian tube.
  - It may provide focus of infection adjacent to Eustachian tube
  - Cause destruction of lymphatics draining middle ear and Eustachian tube
  - Coexistence of adenoid hypertrophy and OME may be incidental also, since both are common below 9 years of age.

- Cleft Palate—It may cause dysfunction of tensor veli palatini and levator veli palatine
- Surfactant deficiency
- Cystic fibrosis and immobile cilia syndrome
- Agammaglobulinemia
- Hormonal changes, such as increased estrogen level, hypothyroidism
- Craniofacial abnormality, e.g. Hunter's, Down's and Hurler's syndromes.

In Adult

- Idiopathic
- Barotrauma: Rapid decent results in decreased middle ear pressure that leads to retraction of TM followed by pain and immobility of TM and ossicles.It may cause conductive hearing loss, transudation of serum and blood.

Treatment

Valsalva maneuver/decongestants—

- Nasopharyngeal carcinoma: It may cause mechanical obstruction of Eustachian tube, infiltration and immobility of Eustachian tube and lymphatic obstruction of middle ear and Eustachian tube
- Radiotherapy: It may cause fibrosis around the Eustachian tube
- Surgical procedures in head and neck region may cause OME
- Patients with diseases related to immune system, e.g. multiple myeloma, polyarteritis nodosa and immune deficiency syndrome, may develop OME.

Clinical Features

The signs and symptoms of OME includes—
- Decreased hearing (97%) is insidious in onset and rarely exceeds 40 dB. Hearing loss may pass unnoticed by parents may be detected during audiometric screening tests
- Feeling of ear fullness and pulsatile tinnitus (60%)
- Recurrent ear infection: Scarring of TM and tympanosclerosis are seen with recurrent infection
- Poor speech development is due to deafness
- Failing performance at the school
- Earache and dizziness are due to fluid pressing on round window membrane.

Otoscopic Findings

Tympanic membrane is dull looking with loss of light reflex. The thin leash of blood vessels is seen along the handle of malleus and at the periphery of TM. TM shows varying degree of retraction and restricted mobility on pneumatic otoscopy. Fluid level and air bubbles are seen through intact and transparent TM. Examination with microscope improves the findings for diagnosis (Fig. 2).

Hearing Assessement

- Tuning fork with 512 cps shows conductive hearing loss
- Audiometry shows conductive hearing loss of mild to moderate degree (20–40 dB). Associated sensory neural hearing loss (SNHL) may be present. It disappears after removal of fluid

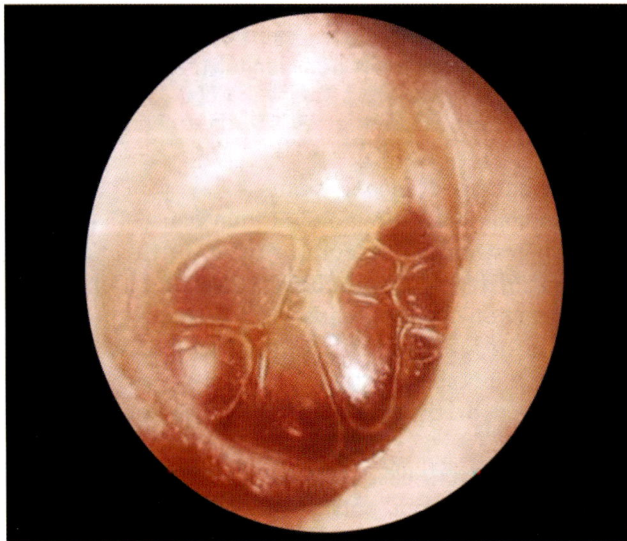

Fig. 2: Otoscopic findings of OME

- Impedance audiometry shows type B tympanogram with a sensitivity of 45% and specificity of 92%. Negative middle ear pressure results in a type C tympanogram (mean air pressure less than -100 daPa)
- Transient evoke otoacoustic emissions (TEOAEs) helps testing of hearing at the age of 4 days. They are effective in detecting patients with normal hearing and with hearing loss more than 25 dB
- Radiology: X-ray mastoid shows clouding of air cells due to fluid. MRI of temporal bone if shows absence of fluid, it does not imply an absence of OME as 1/3rd of patients in MRI show fluid in mastiod but not in mesotympanum. MRI of bilateral temporal bone in patients with nasopharyngeal carcinoma shows 27% has radiological middle ear fluid
- Superfine fibrescopy through Eustachian tube helps direct observation of tympanic cavity as it is reported by Yamaguchi (1994)[7]. The fiberscope is flexible having diameter of 0.6–0.8 mm. It is used under local anesthesia. The findings are recorded on video tapes.

Management of OME

Aim of management is the aeration of middle ear cleft. It is directed at—
- Alleviating hearing loss
- Preventing sequelae
- Preventing recurrent OM.

Medical Management

Medical management includes—
- Watchful waiting
- Control of environmental risk factor
- Antimicrobial therapy.
  OME usually resolves within 3–6 months if hearing loss is mild. Therefore, watchful waiting is an appropriate therapy. It is observed that the season of attendance (i.e. July to December) and a bilateral hearing loss of more than 30 dB make spontaneous resolution unlikely. Antibiotics help about 15% of patients to clear effusion within a 1 month period. Antibiotics that are effective on beta-lactamase producing organisms are preferred, as there is a high incidence of resistant strain. A significant delay in speech and language development needs immediate intervention. It has been found that use of topical and systemic steroids gives short-term benefit in hearing but not long-term benefit. Thus steroids are not recommended in treatment of OME. Again, there is no support to use of decongestents, antihistaminics and mucolytics for the treatment of isolated OME. Autoinflation by performing Valsalva maneuver gives improvement of 50% and it is recommended in

treatment before surgical management of OME. It is of less value in chronic cases.

Surgical Management

Surgical options include—
- Tympanocentesis
- Simple myringotomy
- Myringotomy with tympanostomy tube insertion (Grommet)
- Adenoidectomy with myringotomy and grommet insertion
- Treatment of other nasal and sinus surgery.

Surgery is recommended for persistent disease with significant hearing loss.
- Tympanocentesis is the transtympanic needle aspiration of fluid from mesotympanum. The procedure helps to perform culture sensitivity to identify organism in the middle ear fluid of children who are unresponsive to antibiotics
- Myringotomy is the incision in the TM. It allows drainage of middle ear fluid. It is unusually indicated in purulent OM, e.g. sever otalgia meningitis or facial palsy. In OME myringotomy, without ventilation tube insertion gives short-term benefit and is not recommended
- Now Carbon Dioxide laser myringotomy is used as a low-pain procedure for middle ear ventilation for OME. It is done under local anesthesia to create a 2 mm circular perforation to provide ventilation of middle ear for about 3 weeks. The CO_2 laser otoscope is a new application to reduce the complexity of surgery
- Myringotomy with insertion of tympanostomy tube (Fig. 3): It was advocated by Politzer in 1883[9] and Armstrong in 1954[9]. After insertion of tympanostomy tube or ventilation tube (VT), hearing comes to an average Air- bone gap (A-B) of 9.5 dB. If 75% closure of AB gap does not occur after inserting VT, it will be assumed that the cause is other than OME (e.g. ossicular discontinuity). Timing of insertion of VT is before winter. Average period before expulsion is 6 months.

There are three main types of tubes (Fig. 4)[1]—
- Short-term tubes (Shepard VT): It may be made up of Teflon or silicon. The tube remains in TM for an average of 6 months
- Midterm tube: It remains in TM for 6–12 months.
  - Shah grommet—It is made up of Teflon. The triangular flange helps to prevent extrusion
  - Reuter Robbin—It is made up of stainless steel or Teflon. It has flange with holes to help the tissue to grow in between them and this helps in anchoring
  - Armstrong—It is beveled VT made up of silicon or Teflon. The angle of the inner flange to the shank helps in easy insertion through a small incision
  - Paperella type I—It is soft silicon tube with a notched inner flange. It requires a small incision for insertion
  - Feuerstein split tube—It diminishes the chances of blockage
  - Linderman-Silverstein arrow tube—The widely flared inner flange helps in anchorage.
- Long-term tube—It remains for several years. It may cause high incidence of residual perforation.
  - Per-Lee tube—It is made up of silicon. It has wide flange that is effective in resisting extrusion
  - Goode T-tube—Silicon tube, the lumen opens into a half tube placed at right angles forming a T
  - Paparella type II and type III are similar to Parparella type I. It is also of soft silicon. They have larger lumens and wider flanges to resist blockage and extrusion.

Indications for bilateral myringotomy and VT insertion are[11]
- Recurrent acute OM (three episodes within 6 months or four episodes within 12 months)
- Chronic OME (The symptoms present for three months with associated hearing loss more than 20 dB in the better ear)
- Poor response to antibiotics
- Chronic retraction pockets of TM
- Barotitis media
- Autophony due to Eustachian tube dysfunction.

Complications of VT are
- Slippage into the middle ear cavity
- Granulation formation which is usually associated with long-term tubes.
- Occlusion of VT—It is treated with 3% of Hydrogen Peroxide/3% Boric acid

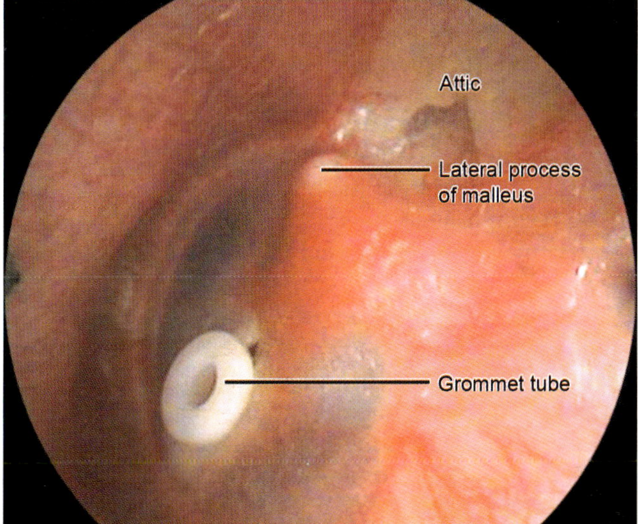

Fig. 3: Myringotomy with tympanostomy tube insertion (Grommet)

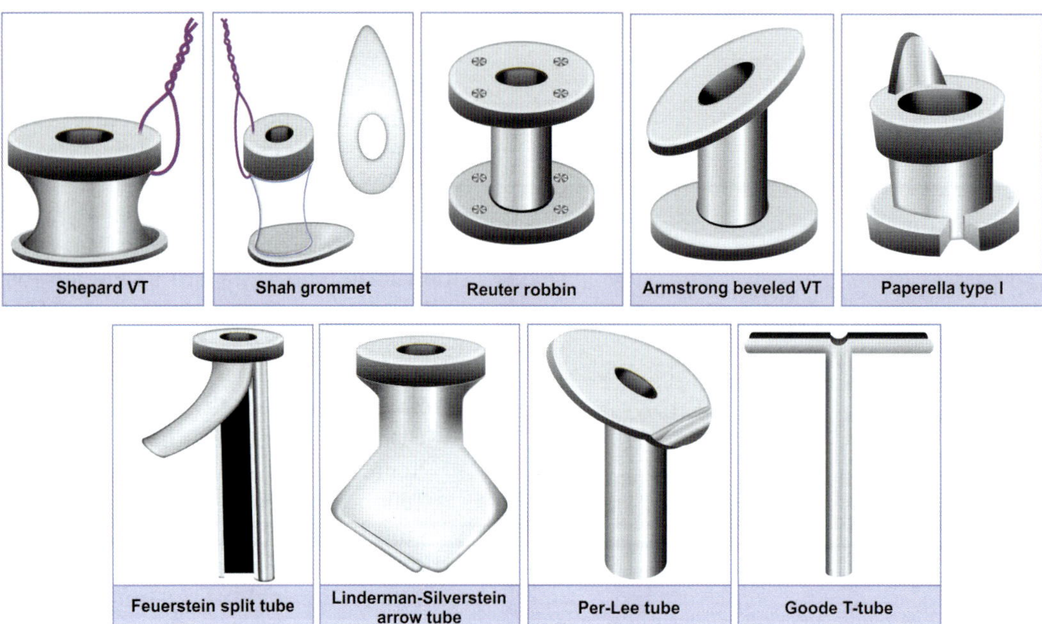

Fig. 4: Ventilating tubes of different materials and designs

- Postmyringotymy otorrhea—Treatment is local toileting
- Tympanosclerosis ⎱ These are associated
- Microatelectasis ⎰ with long-acting tubes
- Persistent perforation
- Cholesteatoma—Less than 1% cases
- Trauma to the ossicular chain resulting conductive/sensorineural hearing loss (SNHL).

Adenoidectomy

Most clinicians prefer adenoidectomy in the treatment of OME. Studies have shown that not only the size of adenoids but the bacterial load in nasopharynx may also be the contributing factor for OME. Adenoidectomy helps by—
- Relieving nasal obstruction
- Improving E-tube function
- Eliminating potential bacterial load.

As adenoidectomy may be associated with potential risks of hemorrhage and sometimes velopharyngeal incompetency, most surgeons like tympanostomy tube insertion alone as the first line of treatment and consider adenoidectomy when repeated tympanostomy tube insertion is required. However, adenoidectomy is to be done only if there is an indication for their removal.

If there is contralateral deaf ear, advices are as follows:
- Little surgery
- Avoid insertion of VT tube
- Hearing aid
- Regular follow-up.

Long-term ineffectiveness of treatment of chronic adult OME, hearing aid is considered as main treatment option[12]. But before prescribing a hearing aid—
- Attic and antrum must be cleared-off granulation by combined approach leaving canal wall and ossicular chain intact
- Exploratory tympanotomy is to be done for chronic intractable stage and silastic sheet is put to maintain air-space between Eustachian tube and round window
- For atrophic drum head—gel foam/fascia underplant procedure is done.

Sequelae may happen as a consequence of the disease process or as a result of effect of treatment.

Sequelae due to severity of disease and duration are—
- Atropic changes in TM and atelectasis of middle ear – in long standing OME dissolution of fibrous layer of TM results thin and atrophic TM. TM retracts into the middle ear resulting atelectasis
- Ossicular erosion—Commonly long process of Incus gets eroded. Next super structure of stapes is necrosed. This may cause conducting hearing loss up to 58 dB
- Retraction pockets and cholesteatoma—Atrophic pars tensa is invaginated to form posterosuperior retraction pockets or cholesteatoma. Pars flaccida is also retracted in attic region resulting in cholesteatoma
- Cholesterol granuloma—It is formed due to stasis of secretions in middle ear and mastoid air cells
- Inner ear symptom—Sensorineural hearing loss (SNHL) is due to absorption of toxic substances via round

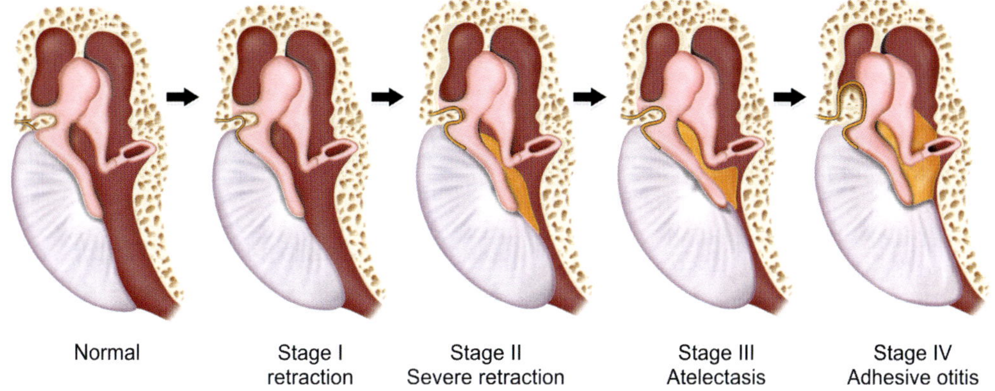

Fig. 5: Pars tensa retraction as per Sade and Berco

window. It is prevented by gel foam pack around round window to decrease permeability

- Developmental and behavioral impairment—Unresolved OME has indirect effects on learning, speech, and behavior of children.

Sequelae Due to the Effect of Treatment

Tympanosclerosis—From studies, it is reported that the incidence of tympanosclerosis is higher in ears treated with tympanostomy tube than ears treated without tube. Explanations for development of tympanosclerosis in relation to VT are as follows:

- Sheering stresses to the fibrils within lamina propria
- Hemorrhage within the layers of the membrane
- High partial pressure of O_2 is toxic.

Tympanosclerosis envelops ossicles resulting in deafness due to stapes fixation.

Secrets of OME

- There is a sharp fall in incidence of OME in children after 7 years of age. It indicates that the improvement of Eustachian tube function and development of maturation of immune system start after 7 years of age
- Unilateral OME in an adult may indicate nasopharyngeal mass obstructing Eustachian tube. It is imperative to examine nasopharynx to rule out neoplastic lesion. Nasopharyngeal biopsies are considered in high-risk cases, e.g. Chinese, Eskimos and positive family history of nasopharyngeal carcinoma.

Middle Ear Atelectasis

It is the collapse of the tympanic membrane. Tympanic membrane is displaced inwards towards the promontory after preceded by chronic secretory otitis media and adhesive otitis media.

Its characteristics are as follows:

- Collapsed drum looks thin, flabby and scarred
- Extent of collapse may be complete or partial
- Pars tensa retractions are basically of posterior TM.

Degree of Retractions as Per Sade and Berco (1976) (Fig. 5)[13]

Stage I—Pars tensa is retracted. There is no middle ear fluid.

Stage II—Pars tensa is retracted. The TM is in contact with long process of Incus.

Stage III—TM is lying over promontory (plastering) but can be lifted. Ossicular chain is intact (Atelectasis).

Stage IV—Adhesive stage. TM is adhered to promontory and draped around the long process of incus and stapes.

Diagnosis: Otoscopy is performed in conjunction with a siegle pneumatic speculum. EUM (examination under the microscope) is useful to confirm the otoscopic findings. TM is thin, transparent and atrophic. It facilitates the examination of middle ear contents. Incus is commonly necrosed and sometimes the stapes crura are also necrosed and surrounded with granulation tissue. Granulation is also seen along the posterior rim of annulus. Tuning fork test and pure tone audiometry show conductive hearing loss. Impedance audiometry shows negative middle ear pressure.

A high-peaked tympanogram type Ad indicates hypermobile TM or ossicular discontinuity.

A type B tympanogram suggests presence of fluid in middle ear in association with retraction.

X-rays shows poorly pneumatized mastoid process.

Differential diagnosis—Adhesive otitis media closely resembles atelectasis.

Careful otoscopic examination with siegle's speculum helps to differentiate an atelectatic tympanic membrane collapsed on to the promontory from adhesion of tympanic membrane to promontory in adhesive otitis media.

Treatment: Aim of treatment is aeration of middle ear cleft. In atelectasis, TM is plastered onto the promontory. It is difficult to find an air-space for insertion of VT. Wright (1969) suggested preliminary politzerization to aerate the middle ear and re-expand the collapsed TM. Long-term ventilation using a Per-Lee tube is considered.

Zöllner (1963) described insertion of plastic tubing along the Eustachian tube. It is now not recommended as it may cause scarring and stricture of Eustachian tube.

House, Glasscock and Miles (1969) advocated tuboplasty techniques using middle fossa approach. Tubal obstruction was removed. The stenosed lining of the tube was excised. A rolled-up silastic sheet was inserted to form the new tube. This procedure has not been established later.

Tympanoplastic procedures are useless in presence of poorly functioning Eustachian tube. Frequent maneuver of gentle inflation by Valsalva technique may give good clinical improvement for long period. Insertion of VT is a surgically tricky procedure as TM is thin and flattened.

Pars Flaccida retractions: Retraction in pars flaccida has four stages as described by Tos et al. (1987) (Fig. 6).[14]
Stage I: The pars flaccida is dimpled and retracted but not adherent to the malleus.
Stage II: Retraction is adherent to the neck of malleus and the full extent of the retraction can be seen.

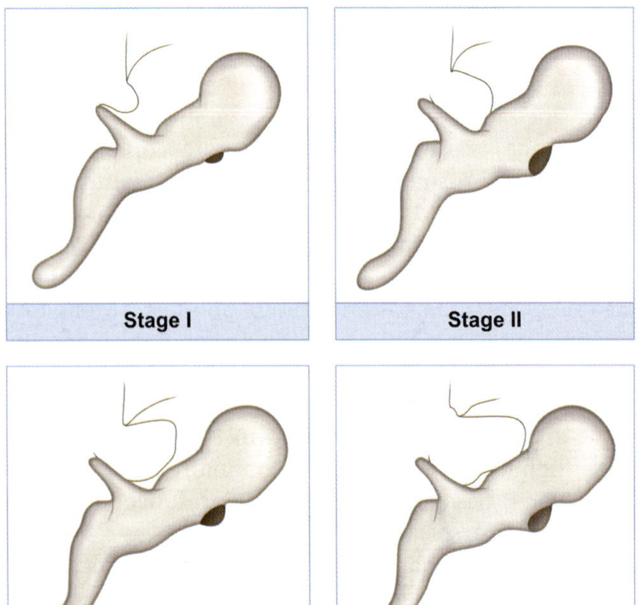

Fig. 6: Pars flaccida retraction as per Tos et al.

Stage III: Partial erosion of bony attic wall and the part of retraction is out of view.
Stage IV: Definite erosion of the attic wall with full extent of the retraction is uncertain as it is out of view.

It is essential to see the fundus of retraction pocket. The retraction pocket is of two types—self-cleaning and nonself-cleaning.

A small clean retraction pocket in pars flaccida or pars tensa seems to be self cleaning. If a retraction pocket progresses in size and configuration, it loses its self-cleaning property and accumulates inactive squamous debris that becomes infected resulting intermittent ear discharge—active squamous COM. TM shows destruction of collagenous middle layer.

Mucosa shows increased mucus secreting cells, edema, granulation tissue that block attic forming cholesteatoma. Erosion of ossicular chain is caused by leukotrienes, osteoclasts, bone resorption factor from granulations and tumor necrosis factor alfa (TNF-α) present in half of the cases.

Long process of incus is commonly involved. Stapes and malleus are also involved.

Management of Inactive Retraction

In Adult Patient

- If AB gap is less than 20 dB (normal hearing) and retraction pocket is self-cleaning, follow-up of the patient on occasional basis is appropriate. If retraction pocket is not self cleaning microscopic suction clearance on regular basis is essential
- If AB gap is more than 20 dB it is surgically managed. A graft with a cartilaginous component helps to prevent recurrence of retraction
- Ossicular disruption needs ossiculoplasty. Defective incus requires malleus and stapes assembly. Defective malleus needs incus + stapes assembly. Stapes alone if is affected—Inverted L-shaped prosthesis, maleus footplate assembly (MFA) is used
- Granulation in attic and blockage of middle ear opening-are managed by removal of granulation via endaural approach or atticoantrostomy/atticomastoidectomy is done by postaural approach.

Children Under 12 Years

- If AB gap is less than 20 dB (normal hearing), no treatment is necessary
- If there is no infection, AB gap is more than 20 dB with middle ear effusion—ventilation tube (VT) is inserted. VT is contraindicated, if there is disruption of ossicular chain

- If retraction is progressing, incudostapedial joint is eroded, surgery is recommended; tympanoplasty with thin cartilage prevents recurrence. Concomitant exploration of mastoid does not improve the outcome in absence of Cholesteatoma.

Tympanosclerosis

Tympanosclerosis is a condition of middle ear characterized by the local deposition of plaques of collagen beneath the lining epithelium resulting conductive hearing loss from impairment of ossicular movement or from ossicular disruption. The plaques are laid down in the substance of TM, in the tympanic cavity and sometimes in mastoid.[15] The term Myringosclerosis is used when the process is confined to the tympanic membrane (Fig. 7). The term Tympanosclerosis is used if the pathology affects the ossicular chain.

Sites of election of these plaques are—
- Stapes—oval window area (most common)
- Subfallopian groove
- Upper promontory
- Long process of Incus, stapes tendon
- Horizontal portion of fallopian canal
- Epitympanum/malleus.

Rare sites of plaques deposition are—Eustachian tube area/Hypotympanum/Round window niche/Mastoid.

Etiology: It represents the sequelae of otitis media in past. Inflammatory episode initiates the release of collagen stimulating factor of unknown origin.

Histopathology: Tympanosclerosis is mesodermal in origin. It affects connective soft tissue. Plaques are located in stratum fibrosum of TM or between the lining epithelium and periosteum in middle ear (Fig. 8).

Two types of plaques are seen under operating microscope.
- Soft creamy type with a rubbery or cartilaginous texture
- Pure white, extremely hard dense plaques adherent to the surrounding bone.

Histopathology shows masses of hyaline material which is devoid of cells and blood vessels and covered by a thin flattened epithelium. Hyaline substance is bi-refringent under polarized light and consists of masses of collagen fibers. Ossicles, usually the incus, looks like moth eaten, porous and demineralized (Fig. 9).

Classification for Tympanosclerosis (Weilinga and Kerr)

Type I—Involvement of TM, either intact or perforated. Sometimes involves the malleus.

Type II—Fixation of malleus-Incus complex in atic with a mobile stapes.

Type III—Fixation of stapes. Malleus-Incus complex is mobile.

Type IV—Fixation of the stapes and malleus-Incus complex.

Biochemical Analysis: It indicates that Tympanosclerosis plaques exhibit the characteristics of carbonate apatite.

Clinical features: Patient is usually presented with deafness and sometimes tinnitus. The condition is usually bilateral

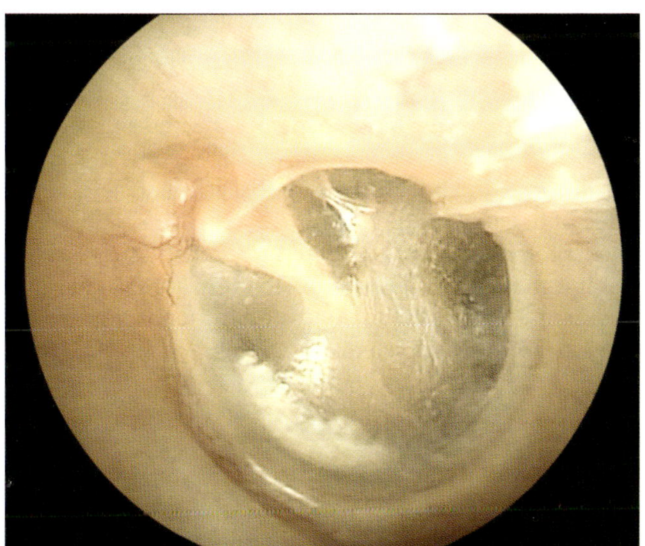

Fig. 7: Myringosclerosis

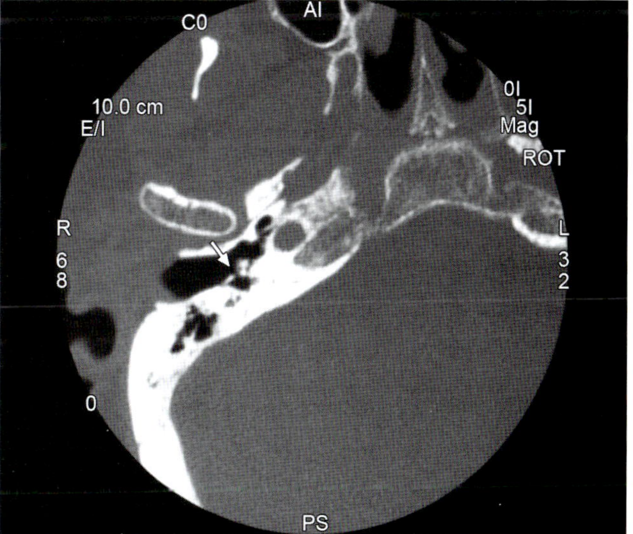

Fig. 8: CT showing calcific foci seen in relation to the tympanic membrane and adjacent mesotympanum (arrow)

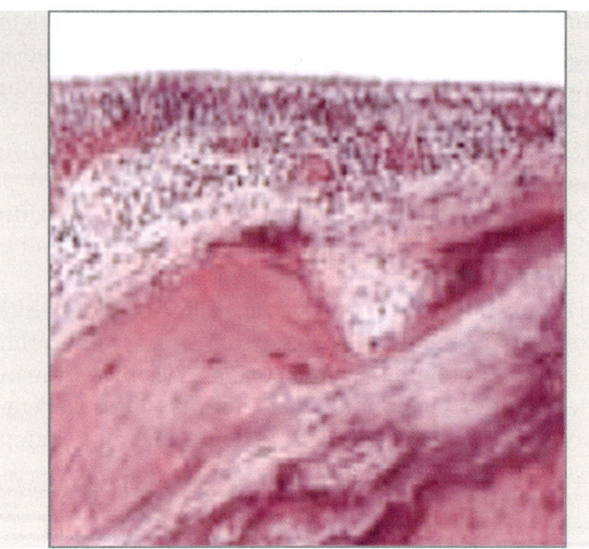

Fig. 9: Histopathology of tympanosclerosis

with past history of otitis media. Otoscopy shows white plaques of hyaline substance present in TM in pars tensa.

A large plaque involves whole anterior half of the TM and is fixed to the bony annulus in front and handle of malleus behind.

Hearing assessment by tuning fork tests and pure tone audiometry shows conductive hearing loss with Air-Bone gap. Impedance audimetry shows flattening of the normal peak due to presence of stiffness. X-ray mastoid shows poor cellularity and sclerotic bone.

Differential Diagnosis

Otosclerosis may be suspected if there is positive family history of deafness/conductive hearing loss, in addition to white plaques in either ear or sclerotic mastoid.

Cholesteatoma is suspected as white plaques look-like localized cholesteatoma. Examination under microscope is essential to solve the problem.

Treatment

Aim of treatment is to improve the patient's hearing. Surgical techniques used are—
- Removal of plaques to restore normal mobility of affected structure, repair of TM and ossicular chain. A bypass is made to overcome the affected area
- In type 1 patient, hearing improvement is satisfactory but in other types improvement varies as short-term to long-term prospect. At short-term hearing improvement, in terms of closer to Air-Bone gap is obtained in a substantial number of patients for mobilization procedures as well as for stapedectomies

- In long-term, mobility improvement shows a gradual deterioration with time. Postoperative sensorineural hearing loss is found in most patients following mobilization procedure and least after stapedectomy. For risk of iatrogenic sensorineural hearing loss, hearing aid is advised in long-term in many of these patients.

CHRONIC OTITIS MEDIA

Chronic otitis media (COM) is the permanent pathology of pars tensa or pars flaccida. It results from AOM, –ve middle ear pressure or OME. The classic term chronic suppurative otitis media (CSOM) is now not advocated as COM is not always associated with production of pus. As per George G Browning, Classification of COM[16] is as follows:
1. Active COM—It is the inflammation of middle ear cleft with production of pus. Active COM is further classified into—
    - Active mucosal COM—perforation with otorrhea
    - Active squamous epithelial COM—Cholesteatoma.
2. Inactive COM—The middle ear mucosa is not inflamed, but there is potential change for the ear to become active. It is also of two types—
    - Inactive mucosal COM—dry perforation
    - Inactive squamous epithelial COM—retraction, atelectasis and epidermalization.
3. Healed COM—There is permanent abnormality of pars tensa without propensity of ear to become active. Pars tensa is intact. There is no significant retraction of tympanic membrane.

Healed perforation (Dimeric membrane)—Loss of lamina propria results in dimeric membrane consisting of epidermis and mucosa.

Tympanosclerosis—It is end result of a healing process where the hyaline deposits of acellular materials are visible as white plaques in tympanic membrane and submucosal layers of middle ear.

Fibrocystic and Fibro-osseous sclerosis—In some cases of healed COM, tympanic membrane is marked by thickening due to proliferation of fibrous tissue. Middle ear and mastoid spaces are overrun by fibrosis and cyst formation—fibrocystic sclerosis and by deposition of new bone—fibro-osseous sclerosis.

Active Mucosal COM (CSOM Without Cholesteatoma)

Active mucosal COM is characterized by intermittent or persistent otorrhea, perforation in tympanic membrane (usually central) and no cholesteatoma present.

Pathology

It is chronic inflammation localized to the mucosa of middle ear and mastoid, usually to the anteroinferior part of middle ear cleft. As in other chronic infection there is varying degrees of edema, submucosal fibrosis, hypervascularity and infiltration of lymphocytes, plasma cells and histocytes.

Ulceration of mucosa with proliferation of blood vessels, fibroblast and inflammatory cells results in formation of **granulation tissue.**

Pathological Changes

- Aural polyp—The mucosal changes progress and coalesce to form aural polyp. It may protrude through perforation and present in EAC. It is pale in contrast to pink, fleshy polyp seen in attico antral disease (Fig. 10)[17]
- Resorptive osteitis of ossicular chain. In active mucosal COM, there is resorption of parts or all of the ossicular chain with replacement of granulation tissue.The long process of incus and superstructure of stapes are mostly affected because of their delicate structure (Fig. 11)
- Bone erosion is a feature of active mucosal and active squamous epithelial COM. The inflammatory process leads to elaborate molecular factors like—
  - Cytokines (Interleukin IL-1, interleukin-6)
  - Tumor necrosis factors (TNF)
  - Protein mediators, e.g. growth factors
  - Nonprotein mediators, e.g. prostaglandins, neurotransmitters and nitric oxide.

These molecular factors initiate recruitment, development and activation of osteoclasts resulting in bone resorption.[18]

Cholesterol Granuloma

Cholesterol granuloma is present in some active COM (both mucosal and squamous epithelial subtypes). It is a special variant of foreign body granulomatous reaction representing a host reaction to cholesterol crystals.

Sites are—Paranasal sinuses/Tympanic cavity/Mastoid aircells/Petrous apex of the temporal bone (Figs 12 and 13).

Etiopathogenesis of cholesterol granuloma is not clear.

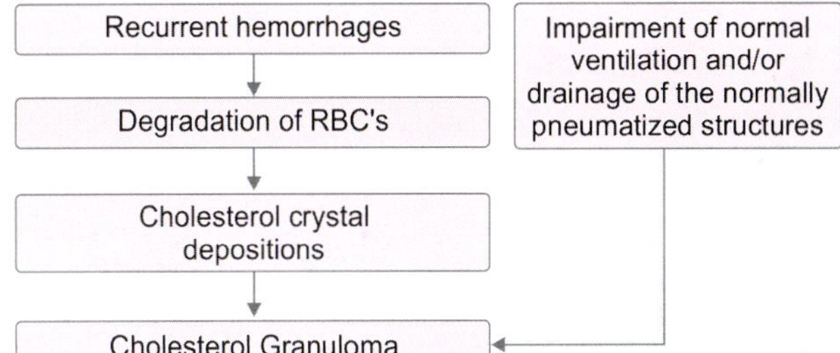

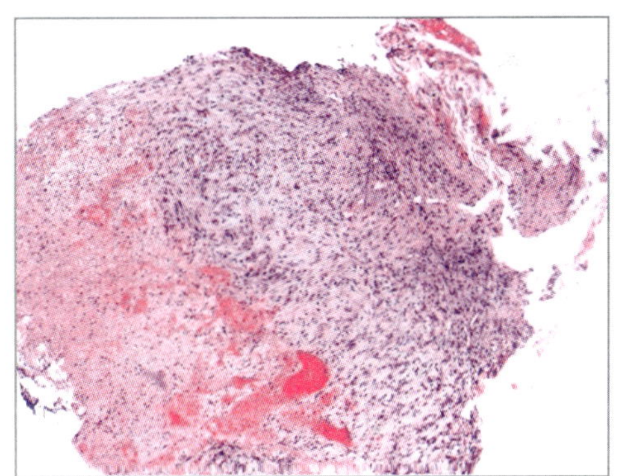

Fig. 11: Histopathology of aural polyp showing fragments of granulation tissue fibrinous exudates

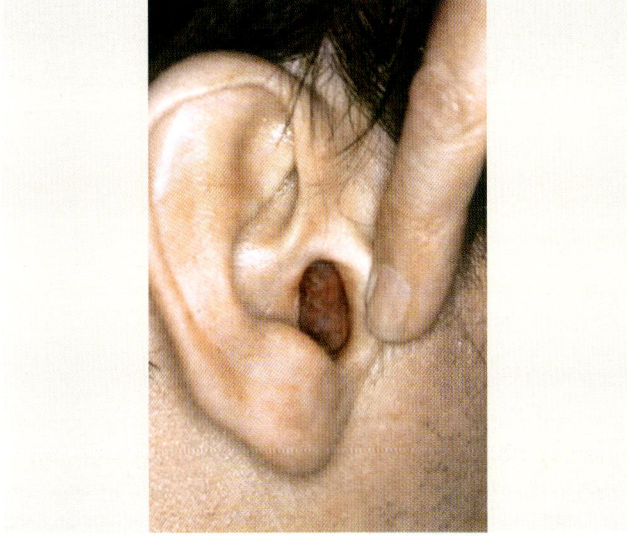

Fig. 10: Aural polyp in right EAC

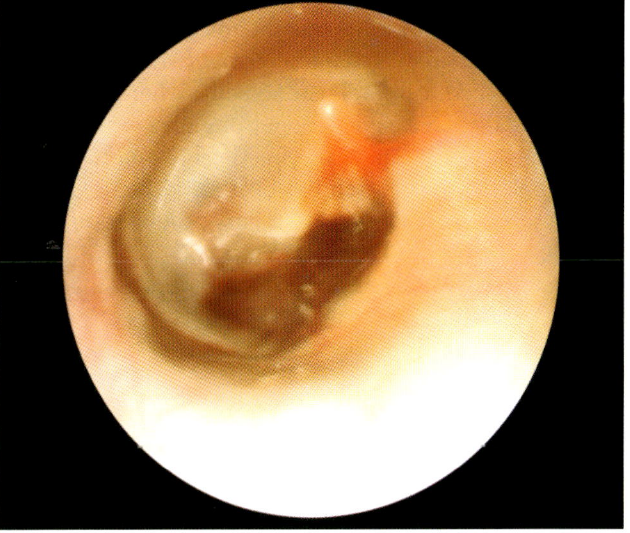

Fig. 12: Cholesterol granuloma behind TM

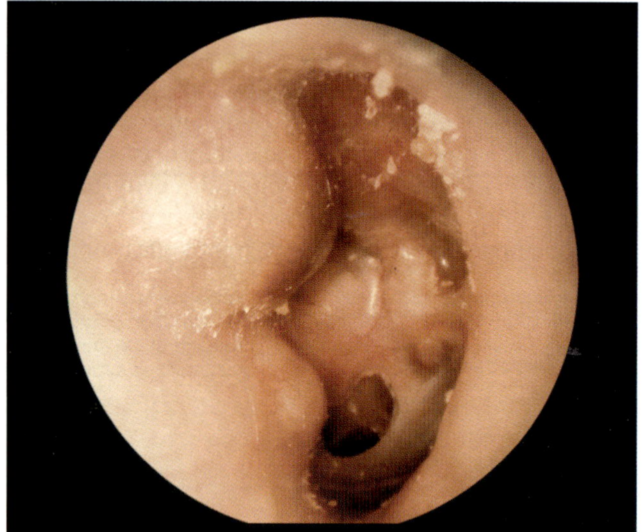

Fig. 13: Cholesterol Granuloma in mastoid cavity

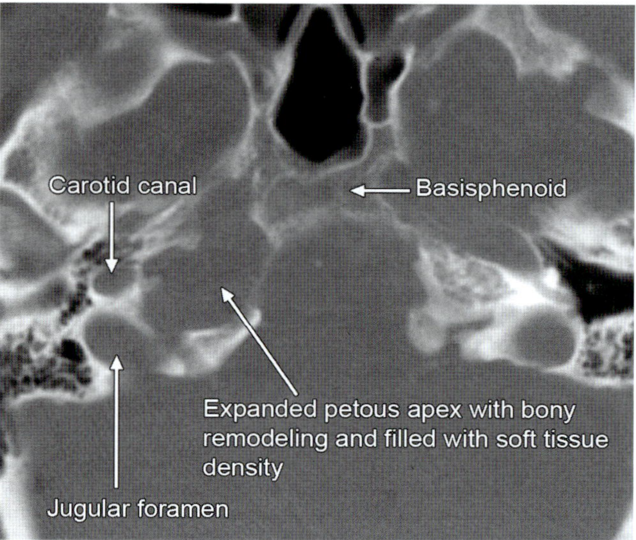

Fig. 14: CT scan of petrous apex cholesterol granuloma

Virtually, any mass within the middle ear cavity may produce mechanical obstruction to ventilation resulting in cholesterol granuloma.

Morphology: When it involves the middle ear space, it generally arises within a fluid-filled middle ear. With an intact tympanic membrane, it appears blue. Grossly, it appears as brown to yellow brown material which may compress adjacent structures. Bone erosion is absent.

Petrous Apex Cholesterol Granuloma

Petrous apex cholesterol granuloma is a sharply demarcated expansile lesion which produces deformity of the internal auditory canal. Local pressure causes destruction of VII and VIII cranial nerve.

In CT scan of petrous apex, cholesterol granuloma shows sharply demarcated rounded mass which is isodense with the adjacent cerebral parenchyma, whereas CT scan of congenital cholesteatoma of petrous apex is hypodense compared to cerebral parenchyma (Figs 14 and 15).

Microscopy shows—cholesterol clefts/hemosiderin/degenerating RBCs/Fibrosis/Capillary proliferation/and a variable giant cell inflammatory response.

Treatment of cholesterol granuloma is the drainage and the evacuation of the lesion (Fig. 16).

Prevalence of COM

It is prevalent in developing countries and in lower socioeconomic groups in developed countries. It is highest in Eskimos, Native Americans and Australian aborigines. It is mostly due to population characteristics and environmental factors rather than uses of antibiotics.

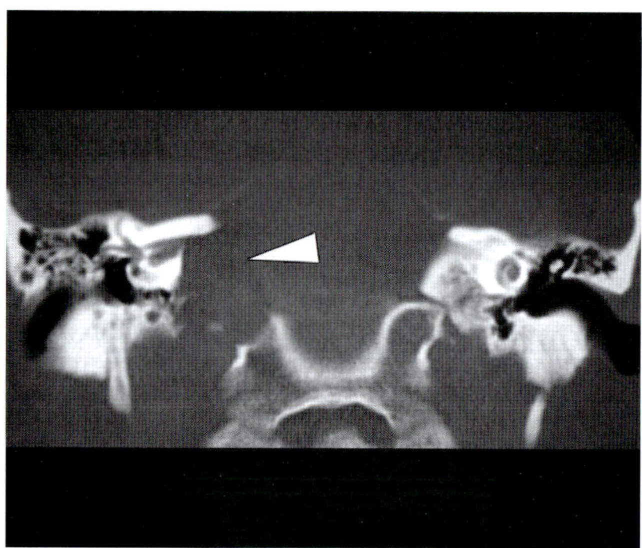

Fig. 15: Coronal CT of Congenital cholesteatoma of petrous apex

Etiologic Factors

As discussed in connection to AOM, some of these factors are equally associated with development of COM.

Bacteriology

Most common bacteria responsible for COM is *P. aeruginosa*. Others aerobic organism include Proteus, *Esch. coli, Staph. aureus, Streptococci, K.pneumoniae* and *H.influenzae.*

Anaerobic organisms are *Peptostreptococcus* and *Bacteroides fragilis.*[19]

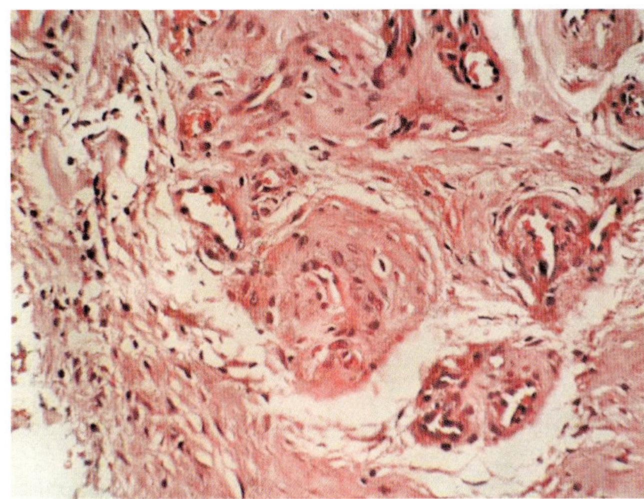

Fig. 16: Microphotograph of cholesterol granuloma—granulation tissue, multinucleated giant cells, clefts of cholesterol crystals and fresh hemorrhages

Otoscopy or examination under microscope (EUM)—shows tympanic membrane perforation.

By definition all perforations of pars tensa are central indicative of tubotympanic disease. It may present anterior, posterior or inferior to handle of malleus. Perforation may be small, medium, large or extending to annulus (Subtotal perforation). By definition, all attic disease is 'attico-antral' and 'marginal'. 'Marginal' means absence of annulus. Annulus is absent in attic or pars flaccida. Annulus is almost always present in pars tensa perforation. Therefore the term marginal perforation applied to pars tensa is confusing and is to be avoided (Figs 17A to F).

In active disease, there is **mucoid or mucopurulent discharge**. If there is an aural polyp or foul smelling discharge, it may indicate the presence of cholesteatoma. After careful suction of discharge middle ear mucosa is assessed through the perforation. Normally, it is pale pink and moist. When inflamed, it looks red and is thickened with polypoid degeneration. The ossicular chain is intact or disrupted. The long process of incus is commonly resorbed. Mobility of incudostapedial joint is assessed under microscope by moving the handle of malleus.

Hearing loss: This is conductive type, although sensorineural hearing loss (SNHL) may occur. The hearing loss is usually 30–40 dB with little complaint from the patient. But in bilateral disease patient becomes significant deaf. Hearing loss in active mucosal COM depends on the size of perforation in pars tensa, presence of granulation tissue, mucous adhesions, tympanosclerosis and ossicular chain continuity. If ossicular chain loses continuity, hearing loss increases to 50–60 dB. Ossicular reconstruction is in need for the patient. Sometimes, patient hears better in presence of discharge than when the ear is dry. This is because of round window shielding effect that helps to maintain phase differential.

Investigation

- A full history and ENT examination is taken
- Examination under microscope is essential
- A rigid endoscope with wide viewing angle gives a good overall view of the anatomy and pathology. Its resolution and color is not as good as microscope. It is helpful if there is an open cavity mastoid and an anterior canal wall bulge for viewing the anterior recess of the tympanic membrane
- Swab for culture and sensitivity to select proper antibiotic drop
- Radiology—X-ray mastoid usually shows sclerotic mastoid but it may be pneumatized with clouding of air cells. CT scan temporal bone with 1.5 mm section in both axial and coronal cuts is an aid to surgical management. In complications of active COM, CT scan gains additional information to guide the management.

Treatment

Plan of treatment of COM is to control infection, stop ear discharge and restore hearing loss by normal functioning of middle ear. This is achieved by medical as well as surgical measures.

Medical Measures are –

- Aural toilet—All discharge and retained debris are removed by suction clearance. Aural toilet comprises 1.5% acetic acid irrigation at body temperature, 3 times a day, with an ear syringe. Acetic acid irrigation removes retained debris, acidifies the external auditory canal and exposed middle ear and prevents growth of pseudomonas and other bacteria[20]
- Ear drop—Topical antibiotic drops (e.g. Ciprofloxacin or ofloxacin preparation) instilled 3 or 4 times daily are helpful to bring infection under control. They are combined with steroids which have local anti-inflammatory action
  Some ear drops, e.g. neomycin, gentamycin are potentially toxic that must be avoided to use
- Systemic antibiotics—Systemic antibiotics have poor penetration of middle ear in COM. They are less effective than topical antibiotics and are of limited use. Quinolone antibiotics have good antipseudomonal activity but they are not prescribed in children because of potential

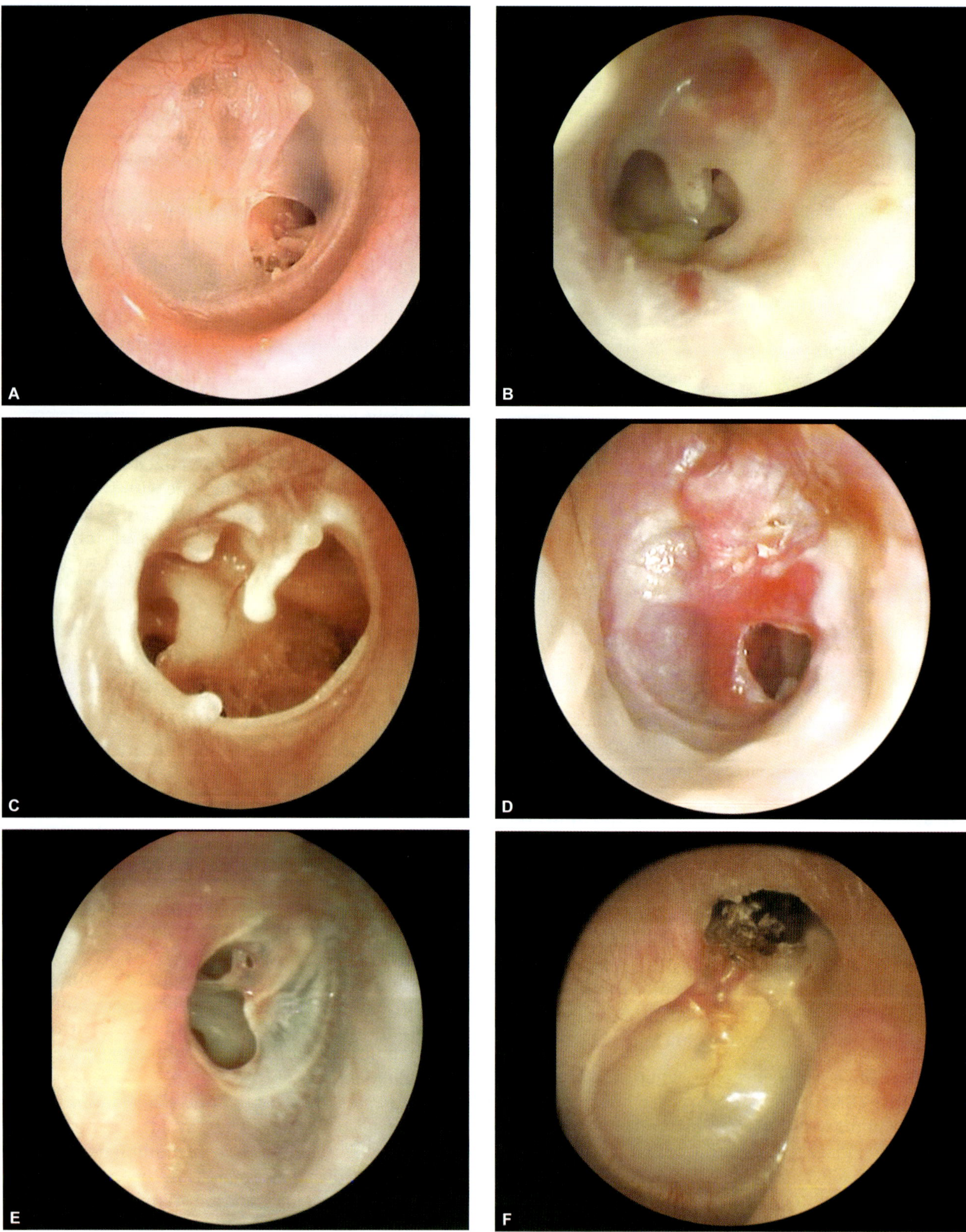

Figs 17A to F: (A) Central perforation in anteroinferior quadrant of pars tensa; (B) Large central perforation of TM; (C) Subtotal perforation; (D) Marginal perforation; (E) Posterior marginal perforation; (F) Attic perforation

risk of arthropathies. Broad spectrum penicillin, such as piperacillin and third generation cephalosporins administered parenterally are recommended in children.[21]

Surgical Measures

Persistent infection needs surgery. An aural polyp or granulation if present is to be removed before aural toilet or topical antibiotic treatment. Aural polyp must not be avulsed as it may arise from stapes, facial nerve or lateral semicircular canal (LSCC).

Tymanoplasty: If ear becomes dry with medical treatment and the middle ear mucosa is healthy, a tympanoplasty with repair of TM and ossicular chain, if necessary is advised.

Tympanomastoid surgery: If ear discharge still persists in spite of medical treatment cortical mastoidectomy with tympanoplasty is recommended.

Cholesteatoma: (Active Squamous COM)

Cholesteatoma is defined as a three-dimensional epidermal and connective tissue structure, usually in the form of a sac and frequently conforming to the architecture of various spaces of the middle ear, attic and mastoid. This structure has the capacity for progressive and independent growth at the expense of underlying bone, displacing or replacing middle ear mucusa and has a tendency to recur after removal. (Abramson—Cholesteatoma, first international conference, Birmingham, 1977)

Cholesteatoma is a bone eroding skin-lined cavity filled with concentric layers of desquamated squamous epithelium (Shambaugh).

Types of cholesteatoma are—
- Congenital
- Primary acquired
- Secondary acquired
- Tertiary acquired
- Recurrent
- Residual.

Congenital Cholesteatoma

It is believed to arise from an embryonic rest of epithelial tissue in an ear without TM perforation, in a patient without a history of ear infection (Derlacki and Clemis)[22]

On Examination

- It appears as a white cyst-like structure within the middle ear (intratympanic) or temporal bone consisting of stratified squamous epithelium with associated keratin debris (Fig. 18). It is most commonly located in the anterosuperior quadrant of mesotympanum
- The TM is intact without any retraction pocket
- No history of otitis media/Eustachian tube dysfunction or trauma
- Hearing is usually normal except when it is in the posterosuperior quadrant.

Course

It can progress if untreated with resultant local destruction of bone and eventual disruption of the tympanic membrane.

Source

It is postulated to be persistence of the epidermoid formation, a derivative of the first branchial groove. This

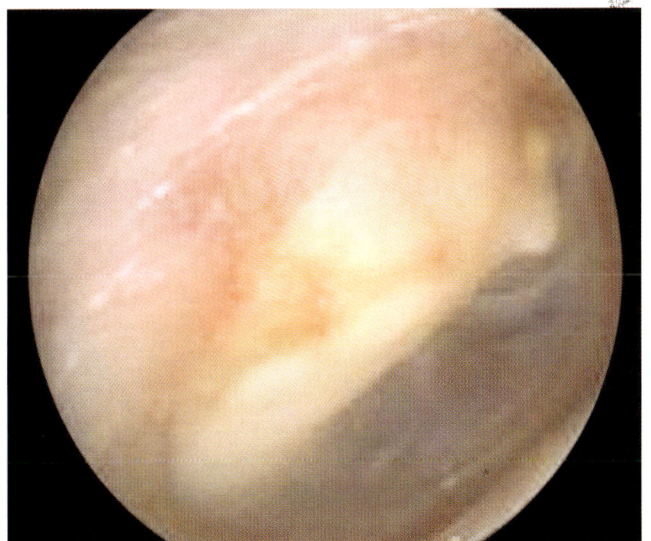
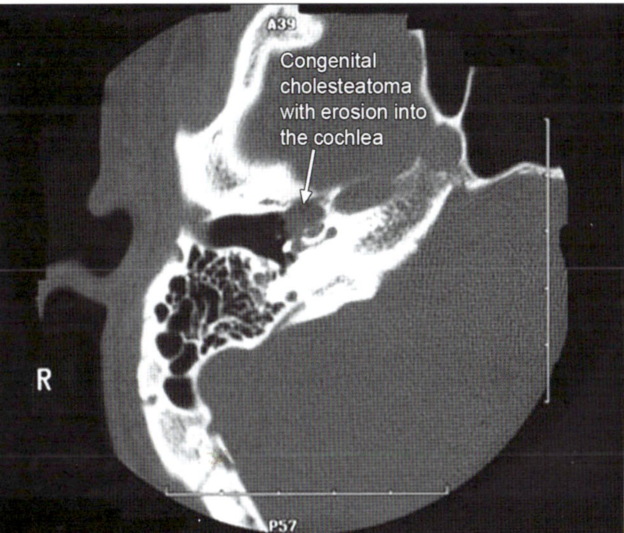

Fig. 18: White cyst-like structures within the middle ear with intact TM

mass of epithelial cells is found at the junction of the Eustachian tube and middle ear. It usually involutes by 33 weeks of gestation.[23,24]

Sites—Congenital cholesteatoma may be seen

- Within TM
- In the middle ear
- In petrous apex of temporal bone.

It may be at times associated with cleft lip and palate.

Treatment

Anterosuperior location (most common)—Extended anterior tympanotomy is recommended. It involves incising the periosteum off the handle of malleus in continuity with the TM.

Posterosuperior quadrant location: Intact canal wall tympanomastoidectomy is advocated.

Primary acquired cholesteatoma is associated with a defect in the pars flaccida. There is formation of a pocket which is unable to clear itself. Perforation usually develops after cholesteatoma formation. It often does not involve the middle ear and leaves the ossicular chain intact. The sac is usually well-defined (Figs 19A and B).

Secondary acquired cholesteatoma arises from ingrowth of epithelium through a perforation of the pars tensa or pars tensa retraction pocket. It is usually associated with marginal perforation (sometimes central) (Fig. 20).

- It invades the middle ear and mastoid and frequently involves the ossicular chain
- The sac is usually ill-defined.

Predisposing factors are

- Infection
- Eustachian tube dysfunction.

Tertiary cholesteatoma is an acquired cholesteatoma which exists behind a normal appearing tympanic membrane (Fig. 21).

It may result from a single chronic inflammatory event of the middle ear.

- Penetrating injury to TM
- Impulsive injury to TM

} Implantation of squamous epithelium in the middle ear.

Chronic infection/Eustachian tube dysfunction are usually not seen in this type.

Residual cholesteatoma is defined as a disease that grows back from viable squamous epithelium that was not removed at the initial surgical procedure.

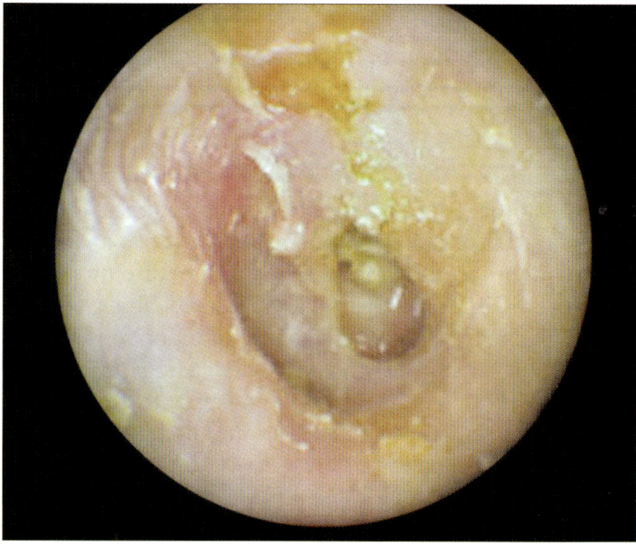

Fig. 20: Secondary acquired cholesteatoma

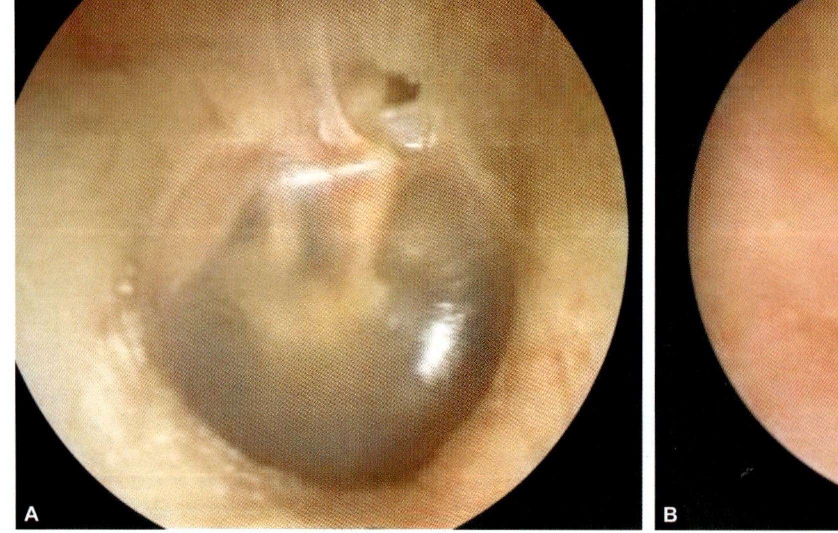

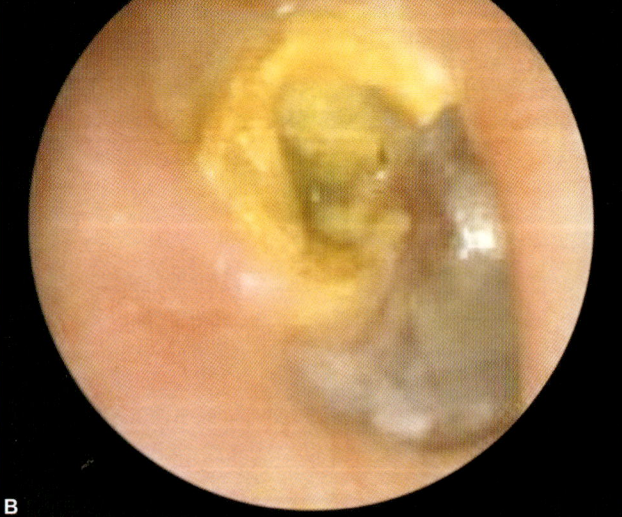

Figs 19A and B: (A) Primary acquired Cholesteatoma in early stage; (B) Primary acquired Cholesteatoma in later stage

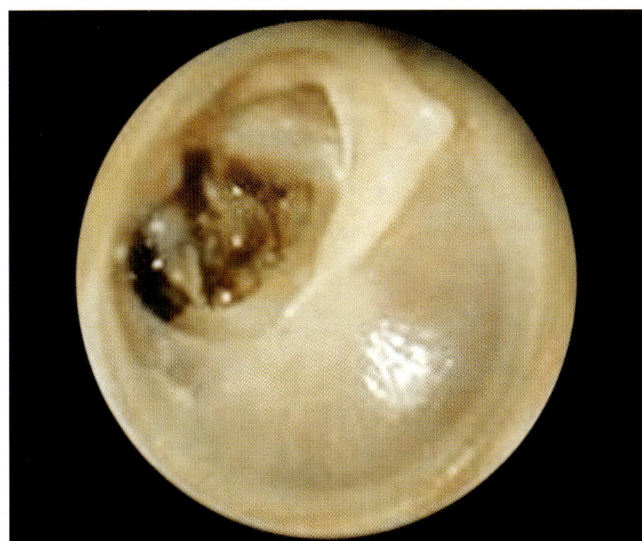

Fig. 21: Tertiary Cholesteatoma—acquired cholesteatoma resulting from a single chronic inflammatory event of middle ear

Recurrent cholesteatoma is a disease that grows back because of the inability of the Eustachian tube adequately to aerate the middle ear, mastoid or both, resulting in a retraction in the ear drum with keratin accumulation and bone reabsorption.

Recidivistic cholesteatoma encompasses all residual and recurrent cholesteatoma and is used in reporting the effectiveness of therapy for this condition. This was introduced because clinically defining the difference between residual and recurrent disease is usually impossible and can only be made by inference.

Theories of Cholesteatoma Origin

Immigration or Invasion Theory (Politzer)

Cholesteatoma develops from epithelium that has migrated through a perforation of the tympanic membrane. The rationale of immigration (invasion) theory is based on—
- Normal direction of canal skin growth is laterally, although medial migration of epithelium has been known to occur
- Temporal bone histology and operative observations especially in cases of marginal tympanic membrane defects have shown that their stratified squamous epithelium lining portions of the middle ear is continuous with canal skin. This was first suggested by Politzer.[25]

Arguments against it are—
- The double layer of mucosa which is necessary for acceptance of the invasive mechanism is not seen on the medial aspect of cholesteatoma

- The coexistence of columnar and keratinizing cells in the wall of cholesteatoma sac is more in favor of a dichotomous development of pleuripotent skin cells in response to an inflammatory or infectious stimulus.

Ex-Vacuo Theory

It was proposed by Wittmak (1930s). Keratinizing squamous epithelium, rather than entering the middle ear as a solid, invasive sheet or plug of tissue, becomes invaginated or sucked-in as a result of persistently reduced middle ear pressure because of Eustachian tube malfunction and then forms a retraction pocket in the epitympanum or posterosuperior part of the mesotympanum.

Therefore, accumulation of debris due to exfoliation of keratin causes a foreign body inflammatory reaction within the walls of sac, resulting in the formation of granulation tissue and consequent bone destruction, thus creating new areas into which squamous epithelium can penetrate. And once inflammation develops, epithelial necrosis can cause a breach in the neck of sac resulting perforation.

Arguments against it are—

The relatively minor alterations from normal pressure cannot by themselves explain the existence of deep retraction pockets (Sade).

Development of a pars flaccida retraction pocket transforming into an attic cholesteatoma is rarely observed in often recurring cases of persistent middle ear effusion (MEE) treated on several occasions by paracentesis.

It is rarely observed at operation that the retraction pockets in the posterosuperior part of the tympanic membrane are clearly seen to obstruct the isthmus tympanicus occurring in association with a separate attic cholesteatoma.

Metaplastic Theory

It is postulated by Sade and Weisman.

It requires existence in the attic of pleuripotent cells which can be misprogrammed by biochemical factors.

Metaplastic changes in mucosa are seen in chronic bronchitis, sinusitis and rhinitis, etc. The middle ear mucosa is also a type of respiratory mucosa which can undergo transformation from one specific cell population into another under inflammatory conditions. Metaplasia of the low cuboidal epithelium, usually found in the middle ear, occurs to keratinized stratified squamous epithelium leading to cholesteatoma in patient with chronic or recurrent otitis media.[26]

In genesis of pars tensa cholesteatoma, squamous epithelium produced by metaplasia in the epitympanum grows inferiorly and medially to the ossicles and eventually extends laterally causing necrosis of the pars tensa leading to a clinically identifiable condition.

Arguments against it are—

- Cholesteatoma is frequently found confined to the mesotympanum without any tympanic extension
- Lack of such a preclinical cholesteatoma is seen in hundreds of thousands of operations on patients with sclerosis/labyrinthine disorders.

Papillary Invagination (Ruedi)

Inflammatory stimulation of the basilar lamina of the squamous epithelium in the pars flaccida or in nearly meatal skin leads to the papillary ingrowths which have the ability to form an expanding mass of squamous epithelium. These ingrowths can later canalize and get filled with keratin product of their own maturation. The papillary invagination with central cornifications enters the epitympanum without tympanic membrane perforation.[27]

Congenital Theory (Derlacki and Clemis)

Congenital cholesteatoma arises as an embryonic rest of epithelial tissue in an ear without tympanic membrane perforation in a patient with no history of ear discharge. The source of the cholesteatoma is persistence of the epidermoid formation, a derivative of first branchial groove found at the junction of the Eustachian tube and middle ear. It normally involutes by 33 weeks of gestation. Cholesteatoma formation depends upon a lamina propria defect of congenital origin in association with an inflammatory stimulus from either middle ear or external auditory meatus.

Implantation and Invasion Theory

The rationale of implantation and invasion theory is based on trauma, ear surgery, ventilation tube insertion. These may cause medial epithelial migration resulting in cholesteatoma.

Pathology of Cholesteatoma

Gross appearance—It is pearly gray or yellow sac-like structure in the middle ear cavity, usually situated in the upper posterior part of the middle ear cleft. It discharges through a perforation of the pars flaccida of the tympanic membrane, usually posteriorly.

Microscopic Findings (Fig. 22)

1. Outer corneal layer of squamous cell epithelium—It consist of dead, fully differentiated anucleate squamous epithelium forming the outer pearly layer.
2. The matrix is composed of fully differentiated squamous epithelium resting on connective tissue.

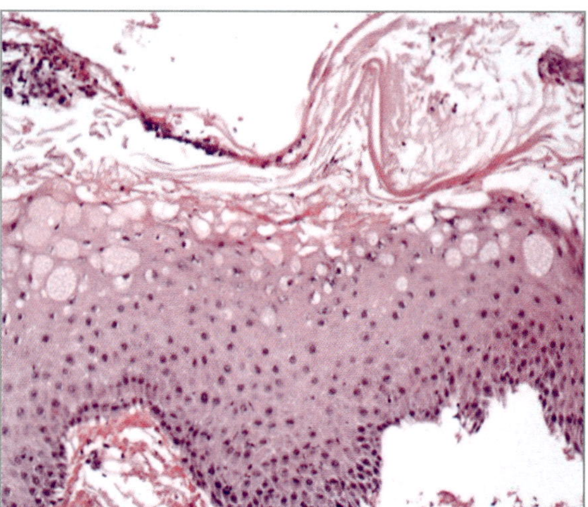

Fig. 22: Photomicroscopy of cholesteatoma

3. Deeper layers of epithelium of the matrix frequently show evidence of activity in the form of down growths into the underlying connective tissue which often separate the cholesteatoma into lobules.
4. Malpighian layer—It is composed of 5–6 rows of cells with intercellular prickles.
5. Basal layer consists of small cuboidal cells.
6. The cholesteatoma is invariably separated from the ossicles and from the trabecular bone of the mastoid cell system by a layer of granulation tissue.

Common sites of cholesteatoma origin[28] are

- Posterior epitympanum
- Posterior mesotympanum
- Anterior epitympanum

Between 3rd and 7th fetal months, four endothelially lined sacs evaginate from the first branchial pouch to form tympanic cavity.

These endothelially lined sacs are—

- Succus medius
- Succus anticus
- Succus posticus
- Succus superior.

Succus medius with contribution from succus anticus forms Epitympanum which is the most common site for cholesteatoma formation.

1. Succus medius breaks into three smaller saccules.
   a. Anterior saccule—It forms the anterior compartment of epitympanum.
   b. Medial saccule—It forms Prussak's space (common path followed by Acquired cholesteatoma) and superior incudal space (it lies above and lateral to malleus head and incus body).
   c. Posterior saccule—It passes medial to the long process of the incus and pneumatizes the petrous

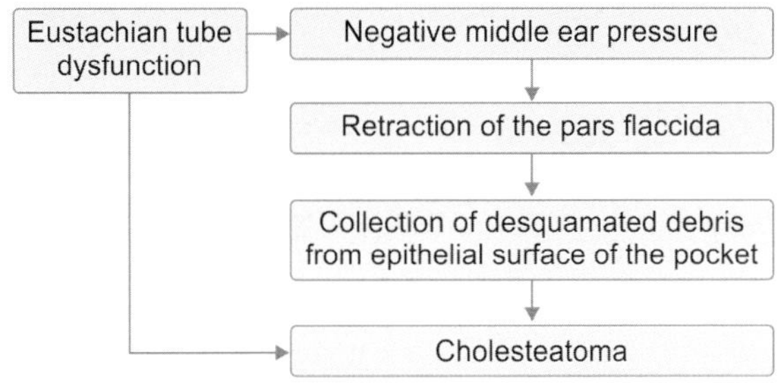

Eustachian Tube Dysfunction (Bezold)

part of mastoid air cell system. Usually, the anterior and posterior compartments of epitympanum are confluent and are separated from the anterior mesotympanum by the tensor tympani fold.

2. The succus anticus forms the anterior mesotympanum and is separated from epitympanum by tensor tympani muscle and fold. But if the growth of the succus medius is slow then the succus anticus forms the anterior epitympanum and the tensor fold remains incomplete (<=10%cases). In such cases, the epitympanum is divided vertically by the superior malleolar fold into anterior and posterior compartments. The anterior compartment communicates with protympanum and Eustachian tube, and posterior compartment is ventilated via the tympanic isthmus and aditus ad antrum.

3. Succus superior passes between handle of malleus and long process of incus. It forms inferior incudal space (beneath the body of incus) and pneumatizes the squamous portion of temporal bone.

The boundary between mastoid pneumatization derived from the succus superior (squamous) and succus medius (petrous) may be evident as a bony plate known as the petrosquamosal lamina or korner's septum. During mastoidectomy, it may mimic the medial wall of the antrum.

4. Succus posticus forms the posterior mesotympanum and hypotympanum. The facial recess, sinus tympani, round window and much of the oval window all are derived from this sac.

Pathways of epithelial migration on the tympanic membrane (Fig. 23) is determined by photography of Bouney's blue (a mixture of crystal violet and brilliant green solution) at weekly interval using a Storz Hopkins rod.

Dye moves posteriorly and superiorly from the pars flaccida region on to the adjacent external canal.

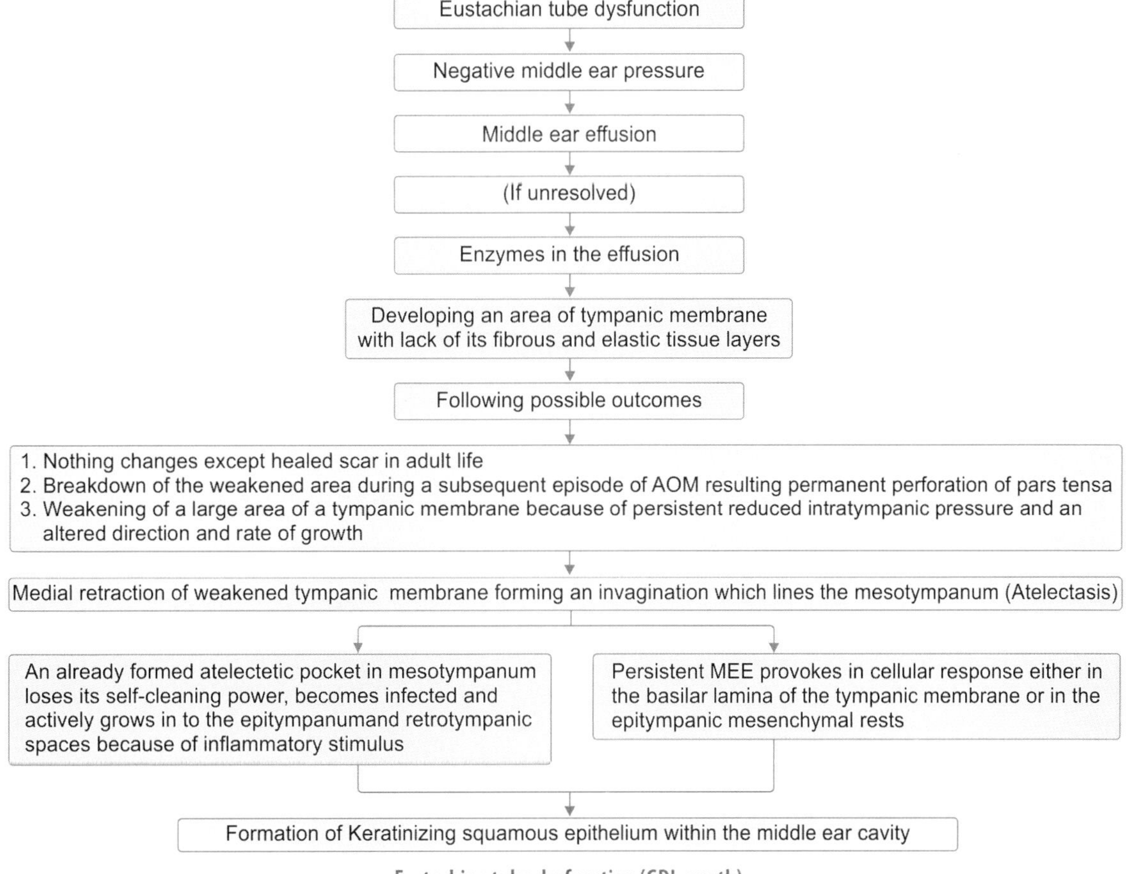

Eustachian tube dysfunction (GDL smyth)

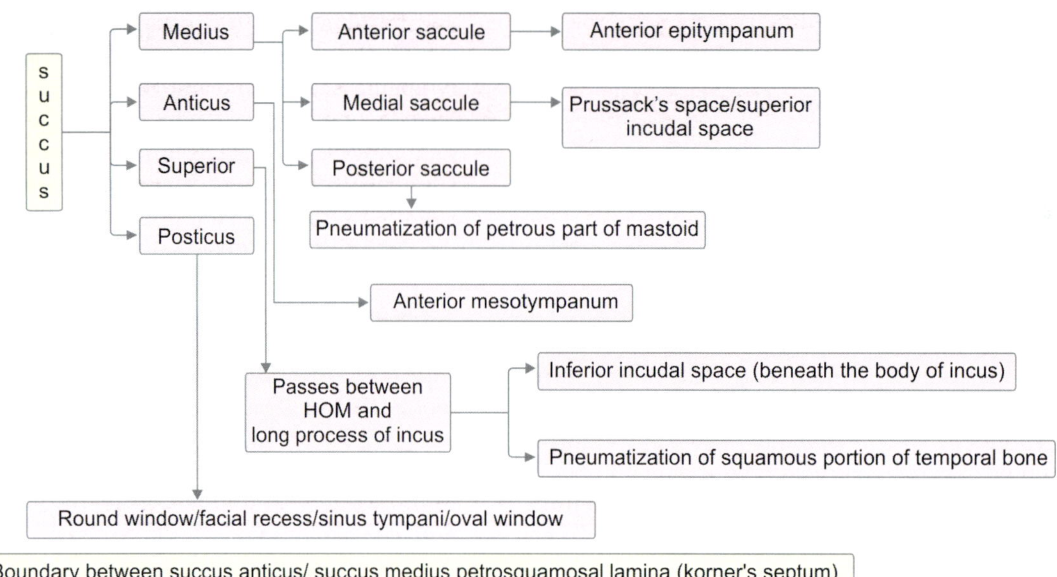

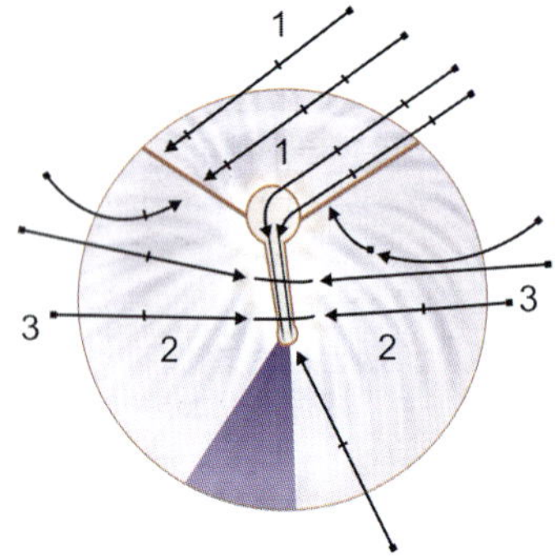

Fig. 23: Pathways of epithelial migration on tympanic membrane. Zone1: pars flaccida region; zone 2: pars tensa region; zone 3: deep external canal

Dye also moves posteriorly and outwards synchronously with pars flaccida daubs if placed on the deep external canal.

Dye placed on handle of malleus moves upwards as far as the lateral process and then moves posterosuperiorly as on pars flaccida.

Dye placed just outside this zone moves away from it to the periphery.

The migratory epithelial movement throughout the life is generated in the same way as elucidates by photographic otoscopy.

Growth Patterns of Cholesteatoma

Most common sites of origin of acquired cholesteatoma by decreasing frequency of occurrence are discussed as follows:

1. **Posterior epitympanic cholesteatoma** follows the embryonic course of succus medius.

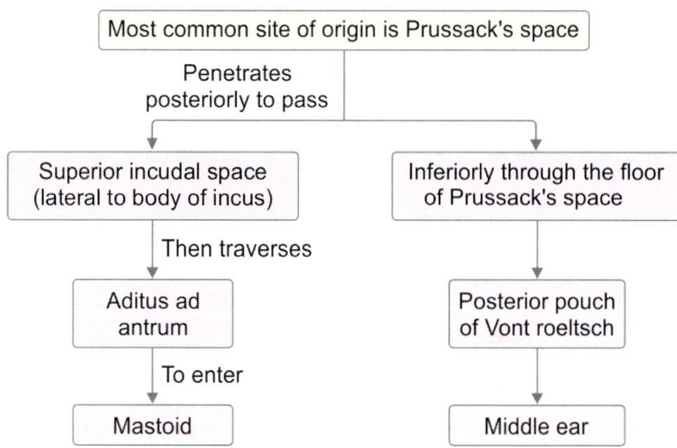

2. **Posterior mesotympanic cholesteatoma** follows the course of succus posticus and succus superior. It commonly involves facial recess and sinus tympani; surgical inaccessibility makes these cholesteatoma more difficult to excise completely.

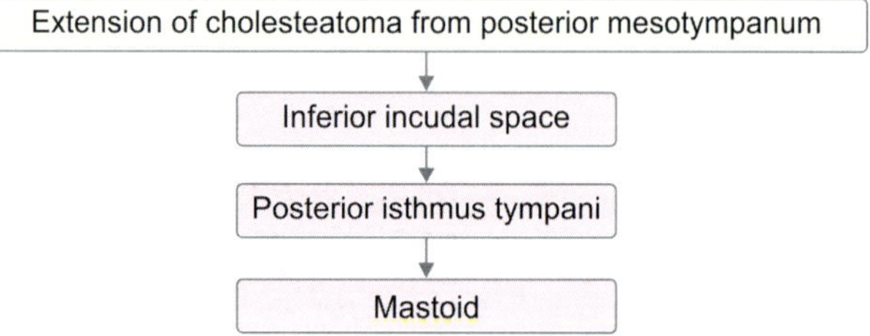

These cholesteatomas pass medial to the malleus and incus in contrast to posterior epitympanic cholesteatoma which passes lateral to the body of incus.

3. **Anterior epitympanic cholesteatoma**—It follows the course of either succus anticus or anterior saccule of succus media.

It results from epitympanic retraction anterior to the head of the malleus.

It can cause facial nerve dysfunction since the floor of the anterior epitympanum is related to the horizontal segment and geniculate ganglion of the facial nerve. Extension—

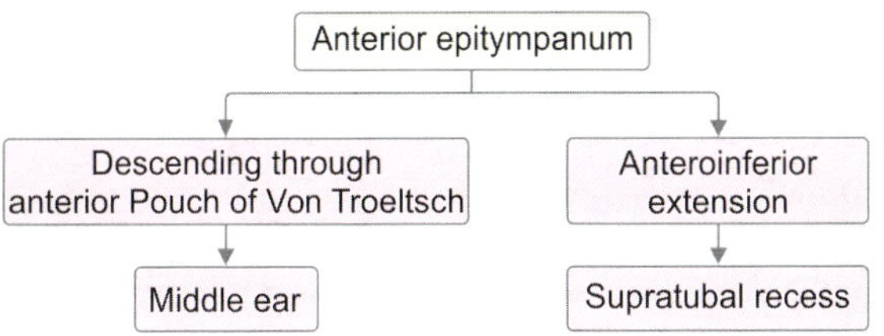

Clinical Features

Symptoms

Otorrhea: Patients having COM with acquired cholesteatoma presents with recurrent or persistent ear discharge. The ear discharge is scanty, purulent with foul smelling due to osteitis. Some patients with cholesteatoma show cessation of discharge from ear, since perforation might be sealed by debris or polyp. Pus may find its way internally resulting intracranial complications.

Hearing Loss: About 80% of patients develop hearing loss. It is usually conductive but mixed hearing loss is encountered later on. Hearing is normal when ossicular chain is intact or cholesteatoma is bridging the ossicular gap caused by the disease.

Tinnitus: It is also common.
Vertigo/disequilibrium may result from labyrinthine erosion by cholesteatoma in few cases.
Facial nerve palsy may result from pressure effect on nerve from inflammatory process (Fig. 24).

Signs

Perforation/Retraction pocket/Cholesteatoma: Attic perforation or a marginal perforation in posterosuperior quadrant of pars tensa is present (Fig. 25). If a small scab is present over attic or upper annulus it is to be removed since it may hide attic or posterosuperior disease. In primary acquired cholesteatoma, retraction in pars flaccida is seen in most cases and retraction of pars tensa is seen less frequently.

Degree of retraction varies, in early stage retraction pocket is shallow and self-cleaning and later on the pocket is deep; it accumulates pearly white flakes of cholesteatoma that can be sucked out.

Aural polypi and granulation: It may be present. These originate from chronic disease within middle ear cleft. Suction clearance and examination under operating microscope are important to assess ossicular erosion, labyrinthine windows and exposed tympanic mucosa. Examination with a rigid endoscope is helpful to know the extent of disease and to decide the management.

In secondary acquired cholesteatoma—If cholesteatoma develops from tympanic membrane perforation, cholesteatoma may be visible through the perforation.

If cholesteatoma develops from implantation of squamous epithelium during surgery or through perforation that is healed but TM may appear normal, Cholesteatoma may once enlarge in middle ear it may visible behind the TM.

Tenderness over mastoid antrum indicates involvement of mastoid.

In all cases, facial nerve (CNVII) is examined to know the erosion of facial canal.

A **fistula test** is performed to consider vestibular dysfunction. Examination of CNS is performed if intracranial complications are suspected.

Radiology: Convention Radiography—Lateral-oblique view of mastoid is carried out to see the cellularity of mastoid and position of the lateral sinus and the middle fossa.

If radiography shows low lying dura or an anteposed sigmoid sinus in a sclerotic mastoid, it helps the surgeon to undertake the proper surgical procedure. Destruction in the attic and the antrum caused by cholesteatoma is seen as a radiolucent area surrounded by an opacity caused by the sclerosis.

CT scan is of great value to delineate the extent of disease. Bone windows axial and coronal cuts of 1.5 mm

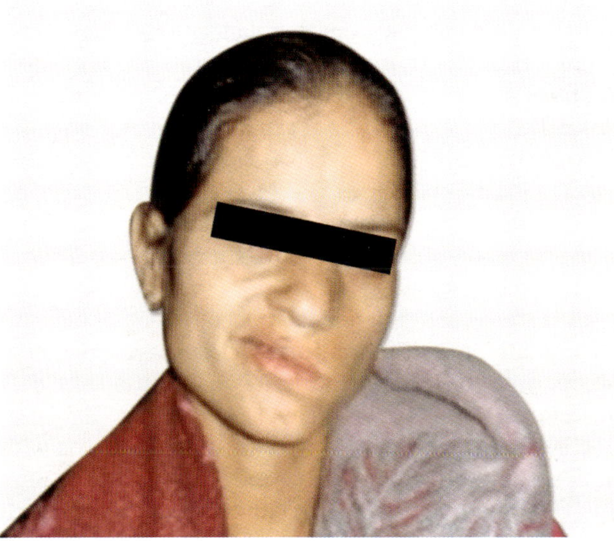
Fig. 24: Left side CSOM with complete facial nerve falsy

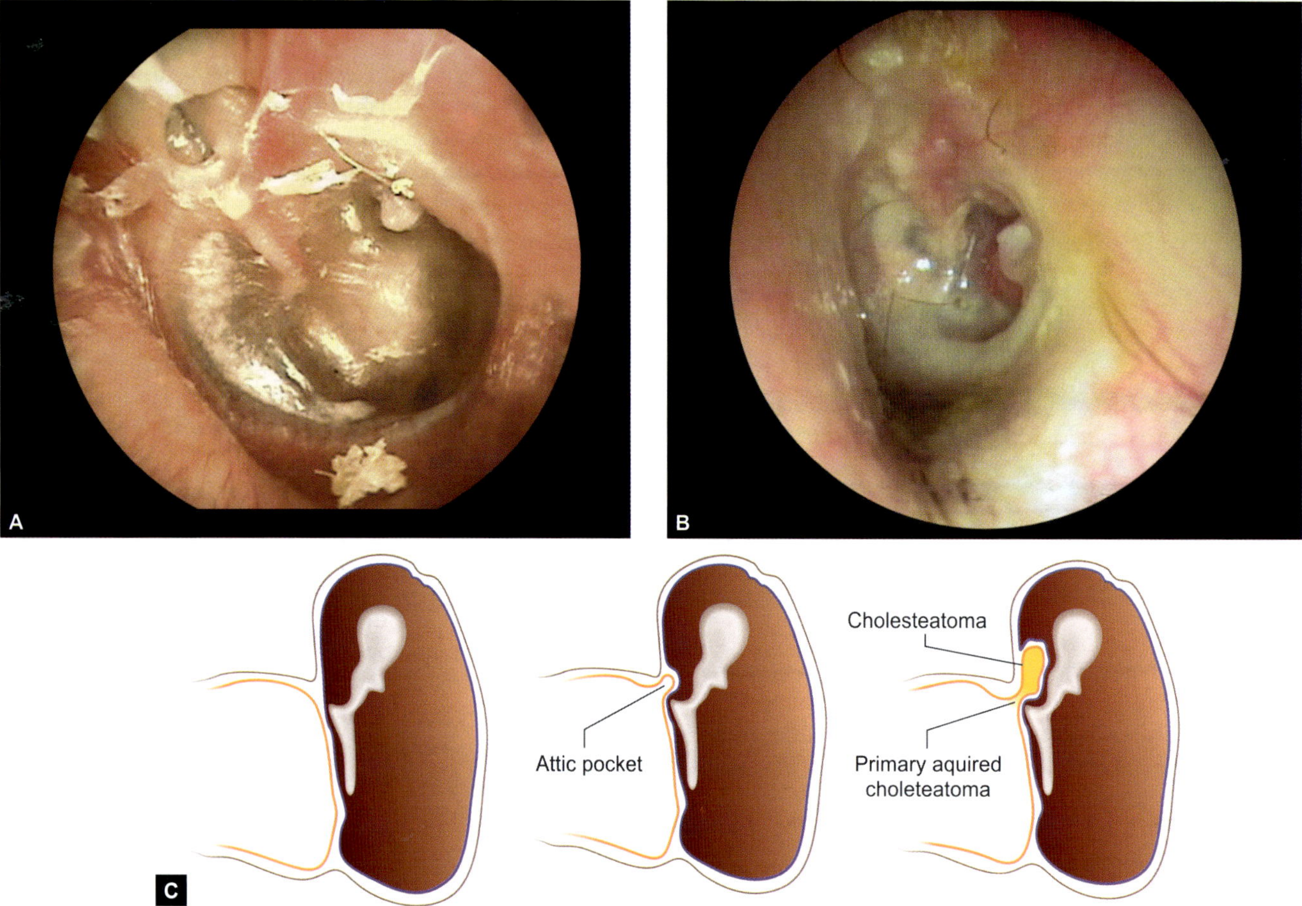

Figs 25A to C: (A) Attic perforation with Cholesteatoma; (B) Marginal perforation in posterosuperior quadrant of pars tensa; (C) Primary acquired cholesteatoma

slices are ideal (Fig. 26). Cholesteatoma appears as a mass of soft tissue density in the middle ear and mastoid that cannot be differentiated from granulation tissue, cholesterol granuloma or other soft tissues or fluid. CT can show bone erosion of scutum, ossicular chain, erosion of labyrinth with fistula and dehiscence of facial canal. Negative CT does not rule out a fistula (10–15% cases). Facial nerve dehiscence is detected in 66% of 29 cases (Fuse T et al.).[29]

CT is not done routinely, specific indications are revision surgery, suspicion of inner ear fistula or possibility of petrous apex disease.

MRI shows better delineation of soft tissue. It helps to differentiate cholesteatoma from other soft tissues, such as a neoplasm or an encephalocele. It is mainly used to assess the lesion of petrous apex (Fig. 27).

Hearing Assessment: Voice test, tuning fork test with 512 cps tuning fork (Rinne, Weber and Schwabach) and pure tone audiometry reveal mainly conductive deafness up to 60 db hearing loss. The presence of sensorineural hearing loss hints the possibility of labyrinthine fistula or recurrent inflammatory process.

Features suggesting complications are—

- Pain—indicating extradural, perisinus or brain abscess
- Vertigo—Indicating erosion of LSCC
- Persistent headache—Suggesting intracranial complication
- Facial weakness—Indicates erosion of facial canal
- Fever, nausea and vomiting—Indicates intracranial infection
- Irritability and neck rigidity—Hints meningitis
- Diplopia—Suggestive of Gradenigo's syndrome
- Ataxia—Indicating labyrinthitis or cerebellar abscess
- Abscess around the ear—Suggestive of mastoiditis.

Differential Diagnosis

- Chronic otitis media without cholesteatoma
- Otitis externa

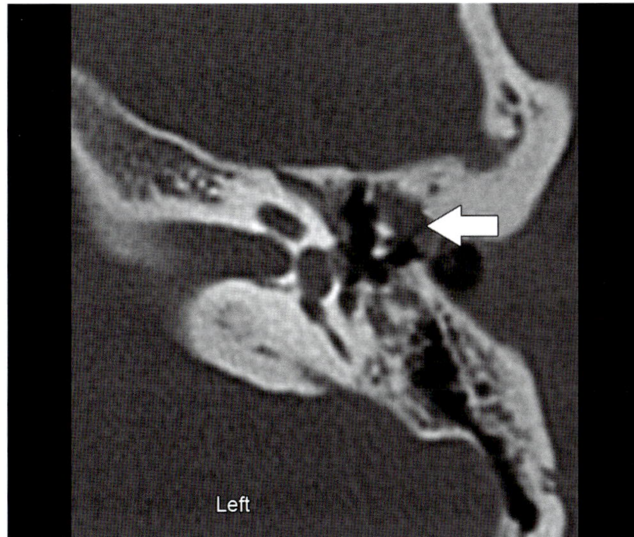

Fig. 26: CT shows cholesteatoma present as a mass of soft tissue density in middle ear with bone erosion of lateral epitympanic wall

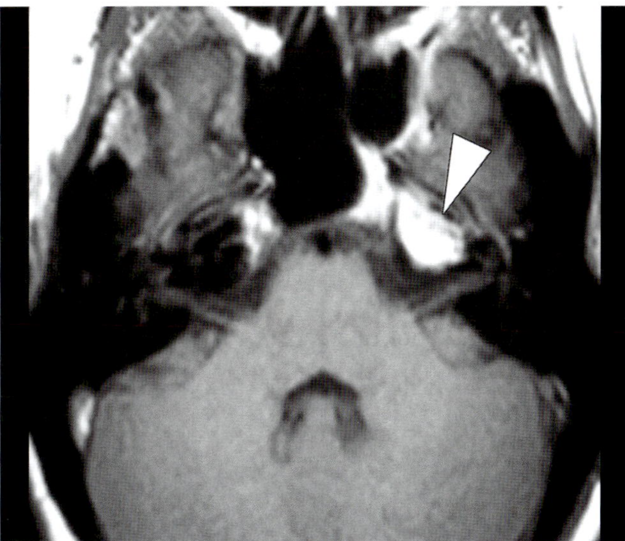

Fig. 27: T1-weighted axial MRI shows cholesteatoma of petrous apex

- Malignant otitis externa
- Squamous cell carcinoma of the ear
- CSF otorrhea
- Tuberculous otitis media.

Treatment

The mainstay of the treatment for cholesteatoma is surgery. The aims of surgery are—
- Complete eradication of the disease
- Creation of a dry, self-cleaning ear
- Restoration of impaired hearing, if possible.

The surgical techniques for active squamous COM are—
- Canal wall down mastoidectomy (open cavity)
- Intact canal wall mastoidectomy (closed cavity).

Canal Wall Down Mastoidectomy (CWD)

The traditional method involves exploration of mastoid using posterior to anterior approach, exenteration of cholesteatoma that is followed forward through aditus into attic and exteriorization of diseased area and mastoid cavity through EAC by removal of posterior bony wall of the canal. Commonly performed operations are—
- Atticotomy
- Atticoantrostomy
- Modified radical mastoidectomy
- Small cavity mastoidectomy (Sade).

The canal wall down technique usually creates a large cavity that may continue to discharge and even if well-epithelialized the cavity does not self-clean.

Recurrent infections of the cavity, pain, granulations or polyp formation are common. Regular care of the cavity by an ENT surgeon is mandatory. The cavity problem may cause nuisance from socioeconomic aspect, employment and marriage.

The main reason for open method is to reduce the incidence of the recurrence of the cholesteatoma. It does not prevent cholesteatoma (Abramson 9%, Gristwood 17%, Sade 20%). Therefore, one should be justified in creating problem by doing open cavity technique.

Small cavity mastiodectomy or atticoantrostomy, anterior to posterior approach is becoming more popular. The surgeon starts removal of cholesteatoma from epitympanum or posterior mesotympanum and follows it backwards. It results a small cavity of mean volume of 1.4 cm^3 compare to larger cavity of mean volume of 2.4 cm^3 following modified radical mastiodectomy.[30]

When cholesteatoma is limited to attic, only atticotomy is performed. The attic wall is closed with tragal or conchal composite cartilage. It is observed that the cavity is actively discharging in 52% cases and dry in 48% cases. Significant changes in active cavity are[31]—
- Incomplete removal of the disease
- High-facial ridge
- Exposed middle ear
- Narrow meatus.

To get a dry ear or to avoid a persistently discharging ear, mastoid and middle ear surgery need following practice.
- Complete removal of the disease, particularly from facial recess and tympanic recess
- Lowering of facial ridge at the level of lateral semicircular canal so that the floor of the external auditory canal (EAC) and the floor of the mastoid cavity lie in the same plane

- Tympanic membrane grafting to obtain a good TM and a mucosa lined air-filled middle ear space
- Ossicular reconstruction to get a good hearing by establishing a connection between the vibrating TM with mobile stapes
- Wide meatoplasty is required to get a wide meatus for self-clearance of the cavity and better postoperative care.

Canal wall down surgery has lower rates of recurrence (5–15%) and the recurrence of disease is easily detected in OPD, thus second look operation is rarely needed. Contraindications for open cavity mastoidectomy are—

- COM without cholesteatoma—Extensive debridement of mastoid or atticoantral infection is accomplished with preservation of posterior canal wall
- Wide exposure of sigmoid sinus, dura and facial nerve caused by the disease.

Close Method or Intact Canal Wall Mastoidectomy (CWVD)

It is done in cases of cholesteatoma confined to attic, antrum with intact sac and mesotympanum. Steps involved are—

- A simple mastoidectomy and removal of polypoid mucosa and delineation of cholesteatoma with its sac in the antrum
- Tympanomeatal flap is elevated. Transcanal atticotomy and widening of bony canal including posterior bony rim to expose sinus tympani
- Total clearance of cholesteatoma and granulation tissue from attic, antrum and middle ear including sinus tympani along with necrosed ossicles is done
- Reconstruction of lateral attic by using a piece of conchal cartilage with perichondrium is done
- Ossicular reconstruction, if any ossicular deficit is present
- Reconstruction of TM by using temporalis fascia—in lay technique.

Advantage of CWU Technique

- It keeps an intact external auditory canal and avoids an open mastoid cavity
- Postoperative hearing thresholds are better.

Disadvantage of CWU Technique

- It is technically more difficult and requires larger operating time
- Incidence of recurrence of cholesteatoma is high (20–50%) so second look operation after 12–18 months may be necessary[32]
- Radical mastoidectomy—It is performed in case of extensive cholesteatoma extends down the Eustachian tube or into the petrous apex or chronic granulation disease involving tympanomastoid region with extension in the Eustachian tube and destruction of entire middle ear mucosa with dead ear
- In these cases, canal wall down (CWD) or open cavity mastoidectomy results in very large cavity. Here healing of the cavity is a big problem. Obliteration of the cavity with conchal cartilage and inferiorly based myoperiosteal flaps is done in most cases where complete disease clearance is achieved. Postoperative ears are almost normal with hardly any cavity problem; the cavity usually heals in a period of 2–3 months depending on the size of the cavity.

Revision surgery is performed in case of—

- Graft failure
- Recurrence of disease
- Stenosis of the EAC
- When there is no improvement of hearing.

In close cavity technique, revision procedures are—

- Canaloplasty for canal stenosis
- Myringoplasty in graft failure cases
- Tympanoplasty for residual cholesteatoma in the middle ear
- Conversion to open cavity for recurrence of cholesteatoma in the atticoantral region
- Tympanotomy with ossiculoplasty in cases of fibrous adhesions, atelectasis and dislocation of ossicle grafting.

In open cavity technique revision processes are—

- Meatoplasty for meatal stenosis
- Revision tympanoplasty with mastoidectomy for recurrence of cholesteatoma and cavity problem
- Tympanotomy for release of fibrous adhesion and ossiculoplasty.

Complications of surgery—are infrequent. Accidental damage to semicircular canals while drilling to find out mastoid antrum especially in a sclerosed mastoid or dislocation of stapes footplate while removing the disease in the oval window and facial canal area may result in total loss of hearing. If facial nerve is injured, nerve grafting by using greater auricular nerve is done. The incidence of dead ear is 2% and that of intraoperative facial nerve palsy is 1% even in hands of expert surgeons. The incidence is higher when surgery is done by inexperienced surgeons.

Complications of Otitis Media

Complications may happen in acute phase of infections (i.e. AOM) or in chronic phase of infection related to bone destruction (i.e. COM with cholesteatoma) (Table 2). With ready access to medical treatment and use of modern antibiotics complications from AOM have reduced. Mastoiditis is the most common complication frequently

Table 2: Classification of complications

Type		Complications
	Middle ear	- Tympanic membrane perforation - Facial nerve paralysis - Ossicular necrosis
A. Intratemporal	Mastoid	- Petrositis - Decreased pneumatization - Mastoiditis
	Inner ear	- Labyrinthitis - SNHL
B. Extratemporal	Extracranial	Subperiosteal abscess - Postauricular abscess - Bezold's abscess - Luc's abscess - Zygomatic abscess - Citelli's abscess (Digastric abscess)
	Intracranial (Extradural)	- Meningitis - Extradural abscess - Lateral sinus thrombosis

	Intracranial (Intradural)	- Subdural abscess
		- Brain abscess
		  • temporal
		  • cerebellar
		- Otitic hydrocephalus

Others		- Developmental problems - Behavioral Problems

seen in children. Nevertheless, intracranial otogenic complication is still life-threatening resulting from COM with cholesteatoma.

Tympanic Membrane Perforation

It is a known complication of untreated OM. It is due to increased pressure in the TM either from purulent matter in mesotympanum or from long standing Eustachian tube dysfunction (Fig. 28).

Mostly TM perforation heals spontaneously in AOM. Some patients are left with persistent perforation. The perforation or defect usually occurs in the pars tensa and is variable in size

Hearing loss associated in TM perforation ranges from 0 to 40 db. Examination under microscope is important to rule out occult cholesteatoma or any ossicular pathology. Closure of perforation and improvement of hearing are seen in 90% of patients.[33]

Facial Nerve Paralysis

Facial nerve paralysis may occur as a result of either AOM or COM. The nerve paralysis is due to bacterial toxins or direct pressure applied to nerve by cholesteatoma or granulation.

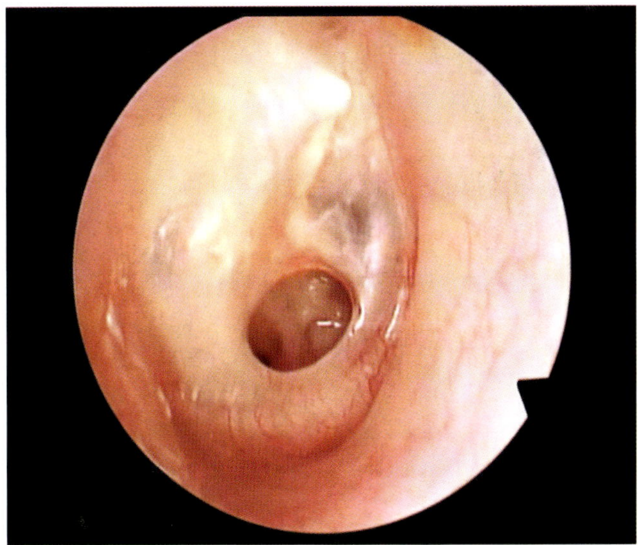

Fig. 28: TM perforation—a complication of untreated AOM

HRCT of temporal bone is essential for evaluation of nerve lesion in OM. Electrical tests of nerve function is seldomly required.

If facial nerve paralysis occurs within the first 10 days of AOM, it is thought to be caused by edema of the nerve within the bony canal of the facial nerve in the middle ear as in Bell's Palsy. Complete recovery is expected with conservative treatment. On the other hand, facial nerve paralysis occurs after 2 weeks of infection, it is believed to be the result of erosion of osseous facial canal exposing the nerve to suppuration. The most common area of involvement is the tympanic segment. IV antibiotics, concomitant corticosteroid together with myringotomy and drainage of pus from middle ear are adequate for resolution of incomplete paralysis. Cortical mastiodectomy is advised for intractable cases.[34]

If facial nerve paralysis occurs in COM, cholesteatoma or granulation tissue results in osteitis and bone erosion to expose the nerve to infection. Urgent facial nerve decompression is indicated. For complete facial paralysis with loss of electrical excitability facial nerve is explored from the first genu to the stylomastoid foramen. Decompression of the nerve is done above and below the area of disease until healthy nerve is seen. Nerve grafting or nerve rerouting and end-to-end anastomosis is done if a dehiscence of nerve trunk is noted.

Petrositis

It is an inflammation of petrous part of temporal bone (Fig. 29). It occurs both in acute and chronic forms. Acute

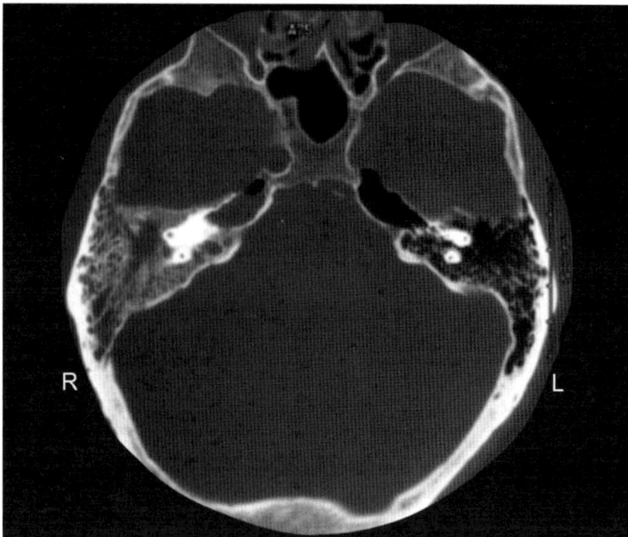

Fig. 29: An axial CT scan of the temporal bone shows inflammation of petrous apex

petrositis results from the extent of infection of acute mastoiditis to pneumatic cells in the petrous pyramid.[35]

Chronic petrositis results from mucosal or cholesteatomatous COM. Pneumatization of petrous apex occurs in less than 1/3rd of petrous bones with cell extending from the middle ear or mastoid to the petrous apex. When it does occur petrositis is an uncommon and devastating complication.

Two cell tracts are present:
- *Posterosuperior Tract:* It starts from mastoid running behind or above the bony labyrinth to the petrous apex
- *Anteroinferior tract:* It starts at the hypotympanum near the Eustachian tube, runs around the cochlea to reach petrous apex.

Infection goes along these cell tracts to the reach to the petrous apex forming epidural abscess that involves 9th cranial nerve and trigeminal ganglion. Because of close proximity of ophthalmic division of the trigeminal nerve and abducent nerve to petrous apex, classical features of petrositis are—
- Persistent otorrhea
- Retro-orbital pain
- Lateral rectus palsy (Gradenigo syndrome).

Less common symptoms of petrositis are—
- Transient facial nerve paresis
- Mild recurrent vertigo and
- Intermittent and low-grade fever.

Diagnosis of petrositis is suspected if persistent purulent otorrhea and deep-seated pain persist in spite of a well done mastiodectomy.

Diagnosis is confirmed by HRCT temporal bone to see bone details of petrous apex and air cells.

MRI helps to delineate diploic marrow of apex from fluid or pus. Gallium 67 and technetium 99m bone scan show increased radioactive uptake on diseased side.

IV antibiotics and surgical drainage are the treatment of choice for petrositis. There are several surgical approaches to the petrous apex in addition to preliminary complete cortical mastoidectomy with skeletanization of the semicircular canals.

Three primary factors that determine the surgical approach to petrous apex include:
- Location of infection
- Pneumatization of temporal bone
- Status of hearing.

In absence of hearing—
- The translabyrinthine approach provides adequate exposure of posterior portion of petrous apex
- The transcochlear approach is done when more anterior exposure is needed. This approach is accomplished without rerouting the facial nerve.

In presence of hearing—
- If anterior drainage is needed
  - Subtemporal approach—it provides wide window of access
  - Infracochlear approach—it provides a very narrow window of access.
- It provides the route for sustained gravity dependent drainage
- If posterior apicitis is present, it is approached by
  - Retrolabyrinthine route
  - Subarcuate route.

Both routes provide adequate access in well-pneumatized bone and keep allowing adequate drainage and better hearing preservation.

Mastoiditis

As there is direct connection between middle ear and mastoid, infection in the middle ear may extent to mastoid hair cell system. In most cases, infection does not progress to clinically apparent acute mastoiditis. In fact, acute mastoiditis is relatively rare. It may progress to acute periostitis due to spread of infection via venous channel or acute osteitis where bony destruction of mastoid air cell trabeculae results in coalescent mastoiditis.

Acute mastoiditis manifests as a complication of AOM in a child. Symptoms of acute mastoiditis are otalgia, postauricular pain and fever. Otorrhea and hearing loss are less frequently noted. The common presenting signs are postauricular tenderness (80% of cases),[36] anteroinferior protrusion of the pinna, postauricular erythema and swelling. The fullness of the posterior wall of EAC is seen on otoscopy.

CT scan of temporal bone characterized by a loss of bony trabeculae is the diagnostic study of choice to detect coalescence mastoiditis (Fig. 30). It also helps to identify occult second complication like an intracranial or neck abscess.

Most of the cases are treated by IV antibiotics and myringotomy with or without VT insertion. Culture and sensitivity should be sent for culture directed antimicrobial therapy. Mastoidectomy is indicated if response is poor even after 2 weeks of conservative management. Aim of surgery is to debride necrotic bone and to prevent intracranial complications.

Masked Mastoiditis

It is subacute mastoiditis due to low grade infection. It results from inadequate treatment of AOM by antibiotics. Symptoms and signs are less severe and more persistent than acute mastoiditis. Ventilation of middle ear and appropriate antibiotics can resolve the infections in most cases. Cortical mastoidectomy is done if above measure fails.

Labyrinthitis

It is most common intratemporal complication of OM due to extension of infection within the temporal bone. Labyrinthitis is of two types—
- Localized, circumscribed or serous labyrinthitis
- Diffuse, purulent or suppurative labyrinthitis.

Serous Labyrinthitis

It results from osteitis of labyrinthine capsule or extension of infection through preformed or acquired pathways. Hematogenous spread of infection of labyrinthine is rare.[37] The preformed pathways are as follows:
- Annular ligament of the oval window
- Round window membrane.

Acquired pathway is the fistula of lateral semicircular canal formed by cholesteatoma.

Vestibular symptoms appear first. It is followed by the cochlear symptoms. It results from depression of sensory response of labyrinth. The symptoms include vertigo, nausea and vomiting. Patient develops spontaneous nystagmus; quick component of nystagmus is towards unaffected ear or healthy side. The cochlear symptom of serous labyrinthitis is high frequency SNHL (Fig. 31).

Treatment: If the cause is early AOM—Systemic antibiotic therapy and myringotomy are done to eliminate the infection.

If the cause is COM with cholesteatoma resulting perilabyrinthine osteitis, mastoid exploration with removal of diseased bone together with IV antibiotics is advised.

Suppurative Labyrinthitis

It follows serous labyrinthitis. In most cases, bacterial invasion to inner ear from middle ear is usually via round window or erosion of bony capsule of inner ear by cholesteatoma provides an alternative route for bacteria to invade the inner ear as to serous labyrinthitis. Sometimes,

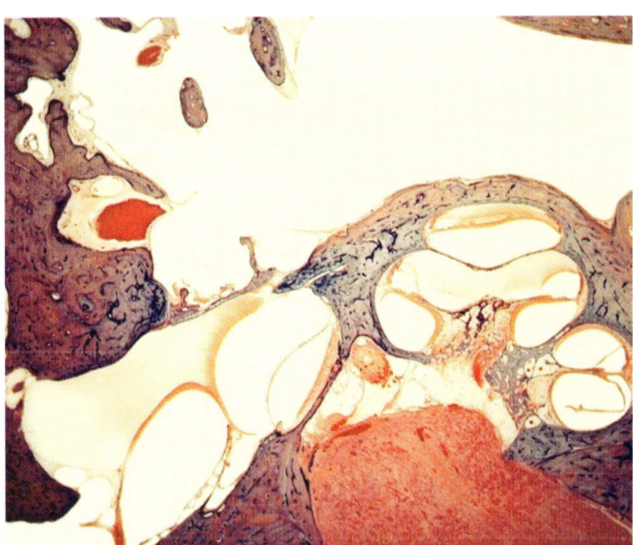

Fig. 30: CT scan showing left acute coalescent mastoiditis

Fig. 31: Presence of eosinophilic staining of the inner ear fluids indicates serous labyrinthitis

it may be the result of generalized meningitis without any prodrome of serous labyrinthitis. The symptoms of suppurative labyrinthitis are severe vertigo, nausea, vomiting and sudden SNHL. The symptoms are more intense and rapid. Caloric response is absent for diseased ear (Fig. 32).

Treatment: Systemic antibiotics and continuous monitoring for symptoms of intracranial extension are important. Surgical labyrinthectomy may be done in case of intracranial spread.

Labyrinthine Fistula

It may be formed as a consequence of infection or neoplastic ear disease or it may be surgically produced. In most cases, erosion of bone by cholesteatoma results in labyrinthine fistula. Patient presents with episodic vertigo. Fistula test is performed to detect fistula clinically either by manual tragal pressure or pneumatic insufflation by siegle's speculum. An increase in ear pressure in EAC stimulates the labyrinthine. A positive test is said when patient feels vertigo or quick component of nystagmus is towards the affected ear (due to ampullopetal displacement of cupula). If negative pressure is applied it would induce vertigo with nystagmus, Quick component of nystagmus is directed to the healthy ear due to ampullofugal displacement of cupula. Mostly fistula occurs in lateral semicircular canal and nystagmus is frequently horizantal.[38] If a fistula is present in superior canal the nystagmus is vertical. When a large (>2 mm) fistula is present it exposes simultaneously the horizontal and superior canals producing rotatory nystagmus.

A positive fistula test indicates that the labyrinthine function is still retained. A negative fistula test does not rule out fistula. Fistula test is negative in more than half of all patients with confirmed fistula.

A false negative fistula test (-ve fistula test in presence of fistula) occurs if fistula is accompanied by localized loss of function of ampulla of the involved semicircular canal or by generalized loss of function of labyrinth or cholesteatoma covers the site of fistula preventing transmission of pressure changes to the labyrinth.

A false positive fistula test (+ve fistula test in absence of fistula) is seen in congenital syphilis due to hypermobile stapes or 25% cases of Meniere's disease due to fibrous bands connecting utricular macule to the stapes footplate, that is Hennebert's sign. In both conditions, stapedial movement causes stimulation of macule of utricle.

Sometimes, patient with labyrinthine fistula experiences momentary vertigo when exposed to loud sound that is known as Tullio Phenomenon.

CT scan of temporal bone is the diagnostic test of choice to find out labyrinthine fistula to help direct surgical management (Fig. 33). In labyrinthine fistula due to cholesteatoma, surgical removal of cholesteatoma is indicated. Fistulae are managed according to the site and size of fistula and the status of hearing. There is always a risk of inner ear damage with loss of hearing in treating labyrinthine fistula (8–56%).[38] Conservative surgery includes canal wall down mastoidectomy with exteriorization of cholesteatoma matrix overlaying the large fistula. Removal of matrix overlying a large fistula involving a single semicircular canal should be avoided as it may result in deafness.

Again in small fistula less than 2 mm in size, cholesteatoma matrix is removed from fistula followed by repair of fistula with fascia, or bone plate. It infection is present, repair of fistula is staged.

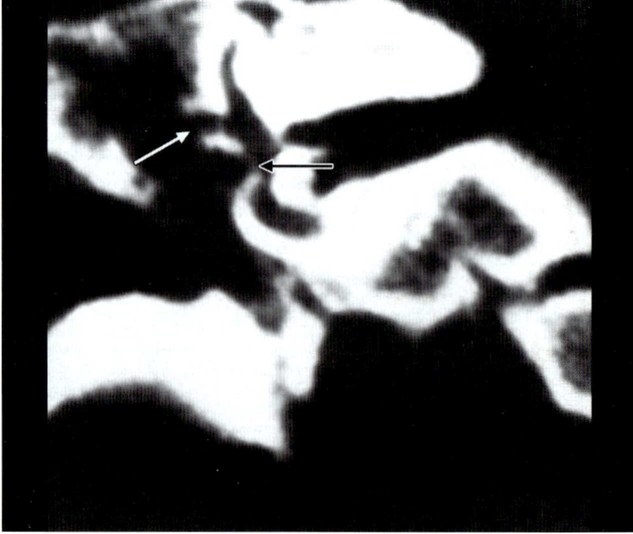

Fig. 32: Suppurative Labyrinthitis resulting from generalized E.coli meningitis

Fig. 33: HRCT temporal bone shows labyrinthine fistula connecting middle ear (white arrow) and oval window (black arrow)

Extratemporal–Extracranial Complications (Flowchart 3)

Subperiosteal Abscess

About 50% of patients with mastoiditis develop subperiosteal abscess. The periosteum in postauricular region is elevated from underlying bone and if mucopus extends to this area from mastoid cavity subperiosteal abscess forms.

Postauricular Abscess (Figs 34 and 35)

- It is the most common abscess formed as a result of direct destruction of thin cortical bone over MacEwen's triangle of mastoid or
- Hematogenous spread through vascular channels.
  It is commonly seen in well-pneumatized mastoids in children and usually associated with cholesteatoma.

Clinical Features

- Ear discharge, acute or coalescent mastoiditis and fluctuant post auricular swelling with pain and fever
- Pinna is displaced outward and forward.

Investigation

HRCT (high resolution CT) of temporal bone detects early abscess formation.

Treatment

Intravenous antibiotics, myringotomy (+/- tube placement) and postauricular Incision and drainage of pus. Pus is sent for culture and sensitivity study. Subsequent mastoidectomy after two weeks of antibiotic therapy is generally required.

Bezold's Abscess

When mucopus breaks through the tip of mastoid process into digastric groove abscess typically forms deep to the sternocleidomastoid (SCM) muscle which is referring as Bezold's abscess. In 1881, Friedrich Bezold described it as a complication of mastoiditis presented with a latero-cervical abscess (Figs 36A and B). This is rare in children and difficult to detect clinically.

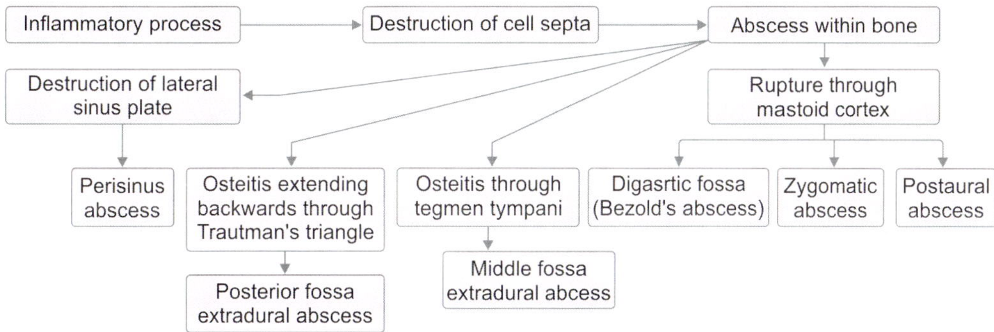

Flowchart 3: Abscess formation in different locations from mastoid

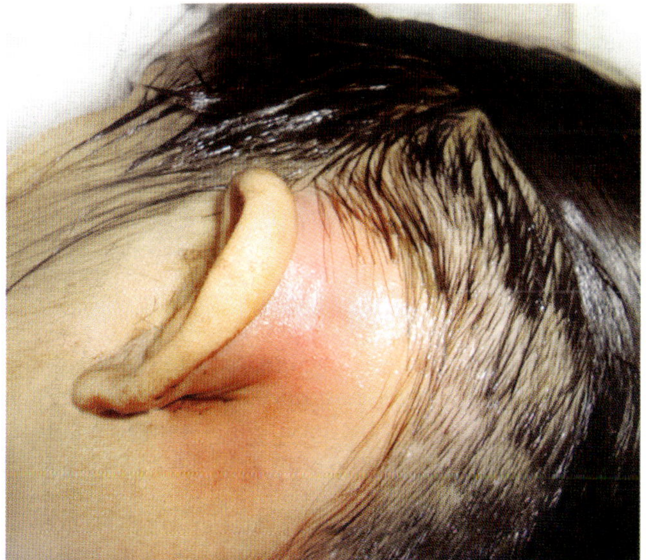
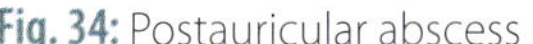

Fig. 34: Postauricular abscess

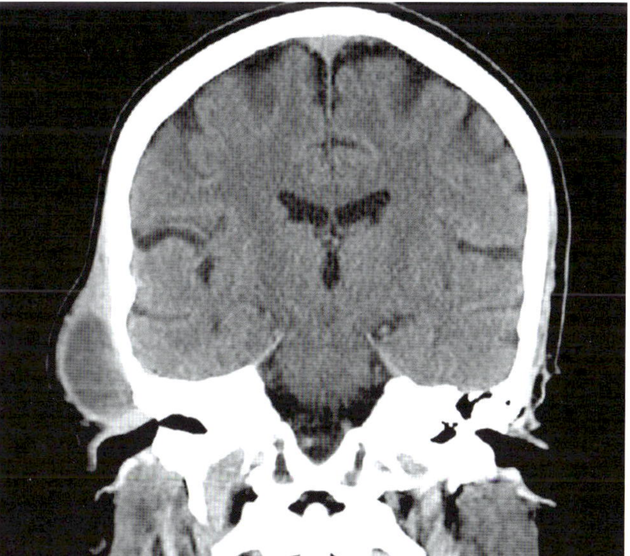

Fig. 35: Coronal CT shows a large subperiosteal abscess

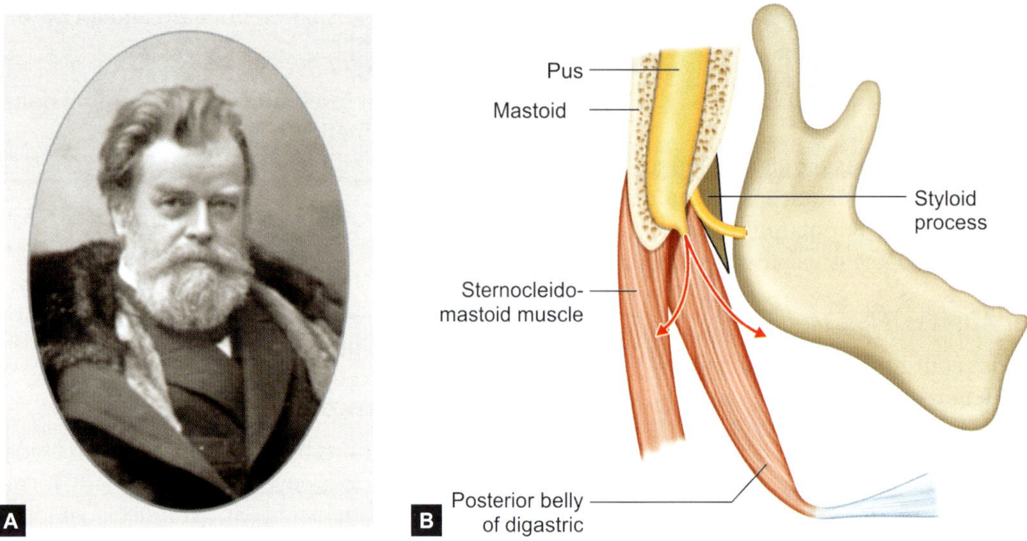

Fig. 36A and B: (A) Friedrich Bezold (February 9, 1842–October 5, 1908) German otologist; (B) Abscess breaks through mastoid tip extending deep to the sternocleidomastoid muscle or into digastric groove—Bezold's abscess

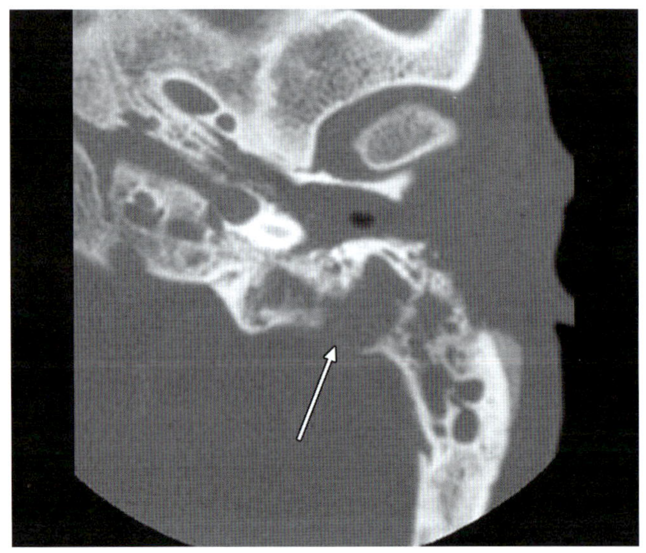

Fig. 37: Axial CECT of temporal bone shows opacification of the mastoid air cells with bone destruction (Bezold's abscess)

Clinical Features

- Patient is usually presented with pyrexia, otalgia, otorrhea, fluctuating neck swelling, restriction of neck movement, neck pain and facial nerve palsy (15 %)
- Infection rapidly spreads to involve carotid sheath, parapharyngeal space, mediastinum and posterior triangle if treatment is delayed.

Investigation

CT scan with contrast media to delineate the full extent of the disease (Fig. 37).

Treatment

- Intravenous antibiotics, incision and drainage of abscess, pus is sent for culture and sensitivity
- Myringotomy (+/- tympanostomy tube) and
- Mastoidectomy in same admition
- Postoperative oral antibiotic is given for 2 weeks.

Luc's Abscess

Infrequently mastoid abscess perforates the bony wall that is lying between antrum and external bony canal and infection runs along the external auditry canal resulting in meatal abscess or Luc's abscess. Henri Luc (1990) first described this abscess (Fig. 38).

Investigation

X-ray mastoid is useful for diagnosis of cholesteatoma in presence of subperiosteal abscess.

Ideal treatment is intravenous antibiotics and modified mastoidectomy with drainage of abscess.

Zygomatic Abscess (Fig. 39)[39]

It is a very rare complication of OM and is described as temporo parietal swelling secondary to mastoid abscess eroding the root of zygomatic process. The pus may present superficial or deep to the temporalis muscle resulting swelling infront of an above the pinna associated with oedema of upper eye lid.

High resolution computed tomography (HRCT) of temporal bone reveals—irregular osteolytic area involving posterior portion of zygomatic process and zygomatico-

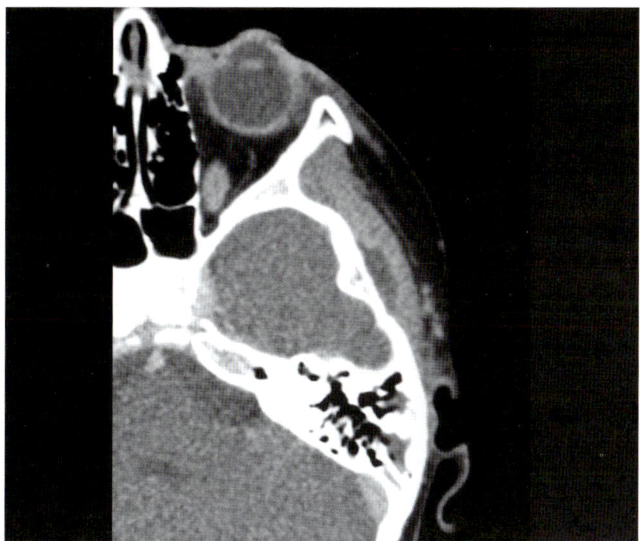

Fig. 38: CT shows low density left subperiosteal temporal collection without any bone erosion (Luc's abscess).

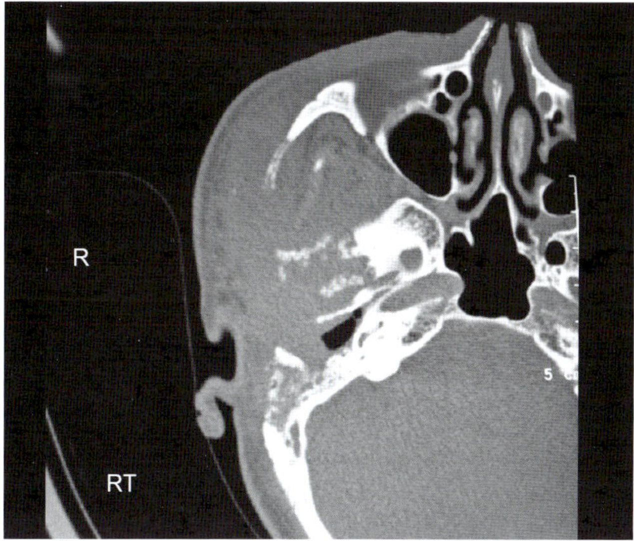

Fig. 40: HRCT temporal bone shows large osteolytic area involving the posterior portion of the right zygomatic process and zygomatico temporal junction, mastoid air cell, and middle ear cavity

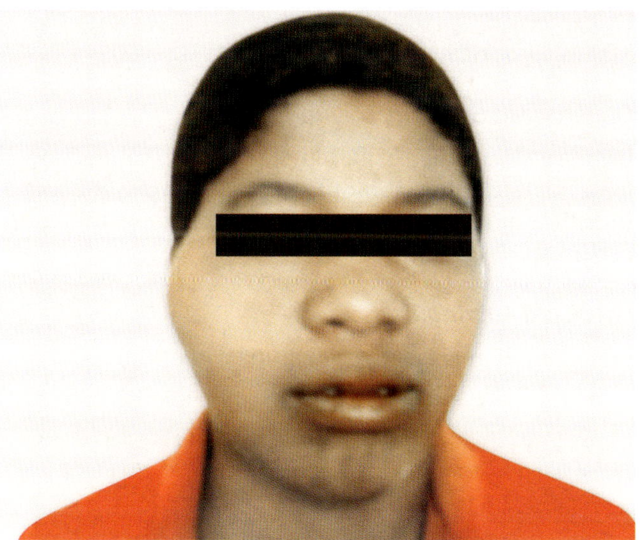

Fig. 39: Zigomatic abscess

temporal junction, mastoid air cells, middle air cavity with erosion of anterior, lateral and superior canal wall. Peripherally enhancing collection is seen around the zygomatic process with ill-defined swelling of soft tissue of temporal region (Fig. 40). Ear swab is sent for culture and sensitivity study.

Treatment protocol—Intravenous antibiotics and modified radical mastoidectomy with drainage of zygomatic abscess.

Citelli's Abscess

Abscess is formed behind the mastoid more towards the occipital bone. Pus may run along the mastoid emissary vein or occipitotemporal suture. It is considered as the abscess of the digastric triangle by some authors.

Parapharyngeal or Retropharyngeal Abscess

It results from infection of the peritubal cells due to acute coalescent mastoiditis.

Ideal treatment option is—suitable intravenous antibiotics. Cortical, modified radical or radical mastoidectomy.

Intracranial Complications of Otitis Media

Intracranial complications develop due to uncontrolled or inadequately controlled ear infection resulting spread of infection from the ear into the intracranial cavity.

Factors influencing initiation of complications are as follows:
- Virulence and antibiotic sensitivity of infecting organism
- Host resistance
- Appropriation and adequacy of antibiotic therapy
- Anatomic routes and barriers to spread infections
- Drainage of pneumatic spaces, either natural or surgical.

In acute middle ear infections common organisms are *Streptococcus pneumoniae, Haemophilus influenzae* and *Moraxella catarrhalis*. The microbiology of acute infections remains more or less constant overtime. Emergence of few antibiotic resistant microorganisms that may vary from one location to another necessitates introduction of newer antibiotics. The microbiology of chronic infection is different. In chronic infection, *Pseudomonas aeruginosa* are more common.[40] Quinolones are reserved primarily for pseudomonas infection.

Patients with immunosuppressive drugs or patients having acquired immune deficiency syndrome (AIDS) are immunocompromised. There are risk of intracranial complications and organisms causing infection are atypical pathogens.

The middle ear cleft has bony partition to prevent intracranial extension of infection. These partitions or barriers are demineralized in acute infection or resorbed by cholesteatoma or osteitis in chronic disease of ear. Demineralization is brought by enzymes that are released in acute infections. Cholesteatoma or granulation tissue causes bone erosion either due to pressure necrosis or halisterisis. Halisterisis is also known as hyperemic decalcification. Fracture of temporal bone creates passage that permits infection to bypass the natural barriers.

Mastoid cavity is about 5cc in volume and middle ear cavity is about 0.9cc in volume. Natural drainage of mastoid cavity occurs through Eustachian tube via relatively smaller middle ear space. Poor drainage causes accumulation of infected secretions that erode middle ear cleft to extend intracranially.

Routes of Intracranial Spread from Middle Ear Cleft

- Preformed tracts (nonanatomical)
  - Fractures of temporal bone
  - Vestibular opening after stapedectomy
  - Fenestration through LSC
- Osteitis and cholesteatomatous erosion—
  - In acute disease osteitis and erosion occur through well pneumatized mastoid
  - In chronic disease ostitis occurs in acellular mastoid.
- Vascular channels—Spread of infection through arterial channel is unlikely. Mostly spread occurs through venous channel.
  - Progressive retrograde thrombophlebitis is the usual route for abscess formation
  - Extracranial and intracranial venous system anastomosis with mastoid emissary vein entering sigmoid sinus that drains into superior and inferior petrosal sinuses
  - All of the dural sinuses are interconnected. Thus sigmoid sinus thrombosis leads to thrombophlebitis of other sinuses.

Thrombophlebitis from the lateral sinus may spread to the cerebellum and from the superior petrosal sinus it may spread to the temporal lobe of brain.

- Preformed channels (anatomical) are—
  - Oval/Round window → internal auditory meatus
  - Cochlear and vestibular aqueduct
  - Dehiscence over dome of jugular bulb
  - Dehiscence of tegmen tympani

- Dehiscent suture lines of temporal bone without the involvement of gray matter of brain.
- Infection may occur directly into the brain tissue through periarteriolar space of Virchow robin. This spread does not affect the cortical arterioles; hence abscess may occur in the white matter without the involvement of gray matter of brain.

Intracranial complications are subdivided into Extradural and Intradural complications.

Extradural Complications

- Meningitis
- Extradural abscess
- Lateral sinus thrombosis.

Intradural Complications (Fig. 41)

- Subdural abscess
- Brain abscess
- Otitic Hydrocephalus.

Meningitis

Meningitis is of the two types.

Generalized Bacterial Meningitis

It is the inflammation of the leptomeninges (Pia-arachnoid) with bacterial invasion of CSF in subarachnoid space. Infection of subarachnoid space may involve the entire cerebrospinal axis.

Localized Meningitis

It is defined as localized inflammation of dura and pia-arachnoid limited to a region adjacent to septic focus

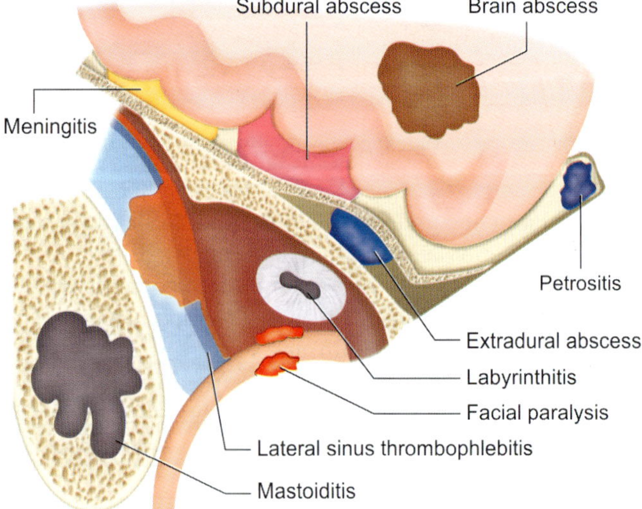

Fig. 41: Intracranial complications

with absence of organisms in CSF. It is most common intracranial complication of neglected OM. In children, it is a complication of ASOM. In adult it is a complication of CSOM.

However, AOM is more likely to cause meningitis than COM.

Major organisms are
- *H. influenzae* type B
- *Streptococcus pneumoniae*
- Proteus/pseudomonas
- Anaerobes.

Polymicrobial infection of CSF from ear is rare (<1% of cases)

Meningitis results from infection spreading from ear via retrograde thrombophlebitis, bone erosion and preformed pathways through round and oval windows.

The mode of extension is via perineural spaces to internal auditory meatus and less frequently via endolymphatic ducts. Meningitis may develop following trauma to the ear with fracture, dural tear, CSF leak and tympanomastoid surgery. Initial inflammatory response is an out pouring of fluid in subarachnoid space with a rise in CSF pressure. Pus initially accumulates in the basal cisterns and more rarely in vertex. Exudate obstructing ventricular foramina impedes free flow of CSF to cause noncommunicating hydrocephalus. Obstruction of CSF flow in subarachnoid space may cause communicating hydrocephalus.

Clinical Features

Complaints	Stage 1 (onset)	Stage II (established)	Stage III (Paralysis)
Headache	Severe	Agonizing	Decreased or absent
Neck	Stiffness	Rigidity	Retracted
Temperature	Raised	High	High/terminal fall
Mental state	Hyperactive, lucid, drowsy	Lucid, drowsy	Delirious comatose
Reflexes	DTR Brisk	Weak, Abdominals	Absent
Photophobia	Sometimes	Absent, Intense	Absent
Vomiting	Sometimes	Usual	Absent
CN palsies	Absent	Absent	Ocular movement (-ve)
Incontinence	Absent	Absent	Present

On Examination

Kernig's sign: It is resistance and painful when knee is extended with hips fully flexed (Fig. 42).

Brudzinski's Sign: It is involuntary lifting of legs in meningeal irritation when lifting a patient's head (Fig. 43).

Patients may also show opisthotonus: Spasm of whole body that leads to legs and head being bent back and body bowed forward.

Diagnosis

Diagnosis is made by CSF findings in otitic meningitis. Any patient with suspected meningitis undergoes lumbar puncture. CSF analysis shows—
- Increased CFS pressure
- Increased White cells
- Decreased glucose level (from 1.7–3 mmol/l to 0)
- Decreased chloride (from 120 mmol/l to 80 mmol/l)
- Bacteria is isolated from CSF
- Increased protein content (2–3 gm/l)
- Polymerase chain reaction is used to detect bacterial DNA from CSF.

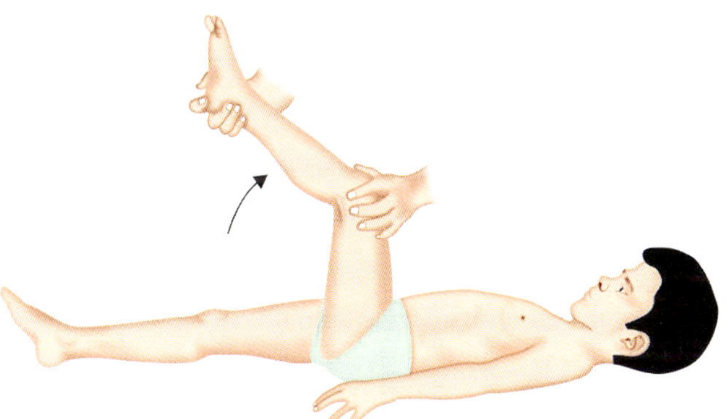

Fig. 42: Kernig's sign

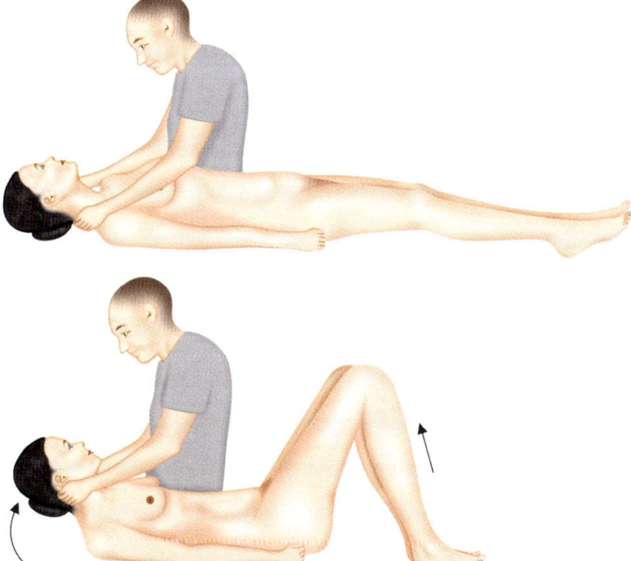

Fig. 43: Brudzinski's Sign—In meningeal irritation flexion of the neck results flexion of hip and knee

- Very high counts of Bacteria in CSF ~ 50000/mm^3 are indicative of a rupture of a brain abscess or subdural abscess into subarachnoid space. But in neither of these is the CSF blood sugar level reduced.

High resolution scan (HRCT) of temporal bone or MRI helps to reveal any associated intracranial lesion.

Management

Medical management—The mainstay in medical management is high doses of IV antibiotics.

- Penicillin is the drug of choice. Streptomycin may also be used as an adjuvant. Chloramphenicol may also be used
- Oral rifampicin works against *H. influenzae* type B
- Azlocillin/Ticarcillin/Ceftazidime acts against gram –ve organism
- Ceftrioxime a 3rd generation cephalosporin is widely used in these days. It has a broad spectrum activity
- Metronidazole IV is used against anaerobes. Systemic antibiotics are continued for at least 10 days after apparent clinical recovery
- Dexamethasone is administered shortly before or concurrently with systemic antibiotics to decrease CSF inflammatory response.

Surgical management—It is deferred for several days until patient's condition improves. After patient recovers from aural problem, effort is made to remove middle ear pathology which is the cause for the disease.

In Coalescent mastoiditis: Cortical mastoidectomy is preferred surgical procedure. In chronic middle ear disease—modified radical mastoidectomy is the procedure of choice.

Extradural Abscess (EDA)

Extradural abscess is the accumulation of pus between dura and tegmen tympani or dural covering of lateral sinus and the bony sinus plate. Routes of spread are given earlier. It is the most common intracranial complication.

Middle fossa EDA may develop lateral to arcuate eminence. It may strip dura extremely with collection of pus resulting in increased intracranial tension, focal neurological signs and papilledema.

Rarely EDA may develop medial to accurate eminence over the petrous apex. It may cause irritation of Gasserian ganglion of 5th and of 6th cranial nerve producing features of Gradenigo syndrome—focal pain, diplopia and aural discharge.

Posterior fossa EDA is limited to groove for sigmoid sinus resulting sigmoid sinus-perisinus abscesses. The perisinus abscess rarely extends into neck through jugular foramen.

Clinical Features

Clinical features are profuse or markedly intermittent otorrhea, earache, headache (ipsilateral), malaise, papilledema, focal neurological sign and low-grade fever of unknown origin following ASOM.

Diagnosis: CT scan shows epidural collection with ring enhancement.

Management

Essentially the treatment is surgical exploration—Tegmen and sinus plates are removed and dura is exposed.

- Enough bone should be removed to expose healthy dura
- Granulation tissue over dura should not be disturbed as there is chance of breaching the dura and spreading the infection to subdural spaces
- Appropriate simple or radical mastoidectomy is done for drainage of abscess
- Appropriate antibiotics are given especially when EDA results from AOM.

Lateral Sinus Thrombophlebitis

The lateral sinus comprises sigmoid and transverse sinuses. It is the largest sinus. When it is filled with suppurating blood clot, it threatens the great risks.

Pathogenesis (Fig. 44)

The pathological process is divided into the following steps:

- Formation of extradural perisinus abscess—Abscess develops in relation to outer dural wall of the sinus

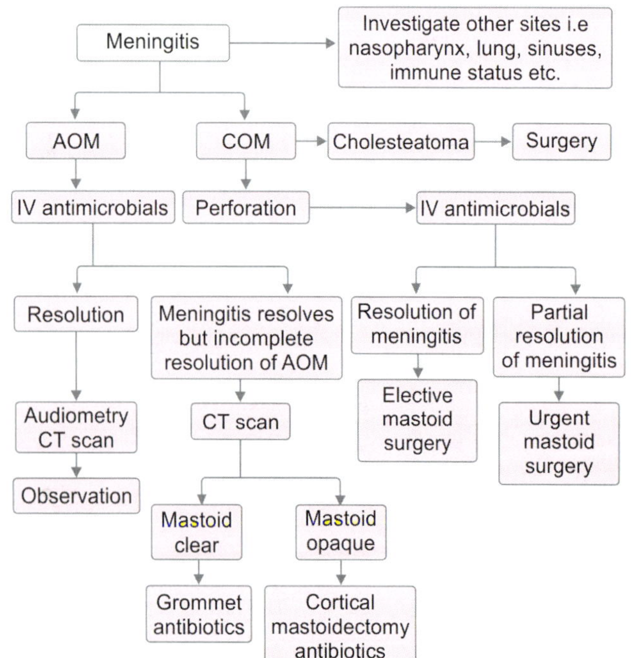

Flowchart 4: Management protocol of otogenic meningitis[41]

- Mural thrombi formation—Inflammation spreads to inner wall of the various sinus with deposition of fibrin and blood cells resulting thrombi formation in the lumen of sinus
- Occlusion of sinus lumen and intrasinus abscess—Progressive extension of the thrombi occludes the lumen. The clot may become partly organized and may be partly invaded by organisms resulting suppuration. Thus, intrasinus thrombi are formed and broken down into systemic circulation causing bacteremia
- Extension of thrombus—It spreads upwards to confluence of sinuses and then to superior sagittal sinus, superior or inferior petrosal sinuses to cavernous sinus, brain substance to form brain abscess
- It spreads downwards to internal Jugular vein and then to subclavian vein.

In earlier days, most cases were preceded by ASOM but now most are associated with CSOM.

Clinical Features

These are as follows:
- Evidence of middle ear infection
- Fever may be high and swinging called picket fence pattern associated with rigors and sweating following fall of temperature
- Tenderness and edema over the mastoid (Griesinger's sign) indicating thrombosis of the mastoid emissary veins—pathogenic sign in lateral sinus thrombosis
- Emaciation with anemia
- Papilledema (in 50%) due to raised intracranial pressure
- Proptosis, ptosis, chemosis and ophthalmoplegia reflecting spread of thrombus to the cavernous sinus
- Tobey–Ayer test (Queckenstedt's test)—The test is done for diagnosis of lateral sinus thrombosis prior to perform a lumber puncture. In normal subject, compression of each internal jugular vein (IJV) results in rapid rise of CSF pressure of 50–100 mm Hg above the normal level and on release of compression there is an equally rapid fall of CSF pressure.

In lateral sinus thrombophlebitis—pressure on IJV draining the occluded sinus causes no rise in pressure of CSF or very slow rise in pressure of CSF (about 10–20 mm Hg).

False negative result is associated with collateral channels draining the dural sinus; False positive result is associated with very small or absent lateral sinus
- Crowe Beck test—Pressure on IJV on healthy side results engorgement of retinal veins as is seen by ophthalmoscopy, on release of pressure engorgement of veins subsides
- Tenderness with cord-like feeling along IJV indicating extension of thrombus to IJV. It results in stiff neck
- Otitic hydrocephalus—It results from involvement of transverse and sagittal sinuses
- Intracranial complications like meningitis and brain abscess expected in ~50% of patients with lateral sinus thrombosis.

Investigation

Blood count shows anemia with raised WBCs count and raised ESR. Blood culture with blood taken as the fever rises at swinging peak shows positive.
- Lumber puncture is done only if CSF pressure is not raised. In uncomplicated cases, WBC count in CSF is low in chronic middle ear disease and increase in acute otitis media. CSF pressure is usually normal
- CT scan with contrast may show filling defect within the sinus, inflammatory enhancement of sinus walls and of the adjacent dura-delta sign (Fig. 45).[42]

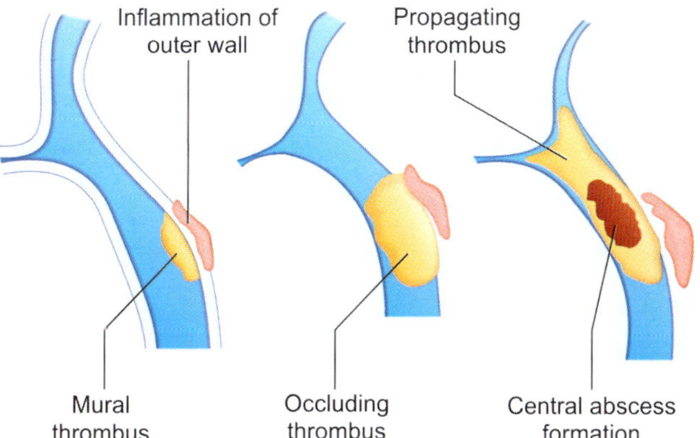

Fig. 44: Pathogenesis of Lateral sinus thrombophlebitis

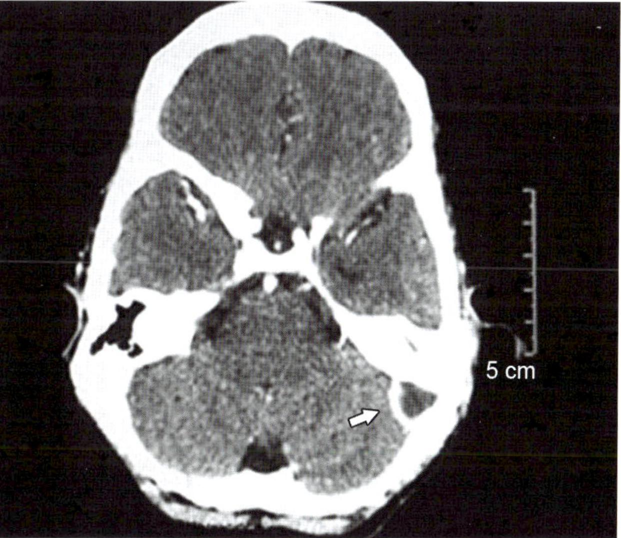

Fig. 45: CT scan showing lateral sinus thrombosis

- Angiography (especially digital substraction angiography) is the definitive investigation. It shows—
  - Obstruction and its site and extent
  - Anatomical arrangement of the individual's venous drainage.
- Radioisotope scanning with gallium can show hot-spots of sepsis.

Treatment

IV antibiotics (a combination of cephalosporin and aminoglycoside) should be started before surgery.

Drainage of the perisinus abscess and removal of clot are done via mastoidectomy. In ASOM with lateral sinus thrombophlebitis, cortical mastoidectomy is performed. Sinus is exposed and needled to confirm the diagnosis. In CSOM, radical mastoidectomy is undertaken. If lateral sinus thrombophlebitis is suspected the sinus plate must be removed and the sinus is examined.

Normal healthy sinus is soft, bluish compressible with a blunt probe. Insertion of a needle through the sinus wall shows free flow of venous blood.

In thrombophlebitis, the sinus appears white and opaque with firm consistency on palpation. It indicates that the lumen of sinus is occluded with fibrosing clot or fibrous tissue. The sinus is open and inspected to confirm the absence of blood or presence of necrotic tissue.

- Necrotic tissue if present, it is evacuated in both directions, upwards towards the confluence of the sinuses and downwards as far as the jugular bulb
- If organized thrombus is present, it should not be removed
- If profuse bleeding occurs the lumen of sinus is obliterated by packing a ribbon gauge impregnated with antimicrobial agents between the sinus wall and the bone.

Internal Jugular vein (IJV) ligation is considered in children showing signs of embolization and in septicemia not responding to initial antibiotic treatment and surgery.

Anticoagulants are not recommended because of increased risk of venous infarction.

Sequelae are permanent papilledema and epileptic fits.

Subdural Abscess (Empyema)

- Subdural abscess is an accumulation of pus between dura and arachnoid. Pus here has a tendency to spread widely and cause multiple abscess
- Infection reaches subdural space through tegmen tympani following localized osteitis with or without EDA formation
- Infection may extend via thrombophlebitis of cortical vein.

Clinical Features

- Severe headache
- Drowsiness/restlessness
- Focal neurological signs of monoplegia, hemiplegia, hemianopia, hemianesthesia, aphasia with involvement of dominant hemisphere and epileptic fit
- (+/-) sign of meningitis
- Papilledema
- Cr nerve palsy.

Diagnosis

CT scan helps in definitive diagnosis but the imaging modality of choice is MRI.[43] Although lumbar puncture shows increased CSF pressure, CSF has normal sugar content and culture is usually sterile (Fig. 46).

Management

- Administration of massive doses of intravenous antibiotics
- Drainage of subdural collection of pus via Bur-hole and irrigation
- In ASOM, myringotomy +/- cortical mastoidectomy
- In CSOM, modified radical mastoidectomy/or radial mastoidectomy
- Antiepileptic medication.

Prognosis

SDA is one of the most serious intracranial complications of otitis media.

Recovery without sequelae is seen only in 50% cases.

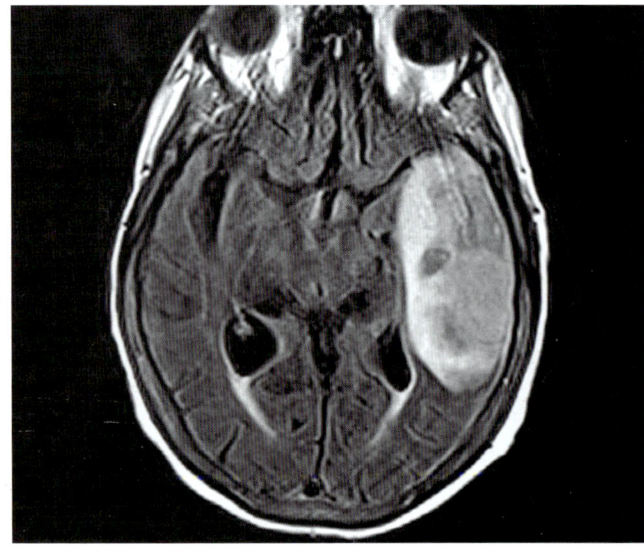

Fig. 46: MRI T1W film shows extra-axial collection hyperintense to CSF- subdural abscess

Otogenic Brain Abscess

- Otogenic brain abscess is a focal intracerebral or intracerebellar accumulation of pus in an area of suppurative encephalitis caused by organisms derived from a middle ear infection of same side
- Temporal lobe abscess is twice as frequent as the cerebellum
- It displays a bimodal age distribution with peaks in the pediatric age group and in 4th decade
- In children, 25% of all the brain abscesses are otogenic whereas it is 50% in adult
- Male to female ratio is approximately 3:1
- COM is much more likely to cause brain abscess than AOM. Cholesteatoma reports for most cases

Even in antibiotic era, mortality rate of otogenic brain abscess is approximately 25%.

Mode of spread—otogenic brain abscesses can result from three paths (Fig. 47).

1. Direct extension through tegmen tympani and dura broken by inflammatory process and cholesteatoma.
2. Preformed pathways like fracture of temporal bone, vestibular openings in stapedectomy, fenestration in LSCC.
3. Venous thrombophlebitis — the venous thrombophlebitis is more common mode of spread than direct dural extension.

Osteitis or granulation tissue causes retrograde thrombophlebitis of dural vessels ending in the white matter of the brain resulting encephalitis. The localized encephalitis progresses to necrosis and liquefaction of brain tissue resulting in focal suppuration. An abscess capsule surrounded by granulation tissue is formed within 2 weeks.

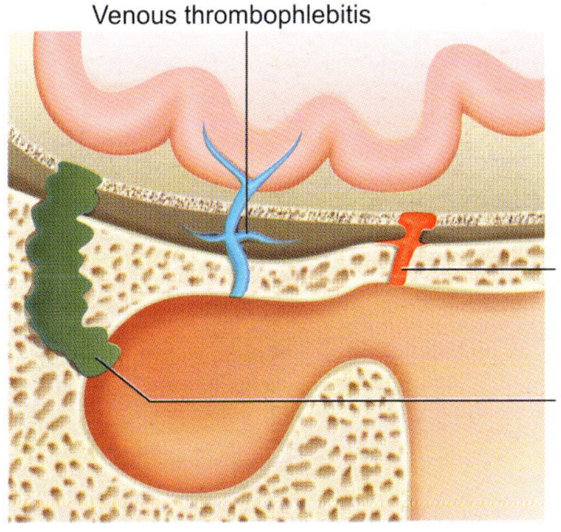

Fig. 47: Spread of otogenic brain abscess

Steps of Formation of Brain Abscess[44]

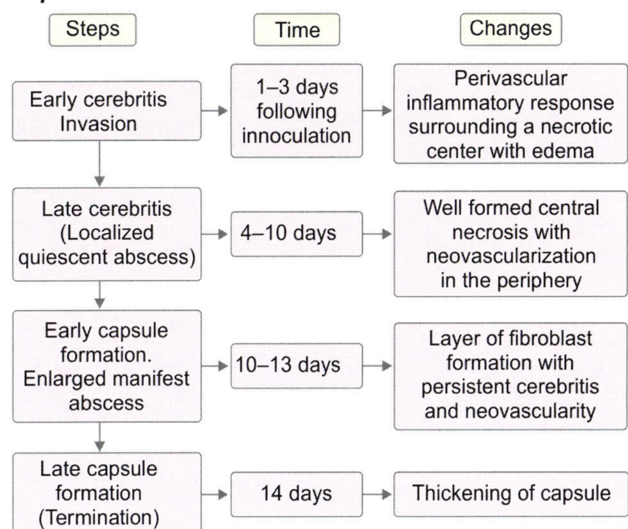

Capsular thickening of an abscess is less on the ventricular side as compared to the cortical side. It explains the more tendency of rupture of the abscess into ventricular system rather than into the subarachnoid space. The maturity of the abscess is directly proportional to local oxygen supply, virulence of organism and host immune system.

Organisms usually present in brain abscess are—

- Anaerobic streptococci (most common)
- *Staphylococci*
- *Streptococci pneumonae*
- *Streptococci haemolyticus*
- Gram –ve bacilli –proteus, *klebsiella, Escherichia coli* and *pseudomonus.*
- *H. influenza* (rare).

Clinical Features

Clinical features are unique to each stage of abscess formation.

Stage I (Local encephalitis)—Patient may present with

- Increased temperature
- Headache
- Listlessness/ irritability
- Focal convulsions.

Stage II (Latent abscess—when pus becomes contained within the developing fibrous capsule)—Patient may present with no symptom or only

- Headache and
- Lethargy.

Stage III (Manifest abscess)—Expanding abscess may cause cerebral compression and increased intracranial tension (ICT). Patient appears weakness, malaise, lethargy, slow pulse, normal or subnormal temperature, headache, vomiting and papilledema.

- Focal signs are nominal aphasia, quadrantic hemianopia, and motor paralysis.
- Cerebellar abscess may provoke ataxia dysdiadoko-kinesia, past pointing, intension tremors, spontaneous nystagmus and vomiting.
- Temporal lobe abscess may result in seizures.
- Lumbar puncture should be avoided if a brain abscess is suspected.

Radiography—Plain X-rays of skull show displacement of calcified pineal gland. They are of limited value.

Carotid arteriography is of value to demonstrate supratentorial masses when CT scan is not available. Upward and medial displacement of the middle cerebral artery indicates temporal lobe mass.

CT scan with and without contrast (I.V lothalamate) is most important investigation for diagnosis of brain abscess. Brain abscess may appear as hypodense area surrounded by an area of enhancement, a picture known as ring sign. CT scan also helps to identify associated complications, e.g. subdural abscesses and lateral sinus thrombophlebitis. Serial CT scanning helps to observe the progress of an abscess during treatment.

MRI is superior to CT scan to detect the slight changes in brain parenchyma and spread of abscess into the subarachnoid space or into the ventricle. But MRI has limitation for delineation of temporal bone configuration. Therefore, a CT scan is required to assess the bony delineation. EEG shows—

- Abnormal delta wave activity
- Accurate localization in 50% of abscesses.

It was useful before availability of CT scanning.

Differential Diagnosis

Differential diagnosis of brain abscess includes meningitis subdural abscess, lateral sinus thrombophlebitis, otitic hydrocephalus and brain tumor.

- In meningitis—typical diagnostic criteria are high sustained fever, neck rigidity and abnormal CSF findings
- A subdural abscess—is suspected if there is rapid evolution of focal neurological signs
- Lateral sinus thrombophlebitis—is suggested by picket fence pattern of fever, chemosis and proptosis of one eye and CT scan findings of enhancement of sinus walls and the adjacent dura
- In otitic hydrocephalous—shows the absence of focal neurological signs, normal CSF biochemistry and raised CSF pressure
- Brain tumor requires exclusion by CT scan appearance with reconstruction in different plane.

Treatment

- Raised ICT is lowered by administration of dexamethasone, 4 mg IV 6 hourly or IV mannitol 20% (0.5 g/Kg body wt)
- IV antimicrobials must be given in large dose for 3–4 weeks. These are chloramphenicol, penicillin (β lactamase resistant), aminoglycoside and metronidazole
- Surgical management includes—
  - Needle aspiration—It involves a small operation and can be done under local anesthesia
  - Burr hole and drainage—It is the current neurological options
  - Primary excision—It offers to decompress the brain immediately but the operation may cause damage to cerebral tissue with incidence of residual neurological damage
  - Open operation—the procedure involves the removal of pus from the abscess cavity under direct vision with less risk of neurological deficit
  - Postoperative antiepileptic medication is continued indefinitely after surgical management of brain abscess as there is high-risk of epileptic seizures
  - Middle ear disease is treated by radial mastoidectomy 10–14 day later.

Otitic Hydrocephalus

Synonym: Pseudotumor cerebri.

Otitic hydrocephalus is a rare syndrome of increased intracranial pressure during or following otitis media, normal CSF findings, spontaneous recovery and no abscess. It is also called benign intracranial hypertension as there is no associated ventricular dilatation.[45]

The etiology is unknown. But it is usually associated with sigmoid sinus thrombophlebitis. The pathopysiology is discussed in Flowchart 5.

Most cases (35%) occur on right side

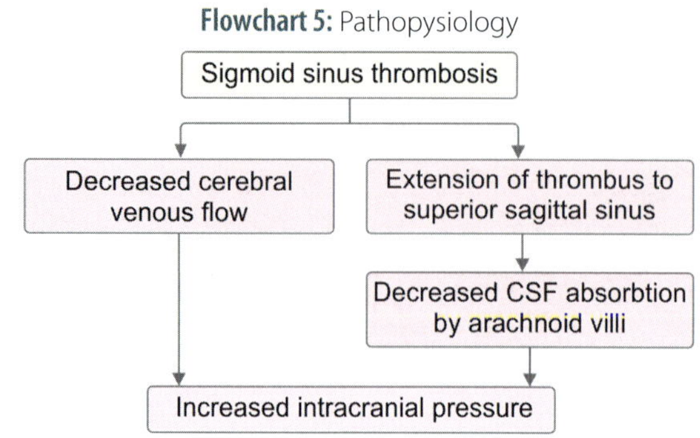

Flowchart 5: Pathopysiology

Clinical Features

Evidence of middle ear infection (ASOM or CSOM) is seen. Right-sided disease is associated with increased incidence of sinus thrombosis.

- Children or adolescents are usually affected
- Headache, drowsiness, vomiting, blurring of vision are leading symptoms
- Papilledema and diplopia are common evident. Diplopia is due to lateral rectus palsy (6th nerve stretching) found one or both sides—it is a false localizing sign associated with increased intracranial pressure
- Optic nerve atrophy may also develop.

Invesigation

Increased CSF pressure with normal CSF biochemistry is typical finding of otitic hydrocephalus.

- Lumbar puncture should be done with caution
- CT scan shows normal-sized ventricle
- MRI is the imaging modality for evaluating the venous sinuses

    Differential diagnosis—is to be done from other causes for increased intracranial pressure, particularly a brain abscess.

Treatment

The aim of treatment is to reduce the raised intracranial pressure and to eradicate the middle ear disease. To lower the intracranial tension, treatment includes—

- Corticosteroids
- Diuretics
- Hyperosmolar dehydrating agents
- Repeated careful lumbar puncture
- Ventriculoperitoneal shunting.

    Optic sheath decompression is also recommended to prevent optic atrophy.

    Decompression of sigmoid sinus is also recommended by Moffat et al (1978).

    Prognosis—Prognosis for survival is good but the treatment may need to be continued for several weeks or months.

TUBERCULAR OTITIS MEDIA (TOM)

Tubercular otitis media is a rare case of chronic suppurative infection of middle ear and mastoid. Typically, patients have a chronic ear discharge, multiple perforations, progressive and profound hearing loss and unresponsiveness to routine therapy. Facial nerve palsy, if present is strongly suggestive to TOM.[46] It is usually considered in a patient with chronic ear discharge of known or suspected tuberculosis, although absence of tuberculosis elsewhere does not exclude the possibility of TOM. Other variable otoscopic findings may be—

- Single perforation with refractory otorrhea and exuberant granulation formation
- Single perforation with minimal otorrhea and absence of granulation formation
- Intact tympanic membrane with middle ear effusion and
- Intact tympanic membrane with tumor like tissue in middle ear.[47]

Etiology

Mycobacterium tuberculosis is the most common causative organism in TOM. Other atypical organisms also causing tubercular otomastoiditis are *Mycobacterium bovis*, *Mycobacterium avium* and *Mycobacterium fortuitum*.

Incidence

In developing countries, Tuberculosis is a common disease, although incidence of tubercular otitis media is low (about 0.37% of COM)[48]. The disease is still to be kept in mind in patients with chronic intractable otorrhea.

Source of Infection

Infection is secondary to pulmonary tuberculosis. The infection reaches the middle ear from the nasopharynx through Eustachian tube. Hematogenous spread may occur from distant foci in disseminated disease. Contiguous spread may involve temporal bone from adjacent intracranial or extracranial infection. Rarely, the infection may come in early life from mother who is suffering from genitourinary tuberculosis.[49]

Clinical Features

- Ear discharge—Watery ear discharge with mild pain or without pain is the usual presentation of TOM. The ear discharge is foul smelling because of underlying bone erosion and fails to respond to usual antimicrobial therapy
- Multiple tympanic perforations are considered to be the hallmark of the disease. Small perforations may coalesce into a single large peroration with abundant granulation tissue formation. Sometimes, intact tympanic membrane with effusion and no granulation tissue are noted[50]
- Preauricular lymph node enlargement without typical systemic features of tuberculosis is present in some patients
- Hearing Loss—is mostly moderate conductive type and results from tympanic perforations and ossicular

erosions. It is progressive and profound in patient with further development of the disease
- Giddiness may occasionally be experienced in TOM
- Tinnitus is pulsatile type and felt in some cases[51]
- Facial paralysis results from granulation tissue eroding the facial canal and damaging the facial nerve. It is common presenting feature in children with TOM[52] Bilateral facial paralysis caused by TOM is reported
- Patient may present with tumor-like mass in middle ear, mastoiditis, postauricular abscess and submandibular lymphadenopathy.

Investigations

Early diagnosis is essential to avoid risk of complications like facial paralysis and irreversible hearing loss. Investigations that help early diagnosis include—
- Pure tone audiometry shows moderately severe mixed hearing loss. Speech discrimination score (SDS) is reduced
- Radiology—X-ray mastoid is nonspecific. It reflects erosions or coalescence of mastoid air cells only.

CT scan of temporal bone reveals multiple soft tissue densities in tympanic cavity with mastoid erosions. Sometimes CT shows presence of soft tissue in mastoid without bone resorption or contrast enhancement. CT also helps to localize the facial canal erosions in patient with facial paralysis, cochlear fistula in progressive disease and intracranial or extracranial tubercular foci, if any (Figs 48 and 49).

Chest X-ray may show the fibronodular lesions in upper lobe in 50% of cases of TOM suggesting concomitant pulmonary tuberculosis.

- Purified protein derivative (PPD) test is considered to be strongly reactive
- Acid fast bacillus stain of middle ear discharge is positive but negative result sometimes does not exclude *Mycobacterium tuberculosis*
- Culturing of ear discharge in Lowenstein-Jensen medium if positive confirms *Mycobacterium tuberculosis*[53]
- Polymerase chain reaction (PCR) on biopsy material is a supplementary test for diagnosis of *Mycobacterium tuberculosis* in a few hours.[54] It is both sensitive and specific test for *Mycobacterium tuberculosis*.
- Histopathological examination shows chronic inflammatory infiltration in connective tissue-multinucleated Langerhans type giant cells, epitheloid cells and round cells.

Treatment

After diagnosis is established medical treatment with antituberculous drug is started as first treatment option for TOM. Mastoidectomy or incisional drainage of abscess with meatoplasty in addition to antituberculous drugs does not show any good result of its effectiveness. Disappearance of ear discharge and granulation tissue, recovery of facial nerve palsy and hearing loss are observed in most of the patients between 1 and 5 months.[55] Antituberculous drugs given are isoniazid, rifampicin, pyrazinamide and ethambutol for 6–12 months. Surgical management like ear surgery or mastoidectomy in addition to antituberculous drug is reserved for medically intractable patients with the idea of complete removal of disease from middle ear and mastoid bone.

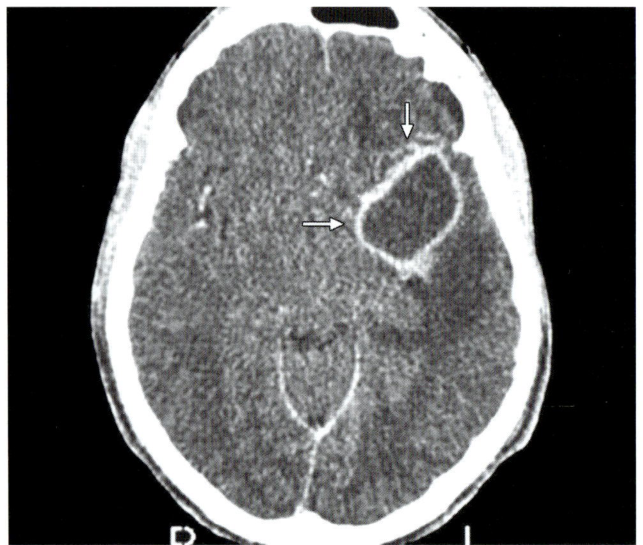

Fig. 48: CECT scan shows a left temporal lobe abscess

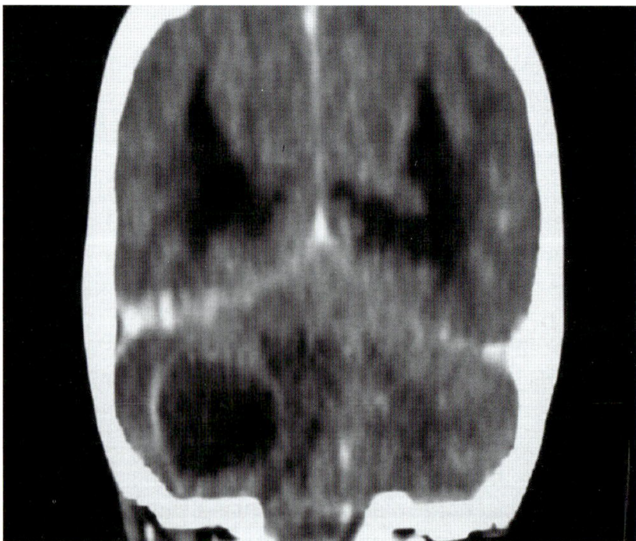

Fig. 49: CT scan shows cerebellar abscess

REFERENCES

1. Philip D, Yates and Shahram Anari, Otitis Media, Current Diagnostic and treatment in Otolaryngology- Head neck surgery. Edited by Anil K Lalwani. Tata McGraw-Hill Publishing Company Ltd; 2008. vol3 p 656.
2. Bruce Proctor. Chronic Otitis Media and Mastoiditis, Otolaryngology. Michael MP et al, 3rd edition. Vol-III (twc) 1991. pp 1363-5.
3. Cambridge R and Stevenson N. Oxford handbook of Ent and Head and Neck Surgery, 1st edition. 2007. p-263.
4. O`Neil P, Roberts T. Acute Otitis media in children. Clin. Evid. 2005;13:227 (Evidence-based review of trials for AOM teratment).
5. Flynn CA, Griffen G, Tu diver F. Decongestants and antivitamines for acute otitis media in children (Cochrane Review) The Cochrane Library. Issue 3, 2001. Oxford update software. [PMID: 11406002] (Meta- analysis of the use of the decongestants and antivitamines for AOM).
6. American Academy of Family physicians- American Academy of Otolaryngology- Head and Neck Surgery. American Academy of pediatrics subcommittee on Otitis Media with effusion. Pediatrics 2004;113(5):1412 [PMID: 15121966] (Practical guidelines for Otitis media with effusion. The online version and updated information can be accessed at http://www.pediatrics.org/cgi/content/full/1131511412).
7. Ruby Udwadia. Brief review of current studies on Otitis media with effusion. Otolaryngology review edited by Shah VH and Karnik PP. 2000. p-46-9.
8. Paparella MM, Jung TTK, Goycoolea MV. Otitis Media with effusion. Otolaryngology Vol II, 3rd edition. In: Michael MP et al. 1991. p-1319.
9. Politzer. A textbook of diseases of the ear translated by Cassels, JP London: Bailhere, Tindall and Cox, 1983. p-375-377. Armstrong, B.W. A new treatment for Chronic Secretary Otitis Media. Archives of Otolaryngology. 1954;59:653-4.
10. Ransome J. Myringotomy, Rob and Smith's operative surgery, Ear, 4th edition. 1983. p 27-37.
11. Douglas HT, Stool SE and Bruce WJ. Otitis media and associated complications ENT secrets, 3rd edition. Jafek and Murrow. Mosby; 2005. P-67-71.
12. Michael CT and C Andrew Van Hasselt. Otitis Media with effusion in adults. Scott-Brown`s Otolaryngology, Head and Neck surgery, 7th edition. Vol 3, p 3393.
13. Sade J, Berco E. Atelectasis and Secretary Otitis Media. Annals of Otology, Phinology and Laryngology. 1976;85:66-72.
14. Tos M, Stangerup SE, Larson P. Dynamics of eardrum changes following secretary Otitis. A prospective study. Archives of Otolaryngology- Head and Neck Surgery. 1987;113l:380-5.
15. Gibb AG. Nonsuppurative Otitis Media, Scott-Brown`s Disease of the ear, nose and throat, 4th edition. Vol 2, 1979. p220-233.
16. George GB. Chronic Otitis Media. Scott-Brown`s Otolaryngology, Head and Neck Surgery, 7th edition. Vol 3. 2008. p 3396.
17. da Costa SS, Paperella MM, Schachem PA, YoonTH, Kimberly BP. Temporal Bone histopathology in chronically infected ears with intact and perforated tympanic membranes. Laryngoscope. 1992;102:1229-36.
18. Jung JY, Chole RA. Bone resorption in COM: The role of the Osteoclast. ORL. 2002;64:95-107.
19. Erkan M, Aslan T, Seviik E, et al. Bacteriology of Chronic suppurative Otitis Media. Ann Otol Rhinol Laryngol. 1994;103:771-4.
20. William H, Slattery III. Pathology and clinical course of inflammatory diseases of the middle ear, 5th edition. 2007. p-429.
21. Yates PD, Anari S. Otitis Media current diagrams and treatment in Otolaryngology- Head and Neck Surgery, Vol-3. edited by Anik K Lalwani. Tata Mcgraw-Hill Publishing Company Ltd; 2008. p-662.
22. Derlacki EL, Chemis JD. Congenital choleasteatoma of the middle ear and mastoid. Ann Otol Rhinol Larynogol. 1965;74:706-27.
23. Michaels l. An epidermoid formation in the developing middle ear; possible source of cholesteatoma. J Otolaryngol. 1986;15:169-74.
24. Michaels L. Origin of Congenital Cholesteatoma from a normally occurring epidermoid rest in the developing middle ear. Int J. Pediatr Otorhinolaryngol. 1988;15:51-65.
25. Sculerati N, Charles D. Bluestone, pathogenesis of cholesteatoma. The Otolaryngologic Clinics of North America. 1989;22(5):859-68.
26. Tumarkein A: A contribution to the study of middle ear suppuration with special reference to the pathology and treatment of cholesteatoma. J Laryngol. 1938;53:685-710.
27. Ruedi L. Cholesteatofin of the attic. J Laryngol. 1958;72:593-609.
28. Jackler RK. The surgical anatomy of cholesteatoma, The Otolaryngologic Clinics of North America. 1989;22(5):883-5.
29. Fuse T, Tada Y, Aoyagi M, Sugai Y. CT detection of facial canal dehiscence and semicircular canal fistula: comparison with surgical findings. Journal of Computer-Assisted Tomography. 1996;20:221-4.
30. Smyth GDL, Brooker DS. Small cavity mastoidectomy. Clinical Otolaryngology and Allied Sciences. 1992;17:280-3.
31. Wormald PJ, Nilsser EL. The facial ridge and the discharging mastoid cavity. Laryngoscope. 1998;108:92-6.
32. Swan LRC. Canter and McKerrow W. Natural history management and outcomes, Scott Brown`s Otolaryngology, Head and Neck Surgery, 7th edition, Vol-3. Edited by Gleeson M, et al. 2008. p 3433.
33. Gross ND, Memenomey SO. Aural complications of Otitis Media, Glasscock-Shambaugh surgery of the ear, 5th edition. 2007. p435-41.
34. Joseph EM, Sperling NM. Facial nerve paralysis in acute Otitis Meda: Cause and management revisited. Otolaryngol Head and Neck Surgery. 1998;118:694-6.
35. Lindsay JR. Suppuration in the petrous pyramid. Ann Otol Rhinol Laryngol. 1938;47:3.
36. Goldstein NA, Casselbrant ML, Bluestone CD, Kurs- Lasky M. Intratemporal complications of acute otitis media in infants and children. Otolaryngol Head and neck Surgery. 1998;119:444-54.
37. Torok N. Tympanogenic Labyrinth. Otolaryngol Clinic North America. 1972;5:45-57.
38. Scheehy JL, Brachmann DE. Cholesteatoma Surgery. Management of the labyrinth fistula- a report of 97 cases. Laryngoscope. 1979;89:78-87.
39. Zygomatic abscess as a complication of otitis media www.ncbi.nih.gov/pmc/articles/pmc 3343403/
40. Feirmesser R, Wiesel YM, Argaman M, Gay I. Otitis external- bacteriological survey. ORL J Otorhinolaryngol Relat Spec. 1982;44:121-5.
41. Levine SC, De Souza C. Intracranial complications of Otitis media, Glasscock-Shambaugh. Surgery of the ear, 5th edition. 2003. p 450.

42. Bunanno F, Moody D, Ball M, Laster D. Computered cranial tomographic findings in cerebral sinovenous occlusion. J Compul Assist Tomogr. 1978;2:281-90.

43. Weingarten K. Subdural and epidural empyema. MR imaging. Am J Radiol. 1989;152:615-21.

44. Ward PH. Setliff RC, Long W. Otogenic brain abscess. Trans Am Acad Opthalmol Otolaryngol. 1969;73;107-14.

45. Foley J. Bengin forms of intracranial hypertension "toxic" and "Otitic" hydrocephalus. Brain. 1955;78:1-41.

46. Kirsch CM. Wehner JH, Jensen WA, Kagawa FT, Campagna AL. Tuberculous otitis media. South Med J. 1995;88(3):363-6.

47. Abes GT, Abes FL, Jamir JC. The variable clinical presentation of Tuberculosis Otitis media and the importance of early detections. Otol Neurotol. 2011 Jun;32(4):539-43.

48. Singh B. Role of surgery in Tuberculosis. Journal of Laryngology and Otology. 1991;105:907-15.

49. Saltzman S, Feigin R. Tuberculosis Otitis media and mastoiditis, Journal of Pediatrics. 1971;79:1004-6.

50. Hushino T, Miyashita H, Asai Y. Computed tomography of the temporal bone in tuberculous Otitis media. Journal of Laryngology and Otology. 1992;108:702-5.

51. www.advancedotology.org/1AOI-3/1AOOCT 2011 p 413-417.Pdf.

52. Ma KH, Tang PS, Chan KW. Aural Tuberculosis, American Journal of Otology. 1990;11:174-7.

53. Farrugia EJ, Ali Raja S, Phillipps JJ. Clinical Records Tuberculosis Otitis Media- A case report. J Laryngol Otol. 1997;3:50.

54. Inoue T, I Leda N, Kurusawa T, Sato A, Nakatani K, I Keda T, et al. [A case of middle ear tuberculosis, PCR of the Otorrhoes was useful for the diagnosis] Kekkakar. 1999;74:453-6.

55. Acuin JM. Tuberculosis of the temporal bone. Scott Brown`s Otorhinolaryngology, Head and neck Surgery, 7th edition, volume-3. Edited by Gleeson M et al.

Facial Nerve and its Disorders

Asok K Saha

ANATOMY OF FACIAL NERVE

The facial nerve is the nerve for nonverbal humanistic expression. It is the nerve of the second branchial arch. It is a mixed nerve having 10,000 fibers. Motor root having 7000 special visceral efferent (SVE), supplies all the mimetic muscles of face. Sensory root (Nerve of Wrisberg) having 3000 sensory and parasympathetic fibres; GVE (general visceral efferent), SVA (special visceral afferent) and SVE (special visceral efferent) fibers, carries taste from anterior 2/3rd of the tongue by the way of the chorda tympani and from palate by the way of the nerve of the pterygoid canal and general sensation from the concha and retroauricular skin.

Sensory fibers are contained in a separate trunk, the nervous intermedius that runs with the 8th nerve in the subarachnoid space. It also carries preganglionic parasympathetic secretomotor fibers to lacrimal, submandibular and sublingual salivary glands.

Embryology

- Nerve of second branchial arch (Fig. 1)
- By 4th week of intrauterine life—facial nerve and its geniculate ganglion appear
- Facial nerve nuclei develop from neural crest cells
- By 8th week—primitive fallopian canal appears in posterior otic capsule
- By 7th week—facial nerve with definitive communicative branches appears
- Fallopian canal has two centers of ossification
- Incomplete fusion results in bony dehiscence
- Facial nerve nuclei appear from neuroblasts in pons; close to 6th cranial nerve nucleus
- Internal genu of facial nerve forms—as brain develops pons expands.

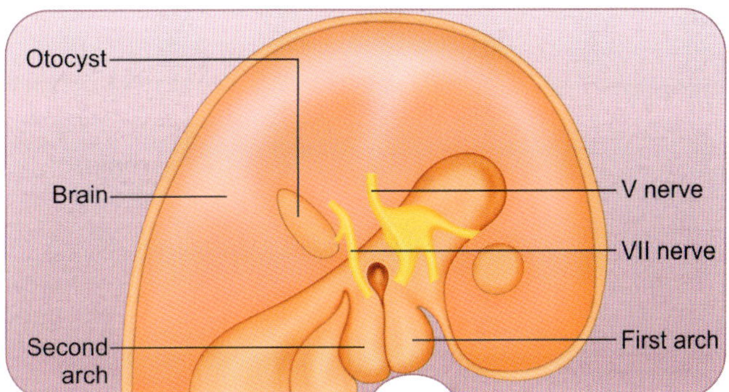

Fig. 1: Facial nerve of second branchial arch developing from neural crest cells

Course of Facial Nerve

It can be divided into following:
1. Intracranial course from pons to internal auditory canal (15–17 mm).
2. Intratemporal course from internal auditory meatus to stylomastoid foramen (22–33 mm).
3. Extratemporal course from stylomastoid foramen to the termination of its peripheral branches (15–20 mm).

Facial Nerve Nuclei (Fig. 2)

- Motor nucleus
- Superior salivary nucleus and Lacrimal nucleus
- Nucleus tractus solitarius.

Motor nucleus is located in the reticular formation of the caudal part of the pons, below and in front of the abducent nucleus. The fibres from the motor nucleus encircle the caudal end and dorsal surface of abducent nucleus occupying the facial colliculus of the floor of 4th ventricle. At the cranial end of abducent nucleus the fibres bend abruptly downwards and forwards, forming

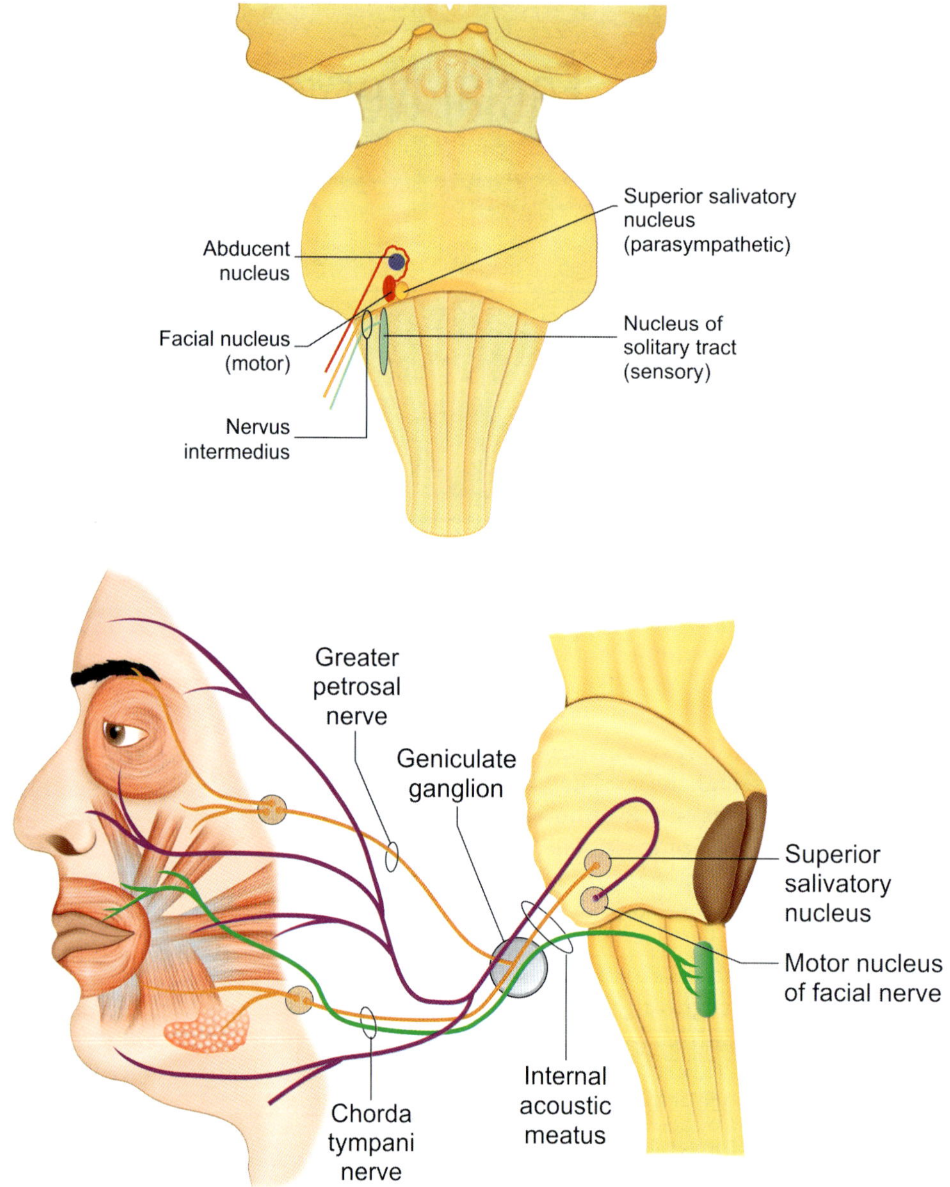

Figs 2: Facial nerve nucleus

an internal genu and emerge at the lower border of pons through the motor root.[1]

Superior salivary nucleus is situated dorsolateral to the caudal part of motor nucleus. The secretomotor fibres arise from this nucleus and emerge through the sensory root.

Nucleus tractus solitarius (NTS) is a series of neuclei present in medulla carring fibres that project to other regions like reticular formation, parasympathetic preganglionic neuron, hypothalamus and thalamus forming circuit concerned for autonomic regulation.

Central Connections (Fig. 3)

Upper part of motor nucleus that supplies the muscles of the forehead and eyelids is controlled by corticonuclear fibers from both cerebral hemispheres.

Lower part of the motor nucleus that supplies lower facial muscles is controlled by the corticonuclear fibers (Pyramidal) from motor cortex of the opposite cerebral hemisphere.

The first order of sensory neurons for taste is located in geniculate ganglion of facial nerve situated in the medial wall of epitympanic part of tympanic cavity that forms an external genu.

The peripheral processes of these neurons pass from anterior 2/3rd of the tongue via the lingual and chorda tympani nerves and extend from the soft palate through the nerve of pterygoid canal and greater petrosal nerve. The central processes of the first order of neurons are relayed into the upper part of the nucleus of tractus solitarius in the pontomedullary junction.

The second order of neurons of the solitary nucleus crosses the middle line and ascends to the opposite side as solitario-thalamic tract to project into the most medial part of ventropostero-medial (VPM) nucleus of thalamus. The fibers of 3rd order neurons from thalamus are projected to the lower part of the post central gyrus (area 3, 1, 2) through posterior limb of internal capsule where taste sensation is perceived.[2]

Infranuclear pathway: The facial nerve after leaving the nucleus travels through the posterior cranial fossa along with the 8th cranial nerve and enters the internal auditory canal (IAC). At the fundus of the IAC, the nerve enters the bony facial canal in temporal bone and then comes out of the stylomastoid foramen.

In bony facial canal, the facial nerve has unique course. In the temporal bone, the total length of facial nerve is 22–33 mm and its course is divided into the following:
- Meatal segment (5–12 mm) within internal auditory canal covered only by piamater
- Labyrinthine segment (3–5 mm) from the fundus of internal auditory canal to the geniculate ganglion. This

is the shortest segment and diameter of the nerve in this segment is also narrowest (0.61–0.68 mm)
- First genu—The nerve from geniculate ganglion takes an acute angle to turn posteriorly to enter tympanic cavity forming a genu
- Tympanic or horizontal segment (10–12 mm) from geniculate ganglion the nerve runs posteriorly on the medial wall of the middle ear above the promontory forwards to backwards. This is tympanic or horizontal segment of facial nerve
- Second genu—Horizontal segment then curves down between pyramid and oval window at an angle of 95–125° forming second genu
- Mastoid or vertical segment (9–16 mm)—It extends from second genu or pyramid to stylomastoid foramen, where the nerve is found more superficial than at the level of second genu.

Branches of the Facial Nerve (Figs 4A and B)

Intracranial
- Greater superficial petrosal nerve—It is the first branch of facial nerve. It arises from geniculate ganglion and carries secretomotor fibres to the lacrimal gland.

Intratemporal Branches
- Nerve to the stapedius muscle—It arises from the mastoid segment at the level of second genu and supplies the stapedius muscle
- Chorda tympani—It arises from the middle of the mastoid segment, passes between the incus and malleus and leaves the middle ear through petrotympanic fissure. It carries secretomotor fibers to the submandibular and sublingual glands and supplies taste from anterior 2/3rd of tongue
- The sensory fibers of the nerve join the auricular branch of vagus and supply the skin of the external auditory canal.

Branches of Facial Nerve in the Neck and Face
- The Ansa Haller (inconstant)—It arises immediately below the stylomastoid foramen. It passes lateral to the jugular vein and anastomoses with the glossopharyngeal nerve
- Posterior auricular nerve—It arises 1-2 mm below the stylomastoid foramen, then winds around the digastric muscle and extends posteriorly upon the anterior surface of mastoid and is joined by a twig from the auricular branch of vagus. It also communicates with posterior branch of the greater auricular nerve and with

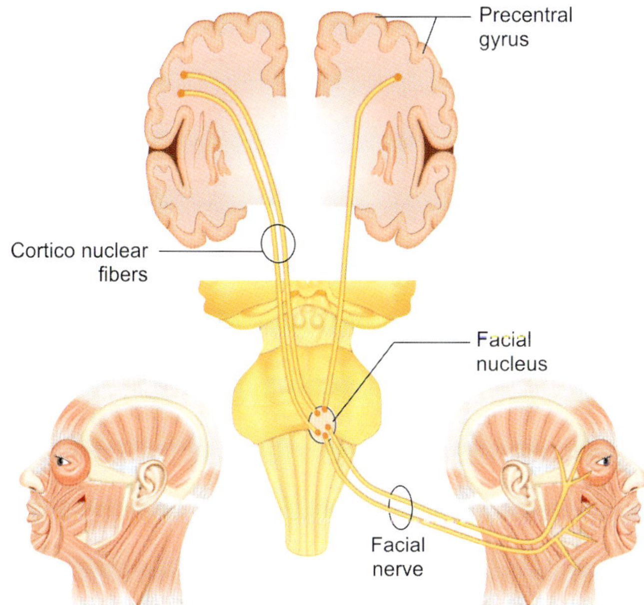

Fig. 3: Central connection

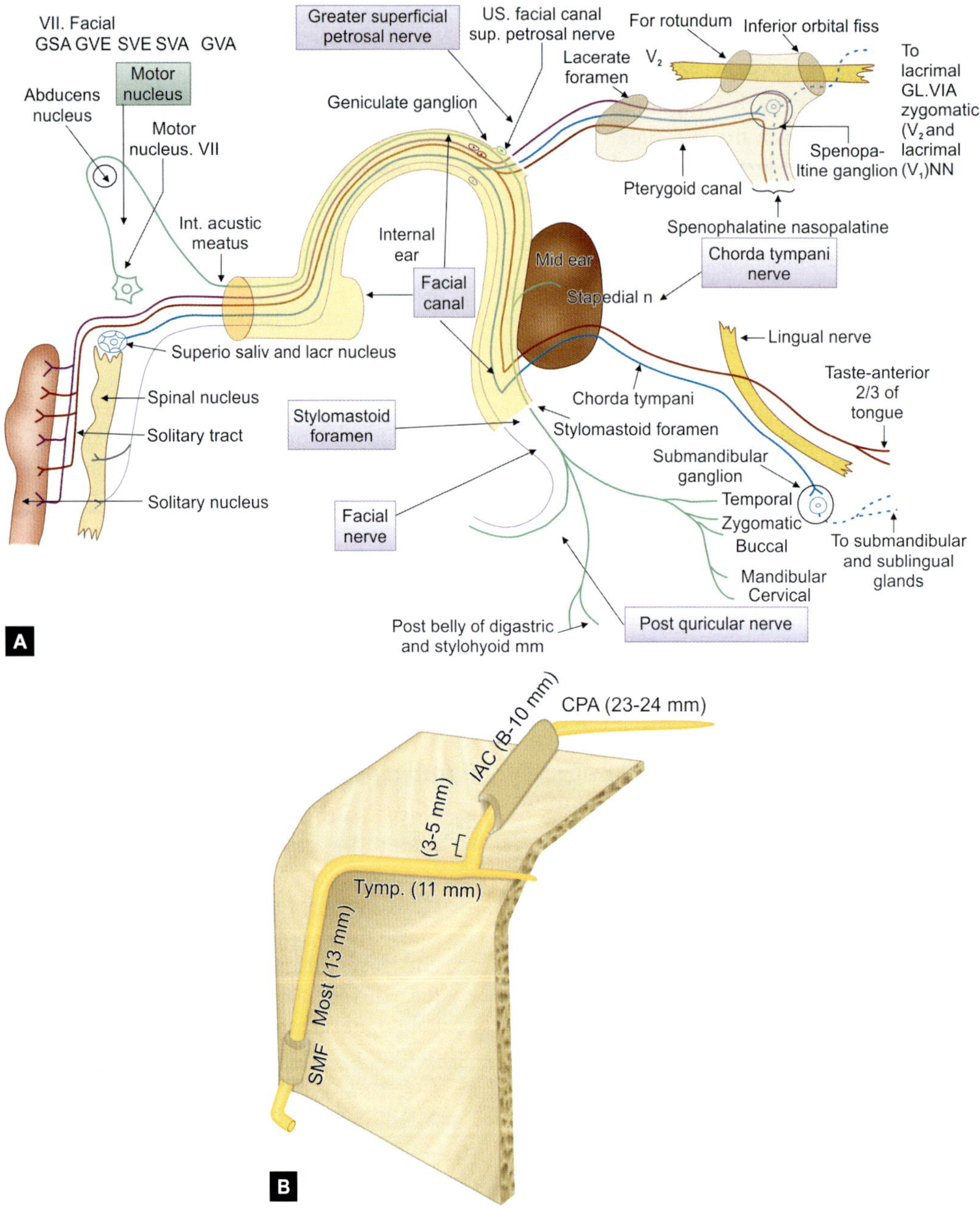

Figs 4A and B: (A) Overview of facial nerve anatomy; (B) Course of facial nerve in temporal bone

the lesser occipital nerve. It divides into auricular and occipital branches between the external auditory canal and mastoid process

- Stylohyoid branch—It arises in conjunction with the digastric branch and enters the stylohoid muscles in its mid position
- Branch to the posterior belly of digrastric muscle
- The lingual branch—It follows the styloglossus muscle and replaces the Ansa Haller.

Branches forming the parotid plexus—The nerve trunk, after crossing the styloid process has two divisions, an upper temporofacial and a lower cervicofacial. These further divide into smaller branches.

- Temporal
- Zygomatic
- Buccal
- Marginal mandibular
- Cervical.

These all together form the Pes anserinus (Goose foot) and supply all the muscles of facial expression.

Internal Auditory Canal and Facial Nerve (Fig. 5)

The length of the internal auditory canal is approximately 1cm. It transmits the facial, acoustic and vestibular nerves, intermediate nerve and internal auditory artery. The transverse crest called the crista falciformis separates the canal into superior and inferior compartments laterally. The inferior compartment transmit the cochlear nerve anteriorly and inferior vestibular nerve posteriorly. The singular canal is a perforate area from internal auditory canal's inferior compartment and contains a branch of inferior vestibular nerve. The superior compartment has a vertical crest of bone (Bill's Bar) which separates the facial nerve anteriorly from the superior vestibular nerve posteriorly[3].

Functional Components of Facial Nerve

- Special visceral efferent (SVE)—Motor supply to 2nd branchial arch striated muscles
- General visceral afferent (GVA)—Sensory input from visceral touch, temperature, pain
- Special visceral afferent (SVA)—Taste
- General visceral efferent (GVE)—Autonomic supply to mucosal, lacrimal, salivary glands
- General somatic afferent (GSA)—Sensory input from somatic touch, temperature, pain.

Functional Components within the Branches (Fig. 6)

- Greater superficial petrosal nerve: GVE, SVA, GVA
- Stapedial nerve: SVE
- Chorda tympani nerve: GVE,SVA
- Posterior auricular nerve: SVE, GSA
- Facial nerve (Terminal branch): SVE.

Blood Supply of the Facial Nerve

The nerve receives its blood supply from

- Anterior inferior cerebellar artery—It enters the internal auditory meatus (IAM) nourishing the nerve of the posterior cranial fossa.
- Labyrinthine artery—Branch of anterior inferior cerebellar artery supplies the nerve in internal auditory meatus.

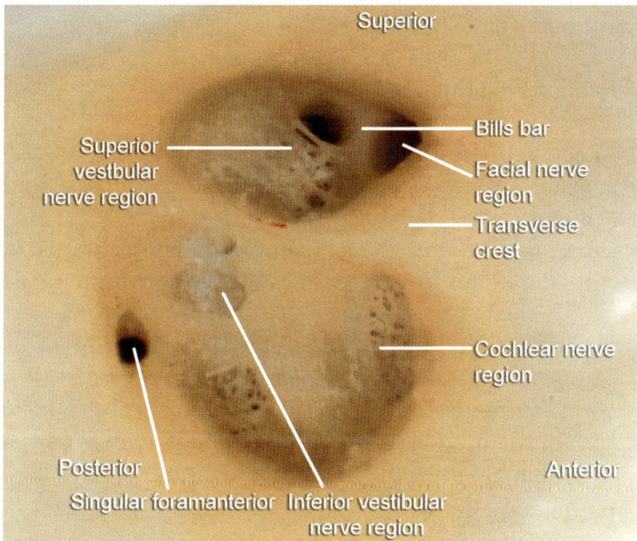

Fig. 5: Internal auditory canal and facial nerve

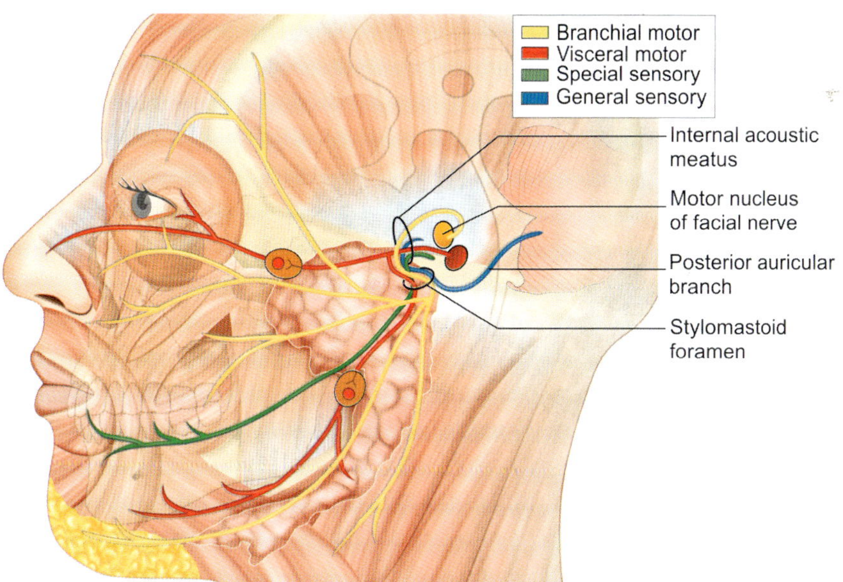

Fig. 6: Functional components of facial nerve

- Petrosal branch of the middle meningeal artery—It runs along the greater petrosal nerve supplying the geniculate ganglion and adjacent region
- Stylomastoid artery, branch of the posterior auricular artery supplying the mastoid or vertical segment of facial nerve.

The veins form a plexus around the nerve from which efferent vessels run, first between the sheath and the nerve and then through sheath to lie on its outer surface. Venous drainage leaves the canal mainly at the stylomastoid foramen and at the second genu. Only small veins accompany the chorda tympani.

The anastomosis between the arterial system is proximal to the geniculate ganglion. This makes the labyrinthine segments vulnerable to ischemia from edema.

Surgical Landmarks of the Facial Nerve (Figs 7A and B)

Landmarks for middle ear and mastoid surgery are as follows:
- The cog—A bony ridge hangs from the tagmen anterior to the head of the malleus. It is useful for localizing the first genu
- Processus cochleariformis—It is immediately inferior to the anterior portion of the tympanic segment. If the processus cochleariformis is inapparent, it is located by Jacobson's nerve on the promontory and tracing it superiorly
- Oval window—The facial nerve runs above the oval window. It is useful guide to the posterior portion of the horizontal or tympanic segment of the nerve
- Lateral semicircular canal—It lies posterior superior to the second genu—a constant landmark
- Short process of incus—The facial nerve lies medial to the short process of incus at the level of aditus
- Retrofacial air cells—They help in locating the medial aspect of the vertical or mastoid segment of the facial nerve
- Chorda tympani nerve—A useful landmark while performing combined approach tympanoplasty
- Pyramidal eminence—The nerve runs behind the pyramid and posterior tympanic sulcus
- Tympanomastoid suture—In vertical or mastoid segment the nerve runs behind the suture
- Digastric ridge—The nerve leaves the mastoid at the anterior end of digastric ridge.

Landmarks for extratemporal parts for parotid surgery.
- Tragal pointer of Conley—The nerve lies medial and about 1 cm inferior to the tragal cartilage
- Tympanomastoid suture line—The nerve lies 6–8 mm deep to the suture line
- Styloid process—The nerve runs lateral to the styloid process at the skull base (Fig. 8)
- Retrograde dissection following a peripheral branch.[4]
  - The ramus frontalis is identified by line from tragus to the lateral canthus
  - The ramus buccalis is identified by a line from tragus to the alae of the nose parallel to the zygoma
  - The ramus mandibularies is situated near the angle of the mandible at a point of about 4 cm from the attachment of the lobule of the pinna.

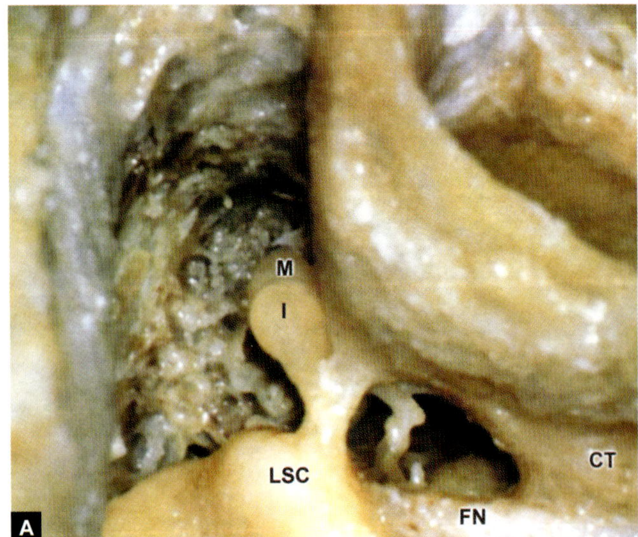

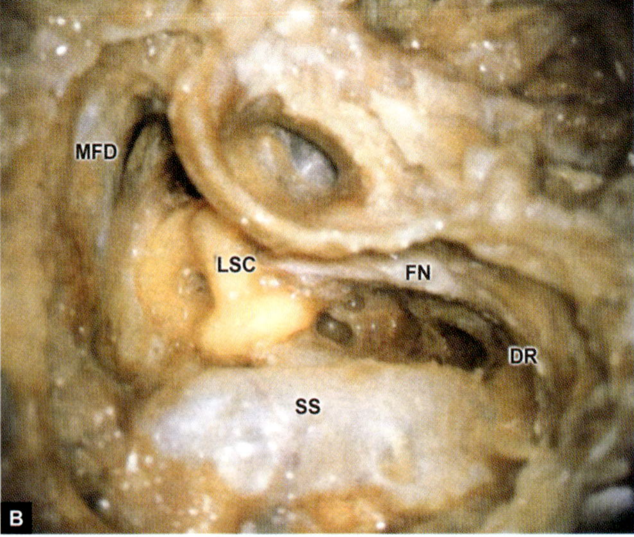

Figs 7A and B: (A) Temporal bone dissection showing Incus (I), lateral semicircular canal (LSC), chorda tympani nerve (CT), facial nerve (FN) and epitympanic recess.[18] (B) Temporal bone dissection showing middle fossa dura (MFD), lateral semicircular canal (LSC), facial nerve (FN), sigmoid sinus (SS) and digastric ridge (DR).[18]

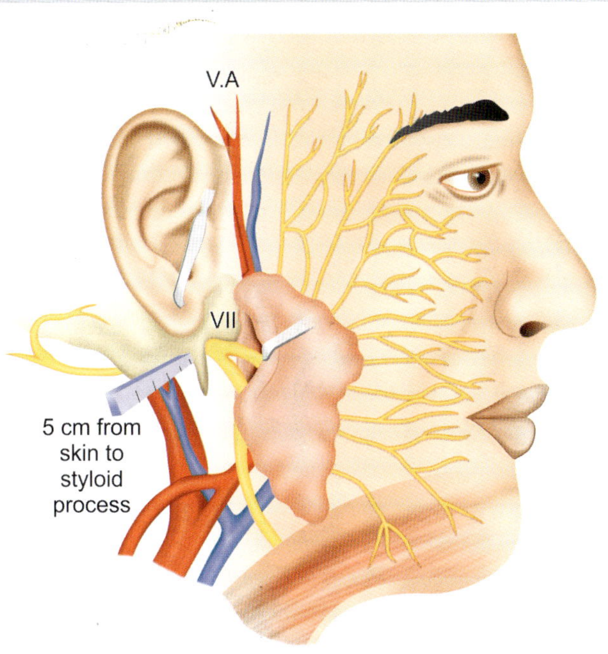

Fig. 8: Landmark of facial nerve with styloid process

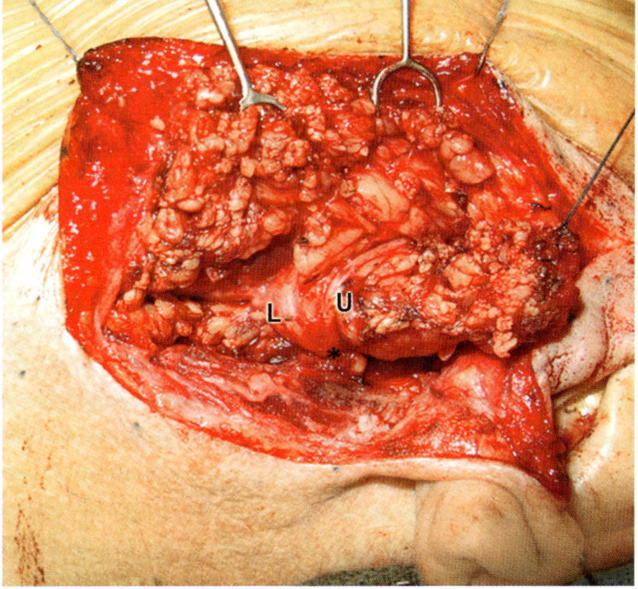

Fig. 9: Facial nerve with upper (U) and lower (L) division in parotid surgery

- Posterior belly of digastric—While tracing the muscle backwards along its upper border to its attachment of digastric ridge, the nerve is seen between it and the styloid process (Fig. 9).

Anatomical Variations of Facial Nerve and its Canal

The facial canal may have following variations:
- Congenital dehiscence of fallopian canal
- Variation of the course of the facial nerve
- Persisting embryonic artery or vein.
    - Dehiscence of fallopian canal—Dehiscence is detected in 55% cases of which 91% are tympanic segment and 9% are in the mastoid segment. In tympanic segment, dehiscence most commonly is located adjacent to the oval window. The variation of tympanic segment is associated sometimes with agenesis of the oval window (Fig. 10)
    - Variation of the course of facial nerve—Dysplasias of the middle ear or inner ear are accompanied by aberrant course of the facial nerve.
- Intracranial segment—The facial nerve may enter the petrous pyramid instead of going through the internal auditory meatus. Then through subarcuate fossa the nerve may run through the centre of superior semicircular canal to the stylomastoid foramen by passing the middle ear cavity. Bifurcation of the nerve may be detected
- Labyrinthine segment—Bifurcation of labyrinthine segment may be present

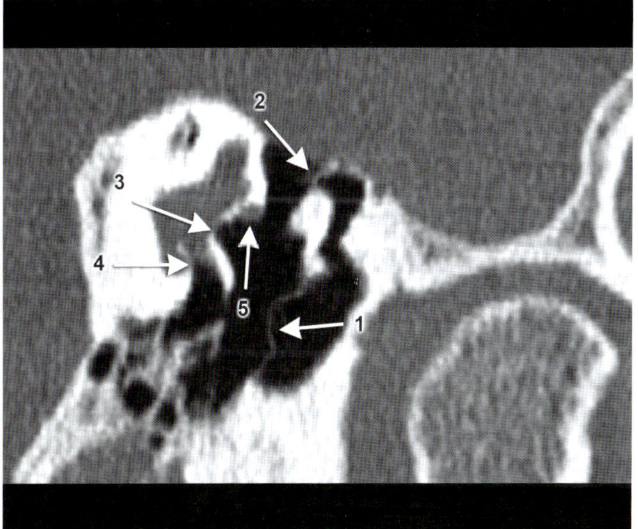

Fig 10: Coronal CT images of a left temporal bone with dehiscence of the facial nerve canal, Tympanic membrane (1), Superior malleal ligament (2), Oval window (3), round window (4), complete dehiscence of the S2 segment of the facial nerve canal (5)

- Tympanic segment—Variations in tympanic segment are:
    - Facial nerve crossing along the superior part of lateral semicircular canal as detected by House
    - Bifurcation of the nerve anterior or proximal to the oval window as noted by Nager and Proctor (1991)
    - Facial nerve crossing horizontally over the oval window

- Facial nerve crossing through the stapedial arch as described by Butler et al. (1968)
- Facial nerve crossing posteriorly between oval and round window as described by Durcan et al. (1967)
- Facial nerve crossing posteroinferiorly to the round window
- Facial nerve coming from geniculate ganglion goes straight downwards over the promontory anterior to both oval and round window and exits through the hypotympanum
- Hypoplasia of the facial nerve as seen by Kodama et al. (1982)
- Mastoid segment—Anomalies of mastoid segment are:
  - Dorsal hump of the canal beneath the prominence of the lateral semicircular canal
  - The nerve may follow posterior, lateral or anterior course
  - Bifurcation of the nerve posterior or distal to the oval window with two branches in separate canals. The separate banches may join into a single trunk before passing through the stylomastoid foramen
  - Hypoplasia of the nerve.

Variation in the Extratemporal Course of the Facial Nerve

Branching pattern within the parotid gland is variable. Five types of branching are classified by Katz and Catalano (1987).[5]

Type I

- Splitting and reunion of the zygomatic branch
- Splitting and reunion of the mandibular branch.

Type II

- Buccal branch fuses distally with the zygomatic branch.

Type III

- Major communication between the buccal branch and the other branches.

Type IV

- Complex anastomatic branching patterns between the major divisions.

Type V

Facial nerve leaves the skull as more than one trunk.
Carotid tympani variety—

- Origin of carotid tympani may vary from 1 mm distal to 11 mm proximal to the stylomastiod foramen
- Bifurcation may occur as reported by Durcan et al. (1967)
- Large chorda tympani may be present.

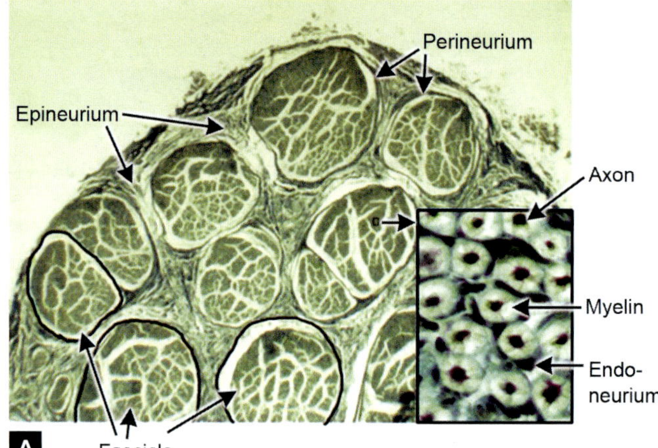

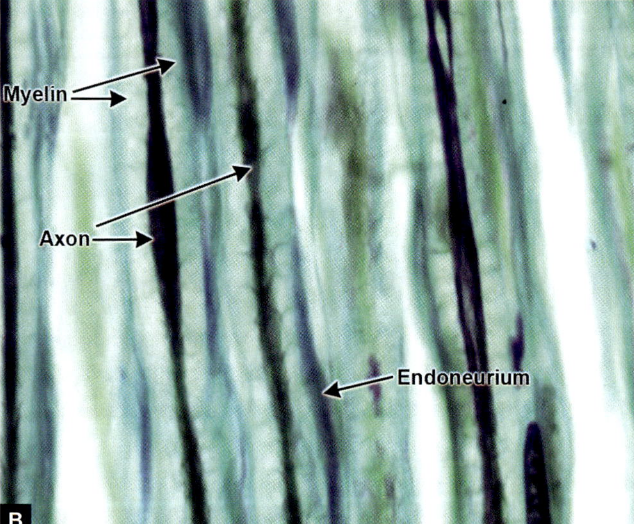

Figs 11A and B: (A) Cross-section of nerve; (B) Longitudinal section of nerve

Persisting embryonic Artery or vein—A persisting stapedial artery occasionally is encountered in tympanic segment of the facial nerve through the stapedial arch.

In rare cases, a large vein joining the nerve near geniculate ganglion is observed. It represents a persistent lateral capital vein.

Structure of Nerve (Figs 11A and B)

A nerve fiber consists of the following:

- Axon
- Myelin sheath
- Neurilemma
- Endoneurium.

A group of nerve fibers is enclosed in a fibrous sheath called perineurium forming fascicle which is bound together by epineurium.

Pathophysiology of Nerve Injury

Nerve injuries are described by Seddon (1943) as—

Neuropraxia: It is the blockage of impulses across the affected axonal segment due to pressure. With this lesion nerve is viable and returns to normal with release of pressure without residual deficit. This is associated with loss of myelin at the sight of pressure but no death and degeneration of the axon. Electrophysiologic testing reveals normal function except that the electromyogram fails to show voluntary motor action potential as they are not conducted across the blockage. This is a reversible conduction block.

Axonotemesis: It is a state of Wallerian degeneration distal to the lesion with preservation of motor axon endoneural sheaths. Electrically, the nerve shows rapid and complete degeneration with loss of voluntary motor units. Regenerations to motor end plates will occur as long as the endoneural tubes are intact.[6]

Neurotmesis: It is characterized by both Wallerian degeneration and loss of endoneural tubules. Electrophysiologic studies yield evidence of complete nerve degeneration. Regeneration is dependent on many factors including the integrity of the endoneurium, perineurium and epineurium and extent of ischemia, and scarring around the lesion.[6]

For assessment of prognosis of recovery of the facial nerve injury in various disorders Sunderland (1951) proposed five degrees of nerve injury based on anatomical structure of the nerve as opposed to the three types of nerve injuries described by Seddon.

- **1st degree**—Partial block to flow of axoplasm, no morphological changes is seen. The injury is reversible and allows complete recovery (neurapraxia)
- **2nd degree**—Wallerian degeneration occurs but endoneurial architecture is preserved; the recovery is complete (axonotmesis)
- **3rd degree**—Wallerian degeneration and disruption of endoneurial architecture occur. There is imcomplete recovery, complicated by functional sequelae. During recovery, axons of one tube can grow into another resulting in synkinesis (neurotmesis)
- **4th degree**—Only the epineurium is intact and recovery is poor. It reflects severe nerve injury (partial transection)
- **5th degree**—It is injury to epineurium in addition to above. It involves complete and total disruption of nerve continuity (complete transection).[7]

House-Brackmann facial nerve grading is widely used to characterize facial paralysis where grade I represents normal function and grade VI signifies complete paralysis. Intermediate grades (grade II, III, IV and V) vary according to function at rest and effort. The grading system predicts recovery of nerve lesion in Bell's palsy (Table 1).

Facial Nerve Testing

a. Topognosis or Site of Lesion Testing:

1. Lacrimal flow rate: Schimer's test (Fig. 12). It is an objective test to test facial nerve:
   - Study of lacrimation. A filter paper strip of 5 cm × 0.5 cm is kept in lower fornix of each eye and the amount of saturation (soakage) produced within 5 minutes is compared from side to side. The test is considered significant, if—
     - Unilateral lacrimation reduces to ≤30% of total lacrimation of both eyes
     - Bilateral lacrimation reduces to ≤25 mm
       - It accurately predicts the side of nerve entrapment in only about 60% cases of Bells' palsy
       - It may be used to determine potential for exposure keratitis.

Table 1: House-Brackmann facial nerve grading system

Grade	Description	Characteristics
Grade-I	Normal	Normal facial function in all areas
Grade-II	Mild dysfunction	Gross: Slight weakness noticeable. On close inspection may have slight synkinesis At rest: Normal symmetry and tone Motion: Forehead—moderate to good function Eye—complete closure with minimum effort Mouth—slight asymmetry
Grade-III	Moderate dysfunction	Gross: Obvious but not disfiguring difference between two sides; noticeable but not severe synkinesis; contracture and/or hemifacial spasm At rest: Normal symmetry and tone Motion: Forehead—slight to moderate movement Eye—complete closure with effort Mouth—slightly weak motion with maximum effort
Grade-IV	Moderately Severe dysfunction	Gross: Obvious weakness and/or disfiguring asymmetry At rest: Normal asymmetry and tone Motion: Forehead—No motion Eye—Incomplete closure Mouth—asymmetric with maximum effort
Grade-V	Severe dysfunction	Gross: Only minimally perceptible motion At rest: Asymmetry Motion: Forehead—no motion Eye—Incomplete closure Mouth—Slight movement
Grade-VI	Total paralysis	No movement at any level and obvious asymmetry at rest

(Adopted from House JW colleagues.[8])

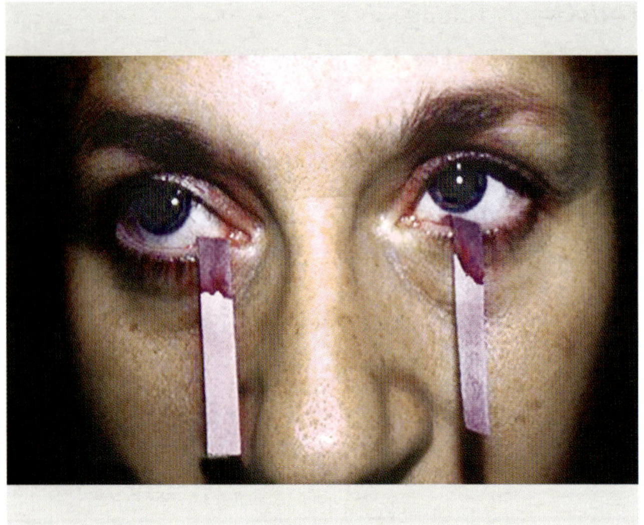

Fig. 12: Schirmer's test

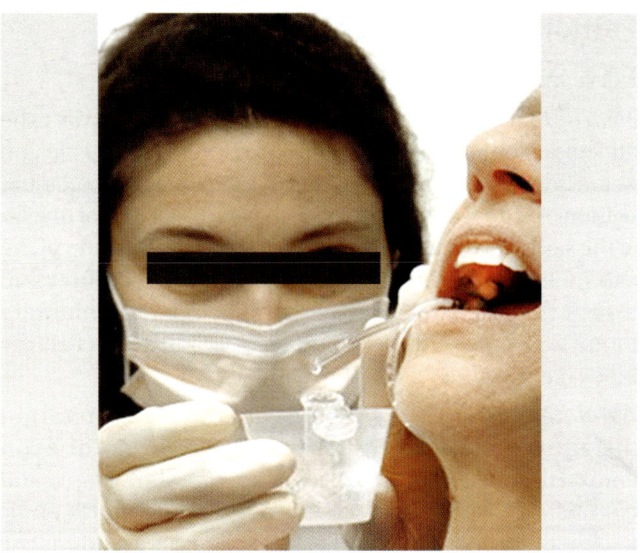

Fig. 13: Salivary flow test of submandibular gland

2. Salivary flow test: It is an objective test of submandibular salivary flow that measures the function of chorda tympani (Fig. 13). A no. 50 polyethylene tube is introduced for about 3 mm into both Wharton's papillae and numbers of drops are monitored over 5 minutes.
   - A 25% reduction between two sides is considered significant
   - It is an unreliable test.
3. Taste testing (Anterior 2/3rd of the tongue): It provides useful information in the diagnosis and management of facial paralysis. It is assessed by electrogustometry. It is also an unreliable test.
4. Stapedial Reflex: It is an objective test that provides easy and repeated assessment by tympanometry. Stapedial reflex is lost in lesions above the nerve to stapedius muscle.
   - It does not offer accurate prognosis in the earliest stages of acute facial palsy
   - However, restoration of the stapedial reflex within 3 week after the onset of facial palsy is associated with a better functional recovery.

b. Electrodiagonostic tests:

These testes are useful for—
- Indicating prognosis of facial nerve recovery
- Assessing time for surgical decompression of the nerve.
1. Electromyography (EMG): It measures electrical responses during needle insertion, at rest and during volitional movement.[9]
   Possible reponses are-
   - Silent resting potential
   It is associated with
   - Normal innervated muscle in a state of rest
   - Severe muscle wasting caused by fibrosis

- Voluntary motor unit potential—It is characterized by diphasic/Triphasic morphology with an amplitude of 50–1500 microvolts
- Fibrillation potentials—It associated with involuntary, invisible contractions of single denervated muscle fiber indicating degeneration of the muscle nerve supply. It has amplitude 10–200 microvolts
- Polyphasic motor units—Precedes recovery of denervated muscle fibers and is seen during nerve regeneration.

Uses of EMG: Help to detect subclinical evidence of early regeneration.
- Help to differentiate birth trauma from an embryogenic etiology.

Demerits of EMG: There is a 14–21 day delay in development of fibrillation potentials after the facial nerve injury. So EMG is not useful in evolution of acute facial paralysis.

2. Nerve conduction time (Latency): It is used to test latency response of a muscle on electrical stimulation. Latency for each compared action potential is the time between onset of stimulus and onset of response.
   Here, EMG equipment is used to stimulate facial nerve near the stylomastoid foramen and record over one of the facial muscle group, e.g. frontalis, mid face or mentalis.
   It is not a reliable prognostic test.[10]
3. Nerve excitability test (NET):
   - Facial nerve is stimulated over the stylomastiod foramen and presence of a twitch response in facial musculature is subjectively determined

- The lowest (threshold) value for eliciting a response on the paralyzed side compared with the threshold value of the normal or contralateral side. Difference more than 3.5 milliampere is associated with poor prognosis
- It is easy to perform, readily available and has a low cost.

Demerits of the test is that, it—
- Presumes the contralateral side to be normal
- Stimulates only the large myelinated fibers
- Patients may have incomplete recovery despite normal NET.

4. **Trigeminofacial (Blink) test:** The Blink reflex is electrodiagnostically assessed by using percutaneous stimulation at the supraorbital foramen and recording EMG response of both orbicularis oculi muscles with the nose at the reference electrode.

It measures conduction in the intracranial and intratemporal portion of facial nerve.

5. **Electroneuronography (ENoG):** Here, bipolar surface electrodes are used for stimulating as well as recording the compared facial muscle action potential. Two techniques has been proposed for positioning of electrodes—
- Standard lead placement (SLP)
- Optimized lead placement (OLP).

OLP is more reliable than SLP. Alae nasi is the optimum site for lead placement.
- The recording electrode is placed at the nasal alae
- The stimulating electrode is placed at the stylomastoid foramen
- After placing the electrode, the stimulus intensity is gradually increased until a smooth biphasic waveform of maximal amplitude is obtained
- The response amplitude of the paralyzed side is compared with that of the normal side and the percentage reduction is calculated
- This percentage reduction correlates with percentage of axonal degeneration and rate of percentage reduction correlates with prognosis.

Electroneuronography is the most accurate prognostic indicator of all the electrodiagnostic test (MST is next best).

Clinical applications
- Bells' Palsy—Surgery is considered, if there is 90% or greater reduction in amplitude within 21 day of onset of paralysis on ENG
- ENoG can document the degree of subclinical facial nerve involvement and prognosis prior to CP angle and skull base tumor surgery
- ENoG—Diagnosis of occult tumors of facial nerve

- Malignant otitis externa—Serial ENoG can be used to monitor prognosis or resolution of an underlying neuritis
- Temporal bone fracture with facial paralysis surgery is considered as soon as the patient's condition permits in cases of immediate paralysis with greater than 90% degeneration by ENoG
- ENoG helps for assessing severity of nerve damage following Iatrogenic injury.

6. **Maximal stimulating testing (MST):** It is defined as a variation of the NET in which the ipsilateral and contralateral facial muscles are stimulated at a level sufficient to depolarize all the motor axons underlying the stimulator. Here, some electrode is used as in NET. Current is initially set at 5 mA (milliamps) and is gradually increased to the level of the patient's tolerance and is assigned a grade of—
- Equal—Associated with incomplete recovery in only 8% cases
- Slightly decreased
- Markedly decreased—associated with poor progression
- No movement.

MST becomes abnormal before the NET and is, therefore, a better progrostic indicator.

Intraoperative Facial Nerve Monitoring (Fig. 14)

The goals of intraoperative monitoring are
- Enhancing early nerve identification

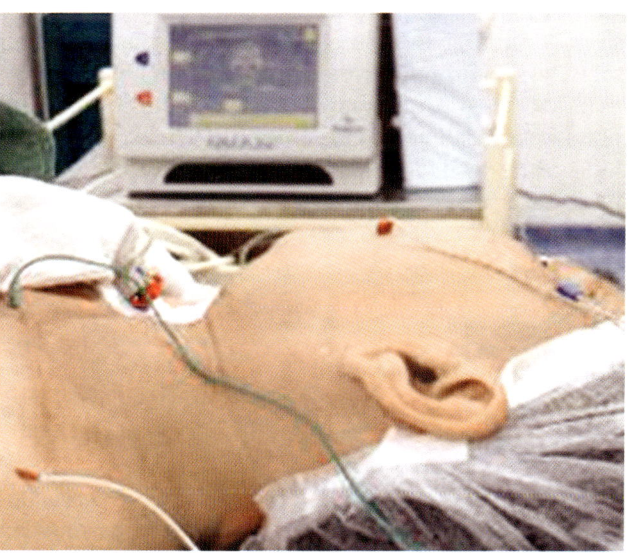

Fig. 14: Intraoperative facial nerve monitoring

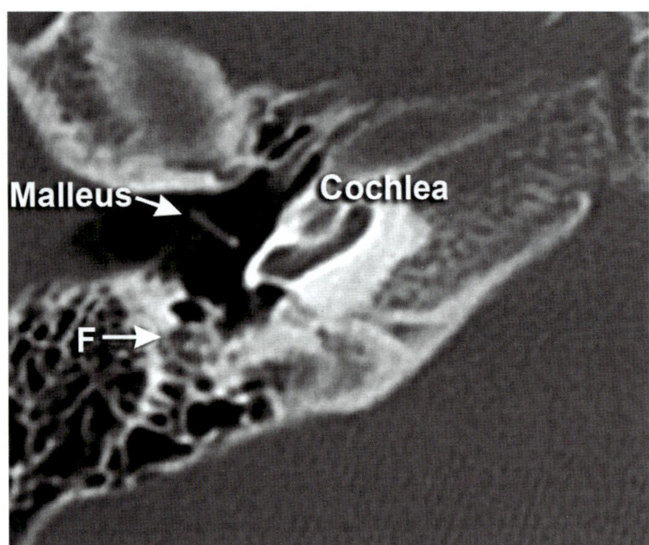

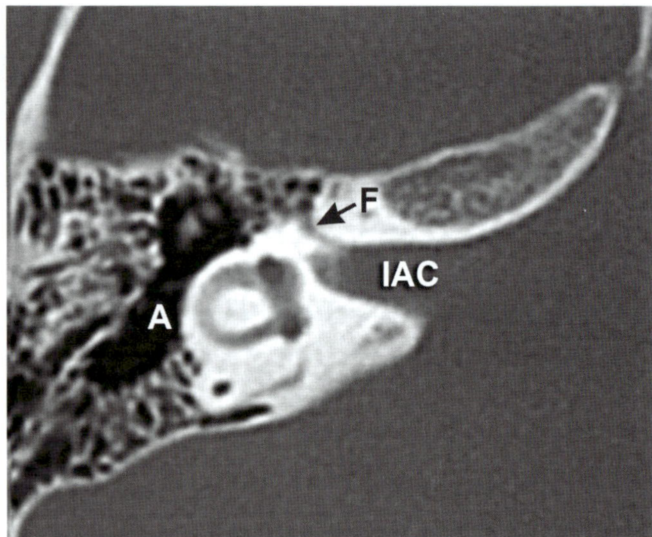

Fig. 15: HRCT of temporal bone (axial cut)
Abbreviations: A, Antrum; F, facial nerve; IAC, internal auditory canal

- Minimizing trauma to the nerve
- Assessing neural integrity after dissection is complete.

Nerve Localization

Two channel EMG recording is done by insertion of close EMG electrode pairs (active/reference) at nasolabial and orbicularis oculi regions.
- Common ground electrode is high at forehead
- Stimulating electrode is monopolar.
    It is used to map out nerve location with respect to tumor mass.

Minimizing Neural Trauma

Blunt trauma gives discrete compound muscle action potential synchronous with the surgical maneuver.

Traction produces asynchronous action potential that may persist for seconds or minutes. These responses indicate the need for change in the dissection technique to decrease facial nerve injury.

Complete transaction of the nerve with sharp dissection may evoke little or no response.

Assessment of Neural Integrity

Assessment of neural integrity is done after the dissection is complete. Facial nerve is stimulated proximal to the area of dissection with a low current level (0.05 mA). During dissection strength of current used is 0.2 mA.

Intraoperative nerve monitoring has a role in cerebello-pontine angle (CPA) tumor surgery, in revision mastoid and parotid surgery, and supervised resident training.

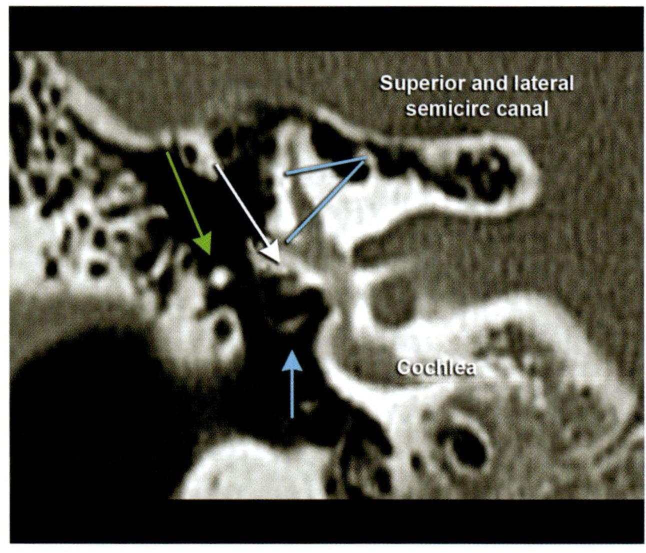

Fig. 16: HRCT of temporal bone (coronal cut) showing the facial nerve above the oval window and below the lateral semicircular canal—white arrow (facial nerve), green arrow (incus), blue arrow (stapes)

Facial Nerve Imaging

HRCT (high-resolution CT) of axial and coronal cut with slice thickness less than 2 mm will display the bony labyrinth, facial nerve canal and the tympanic cavity with its contents. Tympanic portion is best identified on axial CT. Mastoid segment is easier to visualize on coronal or saggital views (Figs 15 and 16).

MRI with contrast may display enhancement of facial nerve because of rich perineural arteriovenous plexus. It

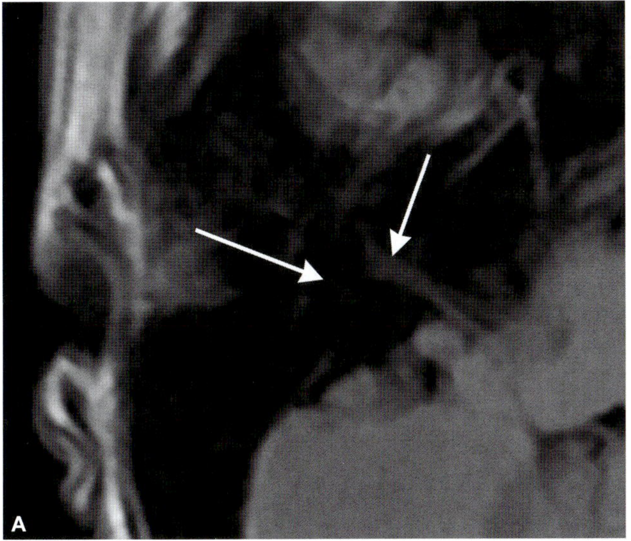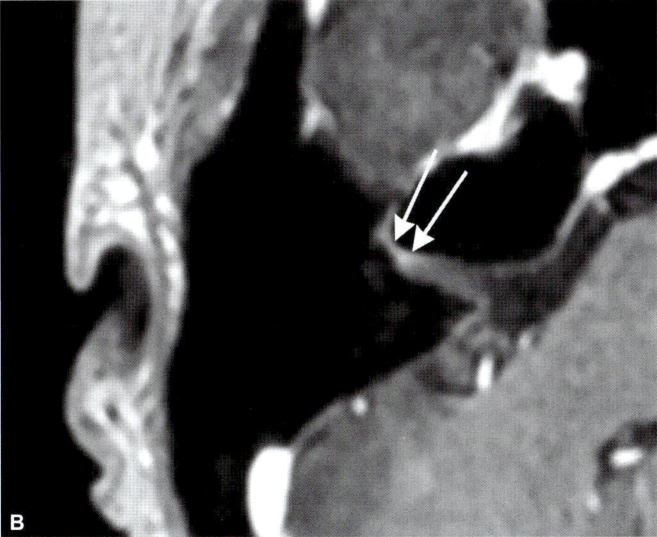

Figs 17A and B: MRI—(A) Precontrast axial image of facial nerve at cerebellopontine (CP) angle. (B) Contrast-enhanced axial image of distal meatal and labyrinthine segment of right facial nerve

is commonly seen in geniculate gangalion and tympanic segment. Enhancement is considered abnormal along the cisternal, canalicular or the extra cranial segment of the facial nerve.[11] It is useful in visualizing neoplastic or inflammatory lesion (Figs 17A and B).

Facial Nerve Paralysis

Facial nerve paralysis is a common problem that involves the paralysis of any structures innervated by the facial nerve. There are number of causes that may result in facial nerve paralysis.

Causes[12]

- Bell's palsy—It is the most common cause of facial nerve paralysis. The lesion is linked to herpes simplex infection
- Peripheral nerve causes (facial muscle paralysis with forehead affected)
  - Lyme disease
  - Otitis media or mastoiditis
  - Ramsay Hunt syndrome
  - Autoimmune polyneuropathy (e.g. Guillain-Barre syndrome, typically bilateral)
  - Head or neck mass lesion (e.g. Cholesteatoma).
- Central/supranuclear causes (facial muscle paralysis with forehead spared)
  - Cerebral mass lesion (e.g. tumor)
  - Cerebrovascular accident (typically with ipsilateral hemiparesis or hemiplegia)
  - Multiple sclerosis.

- Trauma
  - Temporal bone fracture
  - Brain stem injury
  - Penetrating middle ear injury
  - Barotrauma—
    - ◆ Altitude paralysis
    - ◆ Scuba diving
  - Mastoid surgery
  - Parotid surgery.
- Endocrine
  - Diabetes mellitus
  - Hyperthyroidism
  - Pregnancy
  - Hypertension
  - Alcohol.
- Infection
  - Malignant otitis externa (skull base osteomyelitis)
  - Acute or chronic otitis media
  - Mastoiditis
  - Varicella zoster virus (chicken pox)
  - Herpes zoster oticus (Ramsay–Hunt syndrome)
  - Influenza vaccine and influenza
  - Lyme disease
  - HIV infection
  - Parotitis
  - Meningitis or encephalitis
  - Mumps
  - Mononucleosis
  - Leprosy
  - Coxsackie virus infection
  - Syphilis

- – Tuberculosis
- – Botulism
- – Mucormycosis.
- Tumor
  - – Facial nerve neuroma
  - – Glomas jugulare tumor
  - – Primary temporal bone tumors
  - – Meningiomas
  - – Hemangioblastoma
  - – Hemangioma
  - – Pontine glioma
  - – Parotid tumor.
- Birth
  - – Birth trauma (forceps delivery)
  - – Molding
  - – Congenital facial palsy
  - – Mobius syndrome
  - – Cardio facial syndrome.
- Toxic
  - – Talidomide
  - – Tetanus
  - – Diphtheria
  - – Carbon monoxide
  - – Lead intoxication.
- Idiopathic
  - – Myasthenia gravis
  - – Guilain-Barre Syndrome
  - – Sarcoidosis.
- Iatrogenic
  - – Antitetanus serum
  - – Vaccine treatment for rabies
  - – Mandibular block anesthesia
  - – Head Neck surgery.

Bell's Palsy (Fig. 18)

Bell's palsy is the most common cause of facial palsy (80%). It is named after Scottish anatomist Sir Charles Bell who described the disease in 1821.

- It is an acute, unilateral, peripheral facial paralysis resulting in inability to control facial muscles on the affected side
- Although Bell's palsy is defined as idiopathic unilateral facial nerve paralysis, the lesion is linked to a viral. Etiology—herpes simplex infection
- Polymerase chain reaction (PCR) assays done on fresh and stored geniculate ganglions from temporal bone specimens have detected HSV-1
- The hallmark of the condition is rapid onset of partial or complete palsy that often occurs overnight, less than 1% cases it may occur bilaterally resulting in total facial paralysis
- Male or female is equally affected. 5th or 6th decade of life is mostly at risk although any age group may be affected. Right- or left-sided diseases may occur equally. Reccurrence is seen in 10% of patients. Pregnancy increases the risk. About 10% of patients have positive family history of Bell's palsy. A high-frequency of diabetes mellitus is reported in patients presenting with Bell's palsy.

Symptoms of Bell's Palsy

- Sudden weakness or paralysis on one side of the face that may cause it to droop
- Drooling
- Excessive tearing or a dry eye
- Loss of ability to taste (involvement of chorda tympani)

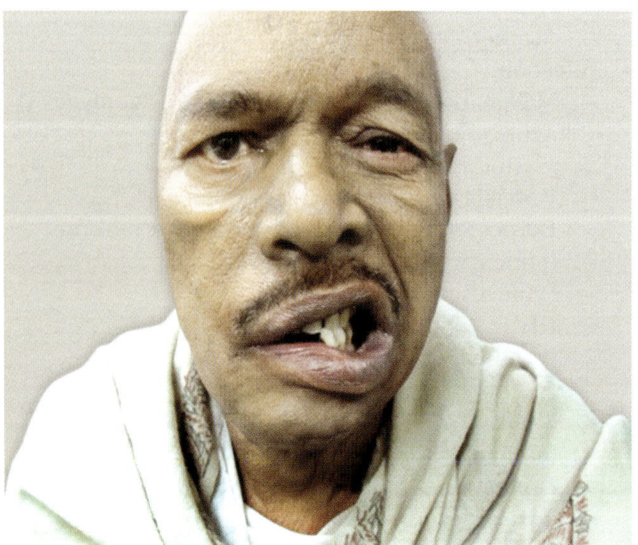

Fig. 18: 60-year-old male with Bell's palsy

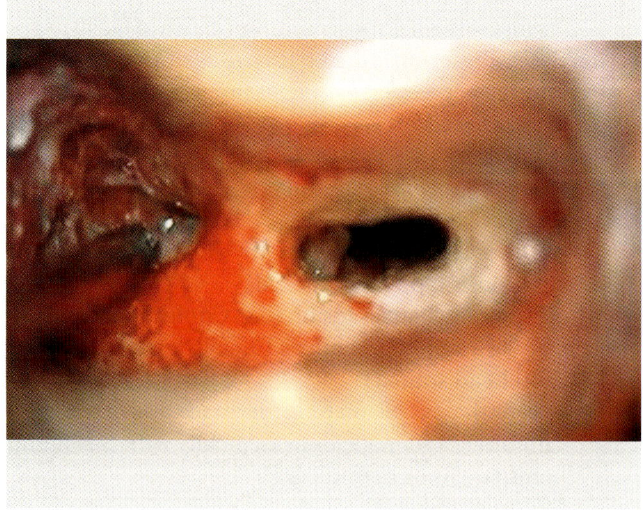

Fig. 19: Facial nerve decompression through transmastoid approach via posterior tympanotomy in a patient with Bell's palsy

- Numbness in the affected side of face
- Increased sensitivity to sound (stapedial paralysis).

Pathophysiology

Pathophysiology of Bell's palsy is an inflammatory condition resulting swelling of the facial nerve within the inelastic fallopian canal. Nerve swelling and compression inhibit flow of axoplasm that results a conduction block or nerve damage. The site of inhibition of nerve impulse is at the narrowest part of facial canal, i.e. the meatal foramen.

On attempted eyelid closure of the affected side with facial paresis or paralysis, eye turns upwards and outwards. This helps in protecting the eye from exposure Keratitis by producing wetting of the globe surface. This is known as Bell's Phenomenon.

Recovery of Bell's palsy is usually beginning within 3 weeks. Full recovery occurs within 6 months. Approximately 15% of patients experience severe deformity with minimal return of facial movement. Prognosis is good in incomplete Bell's palsy (95% complete recovery) and in cases where recovery stars with 3 weeks of acute paralysis (75% complete recovery). All patients with more than 90% neuronal degeneration within 2 weeks of onset are considered MCF surgical decompression of the meatal foramen, labyrinthine segment, geniculate ganglion and proximal tympanic portion. Transmastoid decompression does not have any role in Bell's palsy.

Management Protocol

Management Protocol of Bells' Palsy is out lined below:

Treatment of Bell's Facial Palsy

Medical treatment
- Patients presenting with facial palsy are treated with high-dose of oral corticosteroids
  - Prednisone 1 mg/kg daily for 10 days within the first 2–3 weeks of onset.
- Corticosteroids may improve the recovery of the paralysis via decrease in inflammation. Patient with diabetes mellitus or hyper tension are advised to monitor blood sugar and blood pressure during medication of corticosteroids.

Due to viral etiology of Bell's palsy acyclovir 800 mg 5 times/days or valacyclovir 500 mg 2 times/day is also advised
- Eye care is instituted as needed if improving of facial nerve is delayed
- Electroneurographic testing (ENoG) is repeated every 3 days until more than 90% degeneration is detected, surgical decompression is considered
- Electomyographic testing (ENG) is performed, if facial paralysis persists more than 3 weeks

- Physiotherapy or active facial movements are instituted for return of some movement to the facial muscles.

Surgical Treatment
Criteria for indications of surgical decompression are:[13]
- Complete denervation
- Paralysis for more than 4–6 weeks
- Incomplete return of function in 60 days
- Recurrent facial palsy
- Nerve excitability test shows a difference of 3.5 mA on both the sides
- Schirmer's test shows tear flow is reduced more than 50% on the affected side.

Surgical nerve decompression is controversial. Middle cranial fossa (MCF) decompression provides more than double the chances of facial nerve recovery (HB grade I or II) compared to medical treatment as studied by Gantz BJ et al.[14]

Only this approach (MCF) permits decompression of entire labyrinthine segment, meatal segment and area of meatal foramen.

Periosteum covering the labyrinthine segment is needed to incise from meatal foramen to the geniculate ganglion and dura of internal auditory canal is to be exposed and incised for better result of decompression.

Fibrous band formed around the facial nerve near the meatal foramen needs division for disappearance of swelling of the nerve from distal meatal segment to the geniculate ganglion.

Decompression of the facial nerve through transmastoid approach via posterior tympanotomy is a routine procedure.
- Wilde's postauricular incision with anteriorly based pedicle flap is made
- Cortical mastoidectomy is done
- Mastoid segment of the facial nerve is decompressed
- Incus is disarticulated and translocated in the middle ear, if necessary
- Middle fossa dura is skeletonized and decompression is started proximal to the second genu till the entire nerve is reached.

Following release of nerve various pictures are seen:
- Edematous nerve where steroids are started post operatively
- Congested nerve where acyclovir and steroids are stared
- Thinned or atrophic nerve resulting from disuse atrophy.

Infections

Herpes Zoster Oticus and Ramsay Hunt Syndrome (Fig. 20)

Herpes Zoster oticus is characterized by intense ear pain and erythematous vesicular rash on external auditory canal and pinna. Mechanism of disease is reactivation of dormant

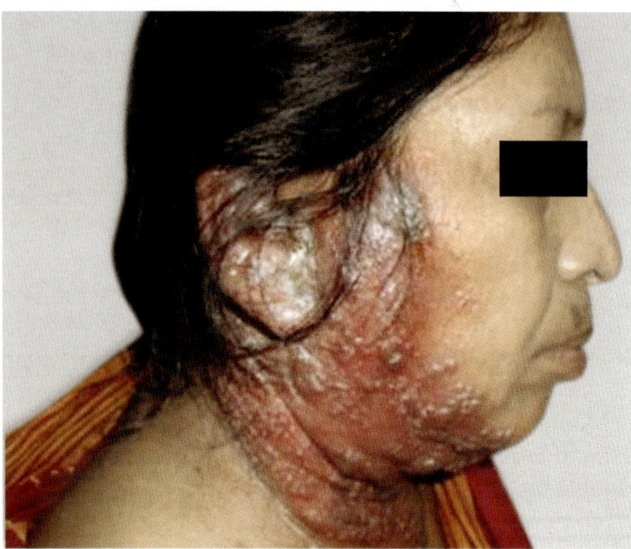

Fig. 20: Herpes Zoster oticus

herpes zoster virus (VZV) in geniculate ganglion affecting sensory afferent neurons. If the viral involvement progresses to involve the efferent motor axons of the facial nerve, then Ramsay Hunt syndrome is developed. The syndrome is characterized by—

- Facial nerve palsy and vesicular eruptions of head and neck in the distribution of the affected facial nerve.

The syndrome may be accompanied with hearing loss, vertigo, and anesthesia of face due to involvement of V and VIII nerve.

Diagnosis is confirmed by rising titers of antibodies to VZV. PCR to detect VZV in ear exudates is highly sensitive and becomes positive before the appearance of vesicles.[15]

Prognosis for Ramsay Hunt is worse than Bell's palsy. Only 10% of patents get recovery following complete loss of functions without treatment.[16]

The recommended treatment includes combinations of—

- Oral steroid (prednisolone 1 mg/kg/day for 5 days followed by 10 days taper) and
- Acyclovir (250 mg i/v t.i.d. or oral acyclovir 800 mg 5 times daily)

There is no indication for surgical decompression.

Besides Bell's palsy and herpes zoster oticus, a variety of infections causing facial nerve paralysis are:

- Acute otitis media
- Chronic otitis media
- Lyme disease and Necrotizing otitis externa.

Lyme disease: It is caused by spirochete Borrelia burgdorferi resulting in wide spread systemic disease. Most common neuralgic manifestation of the disease is facial nerve paralysis. Serology study and CSF analysis to detect IgG and IgM antibodies are done for diagnosis. Treatment includes

antibiotic, e.g. doxycycline, amoxicillin for 2–3 weeks. In most cases, recovery of facial paralysis occurs and surgery is not required.

Necrotizing otitis externa: The disease usually occurs in elderly patients who are immune suppressed or patients with poorly controlled diabetes mellitus. It is commonly caused by pseudomonas aeruginosa. The disease begins in the external auditory canal then extends to involve the temporal bone and skull base resulting in facial paralysis as well as lower cranial nerves also. Diagnosis includes—CT/MRI/gallium and technetium bone scans.

Treatment includes—

- EAC debridement
- Topical antibiotics
- IV antibiotics—Antibiotics to be given till gallium scans show no evidence of infection
- Hyperbaric O_2 therapy

Radical debridement of the temporal bone and skull base is used in resistant cases.

Temporal Bone Fractures

Temporal bone fractures are classified as longitudinal or transverse depending on the relationship of the fracture line to the long axis of the petrous part of temporal bone, although a significant proportion of fractures are mixed. Longitudinal fractures are associated with 20% incidence of facial paralysis. Perigeniculate region is mainly involved. 80% of fractures are longitudinal.

Transverse fractures are associated with higher incidence of facial paralysis (50%). Labyrinthine or mastoid segment are mainly involved resulting in SNHL and vestibular dysfunction. Clinical and radiological considerations which have been discussed by some authors for temporal bone fractures based on otic capsule sparing verses otic capsule violating fractures. Otic capsule involved fractures are:

- Twice more prone to develop facial nerve paralysis
- Four times more prone to have CSF leak
- Seven times more chances to sustain SNHL.[17]

In comminuted, fracture of the temporal bone resulting from head injuries, a combination of the longitudinal and transverse fracture with facial nerve paralysis may happen. The injury is associated with brain edema, pneumocranium and unconsciousness as well as skull base fractures with CSF.

HRCT (high-resolution CT scan) will help to detect type of fracture as well as fracture of temporal bone and other skull base, brain edema, hematoma or pneumocranium (Figs 21 to 23).

ENoG is also helpful for decision making in surgical exploration.

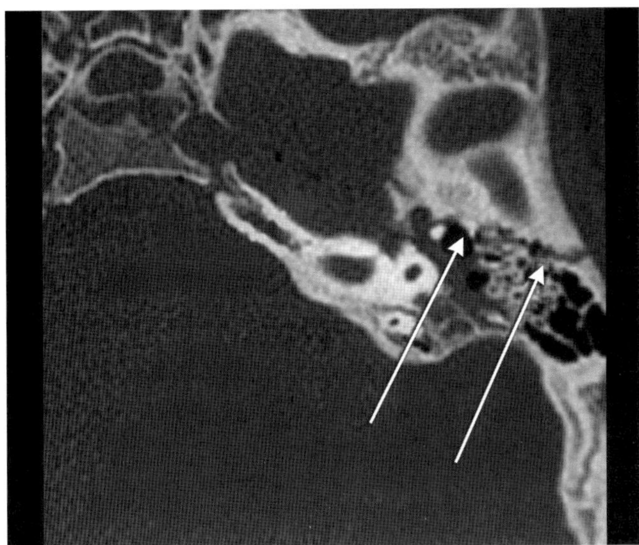

Fig. 21: HRCT Temporal bone (axial cut) showing longitudinal fracture extending through mastoid air cells into middle ear cavity with hemotympanum (arrows)

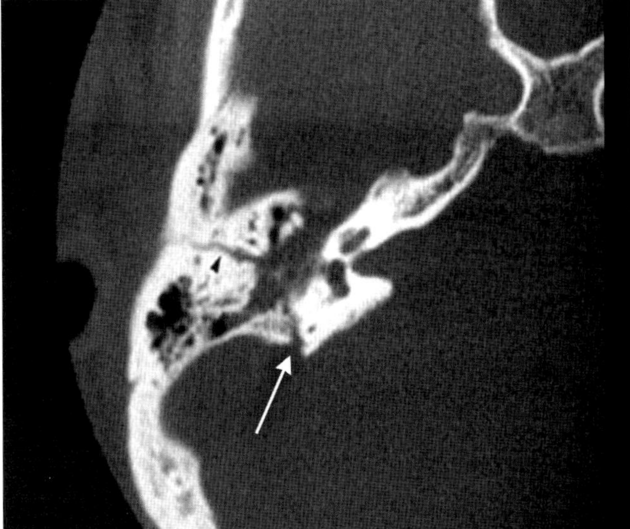

Fig. 23: Axial HRCT scan shows a combination of transverse fracture (arrow) and an oblique facture (arrowhead) of temporal bone

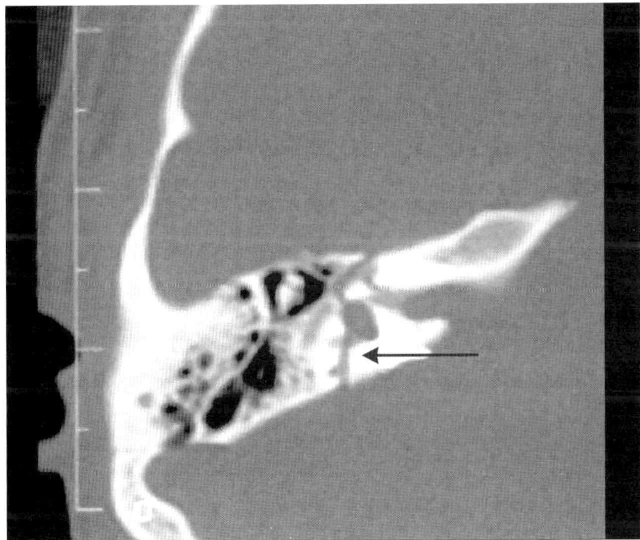

Fig. 22: Axial HRCT scan shows transverse temporal bone fracture (arrow)

Goal of Surgery

- For decompression of nerve to prevent ischemic injury
- For removal of bony fragments impinging on the nerve
- For re-establishing continuity in case of transaction.

Treatment protocol:

For early postinjury case—

- Acute onset incomplete palsy without progression
  - Good prognosis
  - No surgical exploration.

- Acute complete paralysis, if ENoG shows >90% degeneration within 6 days of onset—early surgical exploration is indicated
- Satisfactory recovery is expected if treated within 90 days following trauma.

For late postinjury case—

- ENoG is not helpful after 3 weeks of injury
- CT scan and EMG help to guide for late exploration to remove any fragment of bone and fibrosis that may prevent regeneration. Exploration is done with a thought to gain nerve continuity by—end-to-end anastomosis, interposition grafting or rerouting techniques.
- Surgical approach depends on the site of injury and hearing status of the patients
  - Middle fossa approach is done for longitudinal fractures where hearing is present
  - In mixed fracture or transverse fractures with serviceable hearing, Middle fossa approach is done in combination with transmastiod exploration
  - In severe SNHL, translabyrinthine approach is preferred with less morbidity.

Iatrogenic injury to the facial nerve—It may happen during middle ear or mastoid surgery, parotid surgery, and CP angle tumor surgery. Iatrogenic damage may be avoided by following anatomical landmark and by using good surgical skill. Immediately after operation eye closer alone is not a good guide for estimating facial nerve palsy. Electrical testing like serial ENoG recording if shows 90% of degeneration of facial muscles within 3–5 days surgical exploration is indicated.

Intraoperating facial nerve monitoring helps to avoid nerve injury for any surgery around the facial nerve.

REFERENCES

1. Datta AK. Essentials of neuroanatomy, 3rd Edition. pp 253.
2. Datta AK. Essentials of neuroanatomy 3rd Edition. pp 253-5.
3. Michael E, Glasscock and George E, Shambaugh. Surgery of ear. 4th edition. p 590.
4. Grewal DS and Hathiram BT. Atlas of surgery of the facial nerve, 1st Edition. 2006. p 5.
5. Grewal DS and Hathiram BT. Atlas of surgery of the facial nerve, 1st Edition. 2006. p 13.
6. Bruce W, Jafek and Bruce W. Marrow, ENT secrets 3rd edition. p 146.
7. Glasscork- Shambaugh. Facial nerve injury. pp 434-65.
8. House JW, Brackmann DE. Facial nerve grading system otolaryngol Head Neck Surg. 1985;93:146-7.
9. Crumley RL. Electromyography and muscle biopsy in facial paralysis. In: Graham MD, House WF (Eds): Disorders of the facial nerve. New York: Raven Press; 1982.
10. Esslen E. Investigations on the localization and pathogenesis of meatolabyrinthine Palsies. The acute facial palsies. New York: Springer- Verlag; 1977.
11. Bibas T, Jiang D and Gleeson MJ. Disorder of the facial nerve, Scott- Brown's otorhinolaryngology, Head and neck Surgery, 7th edition. Vol.3 p 3881.
12. Holland. BMJ. 2004;329:553-7, Tiemstra. Am Fam. Physician. 2007;76:997-1002.
13. Marsh MJ, Coker NJ. Surgical decompression of idiopathic facial palsy. Otolaryngologic clinics of North America. 24;675-90.
14. Grants BJ, Rubinstein JT, Gidley P, Wood worth GG. Surgical management of Bell's palsy. Laryngoscope. 1999;109; 1177-88.
15. Murakamis, Honda N, Mizobouchi M, Nakashiro Y, Hato N, Gyo K. Rapid diagnosis of varicella Zoster virus infection in acute facial palsy. Neurology. 1998;51:1202-5.
16. Devriese PP, Moesker WH. The natural history of facial paralysis in herpes zoster. Clinical otolaryngology and Allied sciences. 1988;13:289-98.
17. Dahiya R, Keller J, Litofsky SN, Bankey PE, Bonassa U, Megerian CA. Temporal bone fractures: otic capsule sparing versus otic capsule violating. Clinical and radiographic considerations. Journal of trauma. 1999;47:1079-83.
18. Ahmad R lope ahmad. Anatomy of temporal bone; Dept of Otolaryngology Head Neck Surgery, International Islamic University, Malaysia. www.dc318.4shared.com

Otosclerosis

Asok K Saha

DEFINITION

Otosclerosis is a hereditary and localized disease of bone derived from otic capsule wherein normal lamellar bone is removed by osteoclasis and replaced by woven bone of greater thickness, cellularity and vascularity.[1]

Primary lesion of otic capsule results in stapes fixation with progressive deafness but it may involve the cochlea and other labyrinthine parts.

Otosclerosis is seen in human species only and is basically affecting the growth of collagen.

History

Antonio Valsalva (1741) described ankylosis of stapes while doing postmortem on the body of a dead patient.

The term Otosclerosis was introduced by Adam Politzer (1894) (Fig. 1A).

The term Otospongiosis that refers to active and vascular stage of the otosclerosis was introduced by Sieberman (1912) (Fig. 1B).

Etiology

Races: It is the most common in Caucasians and rare in black people.
Sex: It occurs with equal frequency in men and women.
Age: Age of onset of hearing loss ranges from teen to the forties. Pregnancy and menopause can accelerate the activity of Otosclerosis.[2]
Genetic factor: It has a simple autosomal dominant inheritance with incomplete penetrance.[3] Recent study suggests that Otosclerosis is primarily heterogenetic and 13% of clinical otosclerotic patients shows dominant gene with nearly complete penetrance whereas 40–50% of clinical cases reveals sporadic.

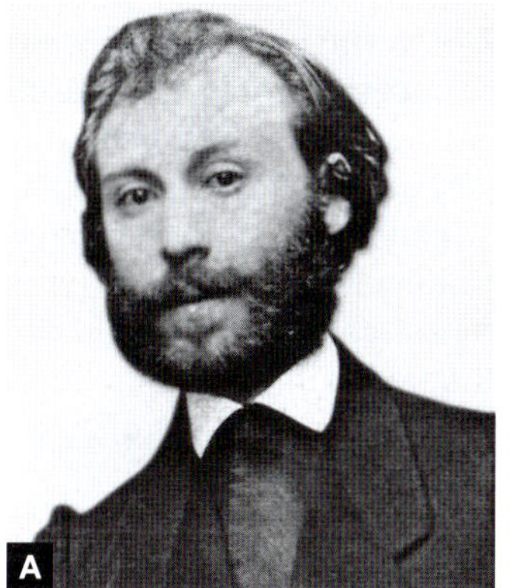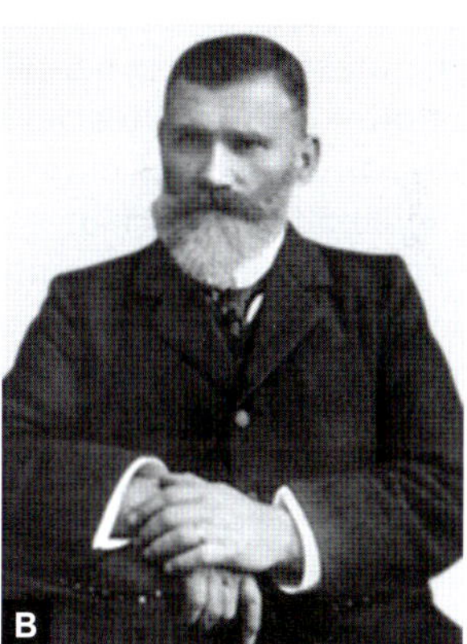

Figs 1A and B: (A) Adam Politzer (1835-1920); (B) Friedrich Siebenmann

It is evident that the clinical Otosclerosis is related to the abnormalities in expression of COLIAI gene that codes for type I collagen, similar to that seen in patients with type I Osteogenesis imperfecta.

Familial aggregation of individuals affected by otosclerosis is well-observed.

Measles: From ultra structural and immunohistochemical evidence it is noted that measles RNA and antigenicity are present in active Otosclerotic lesions, indicating a viral etiology. This is also reported in Paget's disease of bone.

Again higher level of antimeasles antibody has also been noted in perilymph from patients who underwent stapedectomy for otosclerosis as compared to controls, it hints the infective etiology.

Autoimmunity: Increased circulating antibodies to type II collagen in the blood of patients with otosclerosis is demonstrated. It implicates autoimmune disease with humeral autoimmunity to type II collagen.

Biochemistry

There are changes in mucopolysaccharide composition and concentration in fragments of stapes footplate with otosclerosis as compared to control footplate. It is related to active remodeling process rather than intrinsic feature predisposing to Otosclerosis.

Histopathology (Figs 2A to C)

At the time of puberty the normal otic capsule consists of three layers—the narrow endosteal layer, the wider enchondral layer and periosteal layer. The ossification of the enchondal layer is completed at the end of second year of life and no further bone formation takes place so that throughout life the enchondral layer consists of embryonic bone with a very poor blood supply. During or after puberty the otosclerotic process starts in the enchondral layer of otic capsule. Otosclerotic process involves increased osteoblastic and osteoclastic activity with vascular proliferation. This change usually occurs in the anterior part of the oval window near the fissula antefenestram, although lesions may be found to exist independently in other parts of the temporal bone.[4, 5] Other sites of predilection are round window, anterior wall of auditory meatus, within the stapedial footplate. Both temporal bones are affected in about 70–80% cases.

Severe degree of otosclerosis not only fixes the footplate but also causes degenerative changes in the inner ear. It is postulated that a toxic factor diffuses from the focus and acts directly on the organ of corti rather than indirectly by altering the function of other cochlear tissues. The upper basal form can represent a site of predilection for sensorineural degeneration in capsular otosclerosis since anterior focus so commonly expands into this region. A specific audiometric pattern with a low-frequency dip may be characteristics of such cases.[6]

Clinical otosclerosis is about 10 times less than the nonclinical or histological otosclerosis. Histological otosclerosis having ankylosis of stapedio-vestibular joint is about 12% whereas clinical Otosclerosis is about 1%.

Morales-Garcia[7] studied the clinical and histopathological aspects of cochlear involvement in Otosclerosis. The ears with cochlear involvement showed a greater percentage of caloric abnormalities than ears with a pure conductive deafness. In the course of time, the otosclerotic lesions are known to cause a progressive involvement of both cochlea and vestibule thus producing lesions of sensorineural elements. The vestibular involvement may explain the presence of vertiginous crises in at least some of the patients.

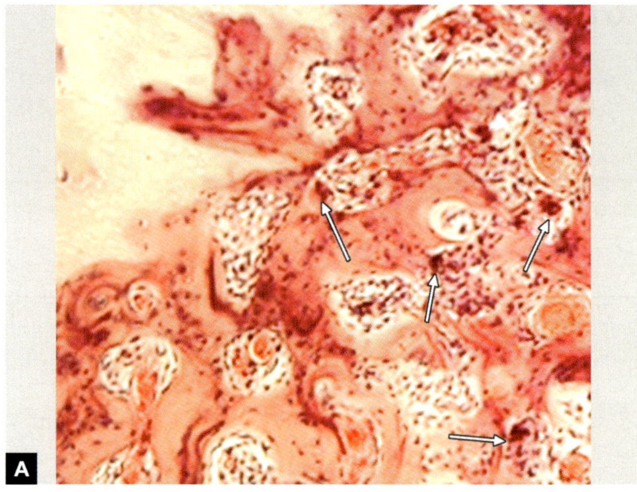

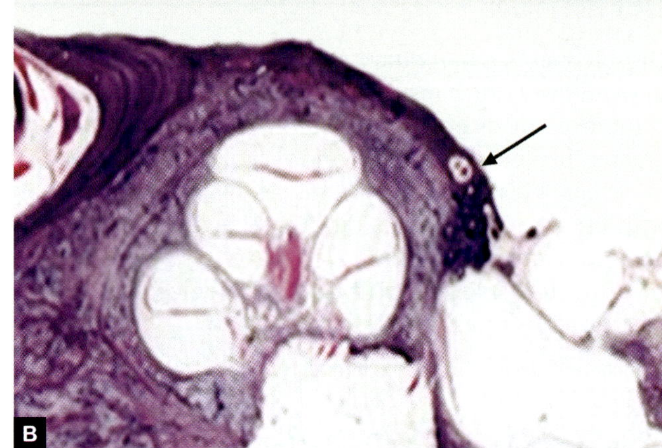

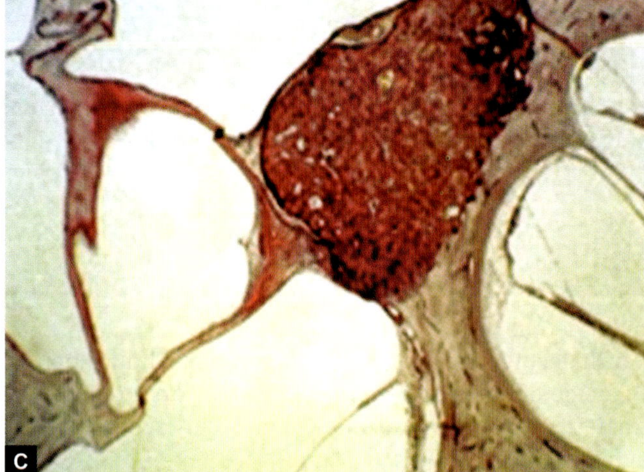

Figs 2A to C: (A) Otospongiotic lesion showing osteoclastic with vascular proliferation (arrows); (B) Histologic otosclerosis with small focus in the anterior oval window (arrow); (C) Clinical otosclerosis spreading across the anular ligament and fixing the stapes (it is ten times less than histological otosclerosis)

Clinical Features

- **Hearing loss**—It is usually bilateral. It may occur slowly at first and then gradually become worsen. The hearing loss is almost equal in each ear but sometimes one ear shows greater loss. Unilateral otosclerosis is seen in 15% of the patients. In some patients, hearing loss occur in plateau forms (or steady form)
- **Paracusis Willisii**—Phenomenon where patient hears better in noisy background. It is noted when conductive hearing loss is present without a sensorineural element. This can be explained as the people with normal hearing raises the voice above the noise level for removing the masking effect of noise, this level of speech is above the patient's threshold of hearing
- **Tinnitus**—Usually indicating sensory neuronal degeneration. It disappears in mature stages of the lesion. It is also seen in patients with pure conductive hearing loss due to increased degree of vascularity of the Otosclerotic focuses
- **Speech**—Patients speaks in a quiet voice with a good tone
- **Vertigo**—It is infrequent transient in nature resulting from the effect of toxic enzymes of the lesion on vestibular labyrinth.[8] Coexistence of hydrops should be suspected in cases of otosclerosis, if there is—
  - Poor discrimination score
  - History of vertigo in recent past.

On Examination

- **Tympanic membrane (TM)**—It looks normal and on siegelization TM is mobile. In active disease, sometimes flamingo flush or Schwartze sign may be seen through the TM due to vascular bone on promontory or prominent blood vessel in the submucosal layer of the mucous membrane of the promontory (Fig. 3)

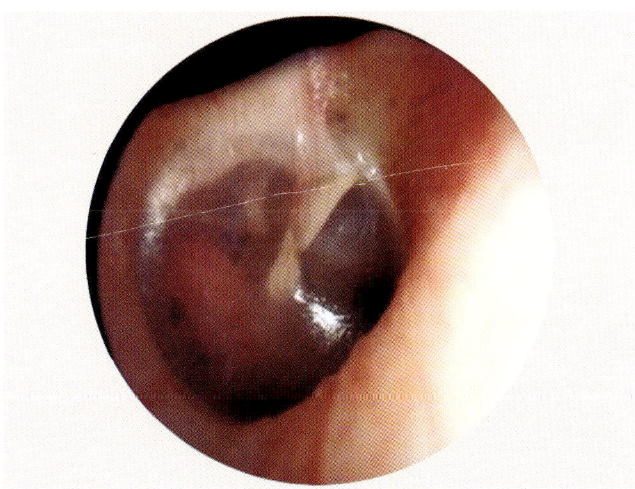

Fig. 3: Schwartze sign (Flamingo flush-active otosclerosis)

- Nose, nasopharynx and throat are normal
- **Tuning fork tests** with 512 cps show conductive hearing loss. With cochlear involvement, mixed hearing loss are present. Pure SNHL may present rarely
- **Gelle tests**—In normal person, when ear pressure in external auditory canal is increased by siegelization or by tragal pressure hearing is reduced by bone conduction because of medial movements of stapes raises the intralabyrinthine pressure resulting in immobility of the basilar membrane. In patients with otosclerosis, no such change in hearing is noted due to the fixity of the stapedeal footplate
- **Audiometry**—Air conduction curve may reveal (Figs 4 and 5)—
  - Low-frequency loss: Rising audiogram configuration (Stiffness Tilt). Hearing loss is confined to frequencies below 1000 Hertz. Higher frequencies remain unaffected
  - Flat configuration of audiogram (near about 60–65 dB)
  - Cookie Bite pattern is associated with greatest hearing loss in mid-frequency range with better sensitivity at low- and high-frequencies. It is associated with cochlear Otosclerosis.

Bone Conduction Curve Reveals

A. **Carhart's notch**—It is characterized by reduction in sensitivity at bone conduction audiometry in patients with stapes fixation caused by any lesion congenital or acquired that interferes with mobility of stapes, most commonly otosclerosis. The maximum reduction in sensitivity is seen at 2 kHz (Fig. 6).

The reduction in sensitivity on bone conduction is about-

5 dB at 500 Hz

10 dB at 1000 Hz

15 dB at 2000 Hz

5 dB at 4000 Hz

Mechanism—One element of bone conduction is the inertia caused by the weight of ossicular chain. It results in the foot plate vibration out of phase with the skull as a whole, when skull is set into vibration by tuning fork or bone vibration. So when the stapes footplate is fixed, it is no longer free to vibrate. Therefore, the inertial component of bone conduction is lost (especially noticeable at 2 kHz).

The carharts notch may disappear after stapedectomy and this phenomenon is then called as an over-closure of air bone gap.[9]

Therefore, the carhart's notch is the results of breaking of normal ossicular resonance which is about 2000 Hz. It indicates mechanical distortion rather than a reflection of cochlear reserve.

B. Mixed or even a pure SN loss may be seen in patients with cochlear otosclerosis.

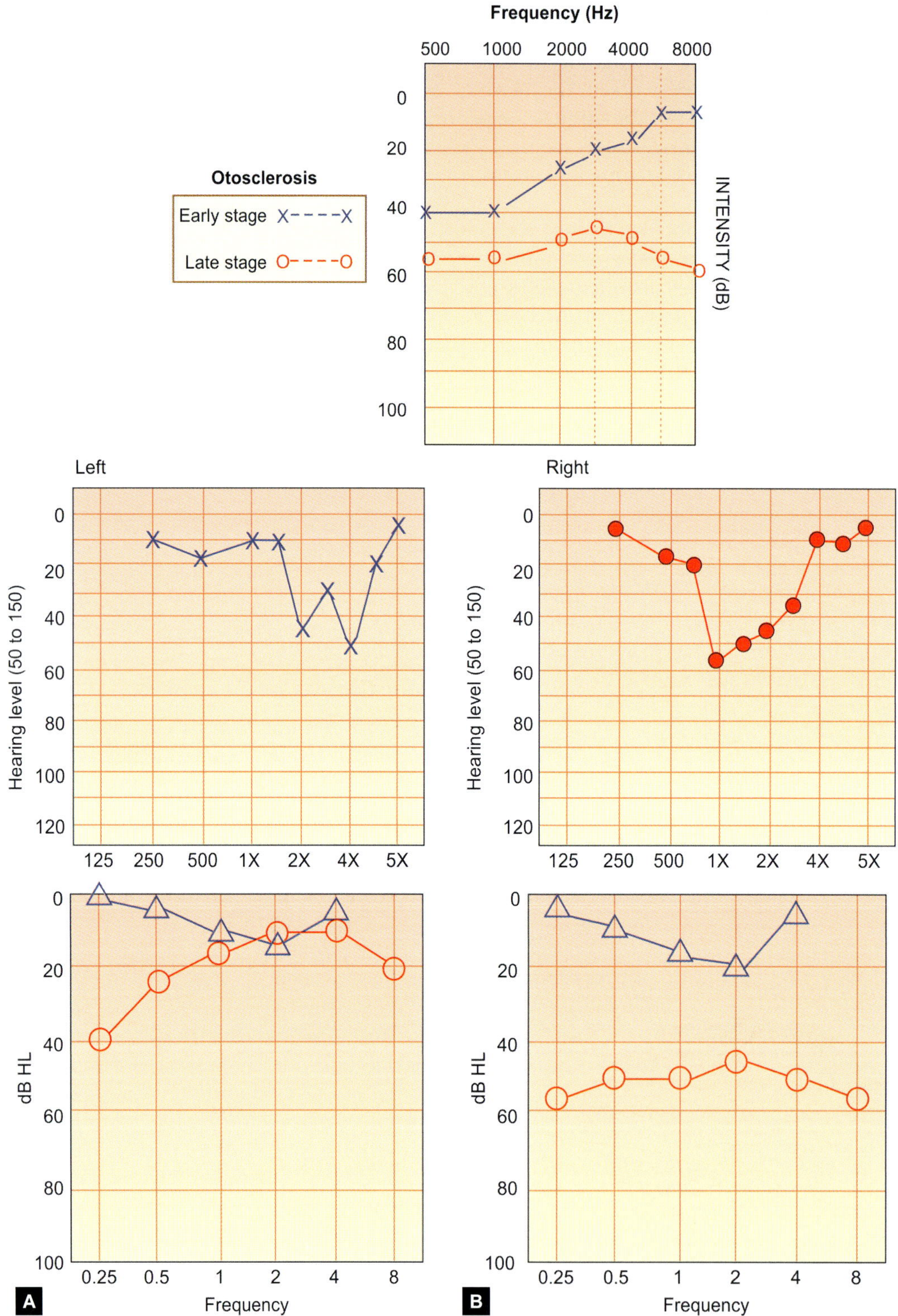

Figs 4A and B: (A) Conductive hearing loss is confined to low-frequencies, high-frequencies are unaffected. (B) As the disease involves entire stapes footplate a flat conductive hearing loss in audiogram is obtained. O—Air conduction (Right ear); Δ—Bone conduction (Right ear)

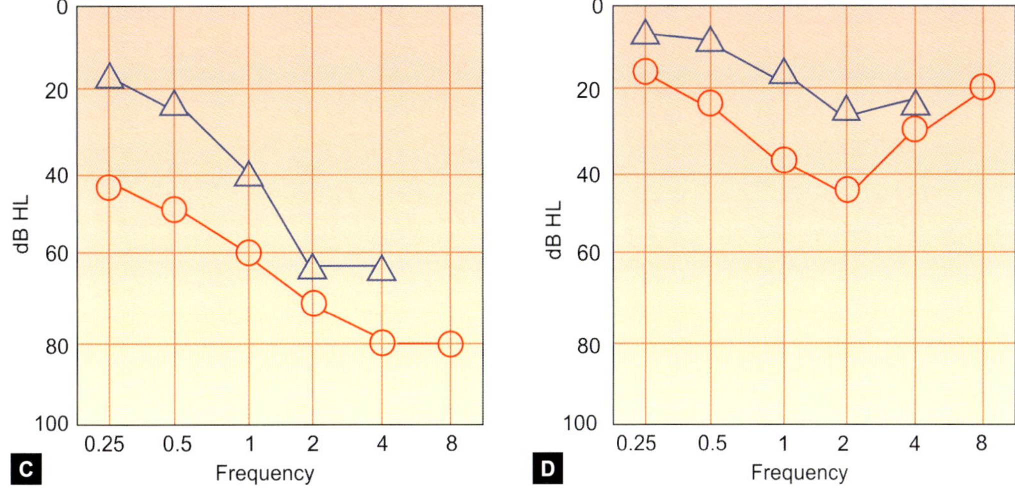

Figs 5C and D: (C) Cochlear involvement results in a mixed hearing loss. (D) Cookie Bite pattern is associated with greatest hearing loss in mid frequencies. O—Air conduction (Right ear); Δ—Bone conduction (Right ear)

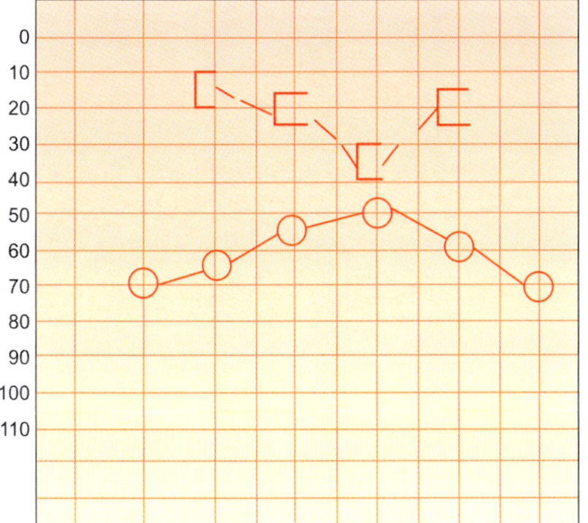

Fig. 6: Bone conduction audiometry shows maximum reduction in sensitivity at 2KHz (Carhart`s notch)

Limitations of bone conduction audiometry are follows:
- False lateralization (this error happen when bone conduction is tested without masking)
- Hyper distractibility (this is due to interference by masking noise)
- Shadow response (the effect of masking the contra lateral ear is ineffective when the hearing loss is severe).

TYMPANOMETRY

Impedance audiometry is not of much value because the results overlap with normal tympanogram as middle ear aeration is not affected by Otosclerosis.
- Normal type A tympanogram is characteristic of early and midstage disease

- As (A short) tympanogram indicates progressive stapes fixation (Fig. 7).

Static compliance—

Static compliance = peak compliance – compliance 200 dPa.

Normal static compliance is 0.3–1.6 cc.

Value <0.3 cc is indicating of increased stiffness in the conductive mechanism. 33% of otosclerotic ears have reduced compliance values.

Acoustic Reflex—In early otosclerosis an unusual diphasic reflex characterized by brief increase in compliance at the onset and at the end of this stimulus is seen. With advancing disease, a reduction in reflex pattern followed by elevation of ipsilateral, then contralateral thresholds and finally absence of acoustic reflex is the pathognomic of otosclerosis.

Imaging Tests

Since the introduction of multidirectional tomography in early 1960s, imaging tests have an important role in diagnosis and management of Otosclerosis.

The tests includes—

Computerized tomography (CT) study: It helps to assess the labyrinthine windows and cochlear capsule in otosclerosis. High-resolution CT of axial and 20° coronal oblique projections is helpful. The axial section shows the cochlear coil and round window. 20° coronal oblique section demonstrates oval window and medial wall of tympanic cavity better than the coronal projection.

In active otosclerosis, margin of oval window shows decalcification. The oval window seems larger than normal.

In mature otosclerosis, when margin of oval window only involves, the oval window appears narrowing.

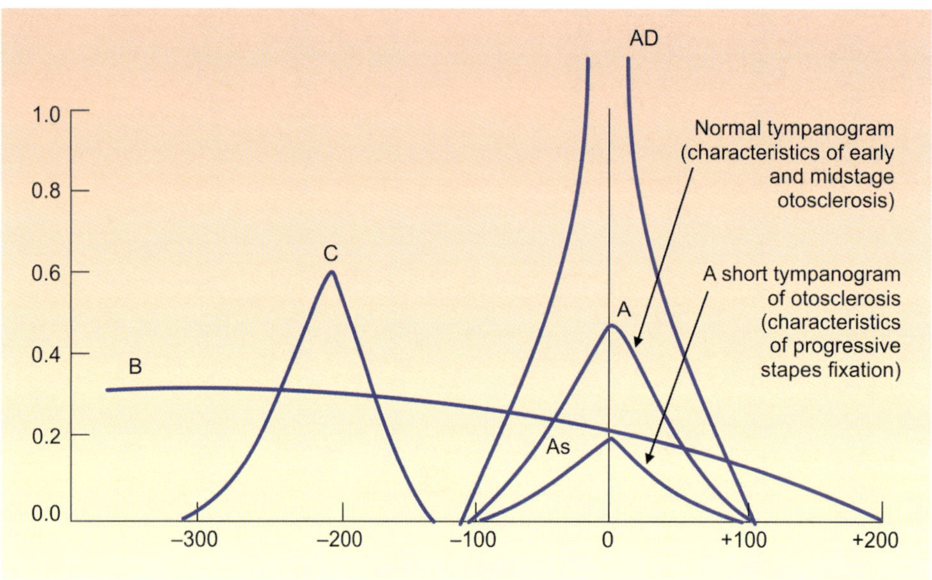

Fig. 10.7: Normal type A tympanogram—characteristics of early and midstage of otosclerosis. Type As tympanogram—characteristics of Otosclerosis indicating progressive stapes fixation

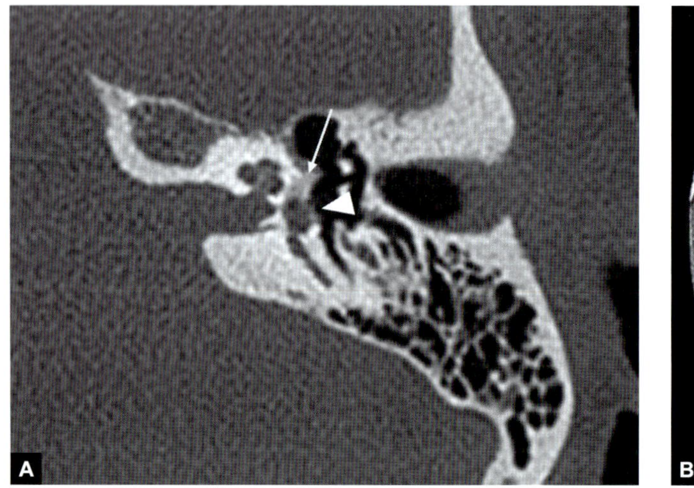

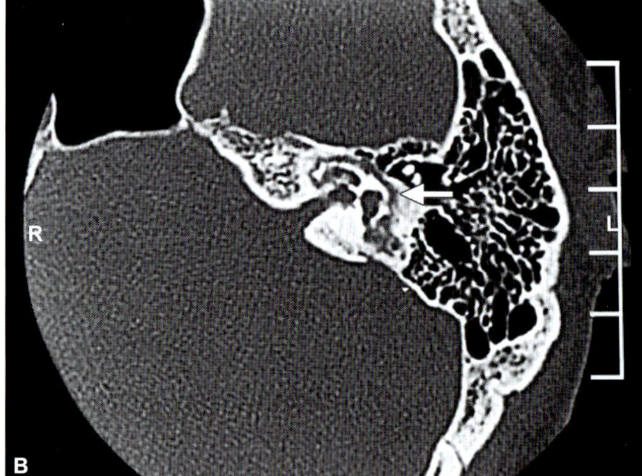

Figs 8A and B: (A) High-resolution axial CT scan of left temporal bone showing anatomy of middle ear and otic capsule with otosclerotic foci involving oval window and footplate; (B) High-resolution CT scan of left temporal bone showing pericochlear spongiotic and sclerotic changes in otosclerosis (arrow)

In diffuse otosclerosis, entire footplate as well as oval window margin are involved, the oval window appears obliterated with a thick bony plate.

In cochlear otosclerosis three factors are considered for radiographic study. These are as follows:

- Otosclerotic foci must be more or equal to 1 mm in diameter
- Density of otosclerotic focus is more than the density of normal otic capsule

- Sclerotic foci can be identified only when the foci are apposed to the periosteal or endosteal surfaces of the capsule (Figs 8A and B)

The pathognomic sign of cochlear otosclerosis is double ring sign seen on CT due to confluent spongiotic foci with the thickness of the capsule.[11]

A mosaic pattern—Area of decreased density intermingled with areas of increased density seen in CT is characteristics of Otosclerosis. CT section especially in 20° coronal oblique cut may show partial or complete reobliteration of oval window by recurrence of the otosclerotic process. It is, therefore, useful in postoperative evaluation.

CT scan is indicated only when patients develop vertigo, tinnitus and sensory neural hearing loss in pediatric patients because of increased risk of congenital malformation of otic capsule of temporal bone.

Magnetic resonance (MR) imaging: MR imaging is useful to detect—

- Congenital anomalies of the labyrinth
- Fibrosis within the cochlea and,
- Activity of the disease.

T1 weight images as thin as 1.5 mm thin obtained through cochlea in axial and coronal planes are acquired prior to and after injection of gadolinium and compared. A faint enhancement or blush within the demineralized area of the capsule is observed. This blush is produced by pooling of the contrast within the numerous blood vessel

and lacunae seen in active otosclerosis focus, thereby correlating between the intensity of the enhancement and the activity of the process.

T2 weight images may detect loss of normal fluid signal from the cochlea resulting from inflammation or obliteration of the cochlea.

MRI is more useful than CT for assessment of cochlear lumen prior to cochlear implant in patients with profound bilateral hearing loss (Fig. 9).

Vestibular Test in Otosclerosis

The vestibular dysfunction results from release of proteolytic enzymes from otoslerotic focus in to the labyrinthine fluids.[12]

Three type of vestibular dysfunction are associated with otosclerosis.

Type I—Mild disequilibrium without a rotational component is present. Caloric tests are normal. Torsion-swing test are indicative of an irritative nystagmus.

Type II—Attacks of acute vertigo (rotational component) are positive, associated with increased tinnitus and fluctuating sensory neural hearing loss. This type is seen in patients with cochlear otosclerosis. Caloric tests may be normal or reduced. Torsion-swing tests are abnormal.

Type III—Coexisting states of cochlear otosclerosis and meniere`s disease. The results of vestibular tests are typical of meniere`s disease.

Classification of Otosclerotic Focus

Gristwood's Classification (Fig. 10)

- Ligamentous fixation
- Anterior polar (small) < 1/2 footplate
- Anterior polar (large) >1/2 footplate
- Posterior polar
- Bipolar
- Marginal/annular

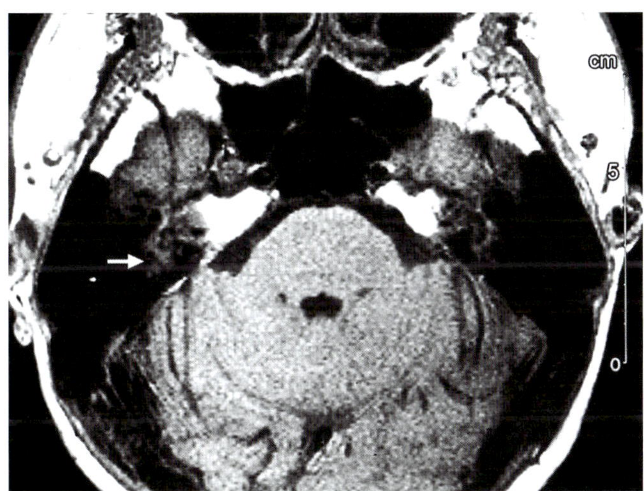

Fig. 9: MRI of cochlear otosclerosis—T1-weighted film showing pericochlear intermediate intensity soft tissue signal (arrow)

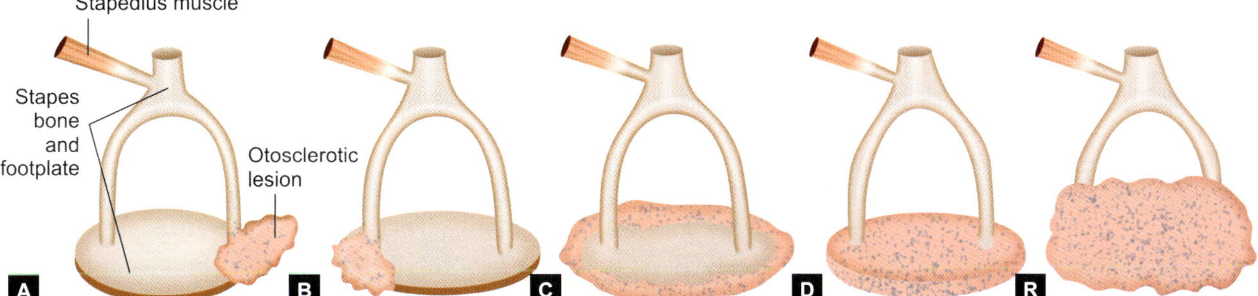

Fig. 10: Types of otosclerotic focus involving stapes footplate: (A) Anterior polar; (B) Posterior polar; (C) Marginal/Annular; (D) Biscuit type; (E) Obliterative focus

Source: Mohan Bansal Diseases of Ear Nose and Throat Head Neck surgery. Jaypee Bros Medical Publishers; 2013. p152

- Diffusely opaque (thin biscuit)
- Solid delineated (thick biscuit or rice grain)
- Solid partly obliterated
- Truly obliterated.

Morrison's Classification

Type I— > 25% footplate area affected.
Type II— >50% footplate area affected.
Type III— >75% footplate area affected.
Type IV— Truly obliterated.

Differential Diagnosis

A. Middle ear lesions causing conductive hearing loss
   – Secretory otitis media
   – Adhesive otitis media
   – Tympanosclerosis
   – Fibro-osseous footplate fixation
   – Congenital footplate fixation
   – Ossicular discontinuity
   – Fixed malleus-incus syndrome: Stiffness or fixation of malleus, incus or both but the stapes is not immediately involved
   – Congenital cholesteatoma
   – Fluid in the middle ear—CSF or perilymh
   – Degenerative footplate arthritis (crural atrophy)
   – Persistent stapedeal artery
   – Paget's disease (osteitis deformans)
   – Osteogenesis imperfecta (vander Hoeve syndrome).
B. Sensorineural lesions
   – Alport syndrome
   – Norrie's disease
   – Meniere's disease
   – Rhinitis pigmentosa
   – Late syphilis of temporal bone
   – Unrecognized ototoxicity.

Treatment

Treatment options of patients with otosclerosis are:
- Observation
- Medical therapy
- Hearing aids
- Surgery
- Each option has its pros and cons that must be explained to the patients before undergoing surgery.

Observation

Patients with unilateral otosclerosis and mild conductive hearing loss may be kept for observation. Hearing assessment by pure tone audiometry is done at least once in a year to see the progression of the disease. If the disease is worsening, surgery is indicated.

Medical Therapy

Fluoride Therapy

Sodium fluoride in moderate doses assists the natural tendency of the focus to become recalcified and inactive.[13] This is evidenced on the basis of following points:
- Schwartz sign becomes negative—fading of the injection of mucous membrane over the active focus
- Progressive SN hearing loss becomes stabilized
- Tinnitus is reduced
- Vestibular symptoms are improved
- Recalcification of focus is seen by X-ray.

Mechanism of Action of Fluoride

Sodium fluoride:
- Reduces osteoclastic bone resorption
- Increases osteoblastic bone formation
- Have antienzymatic action on proteolytic enzymes which are cytotoxic to the cochlea resulting sensorineural hearing loss (SNHL).

Indications of Fluoride Therapy

- Surgically confirmed cases of otosclerosis showing SNHL which is disproportionate to the age of the patient
- Patient with clinical picture of cochlear otosclerosis with pure SNHL
- Radiological evidence of spongiotic changes in cochlear capsule
- Patient with positive Schwartze's sign.

Contraindications of Fluoride Therapy

- Chronic nephritis
- Chronic rheumatoid arthritis
- Pregnancy/ lactation
- Young children (Skeletal immaturity)
- Allergy to sodium fluoride
- Patient with skeletal fluorosis.

Dosage

- In active disease dosage is 50 mg sodium fluoride daily for 2 years
- In very active lesion with positive schwartze's sign dosage is increased to 75 mg daily
- If patient is stabilized or improved with hearing, a daily maintenance dose of 25 mg is given for rest of life.

Adverse Effects

- Gastric irritation
- Increased joint symptoms in rheumatoid arthritis
- Rarely skeletal fluorosis.
  Treatment by sodium fluoride therapy at present is controversial as
- There is no evidence-based support that the fluoridation of drinking water has an impact on the progress of the clinical otosclerosis[14]

- A double blind randomized controlled trial of patients with active therapy and placebo patients for 2 years showed no difference in their air conduction thresholds indicating lack of evidence based support of the use of oral sodium fluoride in otosclerosis.[15]

Bisphosphonates

They are potent antiresorptive agent used in the management of osteoporosis and also in controlling otosclerosis. Bisphosphonates following oral intake are incorporated into bone and inhibit osteoclastic activity without significant osteoblastic bone deposition. Bisphosphonates in clinical use are elendronate, ethidronate and zolendronate.

Adverse effects include—nausea and diarrhea that are dose related. With lower dosage of ethidronate GIT irritation is rarely observed.[16]

Hearing Aids

They are effective in patients with otosclerosis who have pure conductive type of hearing loss where audiogram shows good to excellent bone conduction responses, impaired air conduction responses (60 dB or less) and good speech discrimination scores.

Otosclerotic patients with mixed type of hearing loss with poor speech discrimination score may have significant problem with the use of hearing aids. Patient with successful hearing aid users may avoid the surgery and its risks. Therefore, before surgical intervention otosclerotic patient should be advised for conventional hearing aid trial. The disadvantages of hearing aid as compared to successful stapedectomy include—aesthetic and comfort considerations, poorer sound quality, occlusion effect, ability of hearing only when hearing aid in use.

In far advanced otosclerosis (Hearing loss ~ 90-100 dB and no measurable cochlear reserve on speech discrimination), dual therapy may avoid the need for cochlear implantation. First, stapedectomy is done followed by use of hearing aid. Successful stapedectomy corrects the conductive component of hearing loss. Rehabilitations with hearing aid improve the word recognition score that reflects acclimatization or recovery from auditory deprivation. Therefore, dual therapy helps by improving auditory thresholds and recovering from auditory deprivation.[17]

Bone–anchored Hearing Aids (BAHA) has a specific benefit of subjective outcomes of comfort and sound quality over conventional hearing aid as well as it may avoid the risk of dead ear that may happen following stapedectomy. However, in practice most patients under 60 years of age with cochlear function favor surgery but role of using hearing aid increases with its advancing technology.

Treatment Options: Surgery

Stapedectomy is an operation done in most patients with conducting hearing loss due to otosclerosis. The operation corrects the nonfunctioning stapes and improves the sound transmission of middle ear.

History of Surgery (Historical Background)

- First, operation of stapedectomy was done by Jack of Boston (1891)
- Fenestration operation was started by Jenkins (1914) and developed later by Lampert (1938) who described a single stage endaural approach for otosclerosis surgery
- Stapes mobilization technique was developed by Rosen in New York (1952), but refixation occurred in months
- Anterior crurotomy technique was developed by Fowler (1956) with similar results
- Modern stapedectomy was introduced by John Shea (1958) who reconstructed the sound transmission with prosthesis (Fig. 11).

Indications

- Otosclerotic patients with bone conduction threshold below 25 dB and air conduction threshold below 60 dB in speech frequencies are good candidates for surgery
- Air bone gap of at least 15 dB and speech discrimination score (SDS) of 60% or more are essential for good hearing improvement
- Larger the air-bone gap, greater the improvement of hearing by surgery is expected
- In far advanced otosclerosis (patients with a severe to profound mixed hearing loss), where hearing aid is unserviceable, operative treatment may enable patients

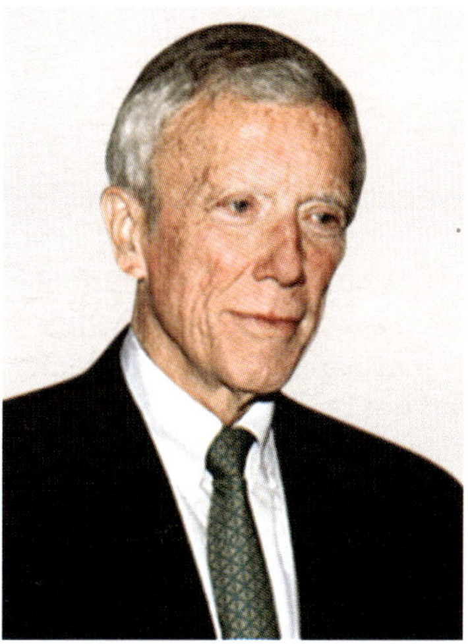

Fig. 11: Dr John J Shea (Father of modern Stapedectomy)

to make hearing aid serviceable. Goal of surgery is to restore available cochlear function.

Contraindications

- General medical illness
- Age >70 years, older age group is associated with increased risk of fistula formation and decreased chance of discrimination scores
- Children are not advised for operation by most surgeons. Sensorineural thresholds deteriorate at a mean of 0.7 db per year
- Conductive losses for other causes, e.g. stapes fixation caused by tympanosclerosis as operation may result high incidences of sensorineural hearing loss (SNHL)
- Presence of otitis externa or a perforation
- Early fixation with a small degree of hearing loss
- Unilateral otosclerosis (+/-). Loss of symmetrical hearing if not accepted by the patients surgery is justified in these cases
- Only one hearing ear (operation is justified unless hearing aid is absolutely useless)
- Meniere's disease, as there is increased risk of dead ear from damage to distended saccule during operation
- Stapedial and cochlear otosclerosis with poor air-bone gap
- Second ear stapedectomy (±) because of risk of immediate and delayed SNHL
- On the other hand to gain binaural hearing and to obtain normally functioning ear operation is justified by some surgeons
- Young adult with positive schwartze sign
- Pregnancy and up to 12 months following delivery
- Occupations like sports and aircrafts personnel
- In bilateral otosclerosis, if there is poor Eustachian-tube function in one ear and the ear with better Eustachian-tube function is advised for operation.

Preoperative Counseling

Merits and demerits of operations should be explained to the patients as alternative method of treatment. A hearing aid in most cases is satisfactory. Patient should be informed that the operated ear may be worsen after an initial good result and this may happen many years later. Violent nose blowing should not be done at all time because of risk of fistula formation. Flying and lifting of heavy weights must be avoided for two weeks following surgery. Possible need for revision surgery must be explained to the patients.

Anesthesia in Stapes Surgery

Local or general anesthesia is used in stapes surgery.

Advantage of Local Anesthesia

- Patient can be asked for subjective improvement in hearing on the table or disequilibrium, if adhesion extends in the vestibule, particularly in revision surgery
- Less tendency of bleeding because of adrenaline mixed with local anesthesia (1% lignocaine with 1:30000 to 1:100000 diluted adrenaline).
  The posterior wall of external auditory canal is infiltrated via the postauricular sulcus. Then four quadrant infiltration of local anesthesia is made in the canal skin at the level of bony and cartilaginous junction permeatally. A tragal injection is also given to reduce pain, if retractor is used.
- Local anesthesia reduces the risk of straining that is seen at the end of general anesthesia.
  Transient facial paresis may occur from local anesthesia that may recover when local anesthetic effect subsides.
  General anesthesia is preferred in children and apprehensive patients.

Advantages of General Anesthesia

- Motionless operative field is obtained
- Hypotensive anesthesia may be given
- Flexibility, if difficulties are encountered.

Approach and Incision

- In narrow canal, Lampert's end aural incision is preferred where as in wide canal Rosen's permeatal approach is indicated. A permeatal incision is made from 12 to 8 o'clock on right side and 12 to 4 o' clock on left side. In revision surgery, the incision is made from 12 to 6 o' clock to give additional exposure to round window enabling to test round window reflex. The incision is like bucket handle, just lateral to annulus at two ends and 6–8 mm from annulus at mid point.
  The idea of incision is to get adequate exposure of critical operation area. Here chorda facial gap and incudo stapedeal joint is the critical operation area
- Tympanomeatal flap is elevated. Chorda tympani is preserved in most cases. If it interferes the vision, it is better to section it rather to stretch it
- Removal of bony annulus—There are three types of posterosuperior bony overhang:
  - Type A—Where the whole view of middle ear is seen (5%)
  - Type B—Incudostapedial joint is seen but pyramidal eminence and area of footplate of stapes are not seen (85%)
  - Type C—Whole view of middle ear is hidden including incus (10%).[18]

The bony annulus is removed by sharp curette or microdrill to expose facial canal, pyramidal eminence and posterior crus of stapes. There should be enough forceps space between chorda and curetted annulus for allowing placement of the prosthesis

- Examination of middle ear—The ossicular chain is inspected and palpated to establish the diagnosis. In most spaces, incus moves but no movements of stapes footplate is seen. Once diagnosis is made, blue reflex is searched in the area of footplate. It is seen where the footplate is thin
- Opening in the footplate—The opening or the hole is made in the area showing blue reflex or in the thinnest area of footplate. This is done before cutting the stapedius tendon or removal of superstructure to prevent floating foot plate. A thin straight needle or a perforator or microdrill is used to make the hole. If perforator is used it should be used with a gentle rotator movement. No suction should be done over the opening or very thin suction needle (23 sizes) should be used
- Cutting of stapedius tendon—In most cases stapedius tendon is cut with a micro scissor. The stapedius tendon can be kept intact that can help to prevent noise trauma in future
- Removal of stapes superstructure—Capsular ligament of incudostapedial joint is divided with a right angle pick. Superstructure is then taken out with right angle hook by fracturing the crura down towards the promontory away from the facial nerve. The division of crura is made by crurotomy saw, scissor or KTP laser
- Measurement of length of prosthesis—It is important. Prosthesis used is 0.25 mm longer than the distance from the undersurface of the long process of incus to the footplate.

  The distance is measured following removal of superstructure. Detailed technical aspect of surgery is discussed below.

Surgical Technique (Figs 12 to 15)

Following techniques are used for otosclerosis:[19]
1. Direct piston technique—Pistons are 0.3 mm, 0.4 mm, 0.6 mm, and 0.8 mm in diameter.
   Pistons used are—Teflon piston (Shea), stainless steel piston (Mc Gee), gold piston, titanium piston, wire Teflon, platinum ribbon Teflon piston.
2. Piston with vein graft interposition technique— Polyethelene strut and vein graft (original shea) Teflon piston on vein graft (Causse).
3. Posterior crus stapedeoplasty/platinectomy (Hough/ Portman)
4. Total stapedectomy
   Fat and wire (Schuknecht)
   Gelfoam and wire (House)

Other techniques are used-
   Stainless steel piston on vein (Robinson)
   Platinum ribbon trapeze on soft tissue (Austin)
   Cartilage on perichondrium (Pfaltz)
   Cartilage on vein (Desai) (Fig. 16)
   Each technique has its own merits and demerits. Surgeon should adapt the technique which is most comfort and satisfactory for him.

Direct Piston Technique

It is widely used at present. The risk of damage to inner ear at operation and long-term perilymph fistula is less if a small fenestra is made in the posterior part of footplate.
Essentials of technique are:
- The diameter of the fenestra
- Position of the fenestra
- Length of piston
- Material used around the piston.

Diameter of the Fenestra

GDL Smyth	0.3 mm
U.Fisch	0.4 mm

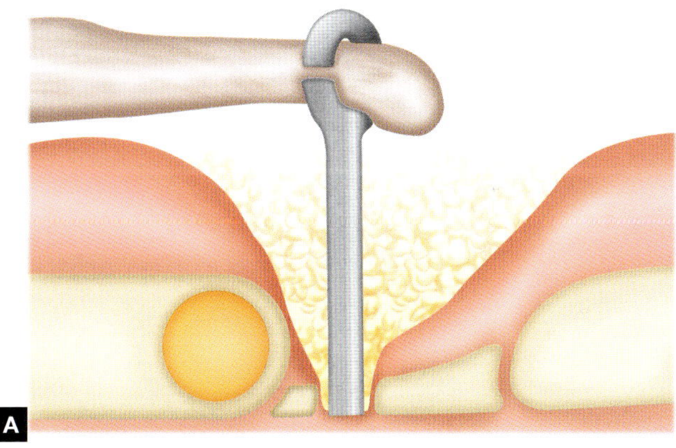

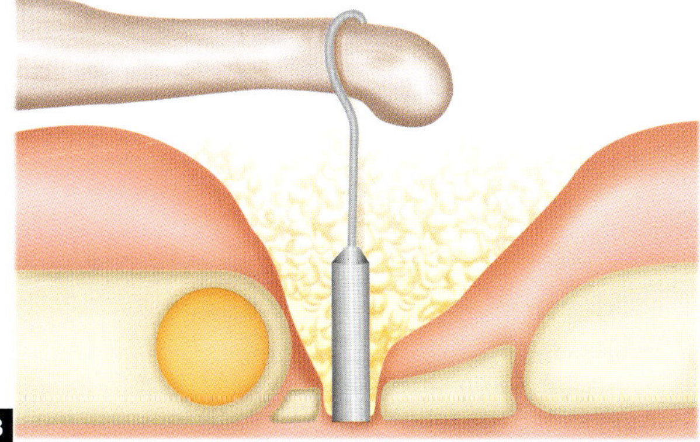

Figs 12A and B: (A) Teflon piston—Shea; (B) Steel piston—Mc Gee.
Source: Scott-Brown`s Otolaryngology 5th edition Otology p318.

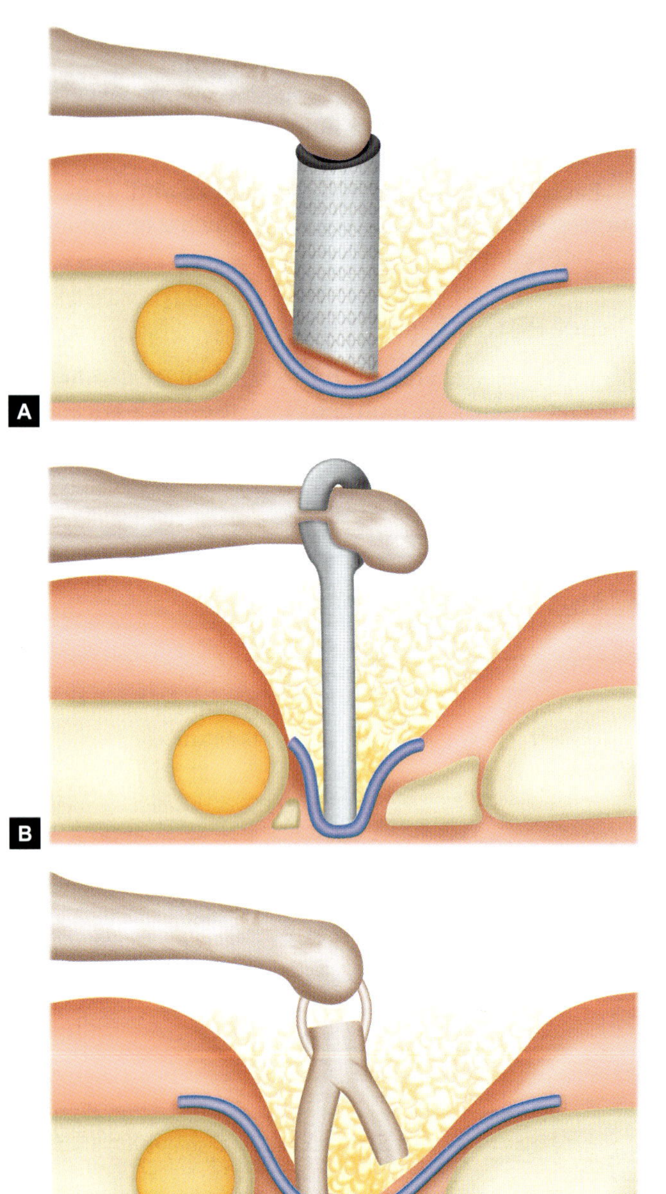

Figs 13A to C: (A) Polyethelene sturt and vein graft (original Shea technique); (B) Teflon piston on vein graft—Causse technique; (C) Posterior rus on Pericondrium (PCOP)—Hough/Portman (From Scott-Brown`s Otolaryngology 5th edition Otology p318)

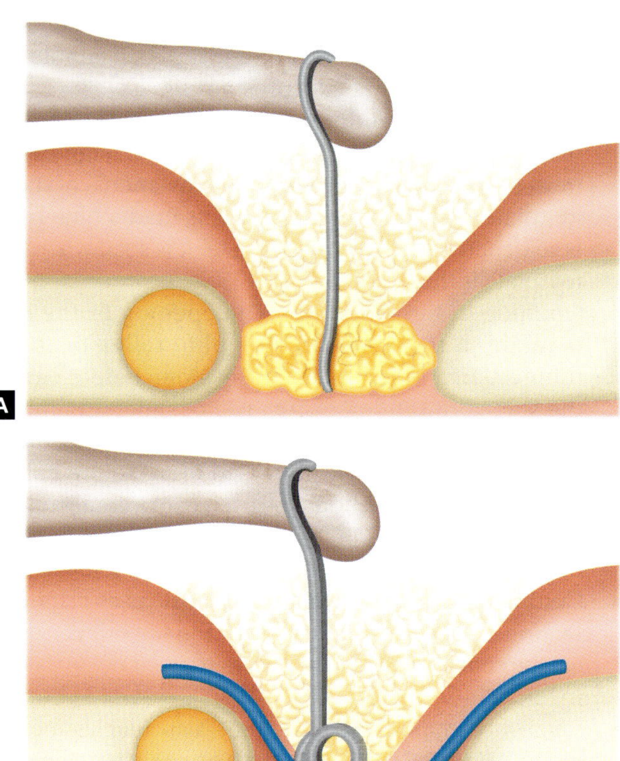

Figs 14A and B: (A) Fat and wire (Schuknecth); (B) Gelfoam and wire (House) (From Scott-Brown`s Otolaryngology 5th edition Otology p318)

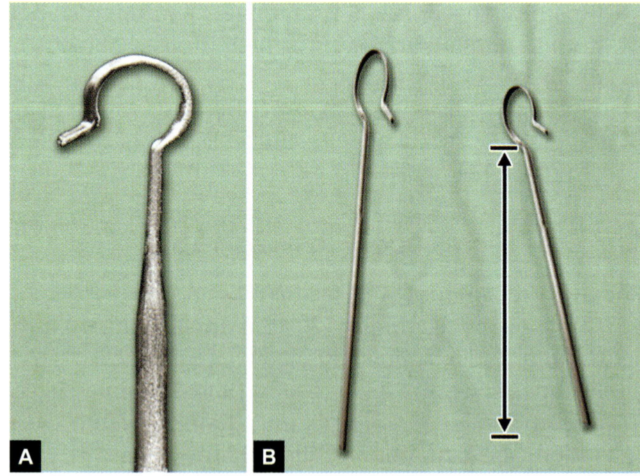

Figs 15A and B: (A) Gold piston; (B) Titanium prosthesis

M Portmann	0.4 mm
J Marquet	0.6 mm
Schuknecht and Gristwood	0.6–0.8 mm

Marquet stated the following advantages of small fenestra stapedectomy:

- There is decreased risk of damage to mucous membrane of vestibule
- Piston does not penetrate more than 0.1 mm into the vestibule. This does not tear or irritate the underlaying membranous structure
- Calibrated hole in the footplate avoids rupture of the annular ligament and vestibular endothelium is not disturbed

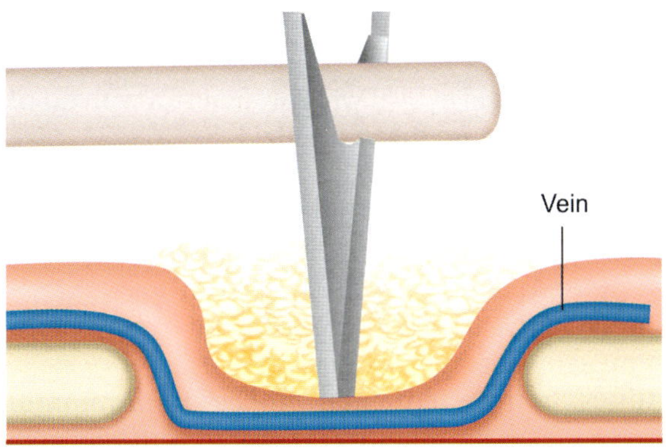

Fig. 16: Cartilage on vein (Desai)

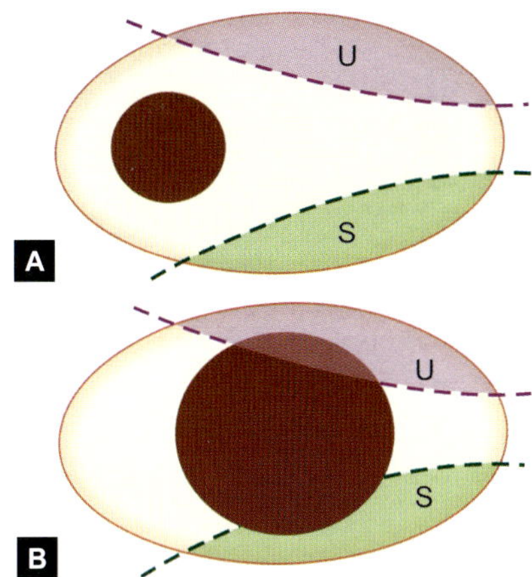

Figs 17A and B: (A) 0.4 mm Teflon piston; (B) 0.8 mm Teflon piston
Abbreviations: S, Saccule; U, Utricle

- Inner ear is sealed rapidly from the middle ear since very small opening is being made is closed by the piston
- Entry of bone dust is prevented by small curvature of meniscus of the perilymph
- Piston is firmly placed so no pendulum movement takes place
- Slender pistons are less effective—a real ratio—surface area of TM/surface area of pistons is more with the slender piston but slender piston moves less perilymph. Therefore, they are less effective.
  Intraoperative audiometry shows that a 0.6 mm piston improves 10 dB better hearing than a 0.4 mm piston and a 0.8 mm piston improves 10 dB better hearing than a 0.6 mm piston
- Slender pistons are safer—Large fenestra means total or subtotal footplate removal , medium fenestra is 0.8–0.9 mm hole and small fenestra is 0.4–0.7 mm hole.

Sensorineural hearing loss

- Smyth compared SNHL with large fenestra versus small fenestra as shown in the Table 1.

Table 1: SNHL comparison

	Immediate SN loss (surgical trauma)	Delayed sudden onset SN loss	Delayed chronic progressive SN loss
Large fenestra(whole footplate out)	1.5%	2%	9.5 db/decade
Small fenestra (0.4mm)	0%	0–0.6%	5.5 db/decade

Large fenestra may cause more damage to inner ear than small fenestra piston technique.

- Results of Fisch (0.4) and Gristwood (0.6-0.8) are compared on SNHL (Table 2).

Table 2: Comparison of SNHL results

	Fisch (0.4)%	Gristwood (0.6-0.8)%
Early dead ear	0	0
Late dead ear	0	0
Early SN loss	0.1	1.25
Late SN loss	1.5	1.4

The above table indicates significant difference in the incidence of early SN loss. It is due to operative trauma related to larger whole. Therefore, use of slender piston gives better result and is safer.

Position of the Fenestra

Posterior part of the footplate is the safe area for fenestration. A 0.4 mm piston that moves in as a result of loud short sound or barotrauma is less likely to strike the saccule or utricle (Fig. 17).

Length of the Piston

The piston should not penetrate more than 0.25 mm in the vestibule. If piston is too long, endosteal membrane has not grown under the piston resulting unsealing off the inner ear whatever seal is put around the piston.

Hanging Test

If piston with a gentle outward pull hangs on the edge of the footplate, the hanging test is positive. The piston is not too long.

Bending Test

If piston in its normal position, on the lateral pressure bends and does not slip up on the edge of the footplate, bending test is positive. Piston is not too short.

Materials used around the Piston

- Smyth—Gelfoam
- House—Blood
- Fisch—blood + connective tissue+ fibrin glue
- Gristwood—fascia
- Marquet—nothing.
  Material used around the piston may result foreign body granuloma. Hence, opinion varies against its use.

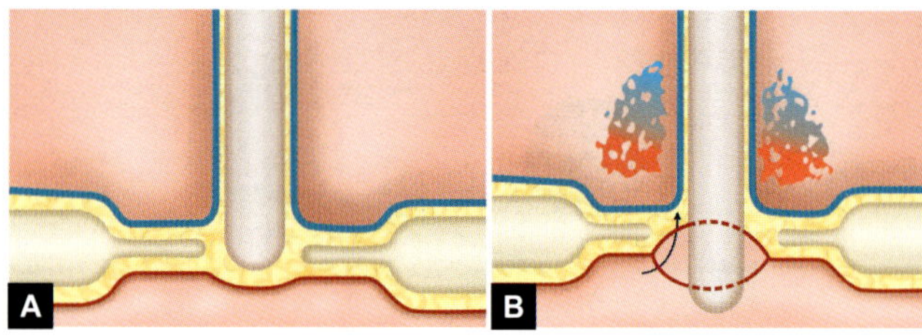

Figs 18A and B: (A) Endosteal membrane has formed; (B) Endosteal membrane has not formed developing perilymph fistula
Source: Otolaryngology Review. 2000. p103

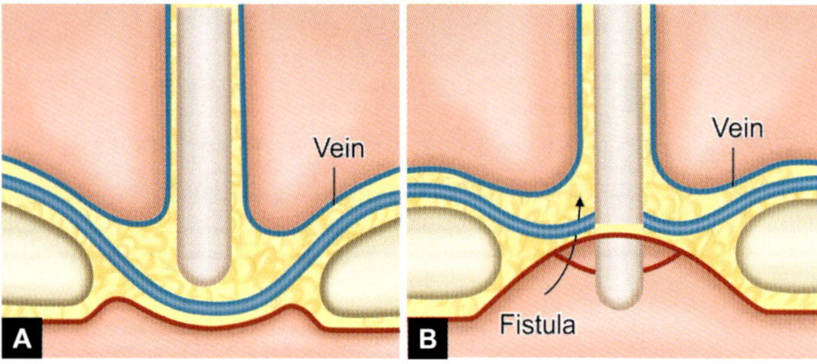

Figs 19A and B: (A) Excessive footplate removal; (B) Late bulging
Source: Otolaryngology Review. 2000. p104

Direct Piston Technique After Healing

The endosteal membrane is formed beneath the piston sealing the inner ear (Figs 18A and B).

The most common cause of fistula and late sensory neural hearing loss is long piston. Perilymph leak is submucous. Therefore, accurate size piston plunging-in is no more than 0.1–0.2 mm into the vestibule. Small fenestra (0.4 mm) or medium fenestra (0.8 mm) technique as judged by bending test and hanging test with reference to the edge of the footplate should be used.

The second cause of fistula is excessive footplate removal. Late bulging of blue membrane that forms will tear resulting in a fistula, even if soft tissue interposition is used (Figs 19A and B).

Crimping the piston is essential otherwise open piston is found lying on the promontory.

Key Points of Direct Piston Technique

- Discreet round fenestra
- Perfect length of piston
- Avoid foreign body granuloma.

Piston with Vein Graft Interposition Technique

JB Causse (1962) performed a technique where he made a 0.8 mm fenestra in the footplate that was covered with a vein graft and a 0.4 mm Teflon piston was put.

Advantages claimed for the modification of Shea Teflon piston are:
- Immediate seal of oval window fenestra with no risk of piston falling into the vestibule
- Tip of piston is protected by soft tissue so there are decrease chances of damage to vestibular membrane
- Strong seal over the oval window fenestra results decreased chances of perilymph fistula
- Immediate seal of window permits accurate monitoring from early postoperative period itself
- Adhesion from lenticular process to promontory is prevented as promontory is covered with vein graft
- Moving surface is 0.8 mm that provides better hearing than with 0.4 mm piston
- If 0.4 mm piston is used sudden movements due to a loud sound or barotrauma will not strike the saccule or the utricle. It results in less chances of dead ear.

Disadvantage of the Causse Technique

Use of microdrill creates osteogenic bone dust that may cause secondary ossification of the vein. Therefore, careful removal of bone dust is essential before placing the vein graft.

Key Points in the Causse Technique

- To get a fenestra of 0.8 mm in diameter a diamond microdrill is used before removing the superstructure
- Both crura are removed with microdrill to avoid removal of a large part of the footplate
- Crura are cut flush with the footplate to allow the vein to lie exactly on the oval window
- 0.6 mm diamond microdrill is used to make fenestra that is enlarged to 0.8 mm. A 0.8 mm microdrill that will plunge in 0.4 mm in the vestibule is not used.

Posterior Crus on Perichondrium Stapedioplasty (PCOP) Hough

Dr Jack Hough used this technique except in obliterative focus where he used the piston (Fig. 20).

Success rate of this technique is excellent (99.8%).

Total or Subtotal Stapedectomy (Large Fenestra Stapedectomy)

Schuknecht (1971) introduced wire and fat graft technique. Advantages of large fenestra operations are:
- Relatively easy
- Immediate seal of oval window by fat graft technique
- Stainless steel wire prosthesis permits accurate placement of the graft.

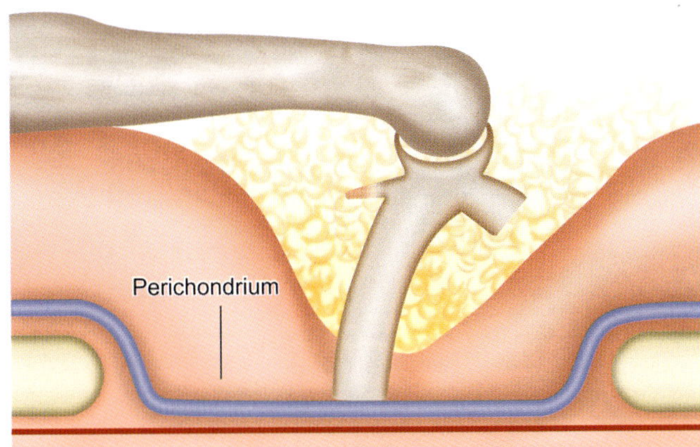

Fig. 20: Posterior crus on perichondrium technique (Hough)
Source: Otolaryngology Review. 2000. p105

Disadvantages of large fenestra operation are as follows:
- More traumatic procedure with greater risk of damage to the underlying membranous structure of the vestibule
- Increase chances of necrosis of the tip of long process if wire crimped very tightly
- Occurrence of oval window granuloma (1.7% incidence)
- Development in some cases of conductive hearing loss due to wondering of prosthesis to the edge of the oval window.

Pfaltz used cartilage on perichondrium whereas Desai used cartilage on vein.

If whole footplate was inadvertently removed as in case of floating footplate, perichondrium or vein graft is advised to place over the oval window and continuity to incus is maintained by cartilage (Pfaltz or Desai technique) or homograft posterior crus stapedioplasty (Hough technique).

Lasers in Stapes Surgery

Lasers are used in surgery of otosclerosis. The purpose of lasers are as follows:
- Making a bloodless fenestra
- No risk of footplate subluxation
- Precise cuts in the footplate.

Various types of lasers are used—CO2, KTP-532, erbium –YAG and Argon. Since 1980 potential risk to membrane labyrinth with lasers are photothermal, photochemical and photoacoustic damage that arise controversy of the choice of the laser type. Ideal laser should have following qualities and objectives to use safely:
- Precise optics for delivery
- Laser tissue interaction without adjacent thermal spread
- No heating of perilymph
- No penetration of perilymph.

Argon laser is preferred in primary cases because of less risk of damage to saccule. CO_2 is used in revision cases as it is well-absorbed by collagen and perilymph to vaporize the adhesion and to make free the prosthesis from its attachment. Uses of micropicks, microdrill and lasers in stapedotomy are reviewed in Marquet's series. It is evident that laser stapediotomy may have less complication rate than traditional techniques.[20]

Intraoperative Problems of Otosclerosis Surgery

- Narrow EAC by exostoses—These are corrected by separate surgery and allowed to heal before going for stapes surgery
- Tear of tympanomeatal flap—Underlay myringoplasty is done to repair the tear
- Dehiscent facial nerve obscuring the footplate (0.5%)— In such cases, surgery may need to be abandoned. The facial nerve canal may also overhang the footplate restricting surgical access that may require adjustment to the angulation of the prosthesis
- Persistent stapedial artery (0.2%) may run from facial canal between the stapedial crura. It can obstruct the surgical access and cause troublesome bleeding
- Perilymph flooding (0.0287%) or perilymph gusher—It is more common in patients with congenital fixation of footplate. Preoperative CT scan may show abnormally patent cochlear aqueduct. If this condition is detected preoperatively, surgery is contraindicated as there is high chance of complete SNHL. If this is encounter intra operatively, fat or muscle graft over the oval window is placed to seal the leak. Postoperatively patient is placed head up position and a temporary lumbar drain is maintained to reduce CSF pressure
- Floating footplate (<1%) this is potentially grave complication resulting dead ear. Preliminary fenestration in footplate before removing the superstructure is a safe precaution to avoid this problem. If it is encountered, a hole is made in the inferior margin of the oval window and then extraction of the footplate fragments is done by fine hook. The perichondrium or vein is placed over the oval window and continuity to incus is made by cartilage (Pflatz, Desai) or posterior crus (Hough). A piston on soft tissue is never used if whole footplate is out. If floating footplate cannot be removed without excessive manipulation, it should be left in place, soft tissue graft is placed over the oval window and operation is abandoned
- Submerged footplate—It is more common than floating footplate. No attempt is made to retrieve the submerged footplate as it can cause complete SNHL
- Blood in the vestibule—Although it has little ill effect, labyrinthine trauma from this cause should not be dismissed

- Obliterative otosclerosis—Gristwood maintained three varieties of the obliterative focus that fills in the oval window niche.
    - Truly obliterated footplate where the rim of footplate cannot be identified and the crura of stapes are buried
    - Partially obliterated footplate in which a rim of delineation is limited to a segment of its circumference
    - Solid delineated footplate or thick biscuit or rice grain footplate is associated with increased risk of floating footplate.

In obliterative otosclerosis footplate is extensively involved with new bone formation. Saucerization of footplate may have increase risk of SNHL. Stapediotomy is done with microdrill and fenestration is wide enough to prevent lateral contact of the piston on to the surrounding bone. In these cases revision surgery should not be recommended because of high chance of SNHL.

- Damage to chorda tympani nerve—during stapes surgery for adequate exposure it is necessary to displace the chorda tympani nerve. The nerve may be cut or stretched. If the nerve is cut permanent loss of taste sensation on the same side may result. If the nerve is stretched a persistent abnormal sensation may happen.
- Narrow oval window niche—Otosclerotic foci around the oval window may lead to narrowing of the niche. Overhanging bone should be removed and then the footplate is seen
- Round window closure because of otosclerotic focus – Attempts to drill out obliterated round window may lead to SNHL and are not advised
- Malleus head fixation (1%)—An atticotomy with silastic sheet interposition to free the malleus head is performed in addition to stapedotomy with vein graft interposition. It is preferred to amputation of the head and using a wire piston from malleus to the oval window (malleostapediotomy)
- Incus problems—if incus is slightly eroded a cartilage is used to connect the malleus and incus to vein on the oval window (Desai technique) for thin plate. If incus is destroyed and obliterative focus a wire Teflon piston from malleus handle to a vein graft on oval window is used and a piece of cartilage is placed between the wire and the drum adjacent to the handle of malleus to prevent extrusion of the wire (Figs 21A and B).

Postoperative Complications of Stapes Surgery

Conductive Hearing Loss

The loss of initial gain in hearing following stapes surgery associated with conductive hearing loss is due to—

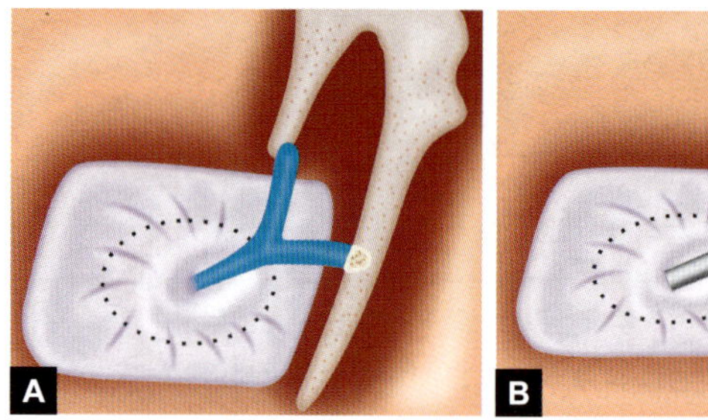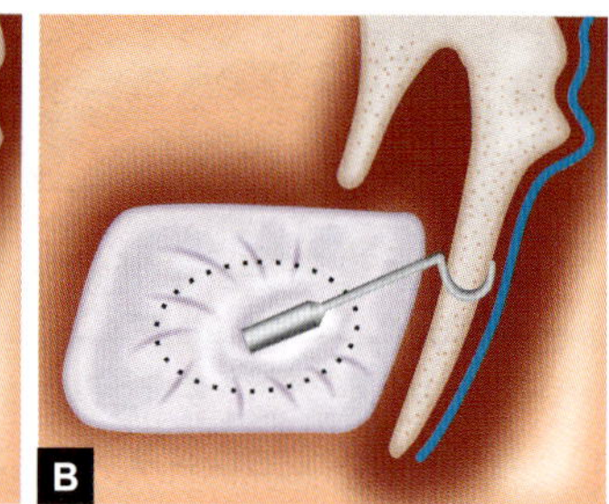

Figs 21A and B: (A) Incus necrosis-cartilage on vein; (B) Incus necrosis-wire Teflon on vein
Source: Otolaryngology Review. 2000. p107

Displacement of Prosthesis Out of Footplate

The possible causes are as follows:

- A short prosthesis that may result from incorrect measurement of prosthesis from long process of incus to footplate
- Distortion of loop around the long process of incus for its variable diameter
- Crimping techniques
- Contracture of connective tissue seal over the fenestration—thicker the oval window seal, greater the lateralization of the prosthesis. A vein graft is more suitable than perichondrium, fat and fascia
- Traction from adhesions between the prosthesis and adjacent structures—less surgical trauma resulting minimal traction force is advised.

Erosion of Incus

- It causes loosening of the attachment of the prosthesis— Incus erosion is due to reduction of blood supply secondary to cutting the stapedial tendon and pressure on the long process from prosthetic loop

Osseous Closure of Oval Window

- Bony regrowth over fenestration is found in 1–24% of cases 20. It is more common in obliterative otosclerosis. It is noted within one year to many years following surgery.

Fibrous Adhesions Fixing Ossicles or Prosthesis

- It is reported in 8–24% of revision operation.[21] Such fixation results ankylosis of malleus or incus to attic wall.

Refixation of Mobilized Footplate

- The mobilization procedures are rarely performed nowaday.

Sensorineural Hearing Loss

Dead ear or severe SNHL may be occurred following stapes surgery. It is noted that the occurrence rate of SHNL is less than 1% for SNHL. The hearing loss may be immediate or delayed.

Possible causes of immediate SNHL are—
- Surgical trauma especially extensive drilling associated with obliterative otosclerosis, postoperative suppurative labyrinthitis, floaing footplates and perilymph fistula.
  The cause of delayed hearing loss is unexplained. Causes may include—
  - Increased negative pressure in middle ear and subsequent forcing of prosthesis into the vestibule, e.g. Barotrauma or blast injury
  - Release of active enzymes from the otosclerotic focus into inner ear
  - Reparative ganuloma
  - These complications may influence the surgeons to take decision for surgery on second ear.

Facial Nerve Injury

It is of two types:
a. Temporary facial nerve injury that may be–
  - Immediate temporary facial nerve palsy
  - Delayed temporary facial nerve palsy.
    Immediate temporary facial nerve palsy—it may happen immediately after operation due to infiltration of local anesthesia.
    Delayed temporary facial nerve palsy—it may be described when palsy may develop between 4 and 10 days after operation. It may result from nerve edema due to heating caused by drill or laser or viral reactivation within the nerve. Recovery is expected over days or weeks. Steroid is advised to reduce the edema.
b. Permanent facial nerve injury—it is rare. It is seen in association with—
  - Aberrant facial nerve crossing the footplate
  - Burr injury or
  - Presence of dehiscence facial canal and while removing fibrous tissue from footplate area in revision surgery.

Perilymph Fistula

It is slow leak of perilymph from the oval window following stapedectomy that results immediate or late cochlear loss. The fistulae are reported in 0.25–2.5% following stapedectomy and in 1.5–12% of revision surgery. The fistulae are significantly lower following stapedectomy. Perilymph fistulae are due to:
- Long piston
- Large hole
- Pull in by adhesions between lenticular process and raw promontory
- Use of gelatin sponge to seal a Stapedectomy.
Deafness in perilymph fistulae is due to—
- Diffusion of toxins
- Infection
- Rupture of utricle/saccule.
Symptoms and signs of perilymph fistulae are similar to those of postoperative endolmphatic hydrops—
- Persistent or fluctuating hearing impairment which may be sensorineural, mixed or conductive (71–87%)
- Vertigo or disequilibrium (66%)
- Tinnitus (28–45%)
- Fullness in ear
- Sometimes meningitis—an asymptomatic patient suddenly develops dead ear following URTI, suspicion of meningitis comes. Treatment includes removal of piston and closure of the fistula.
Bone conduction of operated ear is worse than bone conduction of an unoperated ear. A fistula may exist for many years without any sign and symptom.
Treatment of perilymph fistula includes—
- Re-exploration of middle ear
- If prosthesis is displaced, this defect is closed by graft and a new prosthesis is anchored (Causse technique – vein and 0.4 mm piston in small fenestra. Desai technique—vein and cartilage in large fenestra)
- If the prosthesis is still in the vestibule and adhesions of prosthesis with membranous labyrinth are present, it is safer to pack the footplate with fat to avoid the entering in the vestibule.

Reparative Granuloma

It is the granulation tissue formation around stapes prosthesis and the oval window 1-6 weeks after stapes surgery in which gel foam is used to seal the oval window. Its incidence is 0.1% following stapedectomy and 0.07% following stapediotomy.[22] If symptoms of serous labyrinthitis fail to resolve, postoperative granuloma is suspected. Progressive sensorineural or mixed hearing loss, vertigo and tinnitus are the presenting symptoms. On examination, TM shows dull red in posterior-superior quadrant. Early surgical management is advised to remove the granulation tissue and prosthesis or granulation tissue alone. Many surgeons prefer to use steroid and antibiotics followed by delayed surgery if no improvement comes.

Vertigo

Vertigo or transient giddiness is not infrequent following stapes surgery and can be cured by vestibular sedatives. Vertigo combined with SNHL and tinnitus in the first week of surgery may suspect the underlying cause of serous labyrinthitis from which rapid recovery is expected. A delayed onset of vertigo may happen from perilymph fistula, reparative granuloma overlong prosthesis or suppurative labyrinthitis. Neuro-otological examination and HRCT scanning help to diagnose the labyrinthine origin of vertigo. Treatment is shown to improve the outcome. BPPV is reported in 4/63 poststapedectomy patients, all are successfully cured by Epley manoevure.[23]

Discomfort to Loud Noise

It is reported that 35–40% of patients following stapes surgery suffers from this symptom. Discomfort to loud noise is due to improved hearing in the operated ear as normal hearing person experiences the same. Repair of Stapedious tendon reduces intolerance of loud noise and needs surgical expertization.

Alteration of Taste

About 30% of patients following stapes surgery may have injury to chorda tympani nerve while in revision surgery injury is found as far as 80% cases. Damage to the nerve may result in impairment of taste and dryness of mouth lasting for 3–4 months following surgery. Sectioning produces less symptoms than stretching.

Poststapedectomy Cholesteatoma

It is a rare complication. The etiology may be—
- Eustachian tube dysfunction
- Prosthesis extrusion
- An inverted tympano meatal flap secondary to faulty repositioning
- A marginal perforation from annular ligament disruption.[24]

The cholesteatoma is reported in oval window secondary to squamous epithelium implanted during harvesting of fat graft.

Revision Surgery

As revision surgery is associated with great risk of sensorineural hearing loss, most patients should be motivated to use hearing aid before revision operation is undertaken. Revision is indicated for all conductive hearing loss developed following early or late surgery with the hope of useful hearing improvement. The reason for failure of primary surgery may be—
- Aseptic necrosis of the tip of long process of incus
- Slippage of the prosthesis from the long process of incus
- Gradual adherence of the prosthesis to the edge of the oval window
- Poorly positioned prosthesis—too short prosthesis or displaced prosthesis
- Ankylosis of incus and/or malleus to the attic
- Osseous closure of the oval window.

Following points should be looked for before revision surgery:
1. Examination of other ear and relative function of the two ears in relation to adequate hearing.
2. Amount of air-bone gap by audiometric test that is confirmed by tuning fork test.
3. Discrimination score (SDS) and tympanometry.

Revision surgery is safe under local anesthesia as patient awakes so as to monitor the result of surgery on the table. Technique of revision surgery is almost same as for original operation except tympanic membrane is more fragile and chorda tympani nerve is more vulnerable to injury as it is embedded in adhesion to tympanic membrane. The incus, malleus and oval window may be enmeshed in scar tissue that is best removed by right angle hook or microscissors. During this procedure surgeon should remember the possibility of a dehiscent facial nerve prolapsed over the oval window following primary operation.

Stapes Surgery

Step by step surgery is shown in Figs 22A to O. Surgery is done, under local anasthesia with sedation except in children and apprehensive patients where genral anesthesia is preferred.

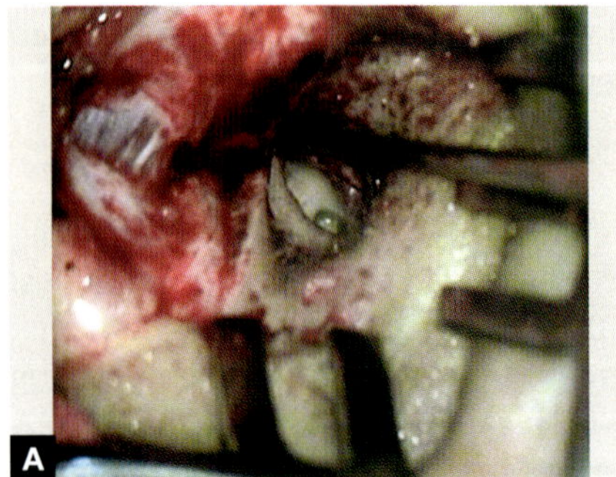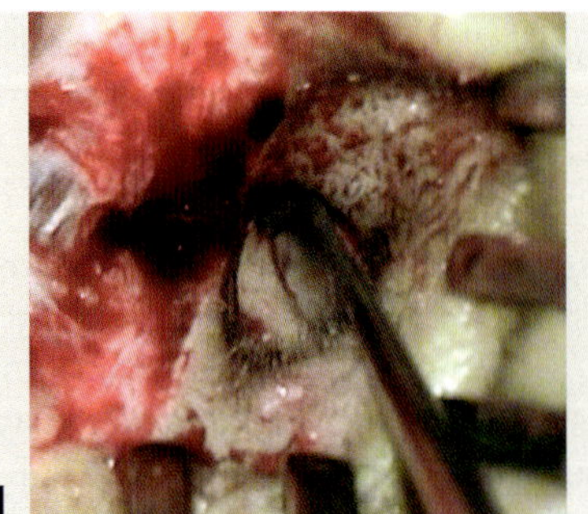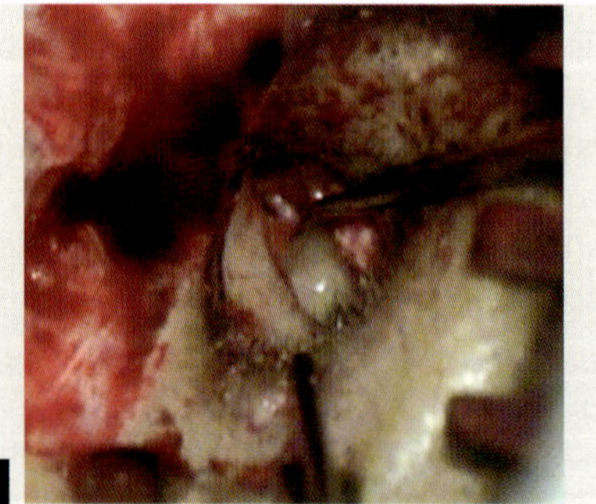

Figs 22A to C: (A) Endaural incision is made and TM flap is elevated; (B) Posterior-Superior bony overhang is assessed; (C) Chorda is separated

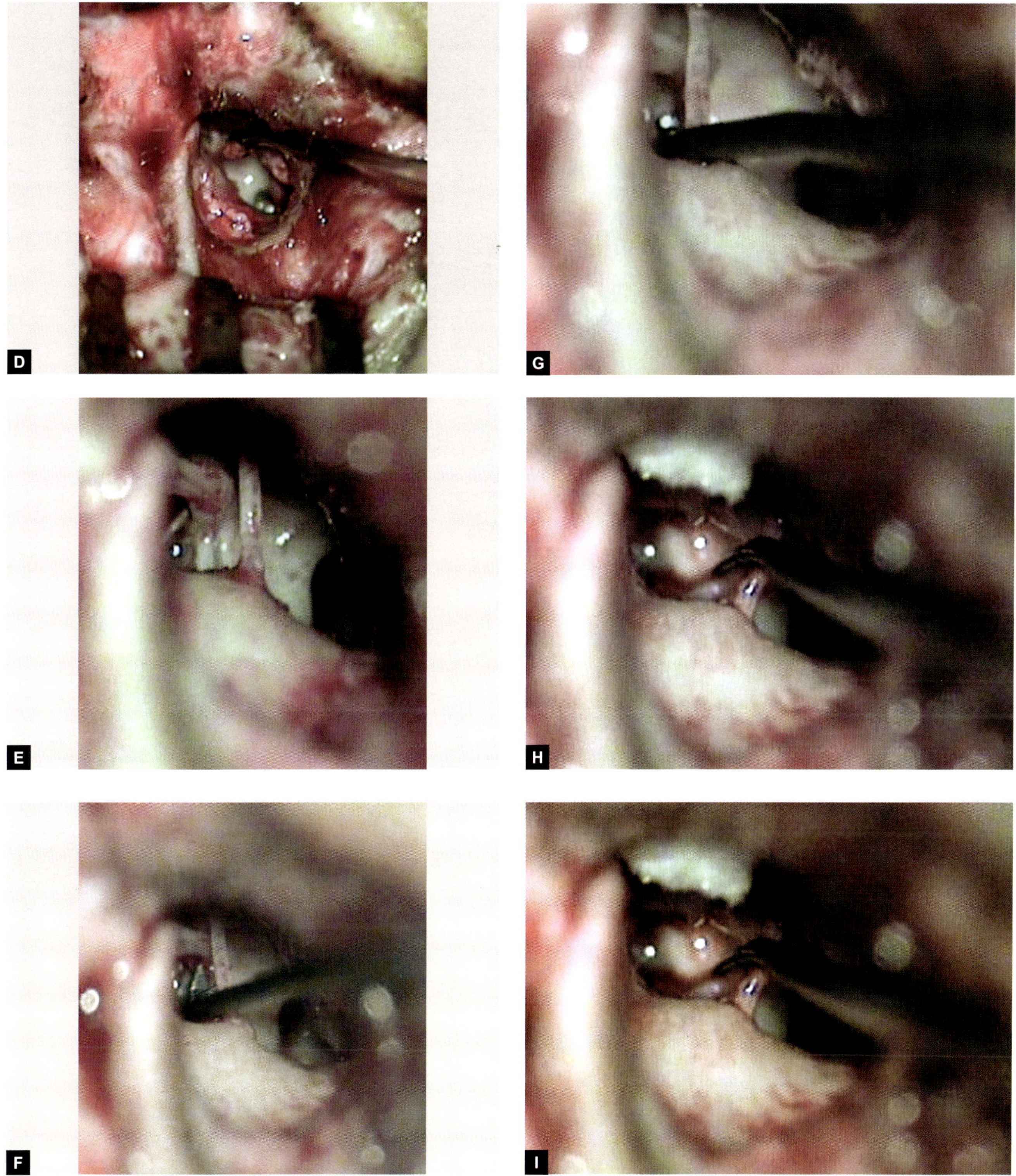

Figs 22D to I: (D) Bony overhang is curetted; (E) Picture showing IS joint, Chorda and stepedius tendon (F) Measuring of distance of footplate and undersurface of long process of incus (G) Small fenestration is made; (H) IS Joint dislocated and stapedius tendon is cut (I) Posterior crurotomy is done

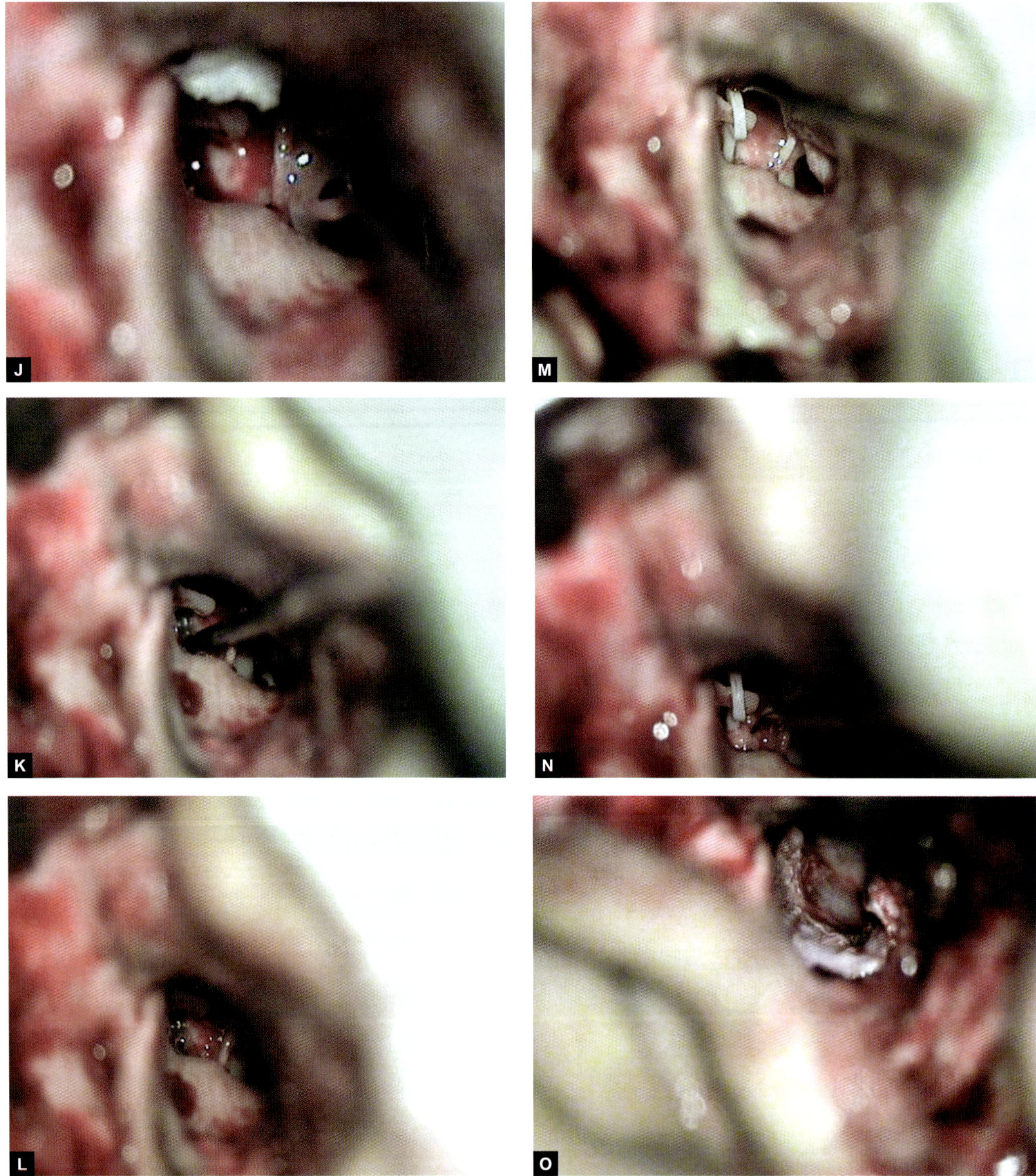

Figs 22J to L: (J) Removal of superstructure of stapes; (K) Widening of fenestrum done; (L) Picture showing fenestrum (M) Placement of Teflon piston; (N) Fat is given surrounding the piston; (O) Reposition of TM flap

Malleostapedotomy

Malleostapedotomy is advised in case of incus erosion or fixation of the malleus and incus. Use of lasers particularly argon laser is better option for clearing adhesions from oval window, for disentanglement of an ankylosed prosthesis from incus, for sculpturing incus or to control bleeding.

Prognosis for maintaining useful hearing following revision surgery is less likely than primary procedure.

REFERENCES

1. Beales PH. Otosclerosis. In: Kerr AG and Groves J (Eds); Vol.3. Scott-Brown's Otolaryngology. London: Butterworth and Con (Publisher) Ltd; 1994. P 301.
2. Linthicum FH Jr. Histopathology of otosclerosis. Otolarygol Clin. North Am. 1993;26:335-52.
3. Morrison AW, Bundey SE. The inheritance of otosclerosis. J Laryngol. 1970;84:921-4.
4. Guild SR. Histologic otosclerosis and Annal otolaryngol. 1944;53:246-66.
5. Ruedi L. Otoscleritic lesion and cochlear degeneration. Arch otolaryngol. 1969;89:364-71.
6. Johnsson LG, Hawkins JE, Linthicum FH. Cochlear and vestibular lesions in capsular otosclerosis. As seen in microdissection. Ann Otol Rhinol Laryngol. 1978;87(suppl. 48):1-40.
7. Morales–Garcia C. Cochleo vestibular involvement in otosclerosis. Acta Otolaryngol. 1972;73:484-92.
8. Causse J, Chevance LG, Bretlau P, Jorgensen MB, Uriel J, Berges J. Enzymatic concept of otospongiosis and cochlear otospongiosis. Ciln Otolaryngology Allied Sci. 1977;2:23-32.
9. Beales PH. Otosclerosis. In: Kerr AG and Groves J (Eds); Vol.3. Scott-Brown's Otolaryngology. London: Butterworth and Con (Publisher) Ltd; 1994. P 301.
10. John W House. Otosclerosis, the otolaryngologic clinics of North America. 1993;26(3):375-6.
11. Galdinoe Valvassori. Imaging of otosclerosis laryngologic clinics of North America. 1993;26(3):362-4.
12. Causse JR, Causse JB. Clinical features and epidemiology of otospongiosis – otosclerosis. In: Wiet-R. Causse JBn Shambaugh G, et al (eds): otosclerosis (otospongiosis). Alexandria, VA, American Academy of otolaryngology – Head and neck surgery foundation: 1991. p-56.
13. Philip H Beales, Scott Browns Otolaryngology. 5th edition, Otology. pp 314-6.
14. Vartiamen E, Kazalainens, Nuttinen J Suntioinen S, Pellinen P, Effect of drinking water fluoridation on hearing of patients with otosclerosis in a low fluoride area: a follow-up study. American Journal of Otology. 1994;15:545-8.
15. Bretlau P, Causse J, Causse JB, Hansen HJ, Johnsen NJ, Salomon G. Otospongiosis and sodium fluoride. A blind experimental and clinical evaluation of the effect of sodium fluoride treatment in patient with otospongiosis. Annals of otology, Rhinology and Laryngology. 1985;94:103-7.
16. Kofio D, Boahene MD and Colin LW, Doriscoll MD. Otosclerosis, current diagnosis and treatment in otolaryngology – Head and Neck surgery. 2008;3:678.
17. Lippy WH, Burkey JM, Arkis PN. Word recognition score changes after stapedectomy for far advance otosclerosis. American Journal of Otology. 1998;19:56-8.
18. Kacker SK. Stapedectomy- Current status. Otolaryngology review 2000. Edited by Vinod H Shah and Prabodh P Karnik. P 96-100.
19. Desai ABR, Desai AA. Stapes surgery today. Otolaryngology review. 2000;101-10.
20. Somer ST, Marquet T, Goverts P. Offeciers Earyngo statistical analysis of otosclerosis surgery perform by Jen Merquet. Annal of otology, Rhinology and Laryngology. 1994;103:945-51.
21. Rea PA and Tange RA. Management option—surgery. Scott-Brown's Otorhinolaryngology, head and neck surgery, 7th edition. page-3475.
22. Seicshnaydre MA, Sismanis A, Hughes GB. Update of reparative granuloma: survey of the American otological society and American Neurotology society. American journal of otology. 1994;15:155-60.
23. Atacan E, Sennaroglu L, Genc A, Kaya S. Benign paroxysmal positional vertigo after stapedectomy. Laryngoscope. 2001;111:1257-9.
24. Feruson BJ, Gillespie CA, Kenan PD, Farmer JC Jr. Mechanisms of cholesteatoma formation following stapedectomy. An J otol. 1986;7:420-4.

Meniere's Disease

Asok K Saha

DEFINITION

American Academy of Ophthalmology and Otolaryngology (AAOO), in 1972 defined Meniere's disease (MD)—a disease of the membranous inner ear characterized by deafness, vertigo and usually tinnitus and its pathology correlates to endolymphatic hydrops (ELH). The additional symptom of aural fullness has been added to the current definition. The deafness and vertigo are characteristics.

The deafness is SN in type, fluctuating and usually unilateral and progressive.

The vertigo is well-defined and episodic. The definitive spell is prostrating, often accompanied by nausea and vomiting and persisting for a prolonged period of time (20 mintues to not more than 24 hours).[1]

The AAOO report (1972) also defined two subvarieties. Cochlear and Vestibular Meniere's disease

- Cochlear type is typical fluctuating progressive sensorineural hearing loss (SNHL) without episodic vertigo
- Vestibular type is typical episodic vertigo without hearing loss.[2]

In 1985, American Academy of Otolaryngology and Head and Neck Surgery (AAOHNS) revised these guidelines and suggested that the term MD should be—"restrictive and include only those cases with full complement of classic symptoms and findings of the disease presumed to result from idiopathic endolymphatic hydrops".[3]

Historical Reviews

In 1861, Prosper Meniere (Fig. 1) in Paris first described this disease as a group of symptoms comprising—
- Episodic vertigo
- Fluctuating SNHL
- Tinnitus
- Aural fullness.

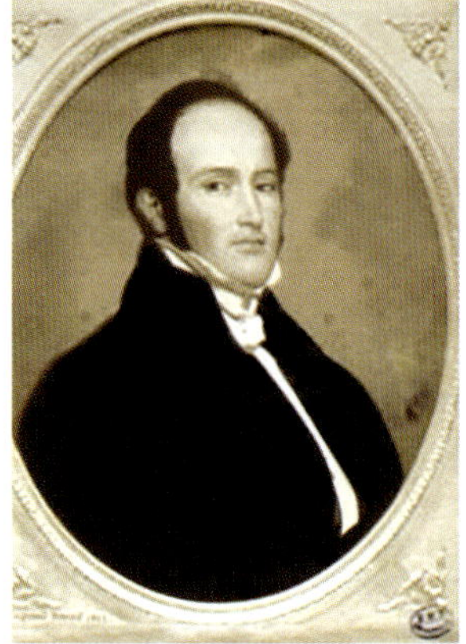

Fig. 1: Prosper Meniere (1799–1862)

At that time, the general terminology used for vertigo was—Apoplectic cerebral congestion which is associated with brain disorder. Meniere first proposed that the disease is a peripheral end organ disorder and not a disease of brain.[4,5]

Flourens (1842), Professor of Anatomy, experimented on Pigeons and confirmed that semicircular canals are related to vertigo.[6]

Parry (1908) performed first vestibular neurectomy for relief of vertigo.[7]

Guild (1927) identified the stria vascularis as the principal source of endolymph and endolymphatic sac as the site of endolymphatic outflow.[8]

Portmann (1927) described endolymphatic sac surgery for the treatment of vertigo.[9]

Dandy (1928) suggested vestibular nerve section (VNS) as the treatment of vertigo.[10]

MENIERE'S SYNDROME

Meniere's syndrome refers to the subjective symptoms of episodic vertigo, fluctuating SNHL, aural pressure and tinnitus, without pathological basis, while the term Meniere's disease implies the presence of endolymphatic hydrops and that this pathology is the cause of the clinical symptoms.[2]

Endolymphatic hydrops is associated with—

- Meniere's disease
- Congenital malformation of ear
- Syphilitic and viral labyrinthitis.

Incidence

- In India, MD comprises 0.5% of patients at ENT clinics
- In UK, the incidence is 0.1%
- A racial variation has been suggested but in a large survey, the incidence is the same in caucasians and blacks
- In Sweden, there is a female preponderance; female: male is 3:2
- In Japan, there is a 3:2 male preponderance but more rigorously repeated survey found no sexual preponderance
- A familial tendency is described in MD with positive family history is up to 20%
- Age of onset is 35 to 60 years. Peak age is 5–6th decade. Right ear ≃ Left ear
- It is usually unilateral, contralateral involvement occurs within 2 years in 50%. Incidence of bilateral disease is 31.8%.

Duration of vertigo:

- Less than 1 hour is 25%
- 1 hour—50%
- 2 hours to 1 day is 25%.

The disease may be progressive and nonprogressive.

In progressive disease, the symptoms worsen in spite of medical treatment and often incapacitate the patient (1 out of 4) requiring surgery.

Pathology

- Endolymphatic hydrops (ELH):
  - Endolymphatic hydrops or distension of Endolymphatic system is a consistent finding in patients with MD, involving the cochlear duct (scala media), the saccule and to a lesser extent the utricle and semicircular canals (SCCs)
  - This hydrops is apparently idiopathic. No obvious pathology in the temporal bones is considered as is seen in a variety of other insults to the ear, e.g. Mondini dysplasia, surgical trauma, temporal bone fracture, labyrinthitis, syphilis, etc. The walls of the membranous labyrinth show areas of thinning, outpouching and ruptures. The dilatation of cochlear duct may completely fill the scala vestibuli; marked bulging of Reissner's membrane may herniate through helicotrema into apical part of scala tympani. The distended saccule may lie against the stapes footplate. The utricle and saccule may show out pouching into the SCCs (Figs 2 and 3).[2]
- Vestibular fibrosis: A band of fibrous tissue is formed between the under surface of the footplate and the utricular macula. This occurrence accounts for a positive Hennebert's sign observed in 30% of ears with MD

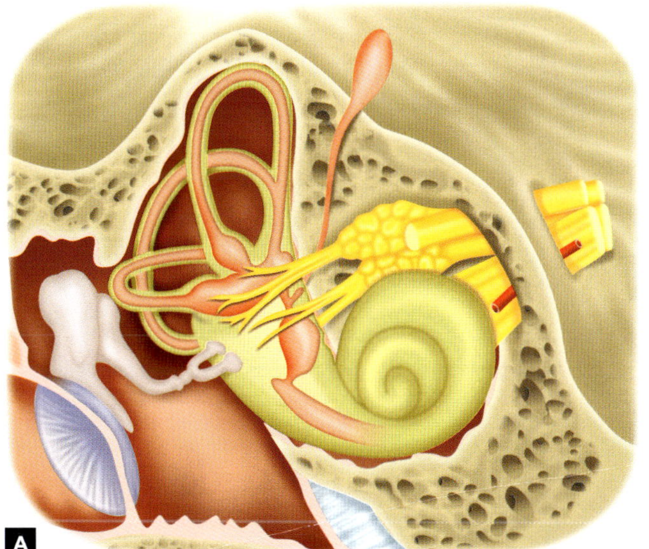
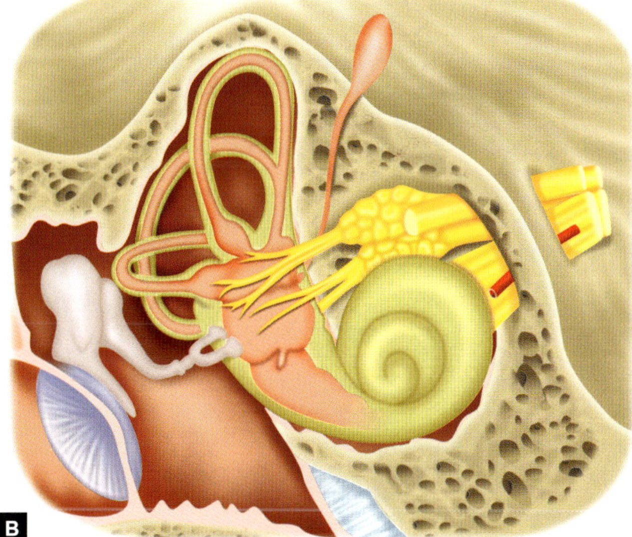

Figs 2A and B: (A) Normal membranous labyrinth; (B) Dilated membranous labyrinth in MD
Source: http://www.dizzinessandbalance.com

- Sensory lesions: There is marked pathologic changes seen in surviving hair cells of cochlea including fusion of cilia, disruption of cuticular bodies and basal ward displacement of hair cells resulting in loss of contact with the cuticular plate
- Neural lesions: Reduction in the number of afferent nerve ending and afferent synapses at the base of both inner and outer hair cells on the affected side is seen in unilateral MD
- Endolymphatic sac and vestibular aqueduct: Hypoplasia of the vestibular aqueduct, hypoplasia of the endolymphatic sac, decreased vascularization of the sac and perisaccular fibrosis have been described in cases with MD or endolymphatic hydrops.

Factors leading to the endolymphatic hydrops include:
- Excessive endolymph production by stria vascularis
- Blocked endolymph drainage by sac
- Ionic imbalance by spirochetal infection, viral infection
- Genetic abnormalities
- Autonomic imbalance
- Allergic phenomena, trauma, endocrine disturbance, psychosomatic disorder and autoimmune mechanism.

Etiology

- Anatomical: Small vestibular aqueduct
- Traumatic: Biochemical dysfunction in the cells of the membranous labyrinth

- Viral infection: *H. simplex* and *Enterovirus* may cause damage to the endolymphatic duct and sac
- Allergy: Food and inhalant allergens
- Autoimmunity: Circulating immune complex may cause direct damage to the endolymphatic sac
- Psychosomatic and personality features: Psychic stresses experienced in childhood and overt neurosis to be more common in patients with MD
- Genetic: The association of both sporadic and familial cases of MD with partial HLA class 1 haplotypes points to a possible locus lying between the HLA-C and HLA-A loci on the short arm of chromosome 6. MD is attributable to a mutation on chromosome 6, designated as M (Morrison et al. 1994).[11]

Pathophysiology of Symptoms

Endolymph moves from cochlea (site of production) to endolymphatic sac (site of absorption) (Fig. 4).

Flow of Endolymph

Stira Vascularis→ Scala media of cochlea→ Cochlea duct→ Ductus reunions→ Endolymphatic duct→ Endolymphatic sac.

Utricle and Semicircular canal   saccule

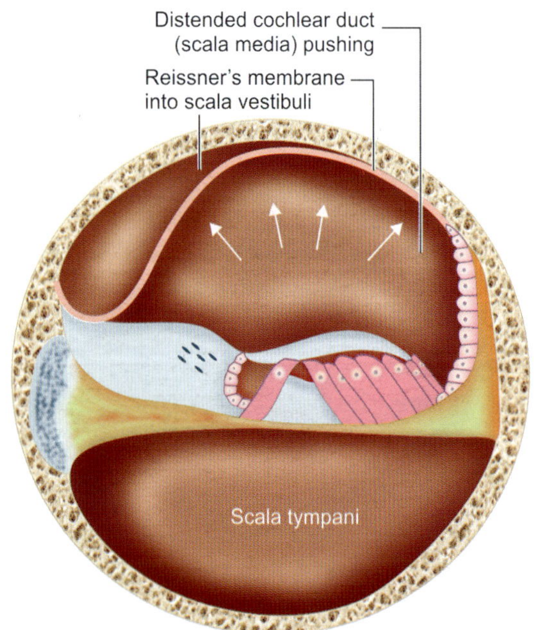

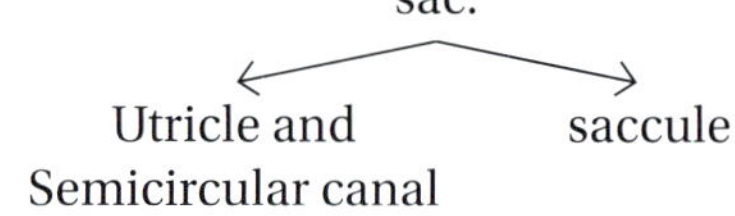

Fig. 3: Dilatation of cochlear duct with endolymph and bulging of Reissner's membrane into scala tympani

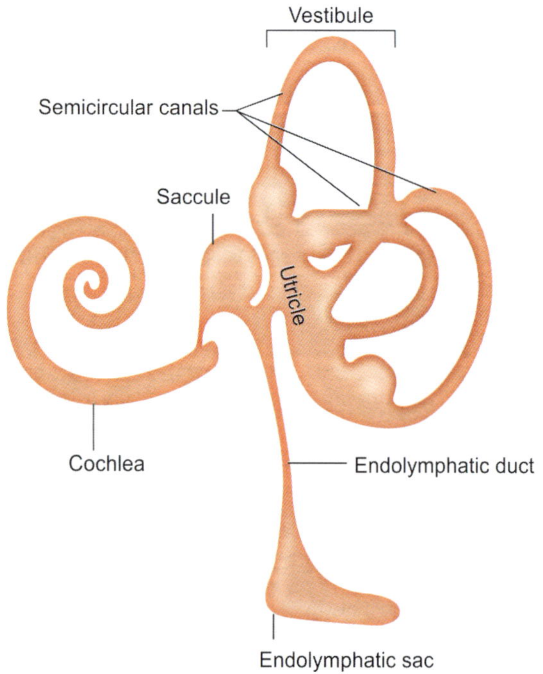

Fig. 4: Membranous labyrinth showing endolymphatic sac and duct

Lake-River-Pond concept of ELH

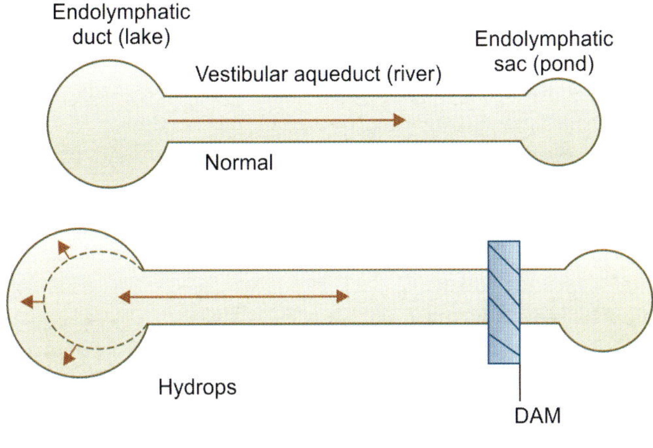

(Lake-River-Pond concept)

Any disturbance in production or absorption causes accumulation of endolymph in cochlea and membranous labyrinth leading to hearing loss and vertigo.

Episodic vertigo and fluctuating SNHL: In presence of idiopathic endolymphatic hydrops, a sudden rupture of thin membranous labyrinth results in flooding of perilymphatic space with potassium-rich neurotoxic endolymph, causing paralysis of sensorineural structures which in turn results in a sudden attack of vertigo and/or hearing loss. Healing of the ruptured area permits the symptoms to subside and set the stage for another attack to occur (Schuknecht et al.) (Figs 5A to D).

Chronic disequilibrium and irreversible SNHL: This may be explained as the basis of permanent morphologic changes observed in vestibular end organ, such as atrophy of Cristae, severe distortions of the ampullary walls and distortion with displacement of the utricular macula. The mechanical distortion of the ampullary walls, alters the motion mechanics of cupula resulting in caloric canal paresis (Rizvi).

Tinnitus: Roaring type and fluctuating in nature. It may be explained as a reduction in activity in cochlear nerve fibers in the cochlear apex and then the partition between the relatively inactive apical part and active remaining part of cochlea is rendered by CNS as a sense of tinnitus.

Aural pressure and fullness: The symptoms might be mediated by sensory nerve supplying the middle ear aspect of the round and oval windows that results feeling of fullness.

- Hennebert's sign is the Vertigo and Nystagmus experienced by patient during pressure induced excursion of the stapedial footplate
- Tullios phenomenon is seen in some cases of MD. Subjective imbalance and nystagmus are observed in response to loud, low-frequency noise exposure.

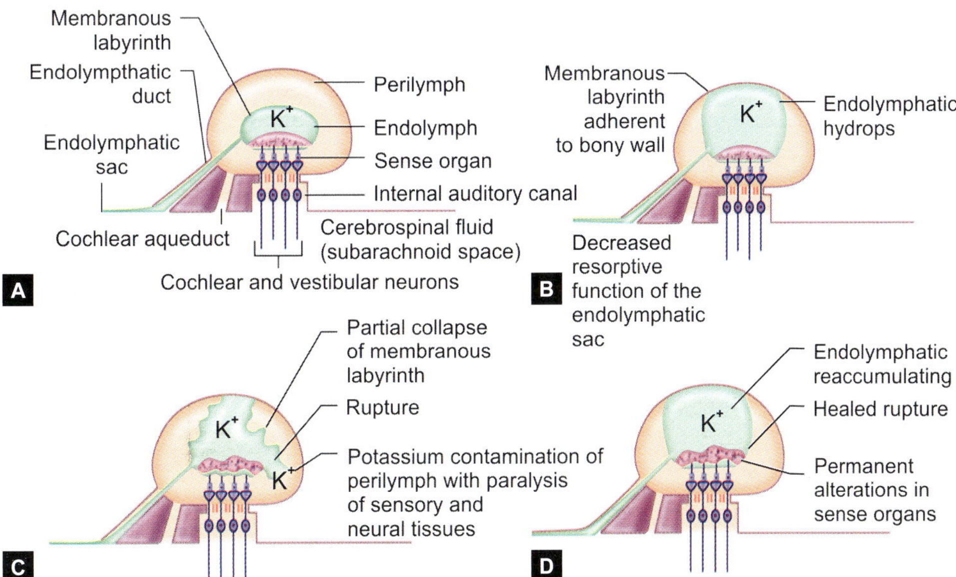

Figs 5A to D: Ruptures of membranous labyrinth leading to neurotoxic potassium contamination of endolymph in the perilymphatic space causing paralysis of sensory neural structures resulting Meniere's symptoms. Healing of rupture allowing to recur hydrops. (A) normal; (B) endolymphatic hydrops; (C) rupture of membranous labyrinth; (D) healed membranous labyrinth allowing distention to recur.
Source: Scott Brown's Otorhinolaryngology head and neck surgery Vol.3 7th edition 2008. p.3697.

Nystagmus

A typical attack has three phases. Each phase is determined on the basis of direction of spontaneous nystagmus.

The first phase (early irritative phase)
- The nystagmus is usually horizontal or horizontal and rotatory, it beats towards the affected side (ipsilateral)
- This phase persists less than an hour.

The second phase (paretic phase)
- The nystagmus beats away from affected ear (contra lateral) because of peripheral vestibular hypofunction
- This phase stays several hours or 1–2 days.

The third phase (late recovery phase)
- The Nystagmus beats towards the affected side (ipsilateral) as peripheral vestibular function recovers and resting activity in the vestibular nucleus is higher than in the unaffected side
- This phase lasts several hours as the second phase.

WATANABE'S CLASSIFICATION OF STAGES OF MD[13]

Type I (Early reversible)
- Mild-to-moderate low-frequency hearing loss (~40 dB)
- It records to almost normal as the patient's condition improves
- Endolymphatic hydrops exists only during the periods when the hearing is impaired.

Type II (Established, fluctuant)
- Moderate flat audiometric hearing loss (~60 dB), fluctuating ($\uparrow\downarrow$) by about 30 dB
- Endolymphatic hydrops is always present but can vary in degree.

Type III (Late nonfluctuant)
- Moderate or severe hearing loss with marked high-frequency loss >60 dB
- Little or no fluctuation of hearing
- Vertigo may lessen as the disease becomes 'burnt out'
- Permanent marked endolymphatic hydrops with wide spread destruction of hair cells in the basal turn.

Types of Meniere's disease

- Classical
- Cochlear (without vertigo)
  - Only fluctuating and progressive SNHL with aural fullness.
- Vestibular (without deafness)
  - Definitive spells of vertigo only
  - Most evolve into the classical variety with time.

- Lermoyez syndrome
  - Sudden SNHL which is followed by an attack of vertigo when hearing may recover.
- Drop attacks (otolithic crisis of Tumarkin)
  - Patient suddenly falls forwards or backwards
  - No preceding aura/or associated vertigo
  - Patient gets up within a few seconds and absolutely normal
  - Acute utriculosaccular dysfunction results inappropriate postural adjustment via vestibulo-spinal pathway.
- MD with migraine
  - About 30–35% of MD sufferers have H/o episodic migraine
  - In basilar migraine, sudden and fluctuant hearing loss may occur and vertigo is the most common symptoms[14]

AAO–HNS (American Academy of Otolaryngology Head Neck Surgery) proposed the diagnostic scale of MD (1995).[15]
- Certain MD
  - MD along with histopathologic conformation.
- Definite MD
  - Two or more episodes of spontaneous vertigo lasting for 20 minutes or longer
  - Audiometrically documented SNHL on at least one occasion
  - Tinnitus or aural fullness in the affected ear
  - Other causes excluded.
- Probable MD
  - One definitive episode of spontaneous vertigo
  - Audiometrically documented SNHL on at least one occasion
  - Tinnitus or aural fullness in the affected ear
  - Other causes excluded.
- Possible MD
  - Episodes of spontaneous vertigo without documented hearing loss or SNHL fluctuating or fixed with disequilibrium but non-episodic.
  - Other causes excluded.

Staging

Staging of MD according to the 1996 guidelines of AAO-HNS based on initial hearing level (Table 1).[16]

Table 1: Staging of MD based on initial hearing level	
Stage	**Four-tone average (dB)**
1	<25
2	26–40
3	40–70
4	>70

Table 2: Classification scheme based on definitive spells of vertigo per month

Numerical value	Class
0	A
1–40	B
41–80	C
81–120	D
>120	E
Secondary treatment initiated because of disability from vertigo	F

Classification Schemes

Reporting guidelines based on definitive spells of vertigo per month after treatment. Numerical value = $(X/Y)*100$.

X = average number of definitive spells per month for the 18-24 months after therapy.

Y = average number of definitive spells per month for the 6 months before therapy (Table 2).[17]

Clinical Features

Acute Attack

- Episodic vertigo
  - Lasting 20 minutes to several hours associated with pallor/diaphoresis/nausea/vomiting
  - No loss of consciousness. Visual blurring caused by nystagmus is always present
  - Patient is usually entirely normal between the spells. No neurological sequelae. Positional vertigo may or may not be present
  - Otolithic crisis of Tumarkin or Drop attacks may be present.
- Auditory symptoms
  - Fluctuating hearing loss, usually unilateral is present (bilateral in ~10%)
  - Tinnitus
    - Nonpulsatile, not affected by pressure on carotids
    - Continuous/intermittent
    - Always present during acute attack
    - Magnitude is proportional to severity of hearing loss
    - Pitch is related to region of most severe hearing loss
    - Diplacusis binauralis dysharmonica (Intolerance to loudness), because of recruitment.
- Aural fullness is present during attacks of vertigo. Pressure all over the head may occur in some patients.

Remission phase—*usually 3–12 months.*
The cycle of activity and remission is irregular. In early stage, the patient is completely asymptomatic in remission phase. With progression some hearing loss and tinnitus become permanently established. Positional vertigo/motion intolerance/momentary ataxia on cornering may or may not be present.

Usually, definitive attacks occur in spells with good health between them.

Investigations

- **Tuning fork test**—show SNHL
- **Pure tone audiometry (Figs 6A to C)**—done at each visit shows SNHL (with fluctuations)
  - In early stages, lower frequencies are affected and the curve is of the rising type
  - When higher frequencies are involved, curve becomes flat or falling type
    - 42%—Flat audiogram
    - 32%—Peaked pattern
    - 19%—Downward slopping
    - 7%—Rising pattern.
- Speech audiometry—Speech reception threshold (SRT) is closely matched with pure tone average in >90% patients. Speech discrimination score (SDS) is 55–85% between attacks, discrimination ability is much impaired during and immediately following an attack.
- Special audiometric tests.
  - Recruitment test is positive in MD
  - SISI score is better than 70% in 2/3rd of patients with MD (normal 15%)
  - Tone decay test is less than 25 dB.

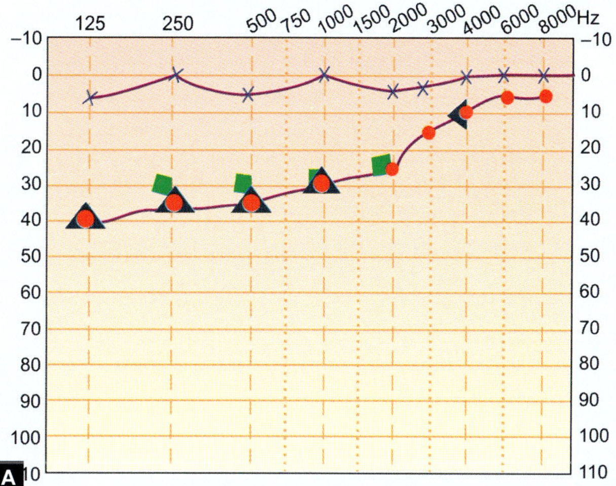

Fig. 6A: Audiogram of early Meniere's disease on the right side (x=left, o=right) showing low tone SNHL and of rising type curve.
Source: http://www.bestpractice.com

Brainstem-evoked Response Audiometry (Bera)

It is the electrical activity occurring in the cochlea and central auditory pathways in response to sound stimuli. It shows reduced latency of wave V. It is an objective and reliable test.

Vestibular-evoked Myogenic Potentials (VEMP)

This is a new diagnostic testing for MD. To obtain VEMP relaxation of sternocleidomastoid muscle (SCM) is measured in response to ipsilateral auditory stimulus. Brief high intensity monaural clicks or tone-bursts generate a large, short latency inhibitory potential (VEMP) in tonically contracted ipsilateral SCM. The VEMP is a vestibulocollic reflex with afferent arises from sound responsive sensory cells in saccule. The afferent signal goes centrally via the inferior vestibular nerve and efferent comes via vestibulospinal tract to produce inhibitory postsynaptic potential in cervical motor neurons. Normal responses have biphasic wave. Altered VEMP reveals saccular dysfunction in MD.[18]

Electrocochleography [ECOG (Fig. 7)]

- It is most sensitive and diagnostic test of MD
- It records the action potential and the summating potential through a recording electrode placed over the round window area
- Normal width of summating potential and action potential is 1.2–1.8 msec. Widening greater than 2 msec is usually significant
- SP/AP ratio is 1:3 = 0.33, Normal <0.4, In MD >0.45—It is diagnostic for MD.

Dehydration Tests

It includes glycerol, urea, frusemide that causes diuresis resulting in decrease of internal ear pressure and thereby, temporary improvement of hearing in patients with MD.

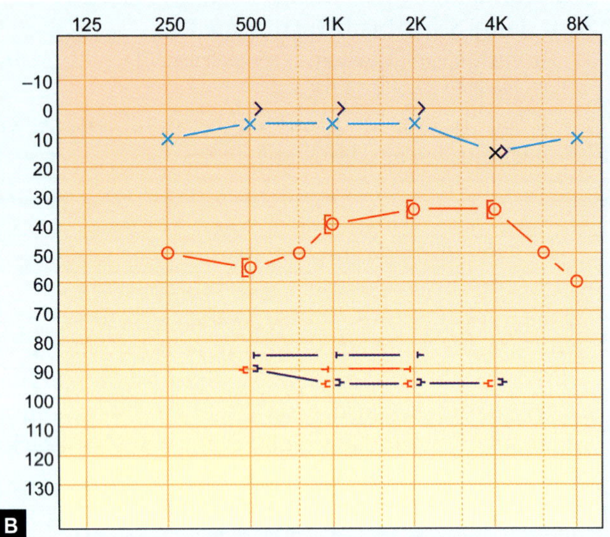

Fig. 6B: Audiogram typical of middle-stage Meniere's disease on the right side showing SNHL at all frequencies, but more so at high-and low-frequencies
Source: http://www.dizzinessandbalance.com

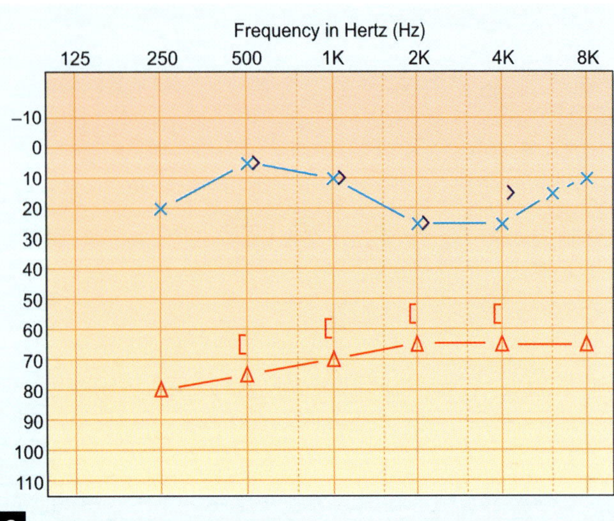

Fig. 11.6C: Audiogram of late-stage Meniere's disease on the right side showing flat curve with SNHL at all frequencies
Source: http://www.dizzinessandbalance.com

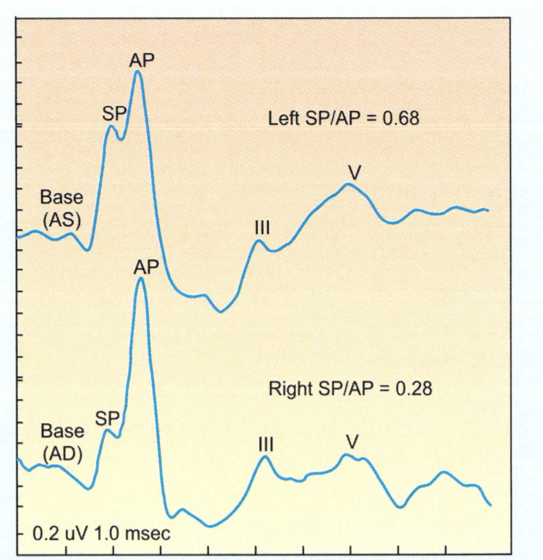

Fig. 7: Electrocochleography (ECoG) recorded with a hydrogel tympanic membrane surface electrode in a patient with Meniere's disease in left ear elicited by an alternating click stimulus presented at 85 dB nHL. SP (summating potential) and AP (cochlear nerve action potential) are measured from prestimulus baseline. Increased SP in the diseased left ear is noted
Source: Otolaryngologic clinics of America Oct 2010 Vol 43 No.5

Negative result does not rule out MD (false negative is 35–50%).

Glycerol Test

Glycerol, a common dehydrating agent when given orally, it produces a decrease in the intralabyrinthine pressure and also improves the cochlear blood flow resulting in improvement of hearing loss or increase in SDS by 10. Glycerol (1.5 mL/kg body weight) mixed with equal amount of orange juice is taken by the patient orally. PTA and SDS are recorded before and 1½ hours after intake of glycerol. An improvement of 10 dB PTA or gain of 10% SDS indicates positive test.

Urea Dehydration Test

It is done with 20 grams of urea mixed with 120 mL of fruit juice given orally. The test is not usually done—because of its bitter taste and rarely effective in patients in severe hearing loss. It is used for only with mild and moderate hearing loss (Table 3).

Both urea/glycerol—causes increase hearing in 50–60% of the patients with hydrops.

Prognostic value of glycerol test
- Negative glycerol test with nonfluctuant hearing loss on serial PTAs indicates decreased chances of improvement following surgery
- Positive glycerol test with fluctuating hearing loss on serial PTAs hints increased chances of improvement.

Caloric Test

In 75% of cases, there is decrease response of caloric test on the affected side. Usually, the test reveals canal paresis on the affected side and sometimes directional preponderance to healthy side. Normal response does not rule out MD.

Electronystagmography

It shows decreased response in 59% patients and normal response in~ 40%. Exaggerated response is seen in 1% cases.

Imaging

Although imaging is not essential for diagnosis of MD, it may give following hints:
- CT scan—Vestibular aqueduct and periaqueductal pneumatization is poorly visualized in hypoplasia of endolymphatic sac and duct

- MRI—shows that endolymph drainage system is significantly smaller in size
- Gadolinium-enhanced MRI—shows enhancement of endolymphatic sac.

Tests for Autoimmunity

Tests are done when MD is bilateral, progressive and responds to steroid therapy as the disease is suspected to be immune-mediated disorder.

The test for autoimmunity includes[1]
- C-RP (C-reactive protein)
- Serum immunoglobulin total complement
- Antinuclear factor
- Tests against antigens in the inner ear, such as lymphocyte transformation/Heat shock protein 70, i.e. Anti-68 kd (cochlear antibody).

Estimation of Hb%, T3, T4, TSH, cholesterol, triglyceride, glucose, VDRL is done to rule out anemia, inflammation, thyroid disorder and syphilis.

Meniere's Syndrome (MS)

Meniere's disease (MD) is an idiopathic condition while MS though resembles MD clinically results from a variety of conditions:

Etiology of MS or secondary endolymphatic hydrops are
- Developmental insult, e.g. Mondini dysplasia
- Abnormal metabolic/endocrine state, e.g.
  - Hypoglycemia
  - Hyperglycemia
  - Hypothyroidism
  - Hyperlipoproteinemia.
- Syphilis
- Chronic otitis media
- Viral infection: Mumps and measles
- Autoimmunity—Cogan's syndrome
  - Interstitial keratitis
  - Vestibular or auditory dysfunction
  - Nonreactive serology for syphilis.
- Otosclerosis
- Abnormal fluid balance—leukemia.

TREATMENT OF MENIERE'S DISEASE

Medical Treatment

Aim of the treatment is to reduce formation or accumulation of endolymph by—
- Low salt diet and decrease of fluid intake (urinary sodium is less than 50 mmol L/day)

Table 3: Mean serum osmolality following glycerol/urea

Glycerol	286	307.5	308.8	305.7
Urea	284	289.5	287.0	290.0
	Resting	1 hour	2 hours	3 hours

- Diuretics, e.g.
  - Hyperosmotic diuretic—isosorbide
  - Acetazolamide- carbonic anhydrase inhibitor
  - Hydrochlorothiazide/Triamterenes (potassium sparing diuretic)
  - Furosemide—40 mg on alternate day with potassium supplement. Furosemide is used in those patients allergic to sulfur and unable to take thiazide diuretics.

    Salt restriction is more useful than diuretics, as diuretic produces unwanted side effects of hypotension and hypokalemia.
- Vasodilators: They increase cochlear blood flow, e.g. inhalation of carbogen (5% carbon dioxide with 95% oxygen inhalation for 15 minutes 4 times per day)
  - Amyl nitrate
  - Betahistine
  - Papaverine hydrochloride.
- Phenothiazines with Antihistaminic properties
  - Cinnarizine- 25 mg 3 times daily
  - Diphenidol.
- Sedative/Tranquilizer: To reduce stress that results in decrease of attacks. Diazepam suppresses the activity of medial vestibular nucleus
- Parenteral aminoglycocides,[19] e.g. streptomycin and gentamicin are used in advanced bilateral Meniere's disease.

Acute Attack

The medical treatment includes:
- Bed rest
- Promethazine/Chlorpromazine intramuscular in high doses
- Intravenous infusion of lignocaine (1 mg/kg body weight at the rate of 6 mg/minute)
- Stellate ganglion block for rapid relief of severe attack to promote remission.

General Treatment includes—avoid smoking/no alcohol/treat infection.

Diet in MD is—Low salt diet/No caffeinated products/No chocolate.

Vestibular Rehabilitation Therapy (VRT)

- Labyrinthine exercises is helpful in long-term management of MD
- Cooksey-Cawthorne exercises are practiced for adaptation of labyrinth.

Intratympanic Gentamicin Therapy (Fig. 8)

It is now used for chemical labyrinthectomy. Gentamicin is vestibulotoxic and used in weekly or biweekly or single injections into the middle ear. Drug is absorbed through the RW and causes destruction of the vestibular labyrinth. Recently, the "low dose" protocol with just one or two injections in 1 month apart, has become the standard. 0.5 mL gentamicin solution is injected/dose with a drug concentration of 80 mg/mL. The total dose of gentamicin is < or = 80 mg, following injection the drug is left in the middle ear for 30 minutes while the patient is on bed, and then an attempt is made to clear the drug from middle ear through the ET tube (with swallowing and "popping" the ear). Total control of vertigo spells is seen in 60–80% of patients. Hearing loss is reported in 4–30% of patients.

Steroids

Intratympanic steroids used in sudden SNHL and potential chance of autoimmune cause of MD have evolved the idea for use of steroids for the treatment of MD. Besides the immune modulating mechanism, steroid may influence the sodium and fluid dynamics in inner ear because of its mineralocorticoid effect.[20] Advantages of steroids includes—
- Low-risk of complications
- Beneficial effect on hearing as compared with gentamicin
- Effectiveness in patient with bilateral diseases.

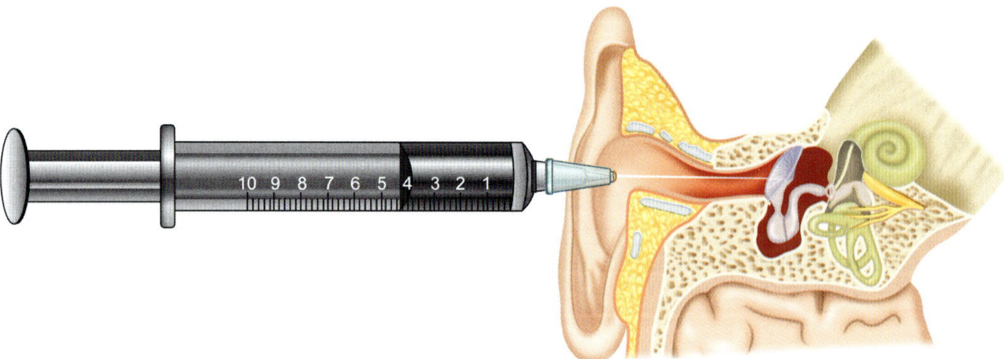

Fig. 8: Intratympanic gentamicin injection using narrow needle in MD

Systemic administration of steroids results in poor accumulation in the endolymph and perilymph because of poor penetration of blood-labyrinthine barrier. Drug accumulates only in the wall of endolymphatic sac. But intratympanic administration results in perfusion of drug in endolymph and perilymph through round window membrane. 1 mL of dexamethasone (16 mL) mixed with 0.5 mL of hyaluronidase (750 units) is injected via two small punctures made into tympanic membrane in the posteroinferior quadrant with one over the round window niche. Patient is advised to lie down with tested ear for three hours. At the same time 1 mL of dexamethasone (60 mL) is given IV. The procedure is repeated for 3 days. 91% of patients are achieving control of vertigo as claimed by some authors.[21] Use of steroids in MD still requires more research to establish its superiority to vestibular neurectomy and larbyrinthectomy.

Surgical Treatment

Surgical procedures are performed to control disabling vertigo refractory to medical treatment. There are various surgical procedures to treat vertigo of endolymphatic hydrops (ELH). Following conditions are considered while selecting an operative procedure:
- Severity of disease
- Surgical status
- Presence of unilateral or bilateral disease.

The surgical treatment is usually more desirable for unilateral disease. In an only hearing ear, the surgical procedure is planned till absolutely indicated because of potential chances of deafness and persisting vertigo.

Conservative Procedures (Hearing Preserved)

Endolymphatic Sac Surgery (Fig. 9)

Endolymphatic drainage procedure is divided into external shunts that help to drain excessive endolymph from endolymphatic sac into mastoid (Endolymphatic sac-Mastoid shunt) or subarachnoid space (Endolymphatic sac-Subarachnoid shunt) and internal shunts that drain excessive endolymph into perilymphatic space (cochlea-saccutomy).

Endolymphatic Sac-Mastoid Shunt (Fig. 10)

Portman (1929)[22] first described the surgery. It was subsequently revised by Paperella and Sajjadi (1994)[23] by using a T-shaped silastic placed in endolymphatic sac.

A routine cortical mastoidectomy via postauricular incision is made and extended to dissect at least 1cm posterior to sigmoid sinus. Posterior fossa dura is skeletonized from sigmoid sinus posteriorly to posterior semicircular canal anteriorly and endolymphatic sac inferiorly. The exposure is then extended towards jugular

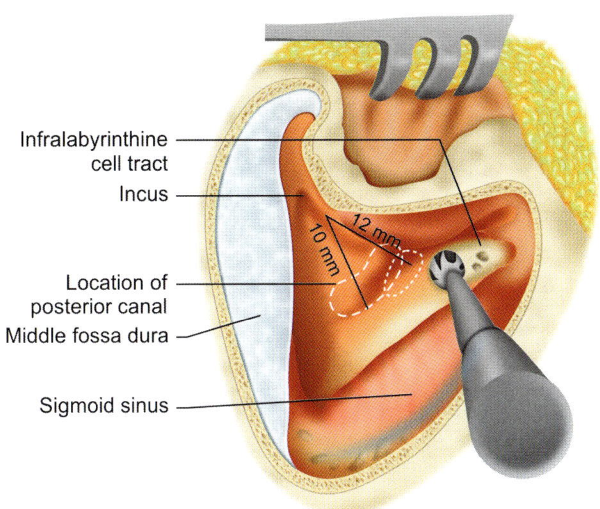

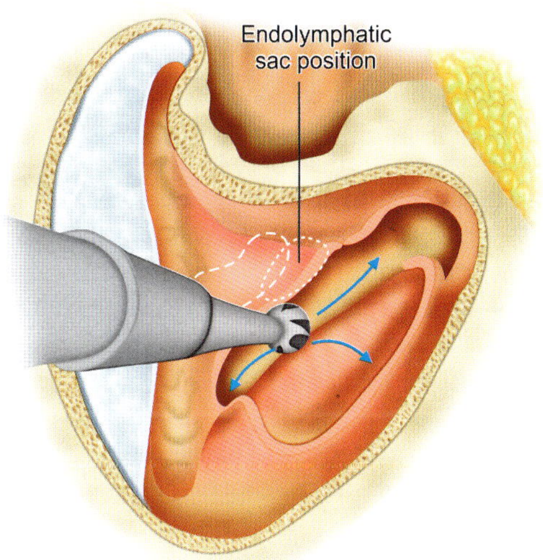

Fig. 9: Endolymphatic sac decompression
Source: Otologic surgery Brackmann et al.1994 p 468

bulb and into retrofacial air cells resulting in adequate decompression of endolymphatic sac. The sac is then opened at its inferior end with attention towards the duct, a T-shaped silastic is placed in the lumen for enhancing sac drainage. The sac is then covered by gelfoam and temporalis fascia, the wound is closed by two layers—subcutaneous layer by absorbing sutures and skinned by silk sutures.

Endolymphatic Sac-Subarachnoid Shunt (Fig. 11)

House (1962)[24] introduced the concept of special shunt allowing drainage of endolymph from endolymphatic sac into subaracnoid space of brain and obtained favorable results. Brackmann (1987)[25] revised the technique of shunt insertion. The shunt is placed anteriorly or posteriorly following incision on the medial leaflet of sac to avoid

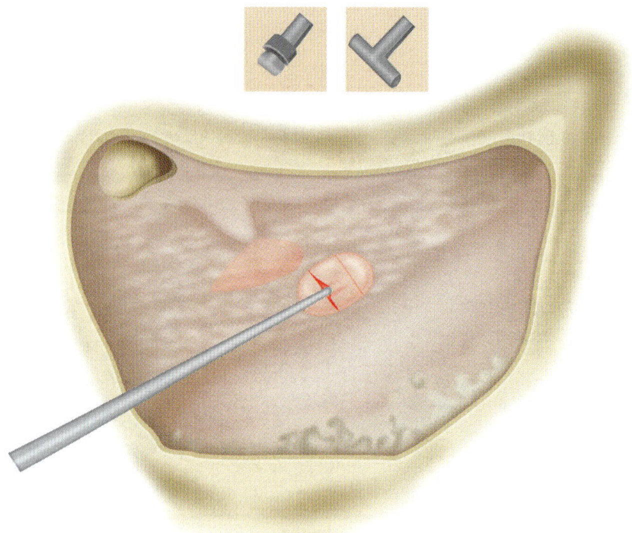

Fig. 10: Endolymphatic sac surgery- Following sac incision T-strut is placed.
Courtesy: House ear institute, Los Angeles, CA

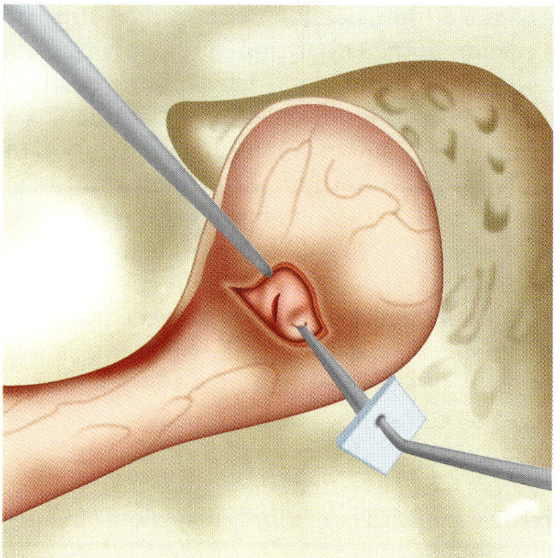

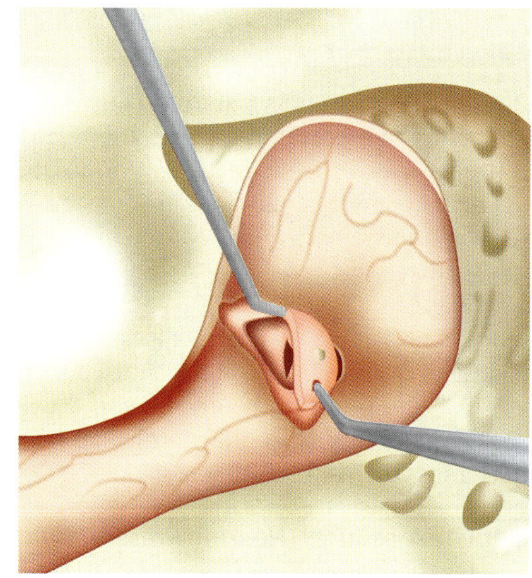

Fig. 11: Endolymphatic sac-subarachnoid shunt with insertion of silicon tube.
Source: Glasscock-Shambaugh Surgery of the ear Fifth edition 2003 p563

injury to the cerebellum. Opening in the sac is sealed with fascia and gelfoam to stop the flow of CSF into mastoid cavity. Pulec (1995)[26] reported a large series of operation of subarachnoid shunts with good results. It is found that efficacy of endolymphatic sac-mastoid shunt and that of endolymphatic sac-subarachnoid shunt has no statistically significant difference.[27]

The results of sac procedure in controlling attacks of vertigo is said to be 55–94% of the patients.

The drawbacks of the concept of these shunt procedures are as follows:[28]

- Endolymph cannot drain against higher pressure of CSF
- Shunts become encapsulated with proliferation of fibrous tissue that makes patency doubtful.

Perhaps the apparent efficacy is due to a nonspecific placebo type effect as reported by Tompson et al.[29]

Endolymphatic Sac Decompression

Endolymphatic sac decompression was first described by Shambaugh (1966).[30] The procedure involves cortical mastoidectomy, exposure of posterior fossa dura posteriorly from the sinodural angle to the jugular bulb along the sigmoid sinus and anteriorly to posterior semicircular canal and inferiorly to endolymphatic sac resulting identification and wide decompression of sac.

Decompression helps by—

- Releasing tight endolymphatic sac
- Revascularization of the perisaccular area
- Passive diffusion of endolymph.

In MD sigmoid, sinus is anteriorly placed. Wide decompression helps to view the obscured sac. It is reported that the result of sac decompression alone are comparable to other shunt surgeries for controlling vertigo in MD and there is no dead ears after the surgery.[31]

Revision Sac Surgery

House (1979)[32] first reported revision sac surgery. Subsequently, Paperalla and Huang (1991) compared the results of revision sac surgery to initial procedure. Failure of initial procedure based on the findings of revision surgery is neo osteogenesis, inadequate bone removal and perisacclar fibrosis obliterating endolymphatic flow.[33, 34]

Vestibular function preservation in revision sac surgery is comparable to initial or virgin procedure and, therefore, revision sac surgery is considered as an option by some authors going for any destructive surgical procedure.

Cochleosacculotomy–Internal Shunt

Schuknecht (1982)[35] first introduced the Cochleosacculotomy procedure for controlling vertigo in MD. The operation is done under local anesthesia and is indicated for patients who are not fit for general anesthesia and are suffering from preexisting severe to profound SNHL, because of risk of SNHL in operating ear (Fig. 12).

The operation consists of the following:

- Anterior tympanotomy to gain adequate exposure of oval and round window
- Usually, a 3 mm right angle pick is introduced through round window without removal of bone
- The pick is advanced through round window membrane in the direction of oval window and passed to the full depth of 3 mm
- This pass will go through the cochlear partition creating a fracture disruption of the osseous spiral lamina and cochlear duct
- The tip of the pick lies at the center of oval window with rupture of dilated saccule
- The pick is withdrawn and perforation of round window membrane is sealed by perichondrium or fat
- Tympanomeatal flap is repositioned and a piece of gelfoam is placed in the ear canal to maintain pressure on the flap. Antibiotic smeared gauze is then placed in external auditory canal.

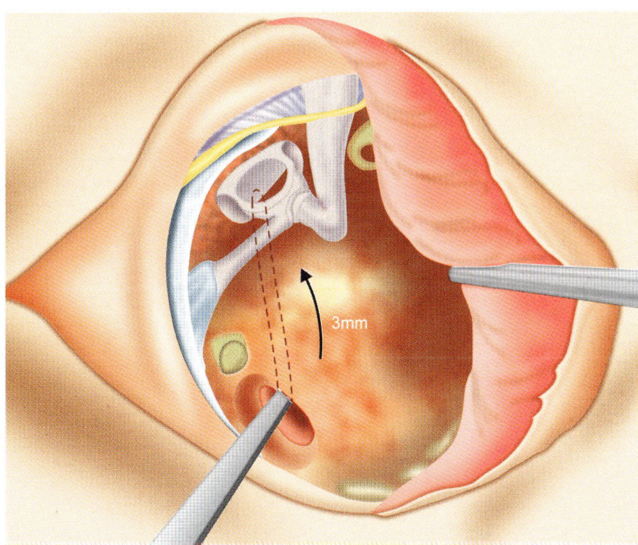

Fig. 12: Cochleosacculotomy—following anterior tympanotomy a 3 mm right angle pick is advanced through round window membrane in the direction of oval window.
Source: Otolologic surgery Brakmann et al 1994 p505

Rarely high jugular bulb blocks the access of round window and it needs to abort the operation. The procedure is not popularized because of high incidence of SNHL.

Partially Destructive Procedure (Hearing Preserved)

Vestibular Nerve Section (VNS)

Vestibular nerve section has been performed by neurosurgeons—Frazier (1912)[36] and Dandy (1941)[37] and they reported cure rate for vertigo is as high as 90% but high-rate of facial nerve dysfunction and of hearing loss avoided the acceptance of the procedure. William House (1961)[38] performed selective vestibular nerve section via middle fossa approach with operating microscope and reported high cure rate of vertigo (>90%) while still preserving hearing and facial nerve function. Drawbacks of the procedure are unfamiliar approach for otologist and required temporal bone lobe retraction.

Silverstein (1987)[39] reported transmastoid retrolabyrinthine approach for trigeminal nerve section where he noted a clear cleavage plane between cochlear and vestibular nerve. Subsequently retrolabyrinthine and retrosygmoid roots has been evolved.

Translabyrinthine Vestibular Neurectomy (Fig. 13)

- A postauricular incision is made above and behind the postauricular crease
- A cortical mastoidectomy is performed
- The posterior bony canal and bone over the tegmen are thin
- Sigmoid sinus is skeletonized
- Sinodural angle is opened as far back as possible. It is necessary to visualize the content of vestibule and helps to identify landmarks for excision of superior vestibular nerve. Matoid tip cells are opened
- Labyrinthectomy is performed by opening lateral semicircular canal, posterior semicircular canal (up to its confluence with superior semicircular canal), superior semicircular canal (along the tegmen) and vestibule
- Internal auditory canal (IAC) is identified by blue lining and is adequately skeletonized
- The superior vestibular nerve enters the lateral and superior ampullae through the perforated area that is carefully thinned
- The superior vestibular nerve is avulsed from vestibular recess and reflected. Facial nerve is visualized. Then inferior vestibular nerve is avulsed with the singular nerve supplying posterior semicircular canal
- Scarpa's ganglion lies midway out of the IAC. The curved ends of the vestibular nerves are reflected and fused nerve are section medial to the scarpa's ganglion and specimen is sent for histopathology examination

- Bipolar cautery is used for hemostasis and dura is closed with 4.0 silk. IAC and labyrinthine defect are sealed with fat obtained from abdominal wall
- The mastoid incision is closed in two layers—first thick periosteal layer with interrupted vicryl suture and skin with 3.0 silk
- Mastoid dressing is applied.[40]

Retrolabyrinthine Vestibular Neurectomy (Fig. 14)

Advantage of retrolabyrinthine approach is to identify the vestibular nerve in CPA (cerebellopontine angle) before it reaches the IAC through mastoid.

- A simple mastoidectomy is done with anteriorly-based postauricular flap
- Bone around the superior and posterior semicircular canals is removed
- Skeletonization of posterior fossa dura anterior to the sigmoid sinus is performed
- For adequate exposure of CPA posterior fossa dura is also exposed posterior to sigmoid sinus that permits extradural compression of sinus
- Anteriorly based U-shaped incision is made in the dura anterior to the sigmoid sinus from sinodural angle to the jugular bulb and then dura is reflected anteriorly

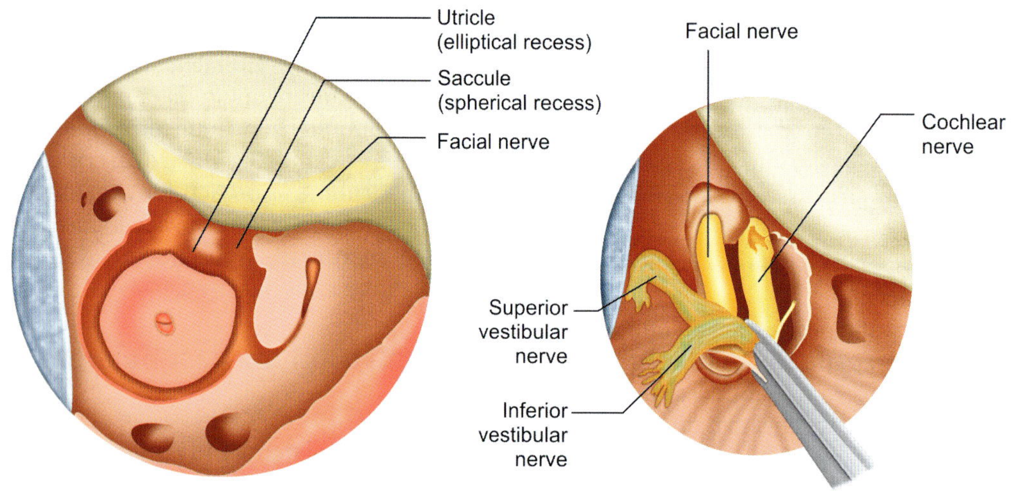

Fig. 13: Translabyrinthine vestibular neurectomy—opening of the vestibule, avulsion of vestibular nerves and section of fused nerve medial to scarpa's ganglion.
Courtesy: Otolaryngologic Clinics of North America October 2010 Vol43 No5 p1096&1099

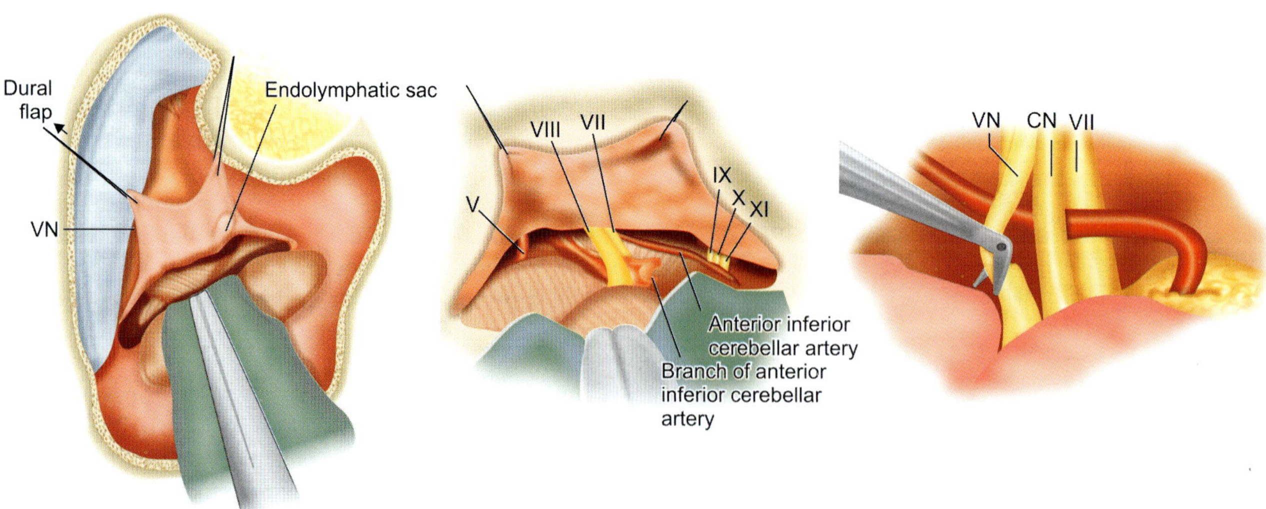

Fig. 14: Retrolabyrinthine approach for posterior fossa vestibular neurectomy
Source: Otologic surgery-Brackmann et al. 1994 p 495
Abbreviations: VN, vestibular nerve; CN, cochlear nerve

- Through dural window content of CPA are exposed. VII and VIII cranial nerves are identified under high powerful magnification of operating microscope
- The vestibular division of VIII cranial nerve is then sectioned if the nerve is seen to retract it confirms complete section of the vestibular fibers
- The dura is then repaired with 4.0 silk suture and mastoid defect is obliterated with abdominal fat
- In MD endolymphatic sac, decompression can be done at the time of vestibular neurectomy in this approach.

Retrosigmoid Vestibular Neurectomy (Fig. 15)

- A posterior fossa craniotomy is done immediately behind the sigmoid sinus
- Cerebellum is retracted to expose the VII and VIII cranial nerves
- The posterior wall of the internal auditory canal (IAC) is removed and dura is incised
- Branches of VIII cranial nerve are exposed. Superior vestibular nerve (SVN) and singular nerve are identified and transected, allowing complete denervation of the vestibular labyrinth without injury of the cochlear nerve (CON). This approach for VNS is most commonly used because of short-operative time. Advantage of this approach are:
  - As mastoidectomy is not performed cavity obliteration does not arise
  - Patients with COM or Sclerotic mastoid require this procedure
  - Anteriorly placed sigmoid sinus suggesting this procedure

  - Chances of CSF leak are less as dura can be closed in a water-tight technique.

Disadvantage of this procedure is that patient experiences postoperative headache because of bone dust arachnoiditis. It can be prevented by using gelfoam to trap the bone dust.[41]

Destructive Labyrinthectomies (Hearing Destroyed)

Destructive surgeries destroy the vestibular and auditory end organs completely. It is only indicated in unilateral MD with incapacitating vertigo and nonserviceable hearing. Usually, following surgical approaches of labyrinthectomy have been described:

Transcanal Labyrinthectomy

Schuknecht and Cawthorne (1957)[42,43] described the transcanal approach for labyrinthectomy on the local or general anesthesia.

- A tympanometal flap is elevated and stapes is then removed as done in stapedectomy
- A right angle pick is then inserted into the vestibule through the oval window. Then the saccular and utricular maculae are removed. The neuroepithelium from the combined lateral and superior ampullary cavity and posterior ampullary cavity is also removed
- The vestibule is then aspirated with a 20 gauge suction tip for ensuring complete removal of the content of labyrinth.

Schuknecht used to fill the empty labyrinth with gelfoam soaked in streptomicin. This is a blind procedure and in most cases, it is not possible to access the posterior structure

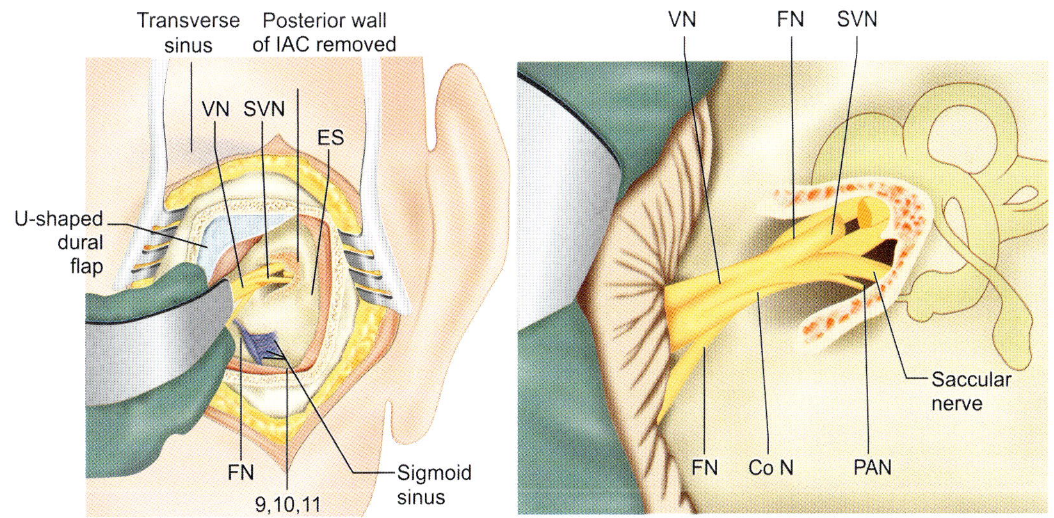

Fig. 15: Retrosigmoid approach for VNS-Transection of dura behind sigmoid sinus
Source: Otologic surgery Brackmann et al. 1994 p 497
Abbreviations: VN, vestibular nerve; SVN, superior vestibular nerve; ES, endolymphatic sac; FN, facial nerve; PAN, posterior ampullary nerve

such as posterior ampullary cavity, resulting in incomplete labyrinthectomy with persistence of vertigo.

Transmastoid Labyrinthectomy (Fig. 16)

This technique ensures more complete and thorough removal of labyrinth than the technique of transcanal approach. The bony labyrinth is exposed following cortical mastoidectomy via postauricular approach. With the help of high-speed drill with cutting bar each of the three semicircular canals is skeletonized. By following the canal to their ampullated ends, the vestibule is widely open and the neuroepithelium is removed from the vestibule under direct vision. Facial nerve should be kept in mind while working because of the risk of thermal as well as mechanical damage.

Other Surgical Procedures

- Cervicothoracic sympathectomy (C3→T3): It corrects microcirculatory failure in stria vascularis through an unknown mechanism. There is no risk of hearing loss. The procedure is suitable for patients having MD in only one functioning ear
- Ultrasonic irradiation: It is an alternative procedure to endolymphatic sac surgeries. Arslan (1953)[44] first introduced ultrasonic irradiation for MD. Ultrasound is applied to the lateral semicircular canal following cortical mastoidectomy to perform selective labyrinthectomy by destroying the cristea of semicircular canals while preserving the organ of corti. Later an alternative procedure is developed by applying ultrasonic probe to the round window via transcanal approach.[45] Ultrasonic irradiation is absorbed, heat is released and dissipates quickly in the fluid of inner ear resulting in selective damage to membranous labyrinth
- Cryosurgery: Wolfson (1966) first applied cold to the lateral semicircular canal via transmastoid approach. Cryoprobe is applied in order to freeze the membranous labyrinth.[46] Later an alternative procedure is evolved

where the cryoprobe is applied to the round window membrane via transcanal approach.[47]

Various other conservative therapies have been advocated for the management of MD. These include isosorbide, adenosine triphosphate, γ- globulin, lithium and anticholinergic drugs which are beneficial for controlling MD. Leuprolide acetate blocks normal sex hormone production and is used for the treatment of MD related to menstrual cycle.[48]

Innover, an anesthetic drug composed of droperidol and fentanyl is used to treat patients with intractable vertigo as an alternative to endolymphatic sac surgery.[49] Hyperbaric O_2 therapy has been evolved for patients with MD.[50] Efficiency of these medications is still not established.

Meniett Therapy

Meniett therapy a minimal invasive, simple and effective therapy for symptoms of vertigo of MD. A standard ventilation tube is inserted before the use of Meniett device (Fig. 17). The device delivers pulses of pressure to the inner ear via the ventilation tube. The micropressure treatment is usually used as a second level therapy when medical treatment fails.[51] The origin of pressure therapy for MD is based on the observation that if ear pressure changes may cause dizziness, then perhaps pressure changes may relieve the dizziness of MD. It is assumed that energy of meniett's micropressure pulse displaces perilymph that stimulates flow of endolymph and reduces it thus relieving dizziness of MD.

Each cycle of therapy takes 5 minutes and repeated 3 times in a day for 6 weeks. If symptoms do not subside, patients with MD may not respond to meniett therapy.

Advantages of meniett therapy
- Portable and convenient therapy takes a few minutes in a day

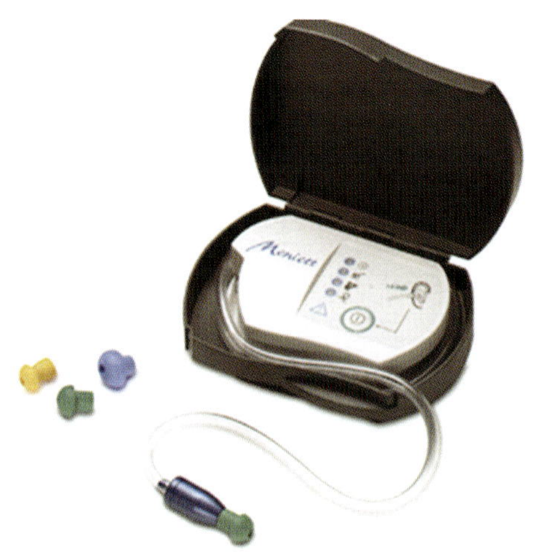

Fig. 16: Transmastoid labyrinthectomy—bony labyrinth is exposed, three semicircular canals are skeletonized, vestibule is widely open and neuroepithelium is removed
Source: Otolaryngologic clinics of North America Oct 2010, vol 43 no. 5 p1096

Fig. 17: Meniett device

- Other MD's treatment may still be employed along with therapy.

Disadvantages of meniett therapy
- Potential risk of infection from tympanostomy tube
- 25% of patients show no benefit.

REFERENCES

1. Alford. Meniere's diseade: Criteria for diagnosis and evaluation of therapy for reporting. Trans Ann Acad Ophthalmol Otolaryngol. 1972;76:1462-4.
2. Merchant SN, Rauch SD, Nadol JB. Meniere's disease–A clinical review Articles by Shah VH and Karnik PP, Review. 2000;114:579-81.
3. Pearson BW. Brackmann DE. Committee on hearing and equilibrium guidelines for reporting treatment results in Meniere's disesse. Otolaryngol. Head and Neck Surgery. 1985;93:579-81.
4. Banerjee S. Meniere's disease- A guide to ENT Practice, complied by Dr S.Banerjee president AOI (2002-2003): 42-50.
5. Meniere P. Maladies de 1oreille interne offrant les symptoms de la congestion Cerebra apoplectiforme. Gazmed de Paris. 1961;16:88.
6. Flowers P. Rherche's experimentales surles proprieties et les Fonctions du system nerveux: dans les animaux vertebres. Paris: JB Bailliere; 1842.
7. Parry RH. A case of tinnitus and vertigo treated by division of the auditory nerve. J laryngol Oltol. 1904;19:402-6.
8. Guild S. The circulation of the endolymph. Am J Anat. 1522-32.
9. Portman G. Surgical treatment of vertigo by the opening of the endolymphatic sac. Laryngoscope. 1965;76:1522-32.
10. Kimura RS. Experimental blockage of the endolymphatic sac and duct and its effect on the inner ear of the guinea pig. Ann Otol Phinol Laryngol. 1967;74:4664-87.
11. Khattar VS, Hatiram BT. Meniere's disease and other causes of peripheral incapacitating vertigo, comprehensive textbook of otology, diagnosis, management and operative techniques. In: Kirtane MV et al. (Eds). 2011. p-297.
12. Bance M, Mai M, Tomlinson D, Rukta J. The changing directions of Nystagmus in acute Meniere's disease: Pathophysiological implications. Laryngoscope. 1991;101:197-201.
13. Wantanabe I. Symptomatology of Meniere's disease. Otorhino Laryngology. 1908;42:20-45.
14. Balol RW, Andrews JC. Migrane and Meniere's disease. In: Harris JP, editor. Meniere's disease. The Hague: Kruger Publications; 1999. P.281-9.
15. Committee on hearing and equilibrium guidelines for the diagnosis and evaluation of therapy in Meniere's disease. American Academy of Otolaryngology- Head and neck foundations. Inc. Otolaringol Head and Neck surgery. 1995;133:181.
16. Committee on hearing and equilibrium. Guidelines for the diagnosis and evaluation of therapy in Meniere's disease. Otolaryngol Head and Neck surgery. 1996;114:236-41.
17. Semaan MT, Megerian CA. Meniere's disease: A challenging and Relentless disorder. Otolaryngologic clinics of North America. 2011;44(2):389-403.
18. Adams ME, Heidenreich KD, Kileny PR. Audiovestibular testing in patients with Meniere's disease. Otolaryngology Clinic of North America, Meriere's disease. 2010;43(5):999-1000.
19. Balyan FR, Taibah A, De Donato G, Asian A, Falcioni M, Ruso A, et al. Titration Streptomycin therapy in Meniere's disease: Long-term results. Otolaryngology- head and neck surgery. 1998;118:261-6.
20. Pondugula SR, Sannerman JD, Wangemann P, et al. Glucocorticoids stimulate cation absorption by semicircular canal duct epithelium via epithelial sodium channel. Ann J. Physiol Renal physiol. 2004;286(b):F1127-35.
21. Bolear–Aguirre MS, Lin FR, Della Santina CC, et al. Congitudive results with intratympanic dexamethasone in the treatment of Meniere's disease. Otol. Neurotol. 2008;29(1):33-8.
22. Portmann G. The saccus endolymphaticus and an operation for draining the same for the relief of vertigo. Arch Otolaryngol Head and Neck Surgery. 1927;6:309-17.
23. Paparella MM, Sajjadi H. Endolymphatic sac enhancement. Otolaryngol Clin North Am. 1994;27(2):381.
24. House WF. Subarachnoid shunt for drainage of endolymphatic hydrops. Laryngoscope. 1962;72:713.
25. Brackmann D, Nissen R. Meniere's disease: Results of treatment with subarachnoid shunt versus endolymphatic mastoid shunt. Am J Otol. 1987;8:275.
26. Pulec JL. Permanent restoration of hearing and vesticular functions by the endolymphatic sac subarachnoid shunt. ENT journal. 1995;74:544.
27. Khattar VS, Hatiram BT. Meniere's disease and other causes of peripheral incapacitative vertigo, comprehensive textbook of otology. Diagnosis, management & operative techniques. In: Kirtane MV, et al. (Eds). 2011;306-12.
28. Schwknecht HF. Meniere's disease. In: English GM (ed) Otolaryngology. Philadelphia: Lipincott; 1989;PP. 1-23.
29. Thompson J, Bretlan P, Tos M, Johnsen NJ. Placebo effect in surgery for meniere's disease. Arch Otolaryngol. 1981;107:271-7.
30. Shambaugh GE Jr. Surgery of endolymphatic sac. Arch. Otolaryngol. 1966;Suppl. 83:305-15.
31. Graham M, Kermink J. Surgical management of Meniere's disease with endolymphatic sac decompression by wide bone decompression of posterior fussa dura. Technique and results. Laryngoscope. 1984;94:680.
32. House WF. Revision of endolymphatic sac subarachnoid shunt for Meniere's disease. Arch Otolaryngol Head and Neck Surgery. 1979;105:599.
33. Paperalla MM. Endolymphatic sac revision for recurrent meniere's disease. Am J Otol. 1988;9:441.
34. Huang T. Endolymphatic sac surgery for meniere's disease. Acta otolaryngol suppl. 1991;485:145.
35. Schuknecht HF. Cochleosacculotomy for Meniere's disease. Theory, technique and results. Laryngoscope. 1982;92:853-7.
36. Frazier CH. Intracranial division of the auditory nerve for persistent aural vertigo. Surg Gynecol Obstet. 1912;15:524-9.
37. Dandy WE. Surgical treatment of meniere's disease. Surg. Gynecol. Obstset. 1941;72:421-5.
38. House WF. Surgical exposure of the internal auditory canal and its contents through the middle cranial fossa. Laryngoscope. 1961;71:1363-85.

39. Silverstein H, Norrell H, Haberkamp T. A comparison of retrosigmoid IAC, Retrolabyrinthine and middle fossa vestiblular neurectomy for treatment of vertigo. Laryngoscope. 1987;97: 165-73.
40. Tenfert KB, Doherty J. Endolymphatic sac shunt, Labyrinthectomy and vestibular nerve section in meniere's disease. Otolaryngol clin N Am. 2010;43:1091-111.
41. Catalono PJ, Witzo J, Post KD. Prevention of headache following retrosigmoid removal of acoustic tumors. Am J Otol. 1996;1(6): 904-8.
42. Schuknecht HF. Ablation therapy in meniere's disease. Acta Otolaryngol. 1957;132:1-42.
43. Cawthorne T. Membranous Labyrinthectomy via the oval window for Meniere's disease. J Laryngol Otol. 1957;71:524-7.
44. Arslan M. Treatment of Meniere's syndrome by direct application of ultrasound waves to the vestibular system. Proc. Fifth Intl. congress Otolaryngol, Amsterdam. 1953b;pp, 629-35.
45. Kassoff G, Wardsworth JR, Dudley PF. The round window ultrasonic technique. Arch. Otolaryngol. 1972;96:113-6.
46. Wolfson RJ, Cutt RA, Ishiyama E, Myres D. Cyrosurgery for Meniere's disease. Laryngoscope. 1968;78:632-42.
47. House WF. Cryosurgical treatment of the Meniere's disease. Arch Otol. 1966;84:161-22.
48. Price TM, Allen TC, Boyer DL, et al. Ablation of luteal phase symptoms of Meniere's disease with Leuprolide. Arch Otolyngol head neck surgery. 1994;120:209-11.
49. Gates GA. Innover treatment for Meniere's disease. Acta Otolaryngol. 1999;199(2):183-93.
50. Fattori B, De laco G, Vannucci G, et al. Alternobaric and hyperbaric oxygen therapy in the immediate and long-term treatment of Meniere's disease. Audiology. 1996;35:322-34.
51. Committee on equilibrium of the American academy of Otolaryngology- head and neck surgery: Micropressure therapy policy statement, March 2008.

Acoustic Neuroma (Vestibular Schwannoma)

Asok K Saha

Acoustic neuroma (AN) is a benign encapsulated neoplasm originating from Schwann cells of the junctional zone of superior vestibular nerve (2/3) or inferior vestibular nerve (1/3) or rarely cochlear nerve in the internal auditory meatus and/or cerebello pontine angle (CPA) with gradual progression towards the brain stem. It is the most common (80%) tumor of CPA. 95% of the tumor is sporadic with unilateral involvement. 5% of the tumor is associated with Neurofibromatosis type ll occurring bilaterally. Sporadic acoustic neuromas usually begin in middle age where as NF_2 associated tumor is seen in younger age.

PATHOLOGY

Acoustic neuroma is extremely slow growing tumor of the 8th nerve. It is usually yellowish white or gray. Some tumors have cystic components. The surface is typically smooth and regular. Vascularity appears on the tumor surface; the vascularity is originating from small vessels of the internal auditory canal (IAC), CPA and brainstem surface.

Microscopically, the tumor shows two hispathological patters—Antoni A and B (Fig. 1).

Antoni A is closely packed cells with small spindle-shaped densely straining nuclei. A whirled appearance of Antoni A is called Verocay body. Antoni B is a looser cellular aggregation of vacuolated pleomorphic cell. In any particular tumor one of the cellular-patterned predominates or both types are admixed. A positive S-100 immunoperoxidase stain is specific for Schwann cell origin. Cytogenetic study indicates that a defect of chromosome 22q is responsible for the development of AN.

GROWTH OF TUMOR

The tumor develops in the nerve sheath (Fig. 2). It compresses rather than invades the nerve. As the tumor

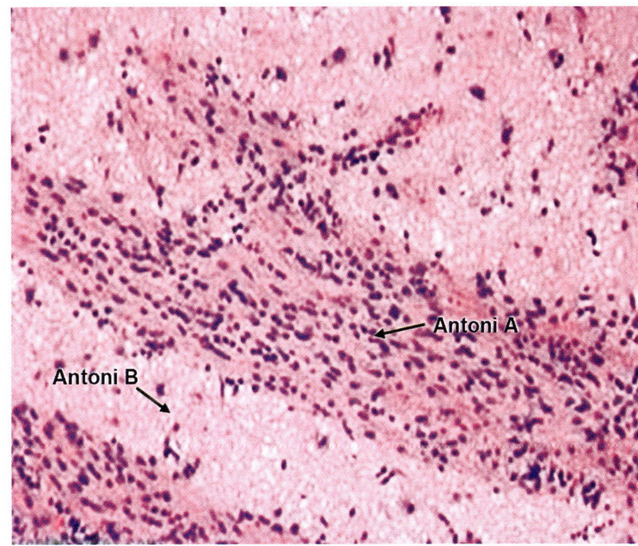

Fig. 1: Histological patterns—Antoni A and Antoni B of Acoustic Neuroma

grows, it gradually fills the internal acoustic meatus and protrudes out of the porus by bone resorption. Degree of bone resorption of internal acoustic meatus varies in AN. Some large and giant tumors have little bone resorption where as some small and medium-sized tumors have extensive bone resorption extending superiorly to the middle fossa dura and inferiorly as far as cochlear aqueduct. Extrameatal extension of the tumor occurs in the CPA where anterosuperior extension causes compression of CN V and inferior extension involves the IX, X and XI CN in jugular foramen. As the tumor grows in size, it displaces the brain stem and compresses the cerebellum leading to increase intracranial tension and hydrocephalus.

Acoustic neuroma is slowly growing tumor. Average growth rate varies from 0.1 to 0.2 cm per year (Figs 3A and B).

It is observed that most of the tumors which are clinically stable over a period of 1–2 years will become remarkable progression over a period of 10 years or more. For this reason younger patient should not be reassured for the growth of the tumor. NF$_2$ associated tumor are usually rapidly growing type. Sudden hemorrhage or cystic degeneration with fluid collection in the tumor results rapid increase in size with mass effect. [1]

CLASSIFICATION OF AN

Classification depends on the size of the tumor.[2] It is based on the measurement taken from preoperative CT or MRI scans to know the size of the largest extrameatal diameter of the tumor.

According to international consensus guidelines grading of acoustic neuroma is provided (Table 1).

SIGNS AND SYMPTOMS

Primarily occurs as a result of pressure effect, while in others are due to infiltration of tumor to nerve and surrounding structures.

- Hearing loss—unilateral, slowly progressive high-frequency SNHL is the most common pattern. There is marked reduction in speech discrimination scores out of proportion to the pure tone loss
- Tinnitus is noted in 10% cases.
  Progressive unilateral SNHL and unilateral Tinnitus if present in any patient, must be investigated to find out AN.
- Vertigo is uncommon due to occurrence of central compensation which results from the slow rate of growth. Disequilibrium or unsteadiness occurs in 50% of patients

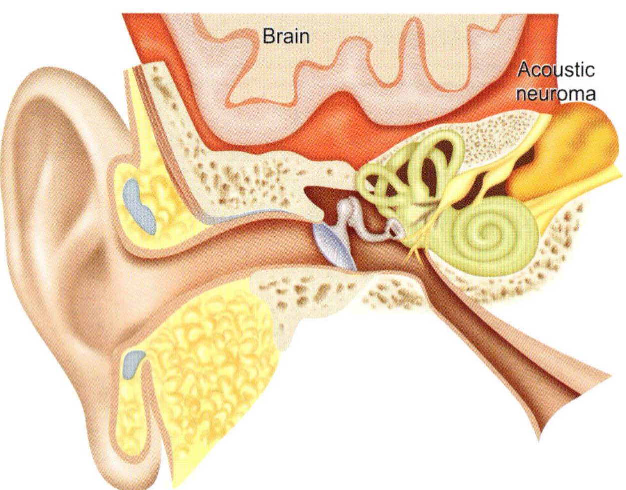

Fig. 2: Acoustic neuroma of internal auditory meatus protruding out of porus

Table 1: Grading of acoustic neuroma (AN)

Intrameatal tumor	Extrameatal size	mm
Grade 1	Small	1–10
Grade 2	Medium	11–20
Grade 3	Moderately large	21–30
Grade 4	Large	31–40
Grade 5	Giant	>40

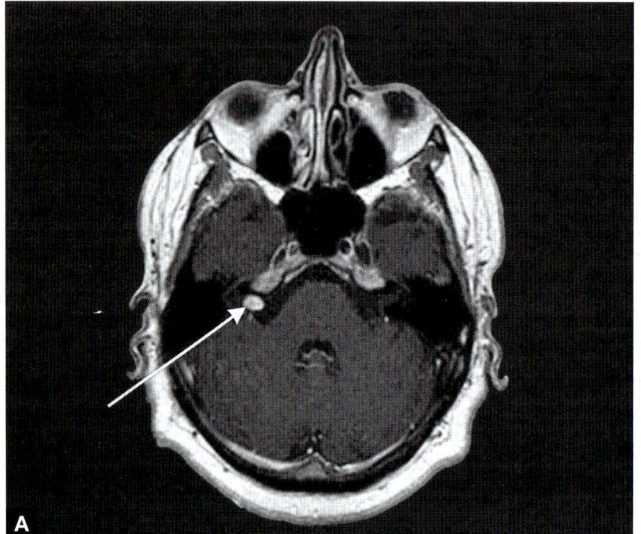

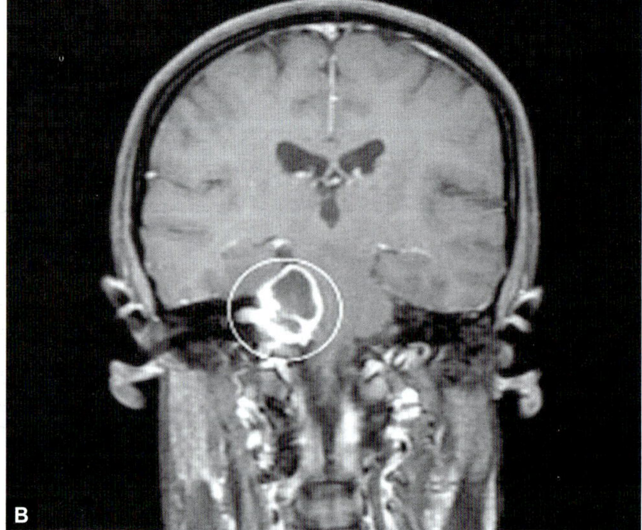

Figs 3A and B: (A) MRI—Small acoustic neuroma in Intrameatal position (horizontal imaging); (B) MRI—Large acoustic neuroma with extrameatal extension (vertical imaging)

- Changes in sensation within the distribution of the 5th Cr Nerve (Trigeminal).

  First extracanalicular nerve to be compressed is the trigeminal nerve root resulting in—

- Absence of corneal reflex
- Hypoesthesia or paresthesia of the face in 15% of the patients.

  Larger tumors can affect motor division of the trigeminal nerve producing atrophy of the temporalis and masseter muscles.

- Facial nerve—Sensory division of facial nerve is affected early while motor division that is resistant to compression by AN is affected late.

Hitzelberger's sign: Anesthesia of the posterior part of external auditory canal which is supplied by sensory fibers of facial nerve. It is the earliest sign to occur. This sign is absent in most cases because of overlapping sensory innervation in this area.[3]

- Schirmer's test—Reduced lacrimation. Facial nerve weakness is found rarely
- Palatal palsy, hoarseness of voice and nasal regurgitation. Very big CPA tumor indicate compression of CN IX or X
- Weakness and numbness of arms and legs with increased tendon reflexes, respiratory difficulty and stupor resulting from brain stem involvement are rarely seen today
- Ataxic gait, finger-nose test, dysdiadochokinesia, positive Romberg's test and Tandem walking (to walk along a straight line with tendency to fall to the affected side) indicate cerebellar involvement
- Large tumor may cause hydrocephalus, headache, blurring of vision and diplopia (CN VI involvement). Fundoscopic examination reveals papilledema/blurring of disc margins.

INVESTIGATIONS

- Pure tone Audiogram—unilateral, high-frequency SNHL but it may also be normal in up to 5% patient
- Speech discrimination—reduced out of proportion to the pure tone loss (i. e. <50%)
- Auditory brain stem response (ABR):
  - Ipsilateral—
    - Absolute wave V latency prolongation
    - I-V interpeak latency prolongation
    - III-V interpeak latency prolongation
    - I-III interpeak latency prolongation (most common and most pronounced)
  - Contralateral—wave V latency prolongation in large tumors with brain shift (off side abnormality)

  A delay of >0.2 m/sec in wave V between two ears is significant.

- Stapedius Reflex—threshold is elevated above normal levels
  - Decay of response declines by more than 50% in 5 seconds at 500 HZ and at 1 KHZ.
- Electronystagmography (ENG)—with bithermal caloric test.
  - Ipsilateral marked hypofunction or absent response is observed in most of cases
  - Positional Nystagmus is noted in occasional cases.
- Radiology (stenver's/transorbital view)—It reveals enlargement of IAC (i.e. enlargement of 2 mm or more of any portion or shortening of posterior wall by at least 3 mm, compared with the contralateral side is suggestive of AN in most cases)[4]
- CT Air meatography and CT with IV contrast—reveal erosion and widening of IAC. Tumor mass is isodense with the brain tissue. CECT has a role for knowing the true nature of the lesion. CN VII and VIII may be individually visualized (Fig. 4)
- MRI with gadolinium—It is superior to CT scan and gold standard for diagnosis of AN. On T1-weighted film tumor is isointense as compared to brain and hyperintense as compared to CSF. On T2-weighted film the tumor is isointense with brain and hypointense with CSF. It can detect ANs which are only a few mm in size (Figs 5 and 6).

Differential Diagnoses of CP angle Lesions

- Acoustic Neuroma—80% of all CP angle lesions arise from investing Schwann cell of the superior vestibular nerve
  - Isodense with the brain substance
  - No extracranial extension.

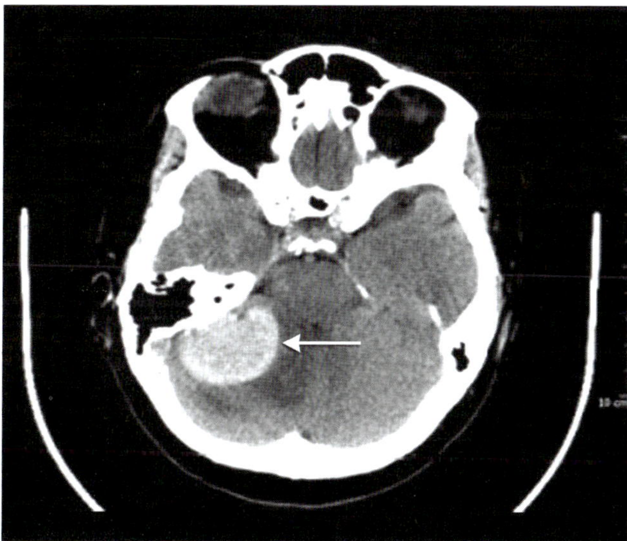

Fig. 4: Axial CT shows vestibular schwannoma in the right CP angle

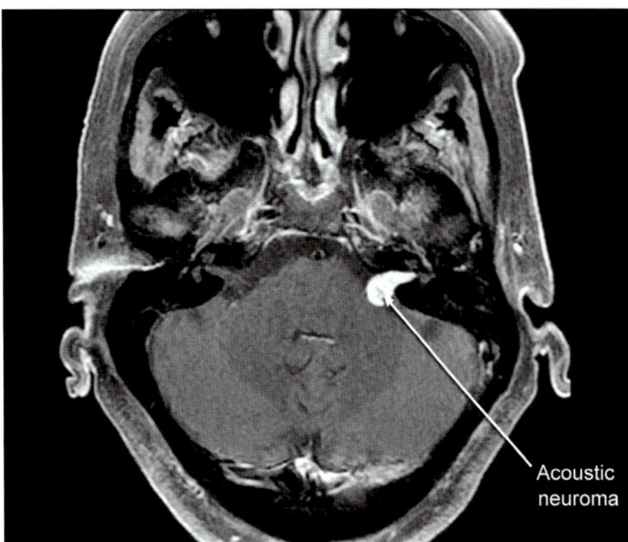

Fig. 5: T_1-weighted MRI with gadolinium of acoustic neuroma

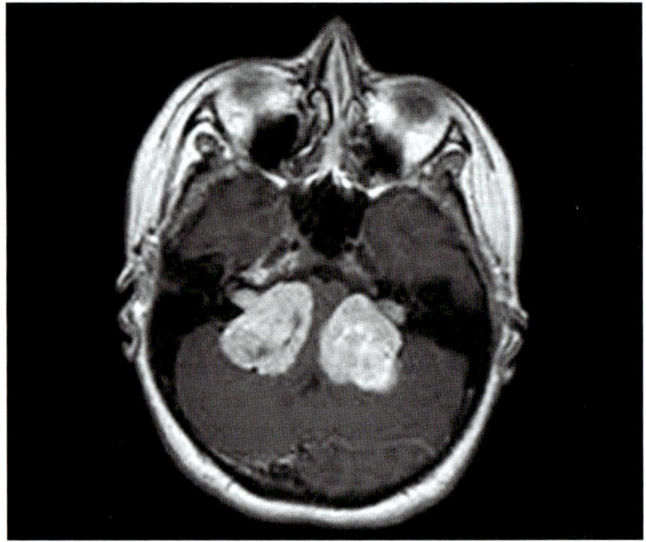

Fig. 6: MRI of bilateral acoustic neuroma (NF_2)

- Congenital cholesteatomas of the petrous apex—These are keratinizing epidermoid inclusion cysts arising from congenital epithelial cell rests.
  - Markedly hypodense compared to surrounding brain substance
  - Abnormalities of Vth and VII CNS are more common.
- Meningioma
  - Hearing is normal
  - Eccentrically placed over the porus acousticus
  - May be associated with extracranial extension
  - May show calcifications.
- Arachnoidal cysts
- A-V malformations
- Hemangiomas
- Lipomas
- Rarely
  - Malignant schwannomas
  - Gliomas
  - Malignant meningiomas.

TREATMENT

Treatment of AN includes—
- Surgical removal
- Stereotactic gamma—irradiation therapy
- Observation.
  Conventional external radiotherapy and chemotherapy have no role in treatment.

Surgery

Surgical approach depends upon size and location of tumor, hearing status, presence of complications and age of the patients. The surgical approaches are—

- Translabyrinthine approach
- Middle fossa approach
- Retrosigmoid approach.

Translabyrinthine Approach

This approach allows wide access to lesion of cerebello-pontine angle (CPA) in patient with poor hearing or absent hearing.

The approach includes following steps (Figs 7A to G):
- Postauricular extended cortical mastoidectomy
- Bony labyrinthectomy
- Bone overlying sigmoid sinus is removed
- Bone removal continues over the middle fossa dura, sinodural angle and posterior fossa dura medial to the sigmoid sinus
- Skeletonization of the jugular bulb that is the lower limit of bone removal is done. Vertical portion of facial nerve is also skeletonized until the sheath is visible
- Internal acoustic meatus (IAM) is skeletonized and intrameatal portion of tumor is exposed
- Posterior fossa dura over the posterior surface of petrous bone is incised. The tumor is removed and dura is repaired
- Abdominal fat graft is used to obliterate the middle ear and petrosectomy defect.

Advantages

- Direct approach to internal auditory meatus (IAM) and intrameatal tumor
- Any size of tumor to be removed
- Minimal cerebellar retraction
- Facial nerve is preserved
- Easy access of facial nerve graft.

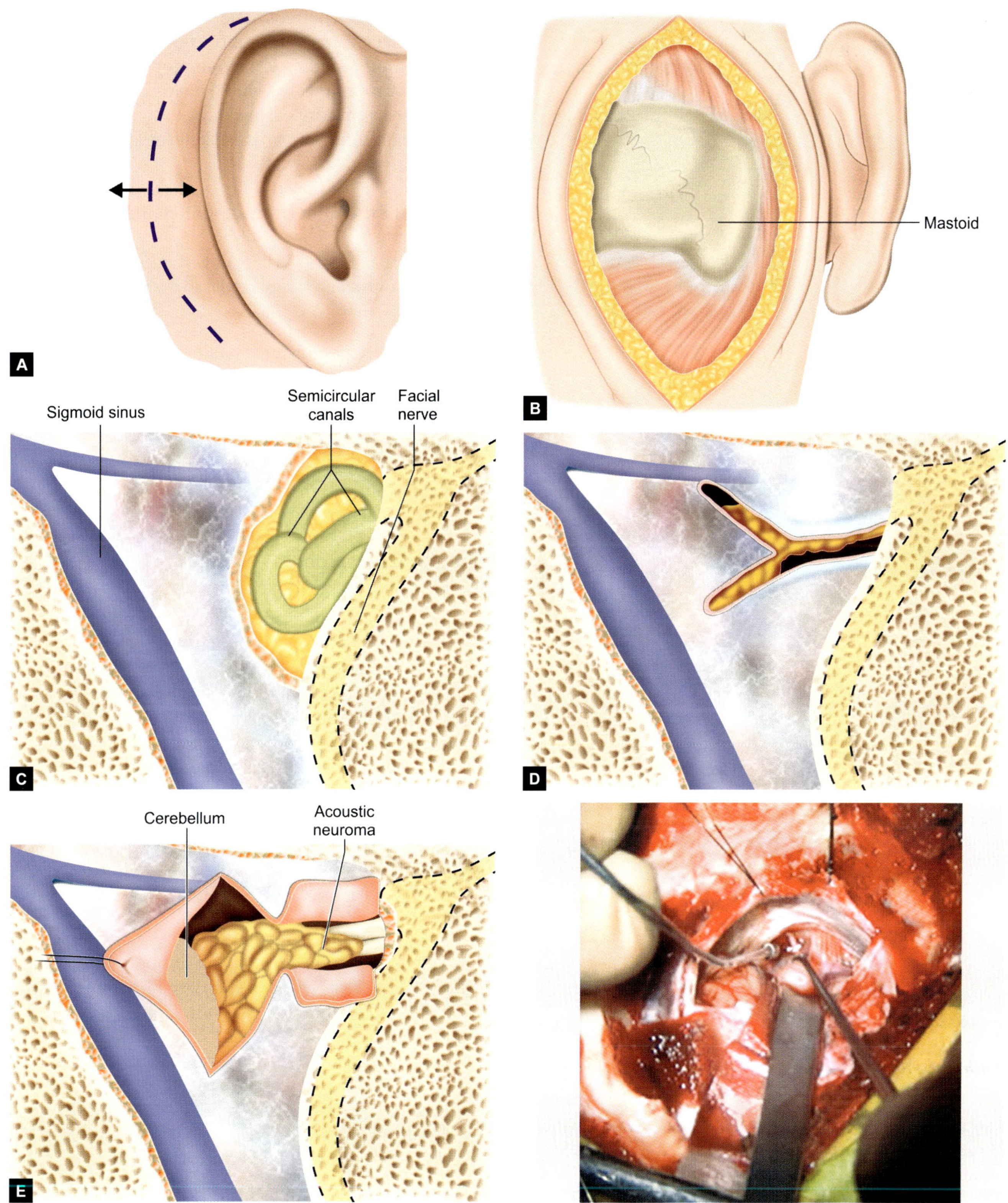

Figs 7A to E: (A) Postauricular incision; (B) Mastoid is exposed; (C) Extended cortical mastoidectomy, bony labyrinthectomy, bone removal over sigmoid sinus, middle fossa dura, sinodural angle, posterior fossa medial to the sigmoid sinus down to the jugular bulb and skeletonization of facial nerve and internal acoustic meatus; (D) Intrameatal portion of tumor is exposed; (E) Posterior fossa dura is incised and tumor is exposed

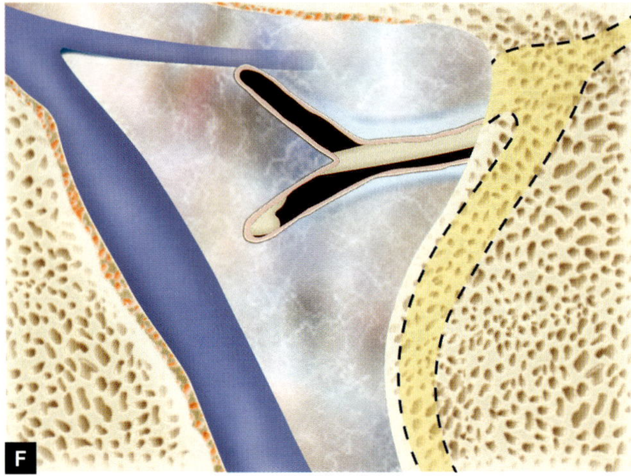

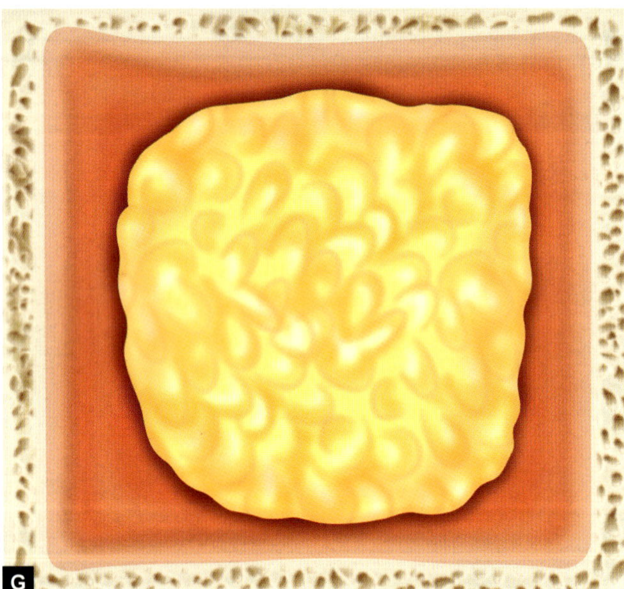

Figs 7F and G: Apposition of dura following tumor removal; (G) Abdominal fat is used to obliterate the defect

Disadvantages

- The procedure causes residual hearing loss, CSF fistula
- Sigmoid sinus, facial nerve, middle fossa dura limit the exposure.[5]

Middle Fossa Approach

The middle fossa approach is an access where internal acoustic meatus is approached extradurally from above through a small temporal craniotomy. It is indicated for small intracanalicular tumor of size 1–1.5 cm.

The approach includes following steps (Figs 8A to F):

- Middle fossa craniotomy is done
- Dura over the temporal lobe is exposed

- Upper surface of petrous bone is exposed by drilling and dura is elevated from the petrous pyramid. Sometimes troublesome bleeding is encountered from the venous plexus surrounding the middle meningeal artery that is controlled with surgical packing
- Internal auditory meatus is skeletonized anteriorly, superiorly and posteriorly
- Facial nerve and vestibular nerve running over the surface of the tumor are identified and the tumor is removed
- The internal meatus is closed with a free muscle plug and free bone flap is replaced.

Advantages

- Possibility of hearing preservation
- Good access to fundus.

Disadvantages

- Temporal lobe retraction
- Cochlea, semicircular canals and temporal lobe limits the exposure
- Risk to facial nerve injury.

Retrosigmoid Approach

This approach has come out from the conventional suboccipital operation used by neurosurgeons for removal of large tumors (CPA tumor >3 cm in size) (Figs 9A to E).

- In retrosigmoid approach, a 5 × 5 cm craniotomy is performed by removing the bone behind the sigmoid sinus and below the transverse sinus
- Dura is open through a U-shaped flap based anteriorly on the posterior aspect of sigmoid sinus and cerebellum is retracted so that surgeon's line of view is along the posterior surface of the petraous pyramid
- Posterior surface of petrous bone is drilled. Contents of IAM and posterior semicircular canal are preserved
- The jugular bulb (JB) present in the inferior aspect of the approach may be high enough to limit the access. Facial nerve and audiovestibular nerve are identified. AICA is noted. Intracranial part of the tumor is dissected off the facial and audiovestibular nerves. Tumor removal continues in medial to lateral direction preserving the facial nerve
- Hemostasis is achieved. Dural flap is repaired and strengthened with fascia. A plate of bone dust and tissue glue sits on the dural repair and fills the bony defect. A separate periosteal flap is made to cover the repair. Skin and subcutaneous tissues are closed in layers.

Advantages

- Possible hearing preservation
- No limit of the size of tumor.

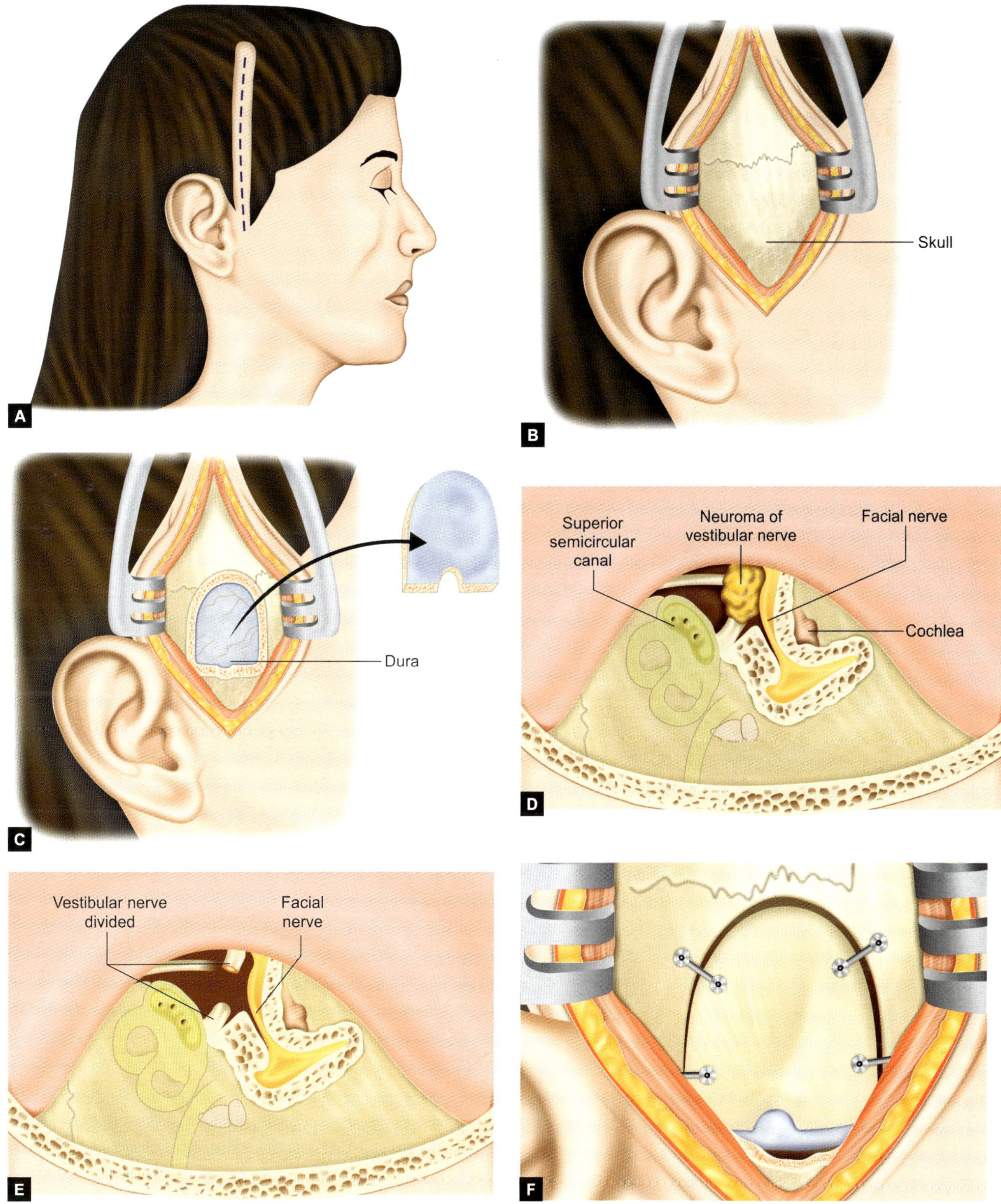

Figs 8A to F: (A) Vertical incision is made above the pinna; (B) Soft tissue is retracted to expose skull; (C) Middle fossa craniotomy and exposure of dura; (D) Facial nerve and vestibular nerve running over the tumor are exposed; (E) Tumor is removed; (F) Following closure of internal meatus with free muscle plug, bone flap is replaced

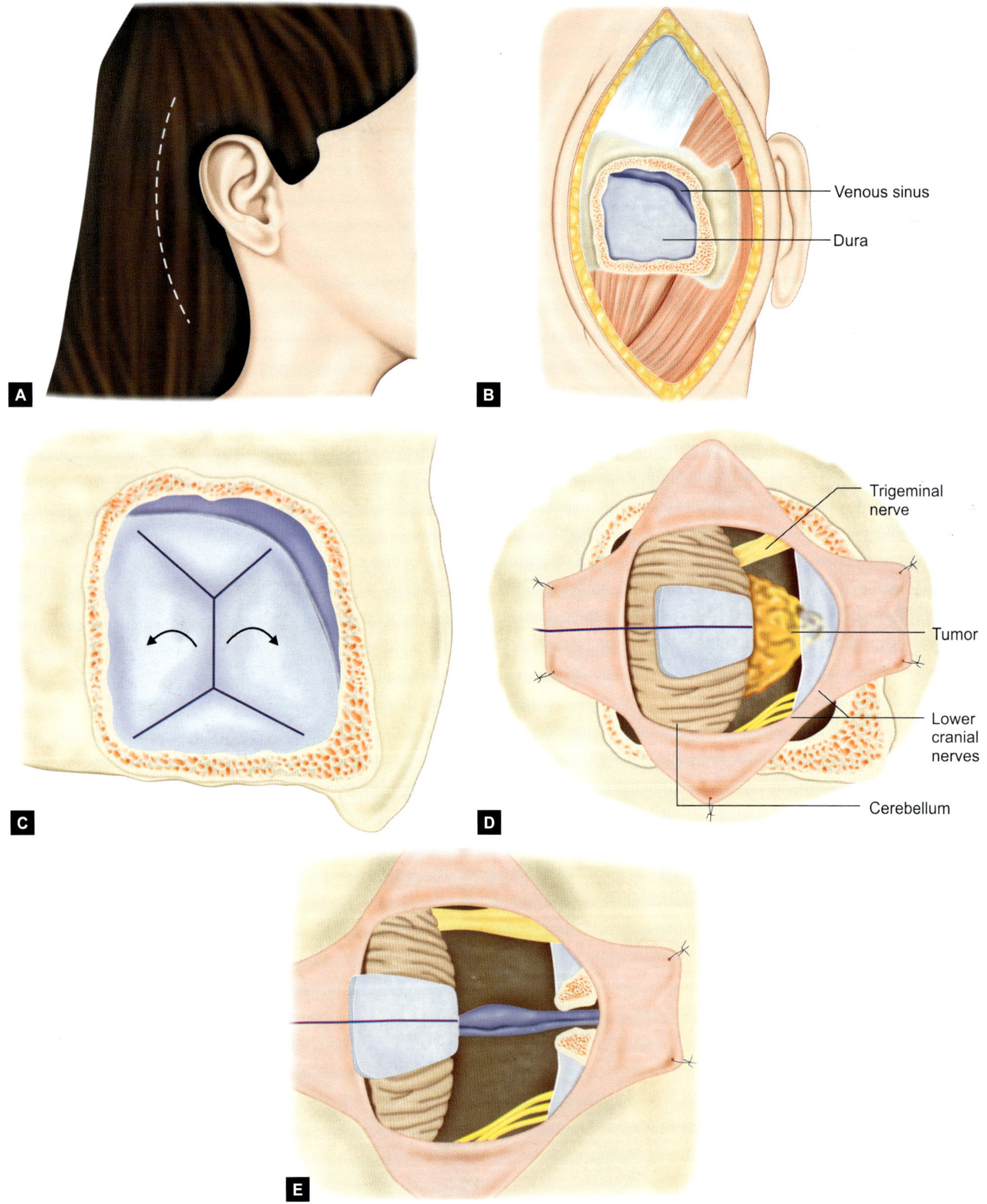

Figs 9A to E: (A) Curvilinear incision is made 3 cm behind postauricular sulcus; (B) Craniotomy is done by removing the bone behind the sigmoid sinus and below the transverse sinus; (C) Dura is incised; (D) Intracranial part of tumor is dissected off the facial and audiovestibular nerve; (E) Removal of tumor from medial to lateral direction with preservation of facial nerve

Disadvantages

- Cerebellar retraction
- Risk of tumor to be left at the fundus
- Facial nerve graft is difficult
- Persisting headache because of bone defect.

Key Points of Surgery

- Microsurgical resection provides complete tumor removal in 95% of patients with low mortality
- Small fragments of tumor if left on the nerve, rarely may lead to recurrence
- Tumor 1cm or less in size underwent middle fossa removal or translabyrinthine approach provides good facial nerve function
- Hearing preservation is not routinely achieved. Translabyrinthine approach for smaller tumours results in residual hearing loss. For middle fossa approach and retrosigmoid approach hearing preservation rates are 16.5% to 65% and 36% to 71%, respectively[6]
- Injury to lower cranial nerves may cause increased morbidity. With large tumor glossopharyngeal, vagus and accessory nerves are at risk
- Surgery should be carried out in a well-equipped center with dedicated team work.

Gamma Knife Stereotactic Radiosurgery

It is a technique that uses single fraction high dose of ionizing radiation to an image defined target. Generally, MRI is used to define the target of pathological structures. The aim is to minimize radiation effect on the surrounding neural tissue and to deliver an optimum radiation to target tissue.

In radiosurgery, a single high dose of ionizing radiation is delivered whereas in conventional radiotherapy fractionated course of multiple low dose radiation is applied.

It is found that 20 Gy dose of radiation as a single-radiosurgical technique is equivalent to 50–110 Gy of radiation in 2Gy fractions.[7]

Targets less than 3 cm in maximal diameter are suitable for radiosurgery.

It is indicated in—

- Patients unwilling for surgery
- Tumor less than 3 cm
- Residual tumor following surgery.

It is reported that gamma knife stereotactic radiosurgery provides[8]—

- Tumor controlled rates of 82% to 98%
- Facial paresis rate ranging from 2% to 53%
- Rate of hearing preservation varying as widely as 20% to 97%.

CONSERVATIVE MANAGEMENT

As the AN is a slow growing tumor in elderly or surgically unfit patients may be kept under wait and watch policy.

REFERENCES

1. Fayad JN, Brackmann DE. Acoustic Neuroma- comprehensive textbook of otology –diagnosis, management and operative techniques. Editors MV Kirtane, et al. Mumbai: Bhalani Publishing House, India; 2010. p.440.
2. Kanzaki J, Tos M, Sanna M, Moffat DA. New and modified reporting systems from the consensus meeting on system for reporting result in vestibular schwannoma. Otology and Neurotology. 2003;24:642-8.
3. Hitseberger WE, House WF. A warning regarding the sitting posting for acoustic tumor surgery (editorial). Arch Otolaryngol. 1980;106(2):69.
4. Richard T. Ramsden. Acoustic Tumors, Scott- Brown's Otolaryngology, 5th edition. Otology. 1987;516-8.
5. Bansal M. Diseases of Ear, Nose and throat. Head neck surgery, 1st edition. 2013. page 276.
6. www.earsite.com/acoustic –neuroma-treatment.
7. Slattery WH III, Brackman DE. Middle forsa approach for hearing preservation and with acoustic neuroma. Neuro Surgery. 1997;7:169-82.
8. Larson DA, Flickinger JC, Loeffier JS. International Journal of Radiation Oncology, Biology, Physics. 1993;25:557-61.

Chapter 13

Vertigo–Approach and Management

Asok K Saha

The term vertigo comes from Latin word 'vertere' meaning 'a sense of turning'.[1] In general, it is the subjective illusion of motion, usually rotational motion. The word dizziness includes a broad range of sensation from severe vertigo to momentary light-headedness. Light-headedness is a presyncopal dizziness rather than vestibular in origin (nonvestibular form of dizziness).

INCIDENCE OF DISEASE

About 30–35% of the population experiences episodes of vertigo by the age of 65 years. It is a common complaint in clinical practice and is seen in about 10–50% of patients attending ENT out patient department. Exact diagnosis of the condition therefore remains a challenge for the family physician as well as among the neuro-otology consultants as good management of the condition depends upon an accurate diagnosis.

TYPES OF VERTIGO

Basically, vertigo is described as rotatory (sense of spinning) or nonrotatory (sense of unsteadiness) type which is subdivided into episodic or prolonged. When it is episodic, it may be short-lasting (less than 1 minute) or long-lasting (hours or days)[1].

Rotatory

- Episodic—seconds or hours
- Prolonged—weeks.

Nonrotatory or Unsteadiness

- Episodic—seconds or hours to days
- Prolonged—weeks to month.

DIFFERENTIAL DIAGNOSIS FOR VERTIGO

Various diseases and conditions may result in sense of vertigo or imbalance if there is—

- Mismatch between the information obtained from afferents—vestibule, eyes or proprioception or mismatch between both vestibules
- CNS (brain stem and cerebral cortex) fails to integrate the afferent information
- Cerebellum fails to generate the motor output
- Defect in motor output system, i.e. in the nerves and muscles of eyes/limbs/trunk/neck.

Peripheral vestibular disorders that may cause vertigo are:

- Benign paroxysmal positional vertigo (BPPV)
- Meniere's disease
- Vestibular neuronitis
- Labyrinthitis
- Vestibulotoxic drugs
- Perilymph fistula
- Syphilis
- Acoustic neuroma.

Central vestibular disorders that cause vertigo are:

- Vertebrobasilar insufficiency (VBI)
- Basilar migraine
- Cerebellar disease
- Multiple sclerosis
- Tumors of brain stem
- Epilepsy
- Cervical vertigo.

APPROACH TO A DIZZY PATIENT

Initial approach to evaluate the dizzy patient is—

- To consider the categories of dizziness in the differential diagnosis

- To determine whether the dizziness is vestibular or nonvestibular in origin.

If vestibular in origin it may be—

- Peripheral—one ear involved or both ears involved
- Central—brainstem or brain[2]

Proper history is taken and a detailed clinical examination is followed by appropriate investigations to come to a correct diagnosis. Many patients may have associated symptoms such as hearing loss, tinnitus, vomiting or nausea. Periods of freedom from vertigo are important to be noted.

History of illness as emergent, acute and chronic helps to clinch the tentative underlying cause of vertigo. Acute vertigo that develops in CNS hemorrhages and infarcts needs immediate intervention. Trauma to inner ear or temporal bone and bacterial labyrinthitis require urgent treatment.

History Taking

It is important to establish the tentative causes of vertigo.

- History of vertigo associated with vomiting, tinnitus and deafness hints to Meniere's disease
- Vertigo only during change of head position indicates BPPV
- History of vertigo and deafness following cold, cough and fever suggests viral labyrinthitis
- Only vertigo without deafness following cold, cough and fever is suggestive of vestibular neuronitis.

Onset of Vertigo

Enquiry about the mode of onset of vertigo is important as it helps in establishing the diagnosis.[3]

- If there is acute onset of vertigo, the patient is asked whether it is first attack or recurrent attack
- If vertigo is recurrent, there is possibility of Meniere's disease, migraine or hypoglycemia
- Nonrecurrent vertigo is suggestive of vestibular neuronitis, drug-induced vertigo or labyrinthitis following ear discharge
- Chronic vertigo indicates brain tumor, diabetes, hypertension, or head injury.

Spell Duration

Hints of causes of dizziness are based on spell duration.
Seconds—BPPV, labyrinthine fistula, cervical vertigo, VBI
Minutes—Transient ischemic attack
Hours—Meniere's disease
Days—Viral labyrinthitis
Variable—Migraine.

Presence of Triggers

Presence of triggers in patient with episodic vertigo is important for establishing diagnosis.[4]

- Dizziness related to head movements, e.g. looking up, lying down or turning over in bed is suggestive of BPPV
- Dizziness triggering by neck movement indicates cervical or vestibulobasilar disorder
- Symptom triggered by loud sounds or Valsalva maneuver suggests Tullio phenomenon due to superior canal dehiscence or labyrinthine fistula
- Dizziness on standing up suddenly hints orthostatic hypotension
- Exercise, alcohol or stress can trigger dizziness in patients with episodic ataxias
- Food like chocolate, cheese or sleep deprivation may trigger migraine associated vertigo.

History taking includes:

- Past history of head injury, operation and fever
- Personal history of blood pressure (high or low), diabetes, alcohol, tobacco, otorrhea, heart disease or arthritis.

Clinical Examination

General medical examination is done. It is followed by specific clinical examination of vestibular pathology that includes:

- Otological examination especially fistula test
- Vestibulo-occular examination
    - Eye movement
    - Spontaneous nystagmus
    - Positional nystagmus.
- Neuro-otological examination that includes—
    - Romberg test
    - Tandem walking with eye open and eye closed
    - Fukuda's stepping test
    - Positional nystagmus test by Dix-Hallpike maneuver to rule out BPPV.

Dix-Hallpike Maneuver (Figs 1A to C)

The patient is seated on the examination table and is advised to keep the eyes open throughout the maneuver so that the examiner can observe the nystagmus. First the patient's head is turned 45° to the right and then the patient is moved swiftly into the supine position with head hanging at the end of the table without rotating the neck. The examiner watches the patient's eye for at least 30 seconds to observe the nystagmus and assists the patient to return to the sitting position. The patient's head is held by the examiner throughout the maneuver. The test is then repeated with

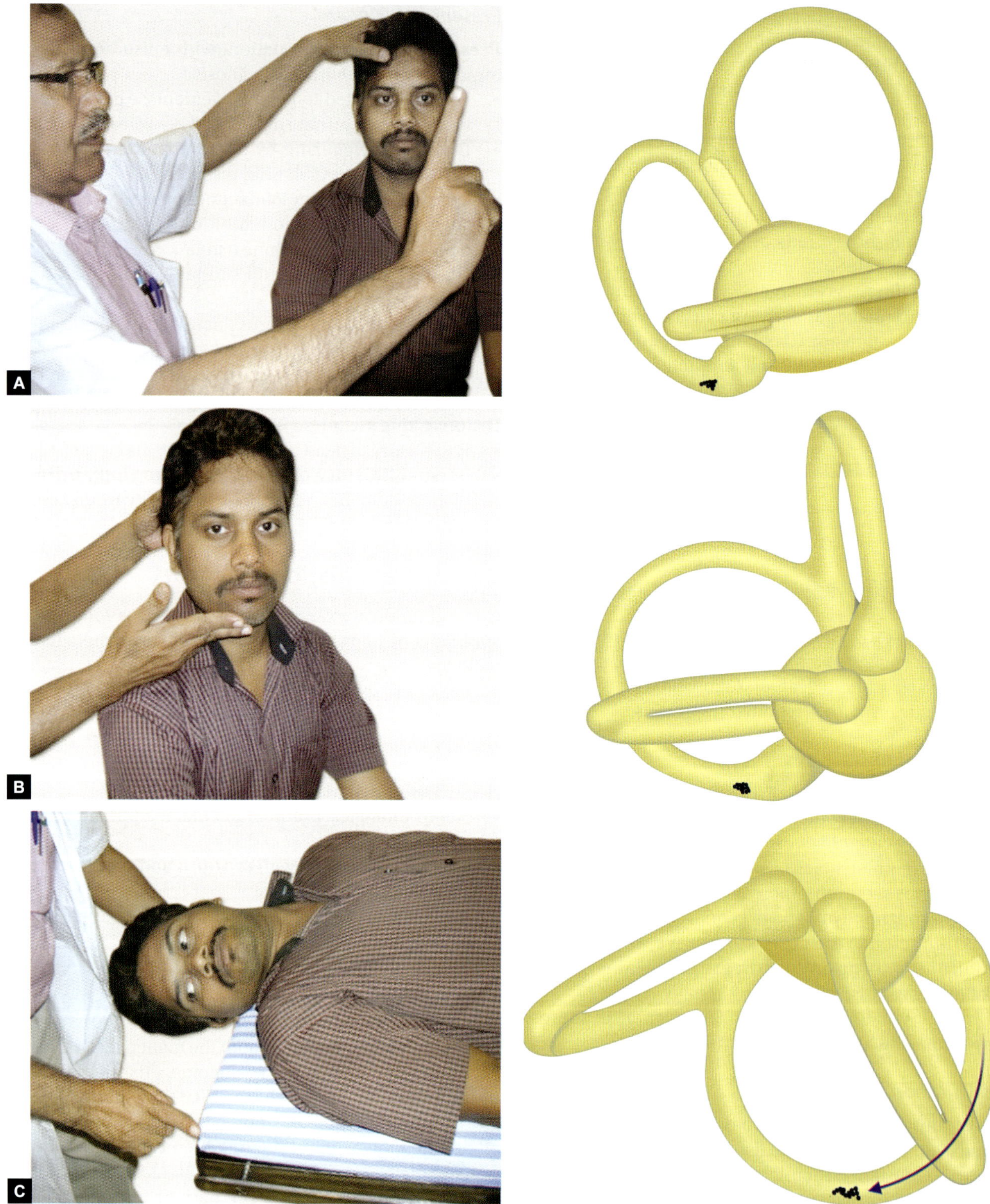

Figs 1A to C: Dix-Hallpike maneuver

patient's head turned 45° to the left. Normal individuals have a few beats of nystagmus during backward movements only but patients with BPPV have burst of intense rotational nystagmus and sense of vertigo that begin several seconds after head hanging position. Nystagmus beats toward the involved (under most) ear. The nystagmus has four characteristic features that are as follows:

- Delayed onset (latency)
- Transient nystagmus fades after less than one minute and reverses direction on sitting
- Fatigable or decreases in intensity on repeated maneuver
- Accompanied by vertigo.

The BPPV indicates malfunction of the posterior semicircular canal and Dix-Hallpike maneuver induces nystagmus which is characteristic of BPPV.

Pathophysiology of BPPV has been explained either by canalolithiasis (free-floating particles) by Hall, Ruby and McClure in 1979 or Cupulolithiasis (particulate debris attached to the cupula) by Schuknecht in 1969.

The term canalolithisis involves deposition of calcium carbonate crystals from degenerated otoliths from utricular macula that float freely in the endolymph of the semicircular canal, usually posterior semicircular canal which is the most gravity dependent canal and rarely the horizontal or superior canal. The free-floating debris is felt to be hyperdense relative to endolymph. Gravitational forces during the change of head position primarily in the plane of posterior semicircular canal (i.e. looking up, bending over, rolling over in the bed, etc.) cause the crystal to migrate inside the canal. This in turn induces a transitory endolymph drag with a consequent cupular deflection resulting in an attack of short-lived vertigo and nystagmus.

The term cupulolithiasis describes that the particulate debris usually attach to the cupula of the posterior semicircular canal rendering it sensitive to positional change. The persistence of nystagmus with positional change is more likely to reflect the phenomenon of the Cupulolithiasis from continued deflection of the cupula.[5]

Cupulolithiasis, however, cannot explain some of the features of the nystagmus including—

- As the cupular displacement happens instantaneously there should be no latency
- Cupular displacement persists as long as head position is maintained but the response disappears usually after 10–30 seconds that cannot be explained
- Fatigability of nystagmus on repeated testing remains unexplained.

In canalolithiasis, the canalith masses during Dix-Hallpike maneuver move along the posterior semicircular canal in upward direction due to inertia. After a short time, they move to more dependent position in the gravitational

Table 1: Findings on Dix-Hallpike maneuver

Cause	Peripheral	Central
Latency	40–60 seconds	None
Severity of vertigo	Severe	Mild
Duration of nystagmus	Less than 1 minute	Usually more than 1 minute
Fatigability	Yes	No
Habituation	Yes	No
Other findings ❑ Postural instability ❑ Hearing loss, tinnitus ❑ Other neurological deficit	Able to walk Unidirectional instability Can be present Absent	Fall while walking Severe instability Usually absent Usually present

plane that explains the latency of the nystagmus. Repeated maneuver results in a smaller and smaller mass effect that may cause decreased dispersion of the conglomerate particle within the endolymph that explains the fatigability of nystagmus. The nystagmus profiles correlate well with the known neuromuscular pathways that arise from the stimulation of the posterior canal ampullary nerves. The canalolithiasis can explain all the features of nystagmus and is the widely accepted theory at present.

Findings on Dix-Hallpike maneuver for differentiation between peripheral and central causes of vertigo are given in Table 1.

INVESTIGATION

Electronystagmography

Electronystagmography (ENG) is the recording of eye movements that allows precise quantification of both physical and pathological nystagmus. Six tests are usually included which are discussed below:[6]

1. Gaze test—Eye movements are recorded by altering the patient's gaze to the right or left or up or down. The central origin nystagmus changes its direction with different gaze positions. The peripheral origin nystagmus has fixed direction in all gaze positions. The tracing is inspected for presence of nystagmus under any of these conditions.
2. Tracking test—Eye movements are recorded while the patient follows a slowly moving a visual target. The tracing is inspected for defects of saccadic eye movements.
3. Saccade test—Eye movements are recorded as the patient looks back and forth between two pairs of horizontal dots placed on the wall and then back and forth between two pairs of vertical dots. The procedure is carried out

to calibrate the recording system. The tracing is also inspected for the defect of saccadic eye movements.

4. Optokinetic test—Eye movements are recorded while the patient watches vertical strips moving at different speeds to the right and to the left. The tracing is inspected for the presence of nystagmus. As the stimulus speed increases, stronger the nystagmus generates. It reveals vestibular asymmetry if nystagmus is stronger in one direction than in the other.

5. Positional test—Eye movements are recorded with patient's eye both open and closed after patient being placed in various position usually sitting, supine, right lateral, left lateral and head hanging. Tracing is inspected for nystagmus following each movement.

6. Caloric test (Fitzgerald and Hallpike maneuver)—Eye movements are recorded using alternate 250cc of hot (44°C) and cold (30°C) water to irrigate each ear for 40 seconds. The position of the patient is supine with head flexed 30° forward. Cold water produces nystagmus to opposite side and warm water to the same side (mnemonic cows→Cold—Opposite, Warm—Same).

Cranio-corpography

Cranio-corpography (CCG) is the photographic recording of patient's head and body movements. It provides the functional measurement of balance that reflexes vestibulospinal function.

Rotatory test (Barany's technique)—Patient is seated in Barany's revolving chair with his head tilted 30° forwards and then rotated for about 20 seconds (Fig. 2). The rotation is abruptly stopped. The nystagmus induced by sudden stop is 10–30 seconds in duration in normal subject that is fairly symmetrical in clockwise and counter clockwise rotation. Gross asymmetries in duration between the responses to clockwise and counter clockwise rotation are taken as a vestibular pathology.

In this test, actually the postrotatory nystagmus is assessed. Nowadays with advent of more precise devices like torsion swing chair for rotating and ENG for recording nystagmus, both prerotatory as well as postrotatory nystagmus are evaluated.

Audiometric Tests

These tests primarily provide information about auditory asymmetry, possible retrocochlear pathology and integrity of external auditory canal and tympanic membrane before caloric test. The tympanic membrane perforation or otitis externa may have contraindication for caloric irrigation of EAC. Audiometric test include[7]—
- Pure tone audiometry

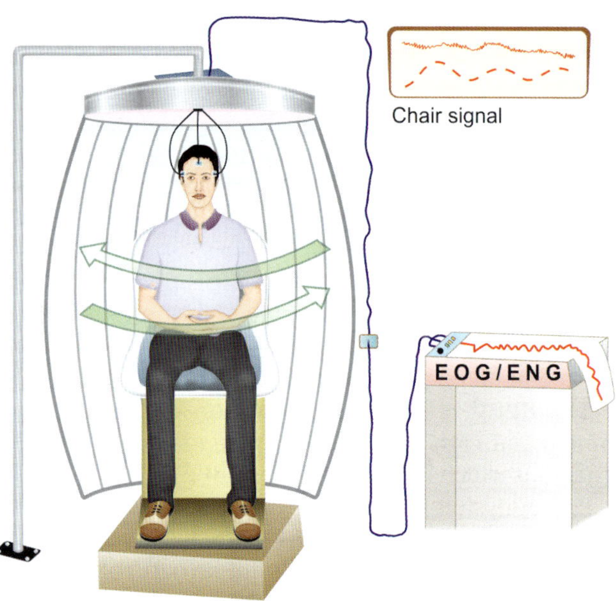

Fig. 2: Rotatory test (Barany's technique)

- Speech audiometry—Speech reception threshold (SRT) and Speech discrimination Score (SDS)
- Acoustic reflex threshold and decay tests
- Speech rollover test.

The difference in pure tone average (PTA) of 15 dB or greater or difference in SDS of 15% or greater between two ears indicates significant auditory asymmetry representing peripheral vestibular or auditory nerve pathology.

- Asymmetric auditory sensitivity is related to specific vestibular disease. Unilateral fluctuating low-frequency SNHL hints Meniere's disease, high-frequency SNHL is the characteristic of acoustic neuroma. Unilateral SNHL with no specific pattern indicates perilymph fistula and labyrinthitis
- Retrocochlear pathology involves lesion at CN-VIII, cerebello pontine angle or root entry of CN-VIII into brainstem. Audiometric findings characteristic of retrocochlear pathology are as follows:
  - Asymmetric high-frequency SNHL
  - Poor speech discrimination score inconsistent with pure tone thresholds
  - Rollover phenomenon—decreased SDS with increase in speech intensity
  - Absent or elevated acoustic reflex thresholds or abnormal acoustic reflex decay.

Brainstem-evoked Response Audiometry

Brainstem-evoked response audiometry (BERA)—an objective test of hearing used for testing the structural and functional integrity of auditory pathway from inner ear to mid-brain by plotting electrical activities in response to auditory or vestibular stimuli.

Vestibular-evoked Myogenic Potential

Vestibular-evoked myogenic potential (VEMP) informs the functional and structural integrity of the vestibulocollic reflex and assesses the function of saccule and inferior vestibular nerve. Vestibulocollic reflex like vestibulo-ocular and vestibulospinal reflexes has important role for balance system and cannot be evaluated by other test. The test records the amplitude of contraction of sternomastoid evoked by saccular stimulation on both sides and if the difference in amplitude between two sides is more than 30% then the side with lesser amplitude of contraction is considered hypofunctioning.

Transcranial Doppler Test

Transcranial Doppler (TCD) is done to assess the blood flow in the vertebral and basilar arteries as well as cerebral and carotid arteries to know the obstruction or stenosis of the vessels supplying different parts of the brain. This test helps to evaluate whether vertigo or imbalance is due to VBI.

Caloric Test (Kobrak Test)

The caloric test as devised by Kobrak who used 2–5 cc of ice cold water to instill into the ear of the patient in a sitting position with head-tilted 60° backwards to bring horizontal canal to vertical position. This initiates vertigo with labyrinthine types of nystagmus in normal subjects.

- If there is no response, 10–20 cc of ice cold water is instilled to initiate nystagmus beating towards the opposite ear indicating canal paresis or hypoactive labyrinth
- No nystagmus or vertigo after 40 cc of ice cold water indicates dead labyrinth.

Radiology

Radiology plays an important role to diagnose the causes of vertigo and dizziness. Multiple radiological tools are available for vestibular and temporal brain disorders which need prior consultation of radiologist for appropriate modality to be employed. Radiology includes—

- Conventional X-rays—These are X-ray mastoid lateral oblique view, X-ray skull AP/lateral and periorbital view, X-ray PNS—Water's view and X-ray cervical spine AP/lateral view
- Computed tomography (CT)
- Magnetic resonance imaging (MRI), MR angiography and digital subtraction angiography.

No imaging findings were available for diagnosis of labyrinthitis before MRI. Enhancement of labyrinth on post-contrast T1W1 helps to diagnose the labyrinthine disorder.

- In acute serous labyrinthitis, MRI finding is negative whereas acute suppurative labyrinthitis may be revealed by MRI with contrast. Precontrast MRI on T1W1 is essential to describe post-traumatic labyrinthitis. In hemorrhagic labyrinthitis low-signal intensity is replaced by high-intensity because of methemoglobin[8]
- Sclerosing labyrinthitis following bacterial meningitis is easily revealed by CT scan showing total 'white out' of membranous labyrinth. High resolution T2W1 shows loss of normal hyperintensity of fluid in membranous labyrinth.[9]

In otosclerosis, CT scan may demonstrate radiolucent focus located just anterior to the oval window, around the margin of oval and round window and sometimes around the basal turn of the cochlea (double ring sign), lateral wall of the internal auditory canal and the promontory. MRI in otosclerosis is less sensitive for these findings.

In Meniere's disease, no imaging technique is specific for the diagnosis. Recently, 3D fluid attenuated inversion recovery (3D–FLAIR). MRI following intratympanic injection of gadolinium DTPA (Gd- DTPA) may delineate the perilymphatic and endolymphatic spaces of inner ear. In Meniere's disease, perilymphatic space surrounding the endolymph is either small or cannot be seen.[10]

Superior semicircular canal dehiscence can be demonstrated by thin section (0.6 mm) multislice CT as a small defect in the bony wall of superior semicircular canal. T2W1 may reveal clear contact between inner ear and brain fluid.

CP angle masses and other pathologies in internal auditory canal may present with vertigo or dizziness. Most common pathologies are:

- Schwannoma
- Meningioma
- Epidermoid cyst or tumors.
  - Most of the vestibular Schwannomas have intracanalicular part. CT scan shows erosion and widening of internal acoustic meatus. MRI on T1W1 shows slightly hypointense to isointense compared to adjacent brain. MRI on T2W1 reveals heterogeneously hyperintense to adjacent brain parenchyma[11]
  - Meningioma accounts for about 20% of intracranial tumors arising from arachnoid cap cells of the meninges. Conventional X-ray skull shows enlarged meningeal artery grooves, hyperostosis or lytic lesion and calcification. CECT reveals homogeneous mass which is hyperdense to adjacent brain. MRI on T1W1 reveals hypo to isointense to brain parenchyma. MRI

on T2W1 shows hypo- to iso- to hyperintense to brain as postcontrast MRI shows intense homogeneous enhancement
- Epidermoid cysts on CT shows hypoattenuating or isoattenuating to CSF. Whereas MRI on T1W1 and T2W1 appear higher signal intensity with heterogeneous and marbled features.

CT and MRI are important tools for investigating vertigo, especially in children.

Hematological study includes—
- Routine blood test—Hb%, TLC, DLC, blood for sugar (fasting and postprandial), serum cholesterol, serum triglyceride
- Serological test for syphilis and HIV I and HIV II, HbsAg and anti-HCV
- Thyroid function test—T4, T3, TSH.

TREATMENT

Treatment involves 3Ps—
- Pharmacotherapy
- Physical exercise regimens
- Psychological intervention.

Pharmacotherapy of Vertigo

It may be symptomatic or specific. The symptomatic treatment suppresses acute symptoms and autonomic complaints where as specific treatment aims to target the underlying cause of vertigo, such as Meniere's disease, migraine and some central vestibular disorders.

Acute vertigo is usually treated by vestibular suppressants and antiemetics. Vestibular suppressants inhibit sensory input at the level of primary to secondary vestibular neurons and vestibular nuclei. In the vestibular nuclei, cholinergic and H_1 histaminergic receptors are the main receptor types and these drugs target receptors along with the GABA –energic system and noradrenergic system. The GABA-energic system inhibits signals from the cerebellar purkinje cells while noradrenergic system projecting from the brain stem to the vestibular nuclei inhibits vestibular activity.[12]

Drugs mostly used in the treatment of vertigo and its associated symptoms are:
- Anticholinergics—These drugs block the action of Acetylcholine (Ach) on autonomic effectors and in CNS exerted through muscarinic receptors. Main drug of this class is **hyoscine hydrobromide** used as 0.3–0.5 mg oral, intramuscular, transdermal patch and nasal spray. It is used for the treatment of vertigo and most effective in motion sickness. **Glycopyrrolate** used as 0.1–0.3 mg intramuscular, 1–2 mg oral is potent and rapidly acting antimuscarinic without central effect. It decreases the severity of vertigo and improves quality of life.

Anticholinergics have side effects like dry mouth, drowsiness, blurring of vision, constipation and urinary retention. They are contraindicated in glaucoma and prostrate hypertrophy. Anticholinergics selective for M_2 subtypes of muscarinic receptors in vestibular system have lesser side effects
- Antihistamines—They include:
  - Meclizine—25–50 mg oral dose TID
  - Dimenhydrinate—25–50 mg oral, intramuscular dose TID
  - Promethazine—1 mg/kg body weight.

These are H_1 receptor antagonists having anticholinergic activity with antivertigo action used in acute vertigo. **Promethazine** has dopaminergic antagonist action also. These antihistamines have side effects of anticholinergic activity along with sedation and drowsiness. Newer nonsedative antihistamines have no role in the treatment of vertigo and motion sickness as they do not enter the central nervous system.

Betahistine is an H_1-receptor agonist and H_3- receptor antagonist. H_1 agonism causes vasodilatation while H_3 antagonism results in increased secretion of histaminergic neurotransmitters to improve neural electrical activity in the vestibular nuclei.[13]

It is evident from study that betahistine decreases the frequency and intensity of vertigo in patient with BPPV but its effect on Meniere's disease has insufficient evidence.[14,15] The dose of betahistine is—8 mg TID for mild vertigo, 16 mg TID or 24 mg BID for moderate to severe vertigo.

Contraindications of betahistine are bronchial asthma, peptic ulcer, pheochromocytoma and concurrent use of antihistamine
- Dopaminergic antagonists—**Prochlorperazine** and **chlorpromazine** are dopamine antagonists with antimuscarinic effects that relieve the patient in controlling nausea and vomiting. Its role in the treatment of vertigo is obscure.[16] They act at the chemoreceptor trigger zone and reduce the neural impulse to the vomiting center. They provide symptomatic relief from vomiting and vertigo, reduce anxiety and morbidity and are effective in managing an acute unilateral vestibular disorder. Prochlorperazine is used as oral doses of 5 mg TID for about 7 days.

Side effects are sedation, extrapyramidal symptoms (EPS), blurred vision and urinary retention. EPS are very rare and practically never occur at the oral doses. It has also injectable form (12.5 mg/mL). It is evident that buccal administration causes less drowsiness and sedation than oral intake.[17]

Metoclopramide is a dopamine antagonist as well as serotonine antagonist. It has gastric emptying effect and centrally acting antiemetic effect. Newer antiemetics are serotonine-5 HT3 receptor antagonists like ondansetron, tropisetron and granisetron. They are used by patients suffering with nausea and vomiting but seldom in vertigo management

- Monoaminergic drugs—These drugs include amphetamines and ephedrine. They are used to potentiate the effect of scopolamine or where single drug therapy is inadequate[18]
- Calcium channel blockers—These are effective in treating vertigo of central and peripheral origin.
  Cinnarizine, a piperazine derivative has antihistaminic and calcium channel blocking action used as vestibular suppressant. It preserves the RBC flexibility by preventing calcium entry into the RBCs and results in improving microcirculation in the brain and inner ear.[19] It also inhibits calcium-induced contraction of vascular smooth muscle resulting in extrinsic anti-vasoconstrictor activity and does not affect calcium dependent tone due to intrinsic myogenic activity.[19,20.] Cinnarizine is effective in vertigo due to vertebrobasilar insufficiency and its combination with dimenhydrinate reduces intensity of vertigo and accompanying symptoms two times more than betahistine. It is used as 20 mg TID or 75 mg OD and side effect is mild sedation. Nimodipine, another calcium channel blocker is seen to be effective in Meniere's disease and is used in treating peripheral vertigo[21]
- Benzodiazepines act as vestibular suppressant through GABA (Gamma–amino–butyric acid)-ergic system and are effective in small doses in managing vertigo. GABA is an inhibitory neurotransmitter in vestibular system and CNS. Benzodiazepines enhance its action and alleviate vertigo and vertigo-associated anxiety and panic disorder. **Lorazepam** is usually used and is effective in vertigo because it has no active metabolites. Side effect like habituation can be avoided in using the dose of 0.5 mg BID or less. For an acute attack of vertigo in Meniere's disease lorazepam is taken sublingually (1 mg). **Diazepam** in low doses 2 mg BID is also effective. **Alprazolam** has restricted use because of potential withdrawal syndrome[22]
- Other drugs—
  - Extracts of ginkobiloba reduce blood viscosity and improve microcirculation in CNS and accelerate central compensation of vertigo[23]
  - Piracetam, a cyclic derivative of GABA is a nootropic agent protecting brain from physical and clinical damage and is used in patients with chronic or recurrent vertigo[24]
  - Trimetazidine, an antianginal drug used in myocardial ischemia is also effective in vertigo management in Meniere's disease in the dose of 20 mg TID for 2–3 months[25]
  - Antiepileptics like phenytoin, gabapentine, carbamazepine and oxcarbazepine are used in the treatment of vertigo. Phenytoin is effective in motion sickness. Gabapentine suppresses nystagmus by enhancing GABA action[26]
  - Antiviral and broad spectrum antibiotics are used in viral or bacterial labyrinthitis
  - Anticoagulants like heparin and warfarin are used in vertigo of thrombotic nature
  - Intratympanic gentamicin is given in advanced Meniere's disease when hearing is lost but vertigo is persistent. It is used for chemical labyrinthectomy and is given in weekly or biweekly or single dose in middle ear. The drug is absorbed through round window and causes destruction of the vestibular labyrinth. 0.5 mL gentamicin is injected with a drug concentration of 80 mg/mL. The total use of gentamicin is less or equal to 80 mg. Total control of vertigo spells is seen in 60–80% of patient. Hearing loss is reported in 4–30% of patients.

Physical Exercise Regimens

Vertigo results from disorders causing asymmetry of electrical discharge of two vestibular labyrinths which is sensed by the CNS. Spontaneous symptomatic recovery from vertigo occurs in most patients due to a complex natural process called vestibular compensation. Symmetry of electrical discharge is achieved either by increasing the electrical discharge from damaged vestibular labyrinth which is not possible or by decreasing electrical discharge from the normal vestibular labyrinth which is possible and effected by CNS through cerebellum. Physical exercise regimen provides habituation and adaptive response of sensory substitution of vestibular system by restructuring of the central vestibular pathways in such a way that the vestibular nuclei of one side in which the vestibular labyrinth is damaged, now gets connected anatomically and functionally to the vestibular nuclei of normal healthy side. Thereby, the system may come under direct control of the vestibular labyrinth of the healthy side.

Vestibular rehabilitation therapy (VRT), therefore, refers to a structural program of treatment aiming at accelerating and enhancing vestibular compensation and rendering dizzy patients asymptomatic such that they return to full occupational and social activity. VRT is very effective in managing patient with chronic vertigo or dizziness related to labyrinth.

VRT Includes

Systemic exercise program as devised by Sir Terence Cawthorne, an otologist (1944) and FS Cooksey, a physiotherapist (1946) comprises a series of exercises for the unilateral vestibular dysfunction which is known as Cawthorne-Cooksey exercises.

Exercises are carried out in following stages:[27]

Stage 1: Eye exercises in bed or sitting—
Active eye movements are practiced by looking up and then down, looking alternately left and right and convergence exercises (Figs 3A to E).
These are the adaptation exercises that help the patient with peripheral vestibular disorders.

Stage 2: Head and neck exercises till in bed or sitting—
Active head and neck movements are carried out by bending forward and backward and then turning alternately to left and the right, at first slow then quick (Figs 4A and B).
These are the habituation exercises to help by conditioning brain through repeated exposure of balance system to mismatched sensory input.

Stage 3: Head, neck and body exercises in sitting position—
Movements of shoulder shrugging and rotating, bending forward and picking up an object from the ground, turning head and trunk alternately to the left and the right are practised (Figs 5A to D).

Stage 4: Exercises in standing position—
Exercises that are practiced in turn are—
- Changing from sitting to standing without support, initially with eye open and then closed (Fig. 6)
- Throwing a ball in an arc from hand to hand and following it with the eyes (Fig. 7)
- These are gaze stabilization exercises retaining the VOR to stabilize images in fovea.

Stage 5: Exercises while walking—These exercises include—
- Walking across the room with eyes open and then closed (Fig. 8)
- Throwing and catching a ball while walking (Fig. 9)
- Walking up and down staircase with eye open and then closed (Fig. 10)
- Playing any game involving stooping, stretching and aiming with the ball, such as basketball playing (Fig. 11).

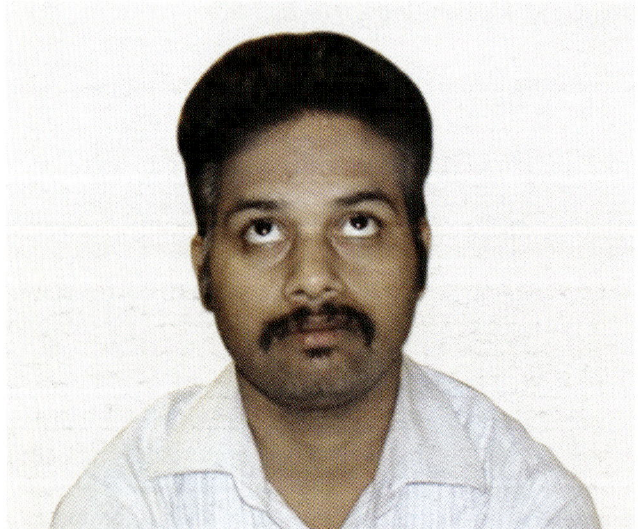

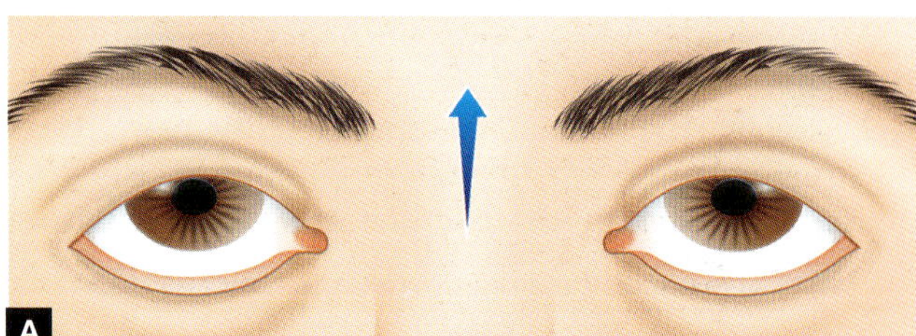

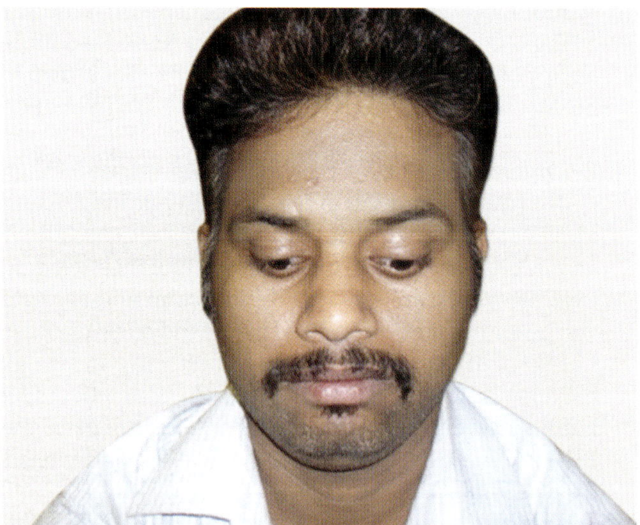

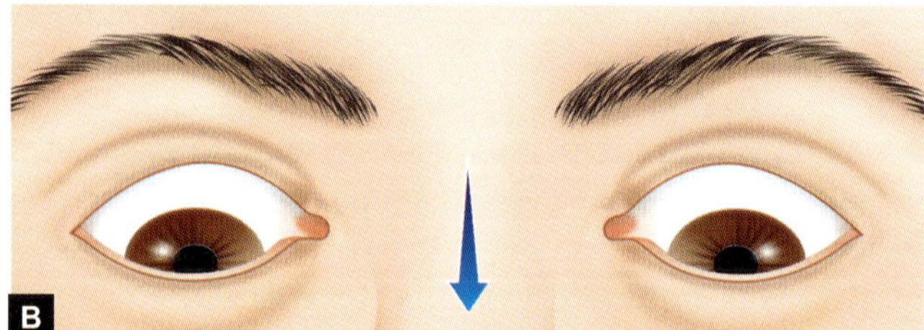

Figs 3A to E: Contd...

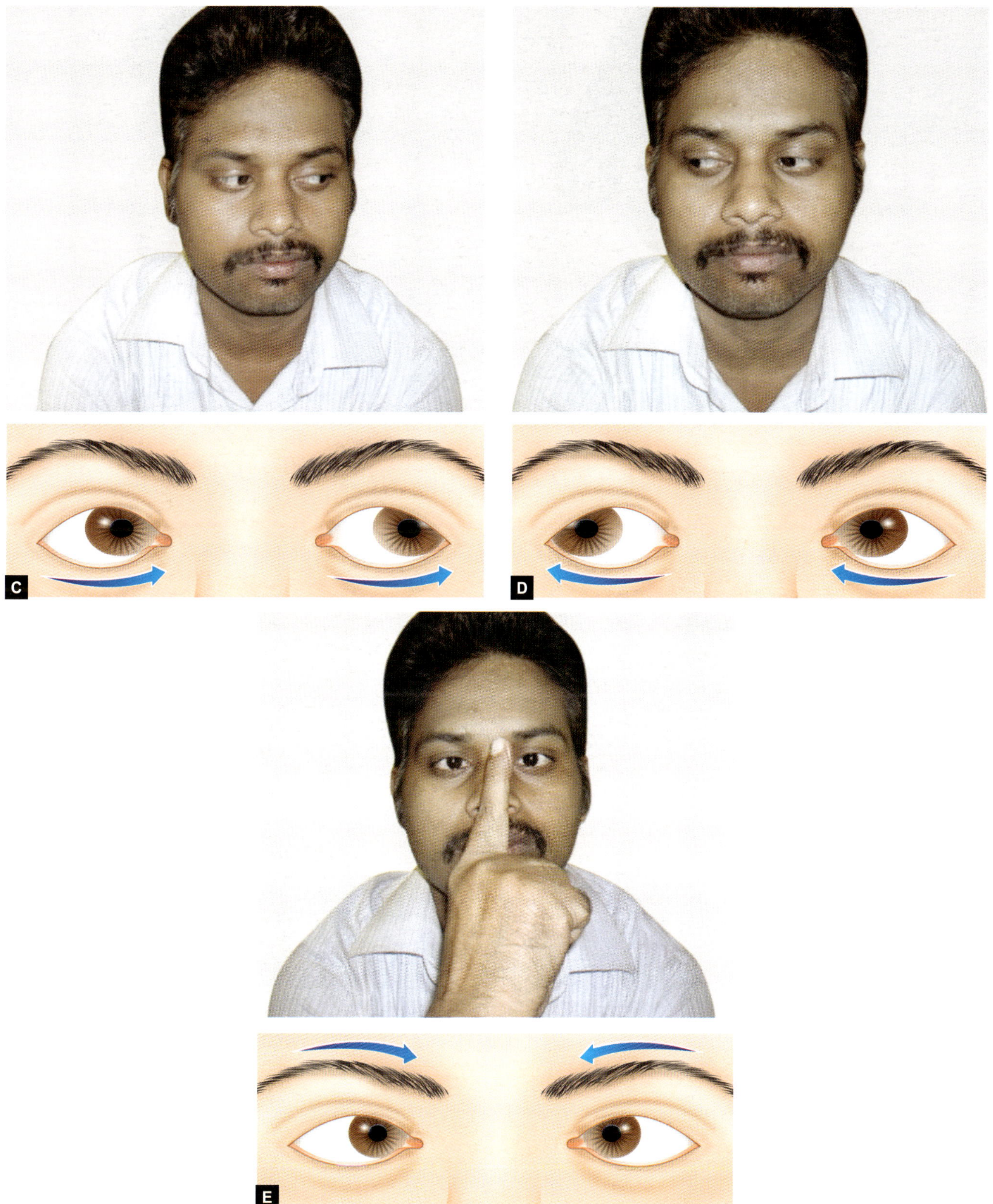

Figs 3A to E: Exercises for unilateral vestibular dysfunction—(A) Looking up; (B) Looking down; (C and D) Looking alternately left and right; (E) Convergence exercise

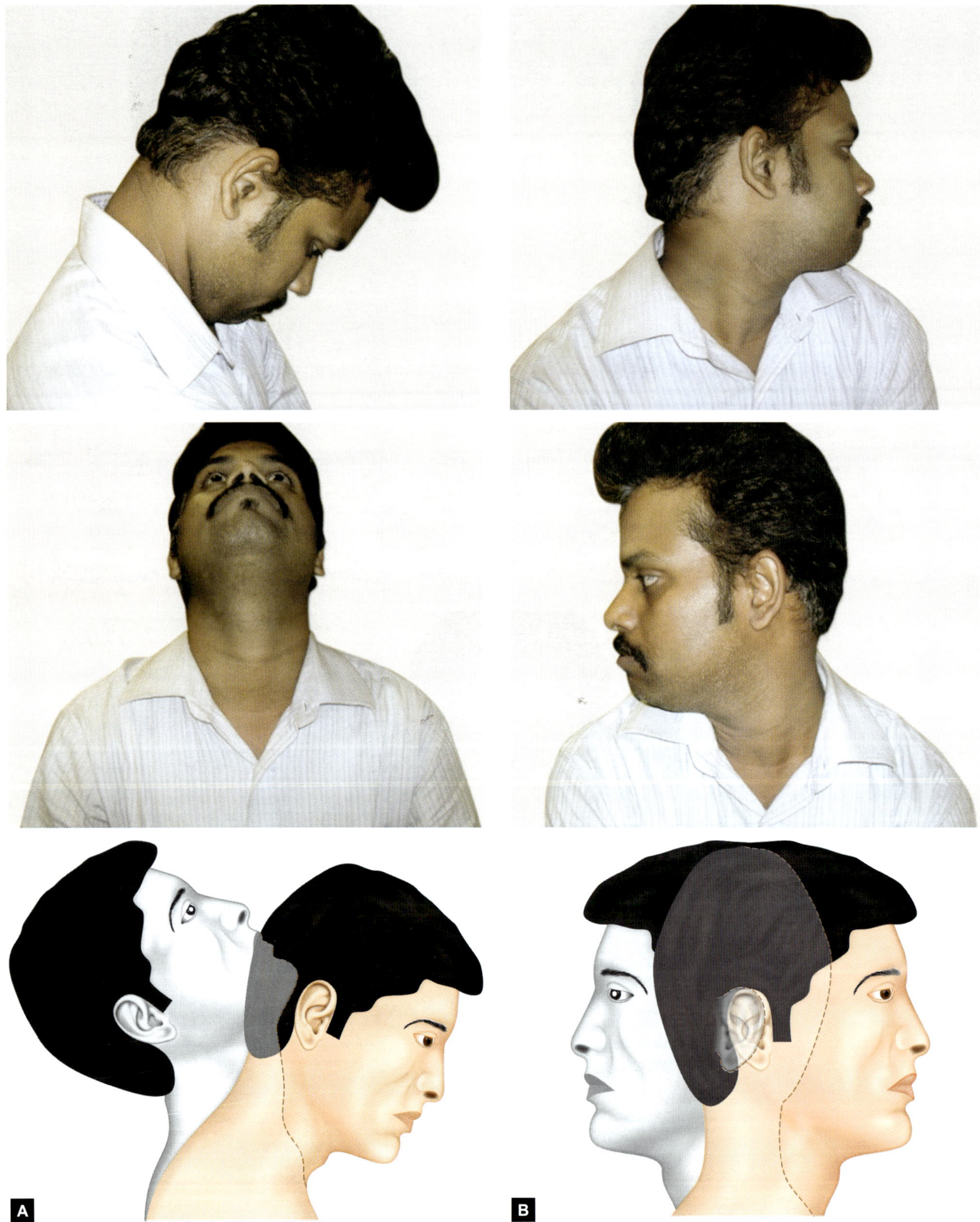

Figs 4A and B: Head and neck exercises—(A) Bending alternately forward and backward and, (B) then turning alternately to left and right

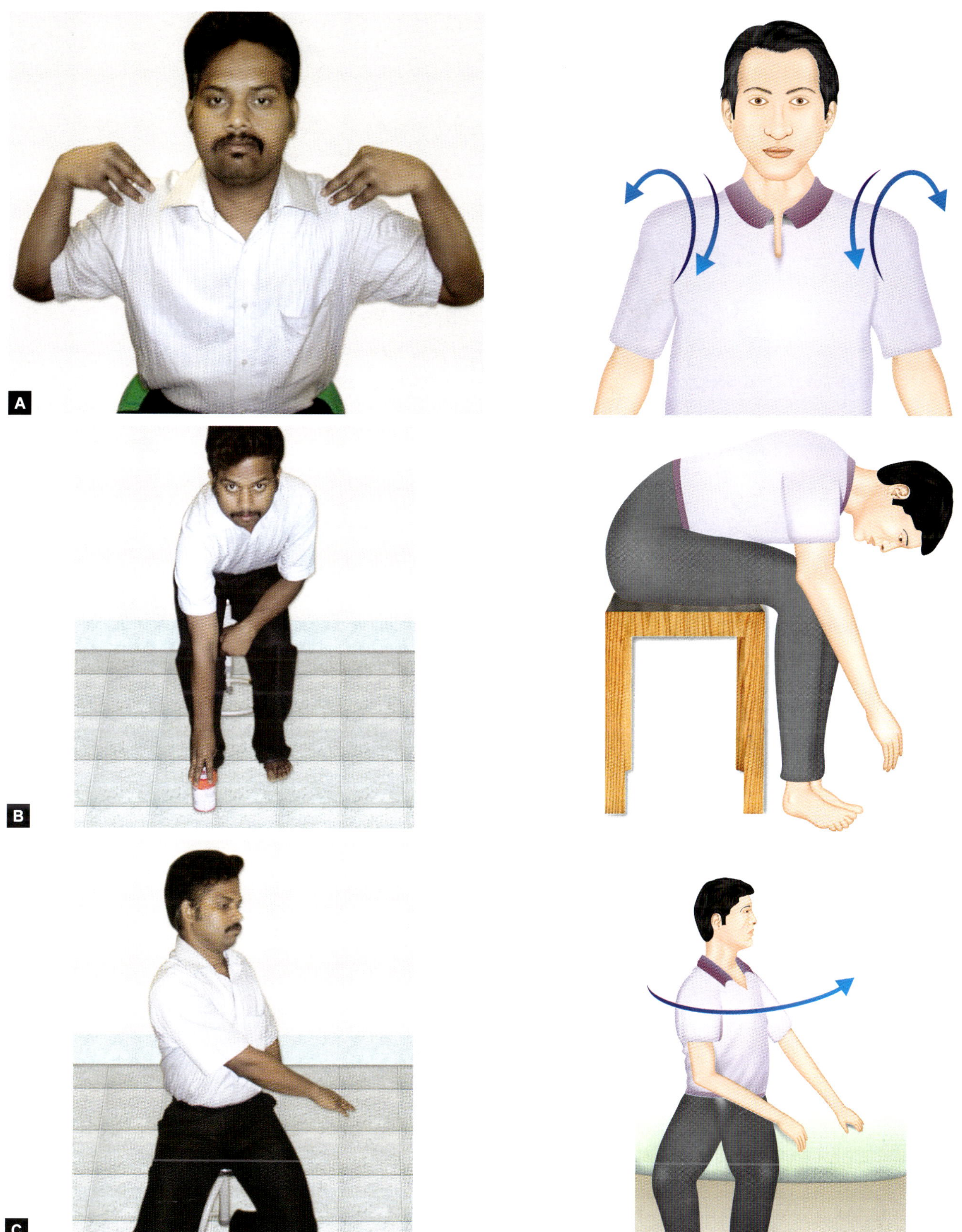

Figs 5A to D: Contd..

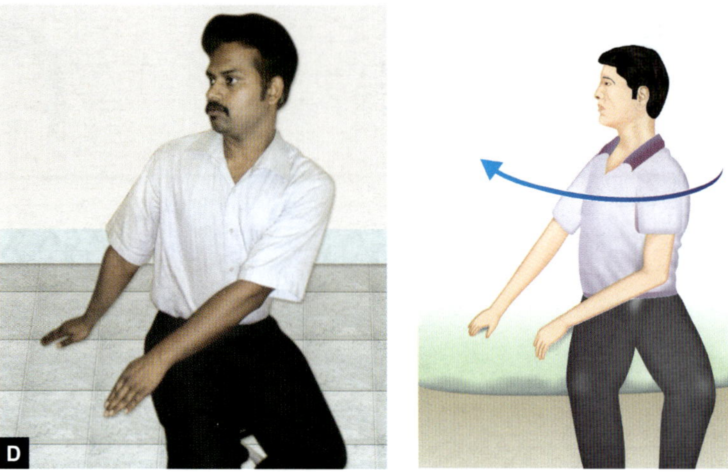

Figs 5A to D: Head, neck and body exercises in sitting position—(A) Shoulder shrugging and rotating; (B) Bending forward and picking up object from the ground; (C) Turning head and trunk to the left; (D) Turning head and trunk to the right

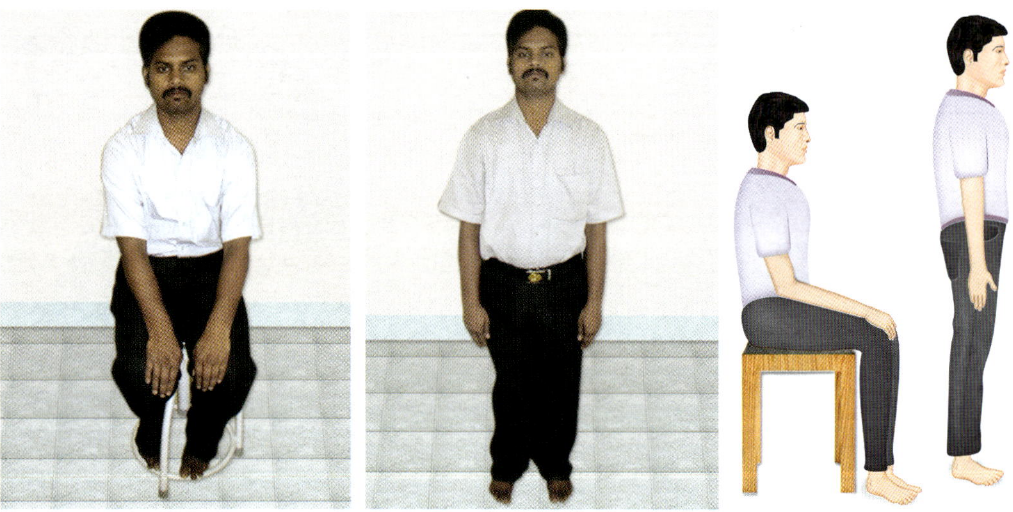

Fig. 6: Changing from sitting to standing, initially with eye open and then closed

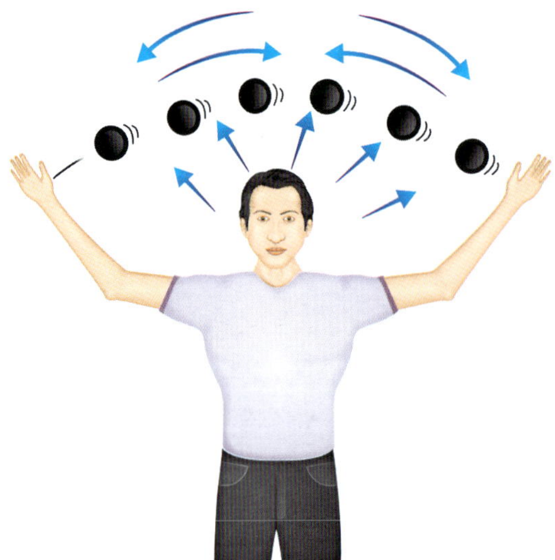

Fig. 7: Throwing a ball in an arc from hand to hand and following it with the eyes

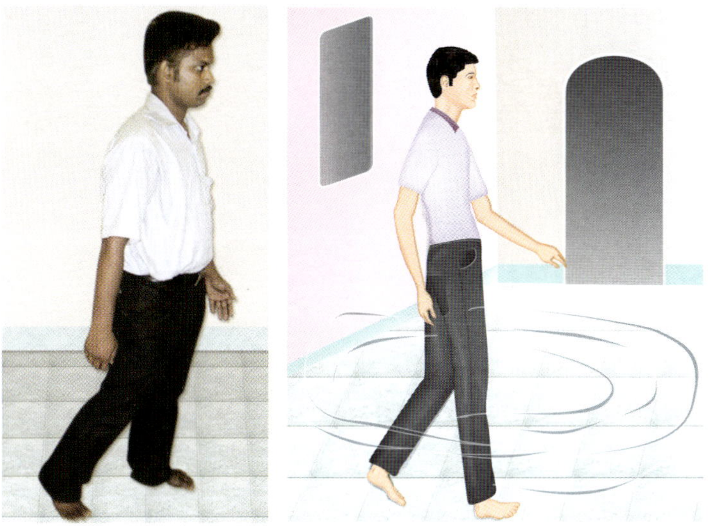

Fig. 8: Walking across the room with eyes open and then closed

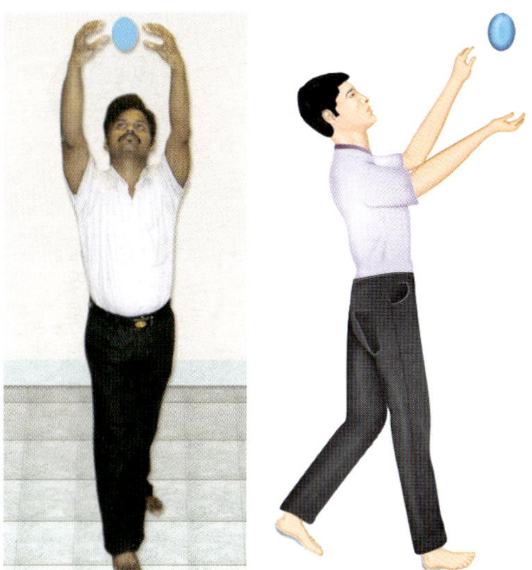

Fig. 9: Throwing and catching a ball while walking

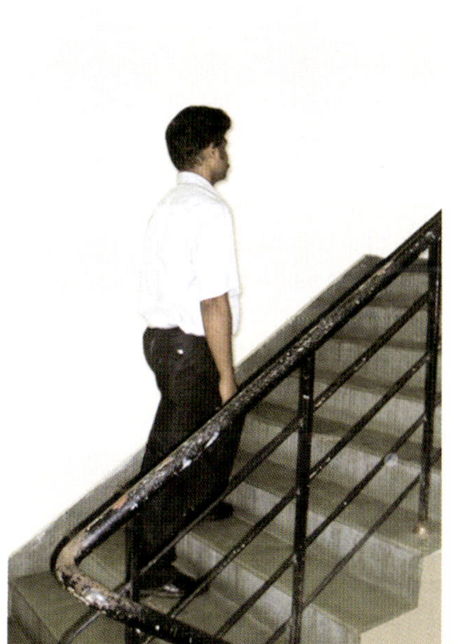

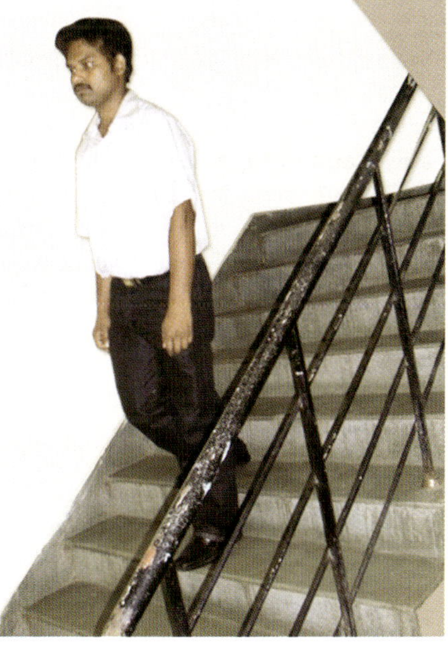

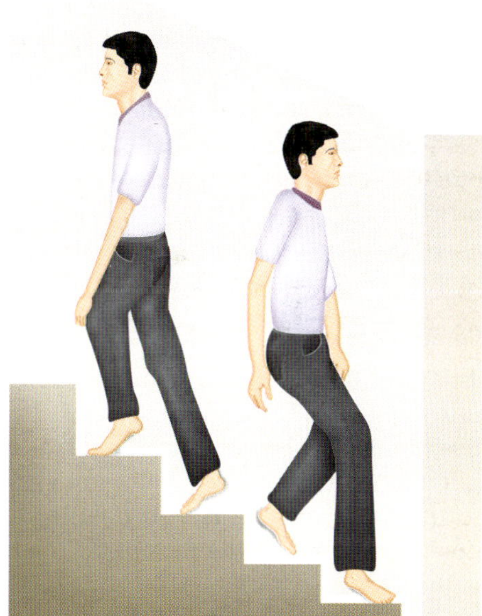

Fig. 10: Walking up and down the staircase with eyes open and then closed

These are the compensation exercises to enhance the visual and proprioceptive inputs to compensate for defective vestibular input.

As these exercises induce vertigo more frequently, brain builds up tolerance mechanism to compensate vertigo more quickly. These exercises should be practiced persistently for 5 minutes, 3 times daily till vertigo persists.

Specific Therapies

Specific therapies are advocated in the treatment of BPPV. These are as follows:

Epley's Maneuver (Canalolith Repositioning Method) (Fig. 12)

This is the office treatment of BPPV.

- The patient is made to sit on the table and brought down with the head turned at 45° to the affected side

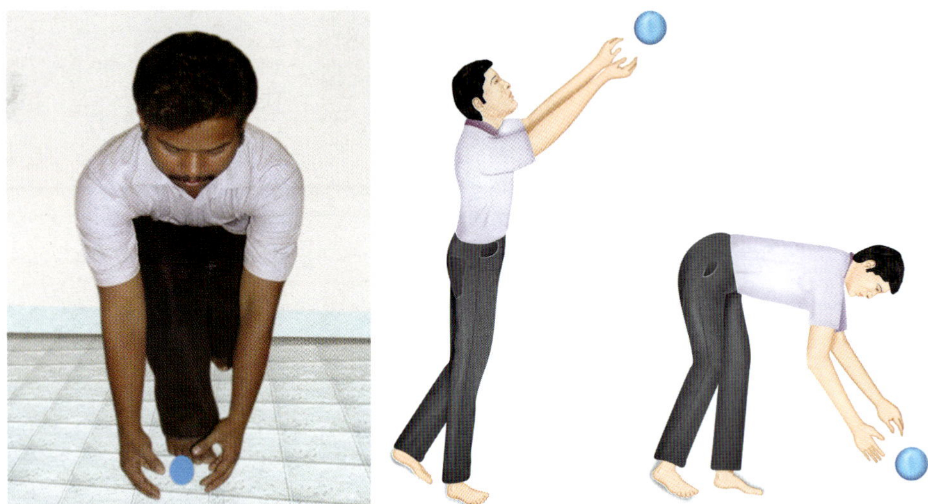

Fig. 11: Playing game involving bending, stretching and aiming with ball

- The head is then turned 90° to the opposite side
- This is followed by rotating the head and body through 90° facing downwards and the patient is brought to the sitting position with the head turned 45° to the unaffected side
- It finishes with the patient in the sitting position, head is turned forward and chin is made down 20°.

The principal of this maneuver involves relocation of otoconia from posterior semicircular canal back into the utricle.

It is evident from the review of literatures that the Epley's maneuver provides good results in the treatment of BPPV.[28]

Semont's Maneuver (Fig. 13)

This is also the office treatment of BPPV. The patient is moved quickly from sitting position to ipsilateral lateral position with the face turned upwards by 45°. After 1–1.5 minutes patient is moved 180° through the sitting position to the contralateral lateral position with face turned downwards by 45°. The patient is then brought slowly up to the sitting position.

A single session of 10–15 minutes is usually needed.

Post-treatment instructions for the patient after office treatment are important.

Patient are advised to sleep in sitting position for 2 nights and then on normal side for next 5 nights to avoid provoking head position that may again induce BPPV.

Semont's maneuver has also been shown to have good results.[29]

Brandt-Daroff Exercises (Fig. 14)

Brandt-Daroff exercises are made for home treatment of BPPV. These exercises start from the sitting position and then the patient is made to lie on the affected side with nose 45° up and remains in this position for at least 45 seconds. The patient then sits up for 30 seconds and then repeats the maneuver in opposite side.

Patients are advised to carry out the Brandt-Daroff exercises 3 times a day for 3 weeks. Follow-up visits are arranged at 2 weeks, 1 month and 3 months. End point is selected as relief of symptoms at 2 weeks with no recurrence of symptoms at 3 months. The results of the Brandt-Daroff exercises are not so encouraging that is evidenced from studies showing about 44% experienced recurrence of symptom after performance of the exercises.[30]

Psychological Intervention

Psychological factors like anxiety state, panic attacks, avoidance behavior and depression enhance the symptoms of the vestibular disorders as well as delay the compensation of vestibular function that cannot be ignored. As in panic attack autonomic symptoms and vertigo are common same as in vestibular disorder anxiety and autonomic symptoms are common. Therefore, there is close interaction between psychological factors and vestibular symptoms resulting in vertigo.

Flowchart 1 shows the interaction of autonomic, psychological and vestibular symptoms.

Again vestibular rehabilitation exercises are not properly carried out in presence of psychological disorders like avoidance behavior and panic attack which need psychiatric consultation and appropriate management of both cognitive and physical symptoms in tandem.

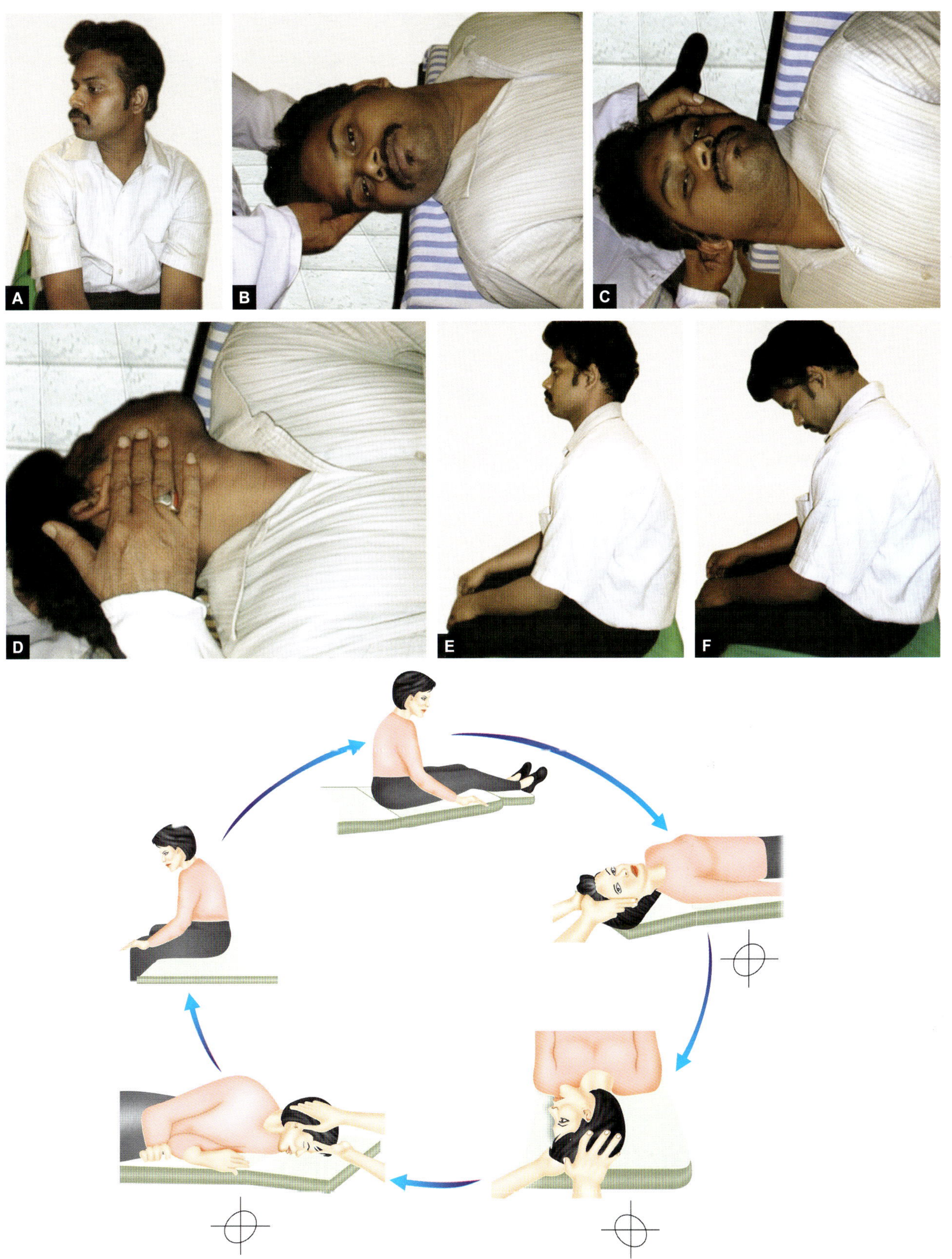

Figs 12A to F: Epley's maneuver

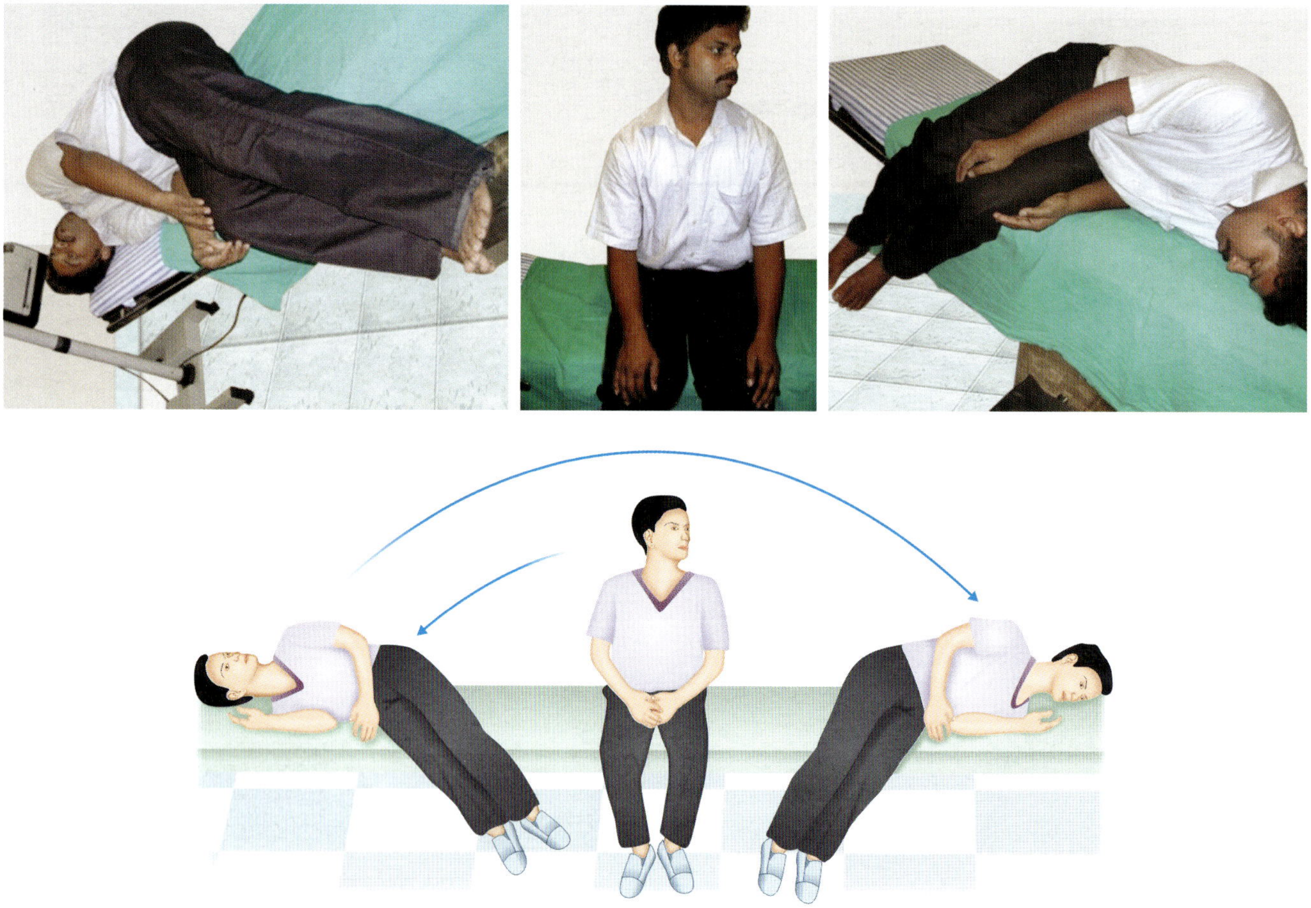

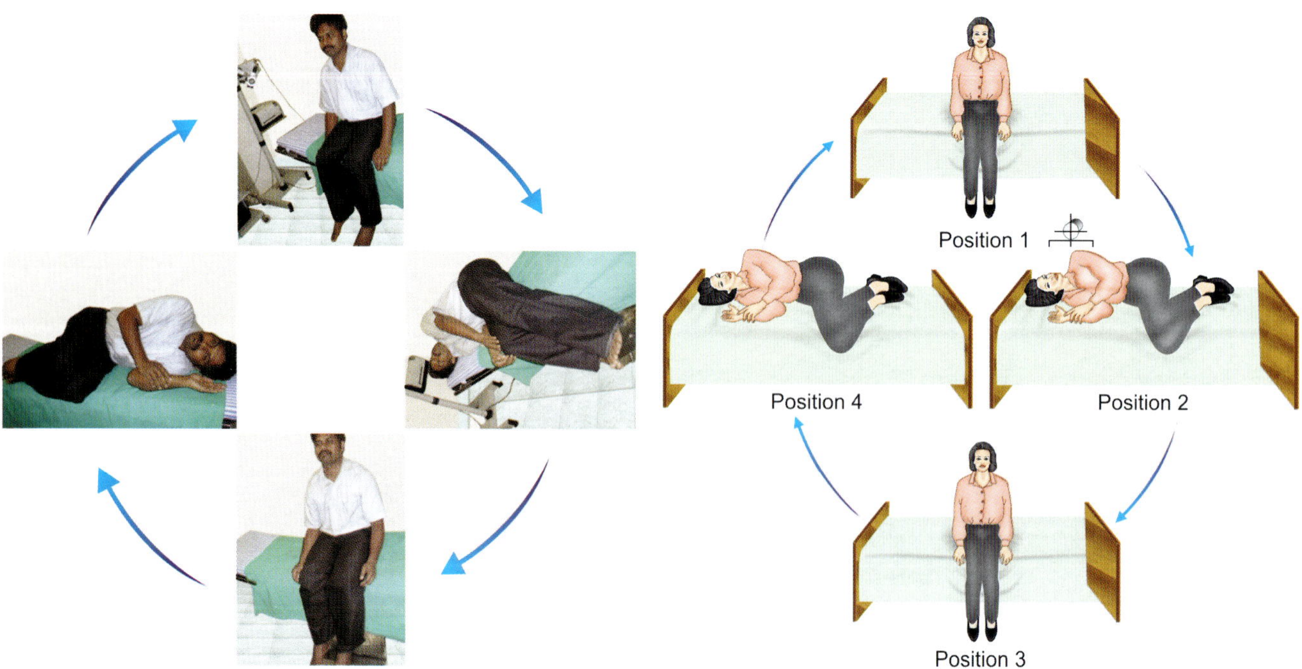

Fig. 13: Semont's maneuver

Fig. 14: Brandt-Daroff exercises

Flowchart 1: Interaction of autonomic, psychological and vestibular symptoms

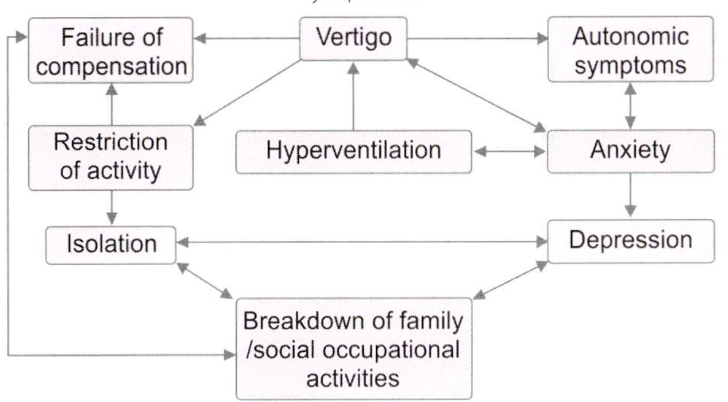

Surgery of Vertigo (Flowchart 2)

Surgical intervention for vertigo is rarely required. Surgeries mainly indicated in disabling vertigo related to—

- Dreadful complications of COM
- Vestibular schwannoma
- Perilymph fistula following trauma

The surgery of vertigo has been discussed in Chapter 11 (Meniere's disease).

Some important points to be remembered about vertigo are—

- Vertigo is a symptom not a disease
- In most vertigo, underlying cause is simple
- Art of history taking for correct diagnosis is essential
- Vestibular rehabilitation exercises help a lot to relieve vertigo.

REFERENCES

1. AG Kerr. Vertigo: Scott- Brown's otolaryngology, 5th edition 1987, first Indian edition. New Delhi: Jaypee Brothers Medical Publishers (P) Ltd. 1994;3:435-43.
2. Foster CA. Evaluation of the dizzy patient, ENT Secrets, 3rd edition. In: Jafek BW, Murrow BW (Eds). Mosby; 2005;73-8.
3. Banerjee S. Vertigo simplified: A guide to ENT practice. Compiled by Dr Santanu Banerjee. 2003-2004; vol 2:42-50.
4. Bronstein AM. Evaluation of balance, Scott-Brown's Otorhino-laryngology, head and neck surgery, 7th edition. 2008;3:3708-09.
5. Zarandy MM, RutKa J. Benign Positional vertigo, Therapeutic Spectrum issue 1: BPPV springer (India) Pvt Ltd; 2010.1-4.
6. Barber HO, Stockwell CW. Manual of Electronystagmography. Saint Louis: Mosby Company; 1976;3-4.
7. Desmond A. Role of audiometry in vestibular assessment. http://hearinghealthmatters.org/dizzinessdepot/2011/the-role-of-audiometry-in-vestibular-testing.
8. Beaumont GD. Radiology and the management of chronic suppurative otitis media. Austalas Radiol. 1980;24:238-45.
9. Patkar D, Yevankar G, Parikh R. Radiology in vertigo and Dizziness, Otorhinolaryngology clinic: An international Journal. May-August 2012;4(2):86-92.
10. Nakashima T, Naganawa S, Sugiura M, Teranishi M, Sone M, Hayashi H, et al. Visualization of endolymphatic hydrops in patients with Meniere's disease. Laryngoscope. 2007;117:415-20.
11. Mulkens TH, Parizel PM, Martin JJ, et al. Acoustic Schwannoma: MR findings in 84 tumors. Am J Roentgenol. 1993;160(2):395-8.
12. ZlatKo Trkanjec, Anka Aleksic- Shibabi, Vida Demarin. Pharmaco therapy of vertigo Rad za medicinske Znanosti, Zagreb, 2007; str: 69-76.
13. Lacour M, Sterkers O. Histamine and betahistine in the treatment of vertigo: elucidation of mechanisms of action, CNS Drugs. 2001;15:853-70.
14. Canty P, Valentine J. Betahistine in Peripheral vertigo: a double-blind, placebo-controlled, cross-over study of serc versus placebo. J Laryngol Otol. 1981;95:687-92.
15. James AL, Burton MJ. Betahistine for Meniere's disease or syndrome. Cochrane data base syst rev. 2001;(1):CD001873.
16. Aantaa E, SKinho A. Controlled clinical trial comparing the effect of betahistine hydrochloride and prochlorperazine maleate for patients with Meniere's disease. Annals of clinical research. 1976;8:284-7.
17. Bond CM. Comparison of buccal and oral prochlorperazine in the treatment of dizziness associated with nausea and/or vertigo, Current Medical Research and opinion. 1998;14:203-12.
18. Shah KU, Shah A. Labyrinthine vertigo treatment with ephedrine nasal douch. J Assoc Physicians, India. 1981;29:819-23.

Flowchart 2: Surgery of vertigo

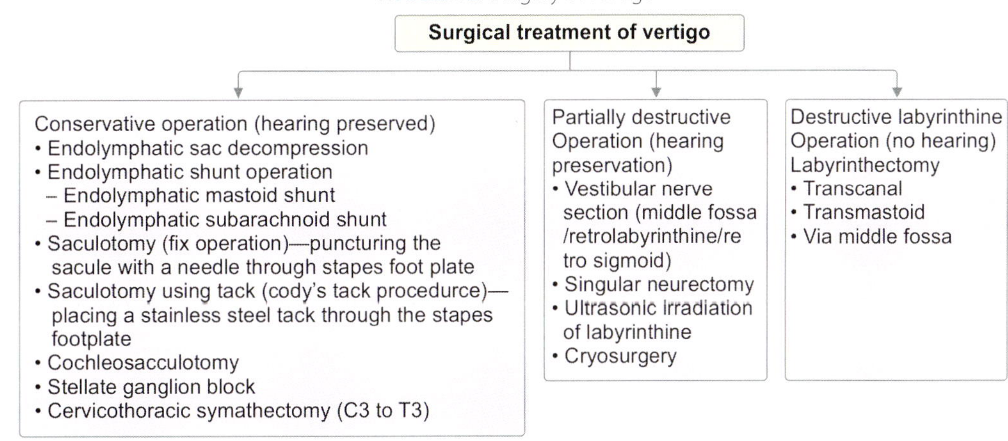

19. Godfraind T, Towse G, Van Nueten JM. Cinnarizine–a selective calcium entry blocker, Drugs of today. 1982;18(1):27-42.
20. Godfraind T, Morel N, Wibo M. Modulation of the action of calcium antagonists in arteries. Blood Vessels. 1990;27(2-5):184-96.
21. Theopold HM. Nimodipine (Bay e 9736) a new therapy concept in diseases of the inner ear? Laryngol Rhinol Otol (stuHg). 1985;64:609-13.
22. Yacovino DA, Hain TC. Medical management of vertigo. Textbook of vertigo – diagnosis and management. In: Dispenza F, et al, 1st edition. Jaypee Brothers Medical Publishers. 2014. P 219-36.
23. Cesarani A, Meloni F, Alpini D, Barozzi S, Verderio L, Boscani PF. Ginkgo biloba (EGb 761) in the treatment of equilibrium disorders. Adv. Ther. 1998;15:291-304.
24. Nicholson CD. Pharmacology of nootropics and metabolically active compounds in relation to their use in dementia. Psychopharmacology (Berl). 1990;101:147-59.
25. Martini A, De Domenico F. Trimetazine Versus betahistine in Meniere's disease. A double blind method. Am Otolaryngol Chir Cervicofac. 1990;107(suppl1):20-7.
26. Hain TC, Uddin M. Pharmacological treatment of vertigo. CNS Drugs. 2003;17:85-100.
27. Dix MR. Rehabilitation of vertigo. In vertigo, edited by Dix MR and Hood JD. Chichester: John Wiley and sons; 1984;P 469-79.
28. Waleem SS, Malik SM, Ullah S, Ul Hassan Z. Office management of benign paroxysmal positional vertigo with Epley's maneuver J Ayub Med Coll Abbottabad. 2008;20(1):77-9.
29. Serafini G, Palmieri AM, Simoncelli C. Benign Paroxysmal positional vertigo of posterior semicircular canal: results in 160 cases treated with semont's maneuver. Ann Otol Rhinol Laryngol. 1996;105(10):770-5.
30. Karanjai S, Saha AK. Evaluation of vestibular exercise in the management of benign paroxysmal positional vertigo. Indian J. otolaryngol head and neck surgery. 2010;62(2):202-7.

Deafness, Assessment of Deaf Child and Rehabilitative Measures

Asok K Saha

- Hearing loss is the diminished sensitivity to sounds that are normally heard
- Hearing impairment or hard of hearing is reserved for people who have relative insensitivity to sound in speech frequencies
- Deafness is defined as a degree of hearing impairment is such a way that a person is unable to understand speech even in presence of amplification. A person is said to be deaf when this hearing loss is more than 90 dB in the better ear or having total loss of hearing in both the ears
- Profound deafness means even the loudest sounds produced by an audiometer may not be detected
- Total deafness—No sounds at all are heard even in presence of amplifications or regardless of the method of production.[1]

WHO classification of degree of hearing loss is based on the Pure tone audiogram taking average of hearing thresholds in speech frequencies (500, 1000, 2000 Hz) with reference to ISO: R389-1970 (International Calibration of Audiometers). Now, it is realized that frequency of 3000 Hz is important for hearing in presence of noise. As per AAOO (American Academy of Ophthalmology and Otorhinolaryngology), average of four speech frequencies (500, 1000, 2000, 3000Hz) is taken during calculation of hearing handicap (Table 1).

- For children below 6 years of age PTA is not possible, free field testing is done
- PTA results, if possible, are supplemented by speech discrimination scores (SDS)
- The term 'disability' is used when hearing impairment affects the ability of performing function in the range considered normal for that individual
- The term 'hearing handicap' is used when hearing disability restricts the duties and roles expected from an individual by the society.

  Therefore, sequence is Disease → Impairment → Disability → Handicap.[2]

DEGREE OF HEARING HANDICAP

Degree of hearing handicap is expressed in terms of percentage for the purposes of compensation.

Method of calculation for hearing handicap in percentage—
- Calculate the average of hearing thresholds in speech frequencies (500, 1000, 2000 Hz) for the ear (say= A)
- Deduct 25 dB (as 25 dB is considered normal) from it, i.e. A-25
- Multiply it by 1.5, i.e. (A-25)*1.5
- This is the percentage of hearing impairment for that ear
- Percentage of hearing handicap of an individual =

$$\frac{(\text{better ear\%} \times 5) + \text{Worse ear\%}}{6}$$

ONLY ONE EAR HEARING

Profound or even total unilateral hearing loss does not produce a serious handicap or affect speech but patient may have following complaints-

Table 1: WHO classification of degree of hearing loss	
Degree of hearing loss	**Average of AC threshold in speech frequencies in the better ear in dB**
No significant	0–25 dB
Mild	26–40 dB
Moderate	41–55 dB
Moderately severe	56–70 dB
Severe	71–91 dB
Profound	>91 dB
NO response	=130 dB

- Impairment of localization of the sound source
- Poor discrimination of speech in presence of noisy background
- Difficulty in hearing when speaker is on the side of the affected ear.

  Proper precaution is to be taken for safety of better ear. Surgeon should be careful while operating on only one ear hearing.

ASSESSMENT OF DEAF CHILD

Approximately one out of every 1000 children is born deaf. The ratio is higher among some populations and in some areas. Socioeconomic deprivation is the key factor behind this. As the children have not heard speech, they do not acquire normal speech and language.

Again another one per 1000 children acquires permanent deafness through illness, mostly meningitis before the age of nine. 99% of deaf children come from hearing families with no previous history of deafness.[3]

Early detection of deafness in children and its early treatment, both are essential for developing better speech and language as well as for improving better social and emotional development.

Prompt management should be started in deaf children before the critical age of language acquisition (before 6 months of age). Delay in the management may result in poor acquisition of speech and language.

Two Types of Hearing Loss

Conductive Hearing Loss

- It affects 4% of all school children
- Most of the cases are due to OME
- Other causes are—atresia of external auditory canal (EAC) along with defects in middle ear structure, congenital conductive deafness often associated with Craniofacial defect (e.g. Treacher Collin's syndrome)
- Conductive hearing loss in children has detrimental effect on language, speech and attention
- Audiologically, it is very difficult to confirm the conductive HL in very small child. Clinical examination of EAC and associated facial deformity help in diagnosis.

Sensorineural Hearing Loss

- It affects 0.3% of all school children
- Can be grouped into four categories—
  - Hereditary or genetic
  - Prenatal, e.g. rubella infection to mother in first trimester of pregnancy.
  - Perinatal, e.g. Kernicterus, hypoxia at the time of birth
  - Childhood acquired deafness, e.g. meningitis or trauma to inner ear (Sensorineural apparatus).
- Children with SNHL may not acquire normal speech and language but may improve the same by proper treatment started before the age of 6 months
- Mixed hearing loss has component of both conductive HL and SNHL.

  Although conductive HL is more common, the majority of permanent deafness is due to SNHL.

ETIOLOGY

Etiology of HL is not always possible to identify. Possible causes are grouped as follows:

Causes Before Birth (Prenatal Causes)

- Genetic reasons—They may affect inner ear alone (nonsyndromic) or may form part of a syndrome (syndromic). Inner ear defects are:
  - Michel aplasia—Complete absence of inner ear (both bony and membranous labyrinth)
  - Bing-Siebenman dysplasia—Complete absence of membranous labyrinth
  - Sheibe's dysplasia—Most common type of inner ear anomaly. Dysplasia is seen in cochlea and saccule (also known cochleosaccular dysplasia). Rest of the inner ear is normal. It is inherited as an autosomal recessive nonsyndromic trait
  - Alexander's dysplasia—Dysplasia involves only basal turn of cochlea resulting in only high-frequency SNHL
  - Mondini's dysplasia—Cochlea has 1.5 turns. Only basal coil is present.
- Maternal reasons
  - Infections—Infections affect growing fetus. They include toxoplasmosis, rubella, Cytomegalovirus (CMV), herpes type 1 and 2 and syphilis (TORCHES)
  - Ototoxic drugs—They cross the placental barrier and damage the cochlea. They include streptomycin, glutamicin, tobramicin, amikacin, quinine and chloroquinine. Thalidomide has teratogenic effect to the limbs, heart, face, lip, palate in addition to ears. Maternal alcoholism may damage developing inner ear of fetus
  - Radiation received by mother especially in first trimester
  - Other factors are nutritional deficiency, diabetes, toxaemia and hypothyroidism.

Causes at Birth (Perinatal Causes)

- Anoxia—Neonatal anoxia damages cochlear nuclei and causes hemorrhage in inner ear. Causes are placenta

previa, prolonged labor, cord compression and cord prolapse
- Prematurity and low birth weight—Born before term and birth weight <1.5 kg may increase risk of being deaf
- Birth injuries—Forceps delivery may result in intra cranial hemorrhage with extravasation of blood in the inner ear
- Neonatal jaundice—Bilrubin >20mg% damages the cochlear nuclei
- Ototoxic drugs used for neonatal meningitis or septicemia may damage the inner ear
- Neonatal meningitis—Causative organisms are *Streptococcus pneumonia* (20%HL) *Hemophilus influenzae* (12%HL) and *Neisseria meningitidis* (5%HL). About 33% of all acquired SNHL are due to meningitis.

Causes in Infancy (Postnatal Causes)

- Genetic—Though deafness is genetic, it manifests later in childhood or adult life. The child may have deafness alone as in familial progressive SNHL or deafness associated with anomalies of other system, e.g. Alport, Klippel-Feil and Hurler syndromes.
- Nongenetic—They are same as adults and include the following:
    - Infections, e.g. measles, mumps, varicella, influenza, meningitis, encephalitis and otitis media
    - Ototoxic drugs
    - Trauma, e.g. fracture temporal bone, middle ear surgery or perilymph leak
    - Noise-induced HL.

Deafness is suspected under following observations:
- Sudden loud sounds or noise fail to awake from sleep and startle the child
- Failure to develop speech in 1–2 years
- Defective speech and poor school performance

Genetic HL (Key points)

- 50% cases of infant HL are genetic in origin
- Of the genetic HL—
    - 75% is autosomal recessive
    - 15–20% is autosomal dominant
    - 1–2% is X-linked
    - Few cases have mitochondrial inheritance.

Risk factors for permanent hearing loss in neonates as recommended by US Joint Committee on infant hearing update in 2000 includes[4]—
- An illness or condition needs admission of 48 hours or more in NICU
- Stigmata or findings associated with a syndrome are known to have a sensorineural and/or conductive HL
- Family history of permanent childhood SNHL

- Craniofacial anomalies including anomalies of pinna and external auditory canal
- Prenatal infections (TORCHES)
  Three major risk factors are:
    - H/O treatment in neonatal intensive care unit (NICU) or special care baby unit (SCBU) for more than 48 hours
    - Family history of childhood deafness
    - Craniofacial anomalies (i.e. cleft palate) associated with hearing loss.
      Above 60% of congenital bilateral permanent hearing loss of moderate to profound degree is associated with one of the three risk factors in the proportions of → 29.3% NICU
      26.7% family history
      3.9% craniofacial anomaly.

Methods of Hearing Assessment in Infants and Children

History Taking

A detailed history taking is an essential part of assessing the baby suspected to be deaf. Prenatal, perinatal or postnatal history, family history, certain clinical tests and investigations related to suspected cause are required for assessing deafness.

Neonatal Screening Procedures

- Arousal test—A high-frequency narrowband noise is presented for 2 seconds to light sleeping infant. A normal hearing infant awakes twice when three such stimuli are presented. The test is suitable for 0–4 months of age
- Auditory response cradle—Baby is placed in a cradle and his behavior like trunk and limb movement, head jerk and respiration are monitored by transducers in response to auditory stimulation.

Behavior Observation Audiometry

- Moro's reflex—It consists of sudden movement of limbs and extension of head in response to sound of 80–90 dB
- Cochleopalpabral reflex—The baby blinks in response to loud sound of 50–70 dB
- Cessation reflex—In response to a sound of 90 dB the baby stops activity or starts crying.

Distraction Techniques

An infant of 6–7 months old turns his head to locate the source of sound. The infant is seated in mother's lap, an assistant distracts the infant's attention, the examiner produces a sound from behind or from one side. Whether the infant tries to locate the sound by turning head or not is noted. Sounds used are high-frequency rattle (8 KHz), low-frequency hum, whispered sound as s,s,s, xylophone, warbled tones or narrowband noise (500–4,000 Hz). If the infant does not turn head to locate the sound, hearing loss is indicated and then a higher intensity of sound is to be applied. This process of hearing assessment is known as free field audiometry.

Conditioning Techniques

- Visual reinforcement audiometry (VRA). The test is usually done in the age group of 7–30 months. It is a conditioning technique. The child is trained to look for auditory stimulus by turning his head. The test is done in a soundproof room with speakers and audiometer. Above or below each speaker is a reinforcing toy which lights up when the child turns to the sound. This reinforces the child's responses and helps to sustain the child's interest in the sound for a long time.[5] A child hearing is normal if he can respond by turning head towards the sound source to a sound of 25 dB for 6–11 months of age, 20 dB for 13–17 months of age, 15 dB for 18–23 months of age and 10 dB for 24–29 months of age (Matkin 1997)
- Play audiometry—In 2–5 years of age, the child is mentally more matured. The child is conditioned or taught to perform an act (e.g. putting a ball into a bowl) each time whenever he hears the sound. Each specific threshold can be measured by standard audiometric technique. Technically, this process is known as Play audiometry. Conditioning is not equally achieved by all the children. Some children stop responding before the threshold is reached. These false responses are not uncommon. The play audiometry is basically a subjective response
- Speech audiometry—The spondee words along with pictures are presented to the child. The child is asked to repeat the word or to point the exact picture. The voice is gradually lowered. In this way, hearing threshold and speech discrimination are tested. Again the child's expressive ability can be tested when he is asked to name the toys or objects.

Objective Tests

BERA for Threshold Estimation

It consists of presenting sound stimuli at gradually increasing intensities and pointing at which minimum intensity of sound stimulus, the wave V of BERA just appears—this is said to be the BERA threshold of the child. The PTA is within 5–10 dB of this intensity level. Advantages of using BERA as a threshold test are:

- The test is objective

- The test can be performed even when the child is sleeping or sedated
- Individual ear can be tested separately.

Limitations

- The test is not frequency specific
- Hearing threshold obtained is in the range of 2,000–10,000 Hz only
- Low-frequency hearing loss, if any is missed by BERA
- Patient related variables like age and sex of the child sometimes alter the wave character
- Identification of the wave is difficult in few patients as muscular contractions caused by movements of the child may cause artifacts
- The test is time consuming. More than 2 hours are required if the child is restless.[6]

Otoacoustic Emission (OAE)

It is the biological sound generated in a normal cochlear. This sound is generated in cochlea either by itself (called Spontaneous OAE) or by sound stimulus presented to cochlea (called evoked OAE).

Transient-evoked otoacoustic emission (TEOAE) is evoked from the cochlea in response to clicks and is used for hearing assessment in children. TEOAEs are absent in ears where hearing loss exceeds 30 dB.

Distortion product emissions (DPOAEs) are absent when hearing loss is more than 50 dB.

If any defect in middle ear or cochlea is present, OAEs are not detectable. Therefore, presence of recordable evoked OAEs means normal functioning middle ear and cochlea.

Impedance Audiometry

Stapedius muscle contracts reflexly in response to a sound of 70–100 dB that can be recorded.

- Absence of acoustic reflex indicates middle ear disorder, retrocochlear HL or severe to profound SNHL
- Absence of acoustic reflex but normal tympanogram-indicates SNHL of severe to profound degree.
- Absence of acoustic reflex but abnormal tympanogram indicates conductive HL.[7]

Universal Neonatal Hearing Screening

Universal neonatal hearing screening (UNHS) is an increasingly popular screening strategy for early detection of hearing loss. The test is done within first 3 months of age. It detects the permanent HL at an average of 3 months. It describes the use of objective tests—Otoacoustic emission (OAE) test Auditory brainstem response (ABR) either singly or in combination to screen the hearing of the whole population of newborns in a particular target region. Only specific target populations within a region say infants in neonatal intensive care unit or with risk factor for hearing loss are screened.

Screening methodology involves two stage processes where screening of hearing is done with either OAE or ABR. Children passing the test need no further assessment but progressive, late onset and acquired hearing loss cannot be ruled out at this time. Children who fail the initial screening test are referred to a second screening assessment with either OAE or ABR. Children failing the second assessment will be referred for diagnostic assessment of hearing. The procedure has some variation from region to region but most follow this basic strategy.[8,9] Screening personnel may vary. In some regions, audiologists are involved; in other regions technicians, nurses or volunteers are involved.

Other laboratory tests for assessing deaf child are:
- Screening for maternal transmitted infection
  - Infant's blood for specific IgM for TORCH and syphilis
  - Detection of virus in urine, saliva, blood or other body tissue within 2–3 weeks after birth for diagnosis of congenital CMV infection. Antibody tests cannot be used to diagnose CMV.
- Genetic testing
  - Genetic factors account for at least half of all the cases of profound congenital deafness. More than 120 independent genes for deafness have been identified
  - Recessive mutation at a single locus GJB2 or connexin 26 accounts for more than half of all genetic cases of deafness. Screening for connexin 26 can provide knowledge to know whether the children will be hearing or deaf even before they are conceived
  - First gene mapped for nonsyndromic deafness is DNFA$_1$. It is identified as causative in a rare form of low-frequency onset progressive hearing loss with autosomal dominant inheritance pattern
  - 35 Del G deletion is responsible for 70% of all connexin 26 mutations. Screening for 35 Del G deletion is available
  - DFNB1—It stands for autosomal recessive nonsyndromic hearing loss, mutation in connexin 26 is associated with prelingual nonprogressive bilateral SNHL
  - Mitochondrial A15559 mutation is related to increase sensitivity to ototoxic effect of aminoglycosides.
- Temporal Bone Imaging
  - Temporal bone anomalies are common in GJB2 related hearing loss.
- CT—Common findings are:
  - Dilated endolymphatic fossa (28%)

- Hypoplastic modiolus (25%)
- Large vestibular aqueduct (8%)
- Hypoplastic horizontal semicircular cannal (8%)
- Hypoplastic cochlea (4%).

CT imaging should be included in routine evaluations of these deaf children.
- MRI—Cochlear fibrosis is detected by MRI but not by CT scans. It is essential for preoperative planning of cochlear implant to assess the cochlear potency, position of facial nerve and presence of auditory nerve. These two imaging modalities are complementary to each other. Facial nerve dehiscence is detected by CT while MRI is normal. Again cochlear fibrosis is detected by MRI but not by CT scans.

PREVENTION

Half of the hearing impairments are preventable.

Preventive Measures

- Immunization against rubella—to reduce congenital infections
- Immunization against *H influenza* and *S pneumonia* to reduce cases of otitis media.

Measurement

There are a number of devices to improve hearing—
- Hearing aids—amplify incoming sound and improve hearing ability but they can never restore normal hearing. They also help in lip reading
- Cochlear implants—They artificially stimulate the cochlear nerve and provide electric impulse substitution for firing hair cells
  - Younger the age of implantations, better are the results of acquisition of effective hearing and speech, particularly if supported by proper rehabilitation
  - Postmeningitis, deafness needs early implantation as delay in procedure faces difficulties of implantation due to cochlear ossifications.

Rehabilitative Measures

Aim of rehabilitation is to develop better speech and language and to improve social adjustment and vocational employment.
- Parental guidance
  - Sympathetic dealing to accept the child
  - Care and periodic replacement of hearing aid
  - Follow-up visits for re-evaluation
  - Education at home
  - Selection of vocation.

- Development of speech and language
  - Auditory oral communication—Hearing aids are given to increase auditory reception and training is imparted in speech reading at the same time. Movements of lips, face and natural gestures of hand and body are read to improve the expressive skill through oral speech. The method is used in those with moderate to severe hearing loss or the children with postlingual deafness
  - Manual communication—It includes use of sign language or finger spelling method. Abstract ideas are difficult to express as general public does not understand it
  - Total communication—This method of communication is used for children with prelingual severe to profound deafness. It utilizes all the sensory inputs, e.g. auditory, visual, tactile and kinesthetic. The children are trained to develop oral speech, lip reading and sign language
  - Vibrotactile aids are useful for children who are deaf as well as blind. The Aids are attached to the hand or sternum of the child. The vibrations of speech are perceived by the child via tactile sensation.[10]
- Education for deaf child
  - For deaf child, there are residential and day school to provide education that is indispensible to achieve higher education
  - Some of the children with moderate hearing loss may be admitted to normal school with preferential sitting arrangement in classroom
  - Now radio hearing aids are available to educate the deaf child. In this device, microphone and transmitter are worn by the teacher and receiver and amplifier is with the child. This system helps the deaf child to hear teacher's speech better avoiding environmental noises.

The World Federation of the Deaf (WFD) advocates, promotes and safeguards educational rights for deaf people of all ages. As for all learners, deaf children have the same right to education and full access to quality education.[11]

REFERENCE

1. Deafness- wikipedia, the free encyclopedia en wikipedia org/wiki/deafness.
2. Dhingra Pl. Disease of ear, nose and throat, 4th edition. page 38.
3. Deaf children- just communication. www.justcommunication.co.uk positive practice pdf.
4. Finitzo T, Sininger Y, Brookhouser P, Epstein S, Erenberg A, Roizen N et al. Position statement: principles and guidelines for early hearing detection and intervention programs. Pediatrics. 2000;106:798-817.
5. Snashall S. Childhood deafness disease of the ear, 6th edition. Edited by Harold Ludman and Tony Wright. 2006. page-164-81.
6. Biswas A. Assessing the deaf child. Otolaryngology Review. Edited by Shah VH, Karnik PK. 2000. page 23-7.
7. Wrighton AS. Universal newborn hearing screening. Am Fam Physician. 2007;75(9):1349-52.
8. Diane C, Heather T, Philips MC, Davis RL, Tracy A, Charles L, Hammer J, Helfand M. Universal Newborn Hearing Screening: Summary of Evidence. JAMA. 2001;286(16):2000-10: d 01: 10.1001/JAMA 286.16.2000.
9. Universal neonatal hearing screening Wikipedia http://ʃfen.wikipedia.org/wiki/universal_neonatal_hearing_screening.
10. Bansal M. Hearing impairment in infant and children. Disease of ear, nose and throat, head and neck surgery. 2013. page 166-72.
11. http:/ʃwfdeaf.org/databank/policies/educations-rights for deaf children.

Asok K Saha

The term tinnitus comes from the Latin word tinnire meaning "ringing". It is described as a sound perceived in one or both ears or in the head in absence of any external acoustical stimulation of the ear. The phenomenon of tinnitus is as old as mankind. Sound perceived includes ringing, buzzing, humming, roaring, hissing, tingling or whistling that are high-pitch in nature. Tinnitus is a symptom but not a disease. It may result from a wide range of underlying causes. In majority of patients with tinnitus may be accompanied with SNHL. It may be side effect of some drugs. But most common cause of tinnitus is the noise induced hearing loss (SNHL).

The prevalence of tinnitus in adult ranges from 10% to 14% and prevalence of clinical tinnitus, i.e. patients is bothered by tinnitus and seeks medical advice is about 7%.[1] Males are affected more than female of similar age.

CLASSIFICATION

Tinnitus is divided into subjective and objective types.

Subjective Tinnitus

The tinnitus is heard by the patient only and the patient perceives sound in absence of any external acoustic stimulus. It may commonly result from otologic disorders.

Objective Tinnitus

Objective tinnitus refers to rare condition that produces sound heard both by patient and the examiner. It may result from varieties of pathological sources which are mechanical in nature, usually vascular or muscular adjacent to auditory system.

Again tinnitus is described as nonpulsatile or pulsatile tinnitus for practical purposes.[2]

Nonpulsatile tinnitus is also known as subjective tinnitus which is more common and has complex pathophysiology

Pulsatile tinnitus (PT) is usually objective in nature and less common. It results from altered blood flow near the ear. Patient experiences sound that synchronizes with the pulse. It may be arterial or venous in origin. It may be subjective phenomenon if it arises due to increased awareness of blood flow in the ear.

CAUSES

Causes of Subjective Tinnitus or Nonpulsatile Tinnitus

Otologic origin and hearing loss:
- Conductive hearing loss
- Otitis externa
- Cerumen impaction
- Middle ear effusion.

Sensorineural hearing loss:
- Noise-induced hearing loss
- Presbycusis
- Meniere's disease
- Labyrinthitis
- Acoustic neuroma
- Mercury or lead poisoning
- Ototoxic drug.

Antibiotics:
- Aminoglycosides e.g. gentamycin, tobramycin, amikacin
- Erythromycin
- Vancomycin
- Polymyxins
- Ciprofloxacin
- Doxycycline.

Analgesic:
- Aspirin

260 Otology and Middle Ear Surgery

- • Nonsteroidal anti-inflammatory drug.

Chemotherapy:
- • Cisplatin
- • Bleomycin
- • Interferon
- • Methotrexate
- • Vincristine.

Loop diuretic:
- • Frusemide
- • Ethacrynic acid.

Others:
- • Chloroquine
- • Quinine
- • Antidepressants
- • Benzodiazepine withdrawal.

Nonotologic origin:
- • Multiple sclerosis
- • Head injury
- • Hyperlipidemia
- • Vitamin B12 deficiency anemia
- • Thyroid diseases
- • Iron deficiency anemia
- • Hypotension
- • Hypoglycemia
- • Epilepsy
- • Migraine.

Psychogenic:
- • Depression
- • Anxiety.

Causes of Objective or Pulsatile Tinnitus

Arterial etiologies:
- • Vascular tumor of middle ear, e.g. glomus tympanicum
- • Carotid artery dissection
- • Persistent stapedial artery
- • Giant cell arteritis
- • Idiopathic intracranial hypertension
- • Dehiscence superior semicircular canal
- • Atherosclerotic carotid artery or subclavian artery diseases.

Venous etiologies:
- • Jugular bulb abnormalities
- • Sigmoid sinus aneurysm
- • Arnold Chiarie malformation
- • Abnormal mastoid emissary veins
- • Stenosis of the sylvian aqueduct resulting hydrocephalus
- • Arteriovenous malformations.

Nonvascular etiologies:
- • Palatal myoclonus arising from muscle spasm that causes clicks around the ear
- • Stapedial muscle and tensor tympani muscle myoclonus.[3]

PATHOPHYSIOLOGY OF TINNITUS

It is now evident that tinnitus is caused by functional changes in CNS as is supported by positron emission tomography (PET) and functional MRI.

- • The function of auditory system is maintained by complex feedback mechanism. The auditory system involves afferent, ascending and efferent descending pathways. It is linked to nonauditory structures also, like—
  - – Reticular serotonergic structure
  - – Somatosensory system
  - – Hypothalamus and limbic system.

The subcortical connections are integrated with CNS network. The afferent pathway provides an input to proximal auditory system and facilitates excitatory processes. Efferent pathway modulates the sound information and facilitates the inhibitory processes. The feedback interaction between the pathways provides a dynamic system where pathological changes at one site may have functional result at other site or sites (Fig. 1). In noise-induced cochlear lesion, there is a decrease in auditory input resulting compensatory disinhibition to

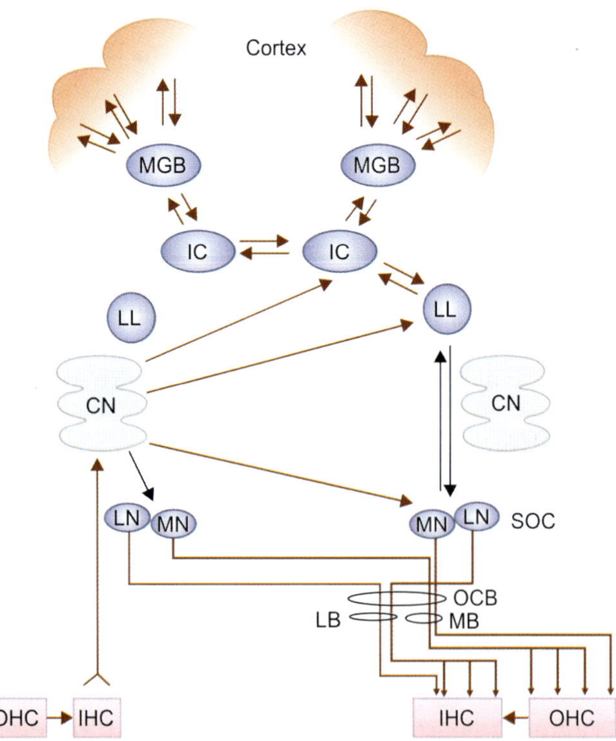

Fig. 1: Afferent and efferent auditory pathways
Abbreviations: OHC, Outer hair cells; IHC, Inner hair cells; CN, Cochlear Nuclei; SOC, Superior olivery complex; LL, Lateral Leminiscus; IC, Inferior Colliculuis; MGB, Medial geniculate body; OCB, Olivocochlear Bundle; MB, Medial Bundle; LB, Lateral Bundle

the proximal auditory system with consequent tonotopic reorganization in long-term.

In most cases, tinnitus attenuates by the process of habituation which is a cortical phenomenon. It involves complex neuronal network and multiple transmitter system as evident by recent functional imaging techniques—single proton emission computed tomography (SPECT), PET, functional magnetic resonance imaging (MRI)

- Modulation of tinnitus in some patients by voluntary acts, such as changes in eye gaze, jaw movements or head neck contraction suggests association of auditory system with somatosensory systems.[4-6] Plastic charges arise in central nervous system with aberrant connections with nonauditory structures including primary temporal and temporoparietal cortical areas, left hippocampus, the right prefrontal network and limbic system[7]
- Intravenous injection of lidocaine changes the tinnitus loudness. It is related to the changes in the neural activity measured by cerebral blood flow in right temporal lobe with PET.

Possible Mechanisms Resulting Tinnitus (Fig. 2)

Abnormal excitation of afferent auditory pathway at the cochlear level

- Spontaneous otoacoustic emissions (SOAEs) are audible in some individual with tinnitus and is an objective correlate of tinnitus. Aspirin can stop both SOAEs and SOAEs relates tinnitus.[8] SOAEs may reflect an increased cochlear gain and auditory disinhibition. SOAEs may interact directly with external sound resulting different auditory perceptions
- Glutamate neuro excitotoxicity—Glutamate has potent excitatory effect as well as neurotoxic effect at cochlear afferent. In acoustic trauma, there is excessive release of glutamate and excitotoxic intracellular Ca^{++} over load, that may lead to tinnitus.

  Glutamate receptors- N- MDA (N- methyl D-aspartate) are selectively blocked by carno verine, an antagonist of their receptor resulting cessation of tinnitus in some patients
- Modulation of NMDA and non-NMDA receptors— In stress, endogenous opoid peptides, disnorphine released by lateral olivocochlear fibers may enhance the sensitivity of NMDA receptors and aggravate-excitation of afferent auditory path resulting stress-induced tinnitus
- Calcium channel dysfunction—Some drugs like salicylates affect intracellular calcium concentration

in hair cell and neurons leading to increase activity in cochlear nerve and contributing abnormal calcium conductance in the generation of tinnitus.

Dysfunction of efferent system/reduction of GABA effect

- Efferent path acts as an inhibitory response within the auditory system and runs in parallel to the afferent path. Medial olivocochlear (MOC) system of the efferent path has been studied mostly and its dysfunction may lead to disinhibition of the auditory system resulting tinnitus[10]
- Degenerative changes of the auditory system related to acoustic trauma, ototoxicity or aging process modulate amino acid neurotransmitter receptors in cochlear nucleus and inferior colliculus of central auditory path. The reduction of GABA effect reduces inhibitory response of the efferent system generating tinnitus.[11]

Alteration of spontaneous activity and reorganization of tonotopic maps

- Noise trauma, ototoxicity or aging may cause reduction in the afferent input and compensatory disinhibition on efferent auditory system, resulting alteration of spontaneous activity and plastic transformation of brain.[12] Tinnitus may arise from auditory system hypoactivity with increase in spontaneous activity induced by pathological alteration. This theory is supported by electrophysiological techniques and functional MRI studies in humans[13]
- Tonotopic organization is the disposition of the cell within the auditory system nuclei according

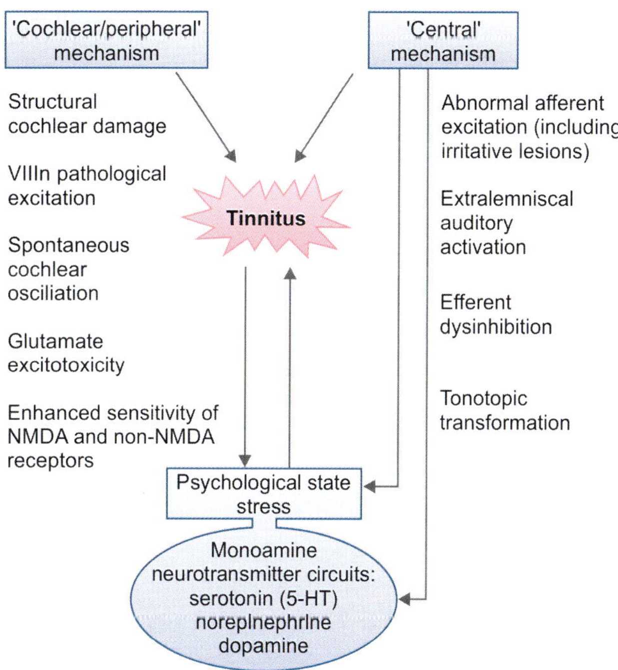

Fig. 2: Peripheral and central mechanisms and stress or psychological factors related to Tinnitus generation

to frequency selectivity indicating the cochlear organization. Following cochlear injury change in tonotopic organization is seen in central auditory structure regenerating Tinnitus. Areas of tonotopic map reorganization are studied through MRI in tinnitus patients.[14]

Stress and psychological conditions

- Stress has some role for generation of Tinnitus. Stress activates the sympathetic-adrenal-medullary system releasing catecholamines (adrenaline and nonadrenaline) and hypothalamic-pituitory-adrenocortical system releasing glucocorticoids (cortisol) that may act on auditory system through various humoral and neural pathways
- Depression, anxiety and mode disorders are associated with distressed tinnitus in some patients through dysregulation of monoamine neurotransmitter circuits involving serotonin, noradrenaline and dopamine; these are central to the process of habituation.[15] Patients with effective disorders suffer from poor habituation with persistent troublesome tinnitus.

INVESTIGATIONS IN TINNITUS

A detailed history taking is important to evaluate tinnitus that includes:

- Subjective description of tinnitus
    - Site and side of Tinnitus—right/left or both ears or centered in head
    - Time of onset, duration, progression, frequency, continuous or intermittent
    - Quality of Tinnitus—loudness/pitch (high or low)
    - Severity—its effect on sleep and daily life.
- Otologic and audiovestibular symptoms, e.g. otalgia, ear discharge, hearing loss and vertigo
- General medical causes like H/O hypertension, diabetes and toxemia
- H/O noise exposure, ototoxic drug and CNS infection
- Past H/O head injury, ear surgery and viral fever
- H/O stressful condition and psychiatric disorder.

CLINICAL EXAMINATION

Clinical examination includes routine ENT examination and detailed neuro-otologic evaluation like—

- Otoscopy to rule out any otologic pathology
- Tuning fork test for hearing assessment
- Gait and nystagmus to detect central or peripheral vestibular lesion
- Cranial nerve test including examination of temporomandibular joint.

Audiolologic Evaluation

- Pure tone audiometry and special tests for hearing, e.g. speech reception threshold, speech discrimination score, tone decay, short increment sensitivity index to know hearing status and site of pathology
- Impedance audiometry and acoustic reflex to assess middle ear function and natural pathway of stapedial reflex
- Otoacoustic emission—spontaneous/evoked/olivo-cochlear suppression test to measure the cochlear status
- Brainstem-evoked response audiometry (BERA) to rule out retrocochlear lesion.

Vestibular Function Test

- Electronystagmography (ENG)—It is an objective test considered for tinnitus patient having vestibular symptoms.

Imaging

- High resolution contrast-enhanced CT of temporal bone has little role in tinnitus patients. It is considered only in tinnitus patients of otic capsule pathology, e.g. otosclerosis and Paget's disease
- A gadolinium-enhanced MRI of temproal bone/posterior fossa is the gold standard method of imaging for tinnitus patients with suspicion of vestibular schwannomas.[16]

Functional Imaging

Functional imaging (e.g. f-MRI and PET) is an objective technique of recording tinnitus related neural activity accompanied by an increase in local blood flow. It helps to localize activation sits in CNS for assessment of tinnitus.

MEASUREMENT OF TINNITUS

It is considered for patients with severe tinnitus who need treatment by masking. Masking is based on comparing tinnitus with external sound.[17] There are four measures of tinnitus.

These are—Pitch, loudness matching, masking and residual inhibition.

Pitch matching: Pitch is the perceptual correlate of the frequency. Pitch matching of tinnitus is the procedure of matching frequency of an acoustic tone or narrowband noise to the predominate pitch of the tinnitus, e.g. high-frequency for noise-induced hearing loss (NIHL) related tinnitus and low-frequency for Meniere's disease.

Loudness matching: Loudness is the psychological magnitude of sound intensity of tinnitus. Loudness matching of tinnitus is the procedure of matching intensity of a pure tone or narrowband noise to a level that is equal to the intensity of the tinnitus. Loudness matching of tinnitus occurs between 5 and 10 dB sound sensation levels (SL).

Minimal masking level: Masking is reduction of tinnitus sound by another sound (masker). Masking is obtained effectively by applying wearable masker either ipsilaterally or contralaterally. By knowing the minimal level of masking required for different frequencies, the tinnitus masking pattern is determined.[18] It is suggested that frequency dependent masking is more consistent with tinnitus of peripheral origin whereas broadband frequency nonspecific masking is matched with tinnitus of central origin.[19]

Residual Inhibition: It is defined as the suppression or complete absence of tinnitus for a temporary period following masking. It is achieved by exposing tinnitus patient to minimal masking level (MML) plus 10 dB for one minute. It refers to forward or central masking.[20]

MANAGEMENT OF TINNITUS

The effective treatment of tinnitus is to treat the underlying cause by medical or surgical measure. In most cases, causes of tinnitus cannot be established. No specific treatment is still available to be satisfactory in all the patients.
Tinnitus management includes—
- Biofeedback or cognitive therapy
  - Taking your mind off from the tinnitus, refocusing and redirecting your thoughts. This type of therapy is used in addition to other modalities
- Hypnosis
  - It removes the negative emotions associated with tinnitus like stress, anxiety and worries, etc. during some session with Hypnotherapies
- Electrical stimulation
  - Electrical stimulation of cochlea through the round window helps to eliminate tinnitus in many patients but it is still not widely accepted procedure
  - Electrical stimulation of external ear—A mild electrical current applied to the external ear helps to suppress tinnitus in some patients. The current is adjusted to patient's own comfort level.[21]
- Relaxation therapy—Tinnitus patient is encouraged to take real interest in relaxation and to understand how it can help the patient to relieve from tinnitus
- Counseling—While meeting the patients with tinnitus, negative counseling is to be avoided. A positive attitude

of doctor to tinnitus patients is important. Patients are reassured about the symptoms and treatment to overcome it. In resistant cases, they should be advised to adopt and habituate with the condition
- Hearing aid and tinnitus masker
  - This is especially useful for patients with tinnitus and hearing loss. Hearing aid amplifies external sounds and reduces awareness of tinnitus. It interferes little with speech and does not produce high-noise level to interfere speech understanding
  - Tinnitus masker is a device that produces noise which is utilized to mask the tinnitus. The masking sound acts as a distracter and is usually more tolerable than the tinnitus. Environmental maskers like running of a fan, low volume music, indoor waterfalls or noisy clock can be helpful at night or in a quiet environment. Wearable tinnitus maskers are behind the ear or in the ear maskers those offer masking sounds to reduce annoyance of tinnitus. Description of the characteristics of tinnitus like pitch, loudness, location, etc. is essential for audiologists to determine what kinds of masking noise are helpful to relieve the tinnitus. If hearing loss is present along with tinnitus masker and hearing aid can operate together as one instrument.
- Pharmacotherapy
  - Tricyclic antidepressants like nortriptyline and amitriptyline are effective for patient with severe tinnitus associated with depression
  - Selective serotonin reuptake inhibitor (SSRI) is effective for elderly patients with tinnitus in whom a down regulation in serotonergic transmission is suspected[22]
  - GABA analogue like benzodiazepines, gabapentin, beclofen are found to be useful in some patients with tinnitus. Aim for use of GABA analogues is a hypothetical dysfunction of the efferent auditory pathways and GABA down regulation.
  Clonazepam (Benzodiazepine) having anxiolytic, sedative and serotonergic properties is beneficial in some patients with tinnitus[23]
- Calcium antagonists—Abnormal calcium channel conductance is responsible in some patients for generation of tinnitus. Calcium channel blockers, Nimodipine and Flunarazine are beneficial for relief of tinnitus in patients where calcium channel dysfunction is the underlying cause
- Antiepileptics like carbamazepine, sodium valproate and lamotrigine are effective in some tinnitus patients in whom abnormal auditory neural activity is the underlying cause. Antiepileptics may cause depression

of neural activity and hyperpolarization of neural membrane

- Prostaglandin analogue—Misoprostol acts as neuro modulators of afferent pathway at the level of cochlea and is effective for relief of tinnitus in some patients
- Lidocain (a sodium channel blocker)—It acts at the central as well as peripheral level of auditory system. Its intravenous use to control tinnitus is most effective. Side effects like disequilibrium, slurred speech and intravenous administration limit its use. Transtympanic application of 4% lidocain is also reported[24]

Surgery

Surgery is needed when tinnitus is associated with otosclerosis, Meniere's disease, pseudotumor cerebri (PC) syndrome, acoustic neuroma, atherosclerotic carotid artery disease and retrotympanic pathology like glomus tumors (tympanicum/jugulare), Jugular bulb/dural venous sinuses abnormalities, aberrant internal carotid artery and carotid body tumor.

Following surgeries are done for the management of objective tinnitus:

Diseases	Surgeries
Carotid artery stenosis	→ Carotid endarterectony
Glomus tympanicum	→ Surgical extirpation
Glomus jugulare	→ Surgical removal, Stereostatic radiosurgery
Arthérosclerotic obstruction of subclavian and internal carotid Arteries	→ Angioplasty
High dehiscence jugular bulb	→ Surgical correction by pieces of mastoid cortical bone and septal, conchal or tragal cartilage
Venous hum	→ Ligation of IJV
Dural AVMs and AVFs	→ Selective embolization
Pseudotumor Cerebri (Venous PT, female, obese)	→ Lumbar-peritoneal shunt
Palatal myoclonus (Tensor tympani and stapedial Myoclonus)	→ Sectioning of the respective muscles via tympanotomy, use of Botulinum toxin
Otosclerosis	→ Stapedectomy/or Stapedeotomy
Acoustic neuroma	→ Surgical removal/sterostatic radiosurgery
Meniere's disease	→ Endolymphatic shunt placement, CN VII or cochlear nerve section

Vestibular nerve section for tinnitus has been criticized by many surgeons as a destructive procedure which has only 40% shown improvement. About 55% of those who have gone surgery through experienced the same symptoms and others claim that it only worsens their uneasiness.

Surgery for tinnitus also includes cochlear implantation following VIII nerve section. Morbidity associated with vestibular nerve section will improve by placing of cochlear implant.[25]

TINNITUS RETRAINING THERAPY (TRT)

It was developed by Dr Pawel Jastreboff in 1980s (Fig. 3). TRT is a form of habituation therapy designed to help patients becoming less aware of the tinnitus TRT uses counseling aimed at reclassification of tinnitus to a category of neural signals and sound therapy aimed at weakening tinnitus related neural activity. If a patient successfully habituated TRT, the perception of tinnitus usually returns to the previous level of awareness before it becomes annoying.

Advantages of TRT

- No side effects
- Patient may have to back for follow-up once in six month
- Consultation may be performed over the telephone
- Hearing aids may provide partial masking effect and group therapy session may alleviate anxiety associated with tinnitus.

TRT works by interfering with the neural activity causing tinnitus at its source in order to prevent spreading to other nervous system, such as the limbic and autonomic nervous system.[26]

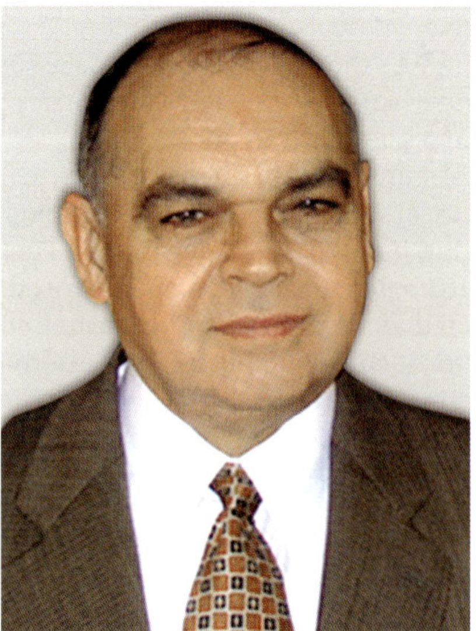

Fig. 3: Dr Jastreboff proposed a neurophysiological model of tinnitus and tinnitus retraining therapy (TRT)

REFERENCES

1. Ceranic B and Luxon LM. Tinnitus and other dysacusis: Scott Brown's Otorhinolarylgology, Head and Neck surgery, 7th Edition. Great Britain: Hodder Arnold Ltd; 2008. page 3597-8.
2. Sismanis A. Tinnitus: Evaluation and Management, Comprehensive textbook of Otology. Editors: Kirtane MV et al. Mumbai, India: Bhalani Publishing house; 2011.pp 355-71.
3. Pulec JL, Hodell SF, Anthony PF. Tinnitus: Diagnosis and treatment. Ann Otol Rhinol Laryngol. 1978;87(6Pt1):821-33.
4. Levine RA, Abel M, Cheng H. CNS somatosensory-auditory interactions elicit or modulate tinnitus. Exp Brain Res. 2003;153(4):643-8.
5. Pinchoff RJ. Burkard RF, Salvi RJ, Coad ML, Lockwood AH. Modulation of tinnitus by voluntary Jaw movements. Am J Otol. 1998;19(6):785-9.
6. Cacase AT, Lovely TJ, Parnes SM, et al. Gaze- evoked tinnitus following unilateral peripheral auditory deafferentation : A case for anomalous cross modal plasticity . In: Salvi RJ, Henderson D, et al (editors). Auditory system plasticty and Regeneration. New York: Thieme Medical Publishers; 1996. pp 354-8.
7. Lockwood AH, Salvi RJ, Coad ML, Towsley ML, Wack DS, Murphy BW. The functional neuroanatomy of tinnitus: Evidence from limbic system links and neuronal plasticity. Neurology. 1998;50:114-20.
8. Penner MJ, Coles RR. Indication for aspirin as a palliative for tinnitus caused by spontaneous acoustic emissions: A Case study. British Journal of Audiology. 1992;26:92-6.
9. Denk DM, Heinz I H, Franz P, Ehrenberger K. Caroverine in tinnitus treatment. A placebo–controlled blind study. Acta Otolaryngol. 1997;117:825-30.
10. Veuillet E, Collet L, Distant F Morgon A. Tinnitus and medical cochlear efferent system. In: Aran JM , Dauman R (eds). Tinnitus 91. Proceedings of the IV international Tinnitus seminar, Bordeaux. Amsterdam, New York: Kregler Publications; 1992:205-9.
11. Caspary DM, Salvi RJ, Helfert RH, Brozoski TJ Bauer CA. Neuropharmacology of noise-induced hearing loss in brainstem auditory structures. In : Henderson D. Prasher D, Kopke R, Salvi R, Hamernik R (eds). Noise-induced hearing loss: Basic mechanisms. Prevention and Control. London: Noise Research Network Publications; 2001:169-83.
12. Eggermont JJ. Physiological mechanisms and neural models . In: Tyler R (ed). Tinnitus handbook. San Diego: Singular; 2000. 85-122.
13. Kalterbach JA. Neurophysiologic mechanisms of Tinnitus. J Am Acad Audiol. 2000;11(3):125-37.
14. Muhlnickel W, Elber T, Taub E, Flor H. Reorganization of auditory cortex. Proc Natl Acad Sci USA. 1998;95:10340-3.
15. Ressler KJ, Numeroff CB. Role of serotonergic and noradrenergic systems in the pathophysiology of depression and anxjety. Depression and anxiety. 2000;12:2-19.
16. Weissman JL, Hirsch BE. Imaging of Tinnitus: A review. Radiology. 2000;216:342-9.
17. Vernon JA, Meikle MB. Masking devices and alpram treatment for tinnitus. Otolaryngoscopic clinics of North America. 2003;36:2007-20.
18. Zwicker E. Masking in normal ears—psycho-acoustical facts and physiological correlates. In: Feldmann H (ed). Proceedings of the III international Tinnitus .seminare, Münster. Karlsruhe: Harsch Verlag; 1987.214-23.
19. Penner MJ, Burns E. Dissociation of spontaneous acoustic emissions and Tinnitus. Journal of Speech and Hearing Research. 1987;30:396-403.
20. Vernon J. Tinnitus causes, evaluation and treatment in otolaryngology. In: English GM (Ed). Otolaryngology. Philadelphia: JB Lippincott Co; 1992:1-25.
21. Sukhtankar VK. Tinnitus. Otolaryngology review. In: Shah VH, Karnik P. 2000. Page-127.
22. Cruz OLM, Kasse CA, Sanchez M, Barbosa F. Serotonin reuptake inhibitors in auditory processing disorders in elderly patients: Preliminary results. laryngoscope. 2004;114:1656-9.
23. Bumby AE, Strephens SDG. Clonazepam in the treatment of Tinnitus–a pilot study. Journal of Audiological Medicine. 1997;6:98-104.
24. Sakata H, Kozima Y, Koyama S, Furuya N, Sakata E. Treatment of cochlear Tinnitus with Transtympanic infusion of 4% Lidocaine into the tympanic cavity. International Tinnitus Journal. 2001;7: 46-50.
25. http://trusted.md/blog/alvinhop/2010/06/02 tinnitus_treatment_surgery_ as a_treatment_for_tinnitus#axzzzvfolhq24
26. Jastreboff PJ. 'Tinnitus retraining therapy. Progress in brain research. 2007;166:415-23.

Tumors of Temporal Bone

Jaimanti Bakshi, Abdul Wadood

Tumors of temporal bone are very rare with benign tumors more common than malignancies. Squamous cell carcinoma of the temporal bone comprises only less than 0.2% of the head and neck malignancies. However, among all the three primordial layers, the neoplasms which arise from the temporal bone vary. However, at the initial presentation they are known to resemble each other and also with other non-neoplastic conditions like Wegener's granulomatosis, fibrous dysplasia or eosinophilic granuloma.

CLASSIFICATION

Tumors of temporal bone can be easily divided to benign and malignant (Table 1). Another better way of dividing the tumors is according to the tissue of origin (Table 2). This is easy to understand and remember.

Clinical Presentation

Early presentation of temporal bone tumors can be very misleading and subtle. They can be easily misdiagnosed as non-neoplastic conditions like chronic suppurative otitis media or eosinophilic granuloma. Initially, the patient may complain of otalgia, otorrhea, hearing loss, tinnitus or imbalance. Usually, these people receive prolonged periods of conservative treatment before the doctor orders a biopsy due to unresponsiveness or when more sinister symptoms like facial palsy or bleeding occur. Biopsy is the only way to confirm the diagnosis.

Advanced tumors present with symptoms of local spread and depend on the site of origin, pattern of spread and aggressiveness of the tumor.

Glandular Tumors

Glandular tumors arise from the glands of the external auditory canal, middle ear and endolymphatic sac. The

Table 1: Tumors of temporal bone

Benign	*Malignant*
Vestibular schwannoma	Squamous cell carcinoma
Glomus tumors	Rhabdomyosarcoma
Ceruminous adenoma	Ceruminous adenocarcinoma
Hemangioma	Chondrosarcoma
Osteoma	Leukemia
Choristoma	Lymphoma
Facial nerve schwannoma	Endolymphatic sac tumors
Chordoma	Malignant melanoma

external auditory canal contains the sebaceous glands and the modified apocrine gland called the ceruminous glands. The tumors of the external auditory canal include ceruminous adenoma and adeno carcinoma, chordoma, pleomorphic adenoma, and adenoid cystic carcinoma.[1]

Ceruminous adenoma arises from the ceruminous glands. They can be either in a solid, cystic or papillary pattern. Ceruminous adenocarcinoma is the malignant counterpart of ceruminous adenoma and is often difficult to distinguish. They grow very slowly like an adenoma and show very little malignant features other than invasiveness. Local recurrence is common after surgery and hence wide local excision is mandated. Radiotherapy has no role in adenoma. However, for adenocarcinoma, postoperative radiotherapy is the best treatment.

Pleomorphic adenoma is similar to any other area. It has to be excised with adequate margin to prevent spillage and local recurrences.

Adenoid cystic carcinoma is slow growing with perineural and perivascular invasion. They can be either cribriform solid or tubular pattern. They can also show significant local tissue destruction. Lymph nodal metastasis is known to occur. Wide local excision with postoperative

Table 2: Tumors of temporal bone based on the tissue of origin

Cutaneous	Glandular	Vascular	Paraganglioma	Bone	Neural	Other
Squamous cell papilloma and carcinoma	Ceruminous adenoma and carcinoma	Hemangioma	Glomus tumors	Rhabdomyosarcoma	Meningeoma	Dermoid
Basal cell papilloma and carcinoma	Chordoma	Hemangiopericytoma		Chondrosarcoma		Teratoma
Malignant melanoma	Pleomorphic adenoma	Leukemia		Ewing sarcoma		Choristoma
	Adenocystic carcinoma	Lymphoma and plasmacytoma		Osteogenic sarcoma		
	Endolymphatic sac tumors					
	Middle ear adenoma					

radiotherapy is considered the treatment of choice. However, bone and perineural involvement are poor prognostic factors. The overall prognosis is poor due to recurrences.

Middle ear adenoma is rare tumor. It primarily arises from the middle ear and it can be easily confused with adenomatous tumors, carcinoid tumors and adeno carcinoma. It usually does not show any local invasiveness or distant metastasis and hence can easily be treated by local excision.

Tumors of the endolymphatic sac are rare tumors previously called the aggresive papillary middle ear tumors.[2] They are very aggressive with local bone destruction and intracranial extension. They usually present as unilateral slowly progressive sensory neural hearing loss. On histopathology, they show a typical papillary structure composed of cuboidal or low columnar cells. Metastatic spread is not reported. Intracranial extension into the posterior cranial fossa is seen. An association between the tumor and Von hippel lindau disease has also been suggested. Surgical excision is the treatment of choice. Owing to the slow growth of the tumor, even partial excision can be tried as the morbidity of radical surgery may be more than the tumor itself and the patient may live his life with the disease. Radiotherapy is used only as an adjuct in inoperable cases or as a palliative therapy.

Sarcoma

Rhabdomyosarcoma is an extremely rare tumor in adults, but more common in children. They arise from the striated muscles and are very aggressive. The overall incidence of the temporal bone sarcoma may be less, but among the head and neck , the ear is the 3rd most common site after nasopharynx and the orbit.[3] As mentioned, they are commonly seen in children, i.e. less than 12 years old. They can present as a mass or polyp in the ear, ear discharge,

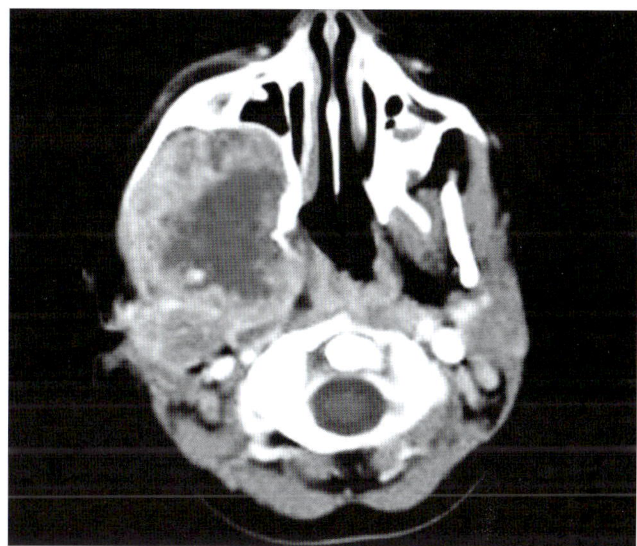

Fig. 1: Rhabdomyosarcoma extending into infratemporal fossa

bleeding from ear, otalgia, hearing loss or facial paralysis. Histologically, they are divided into embryonal, alveolar, pleomorphic and botyroid types. HRCT temporal bone (Fig. 1) would provide the extent of bony involvement and MRI would show the soft tissue involvement. But apart from this, CT chest, bone scan and lumbar puncture are advisable to rule out other system involvements. The Intergroup Rhabdomyosarcoma Study (IRS) has staged the disease into four stages. Stage 1 is localized disease completely resected, stage 2 is grossly resected disease with microscopic residual disease with or without lymph node involvement, stage 3 being those with gross residual disease and stage 4 is the disease with metastasis at the time of presentation. Since temporal bone Rhabdomyosarcoma is detected later, majority falls in stage 3 or 4. The treatment of Rhabdomyosarcoma includes multimodality treatments consisting of chemotherapy, radiotherapy and surgery.

Cutaneous Tumors

Squamous cell carcinoma is the most common malignancy of the temporal bone comprising 80%. Literature gives varied statistics regarding sex predilection with some series mentioning male preponderance and some female preponderance. Most common age of presentation is the 7th decade. There is not much evidence present to support the coexistence of chronic suppurative otitis media and squamous cell carcinoma as an etiological factor. Radiotherapy for nasopharyngeal carcinoma or other intracranial malignancies are also considered as etiological factors.

Clinical Features and Tumor Spread

Since many patients already have coexistent chronic suppurative otitis media,[4] they have long periods of ear discharge. It is only when other complaints like blood stained discharge, pain, facial palsy, growth from the ear (Fig. 2) etc. arise that suspicion of malignancy is made. Further progression of the disease can lead to other symptoms due to local invasion and destruction (Fig. 3).[5] Patients can also present with cervical lymphadenopathy in preauricular or occipital nodes involvement.

Biopsy from the lesion would confirm the diagnosis. HRCT of the temporal bone (Fig. 4) in axial and coronal plane would accurately delineate the tumor extent. All the walls of the external auditory canal, middle ear, the jugular fossa, carotid canal, tegmen, sinus plate, otic capsule and infratemporal bone extension have to be looked for. MR scans with gadolinium DTPA enhancement can help if soft tissue extension like infratemporal fossa, perineural invasion, dural and intracranial extension has to be evaluated.

Staging

There are many staging systems in practice. But the university of Pittsburg classification by Arriga et al.[6] (Table 3) is the most recently accepted.

Treatment

Surgical excision by way of en bloc resection is the treatment of choice even though associated with high levels of morbidity. The type of resection depends on the extent of disease. Even though not proposed nowadays, sleeve resection can be done if only the cartilaginous part of the external auditory canal is involved.

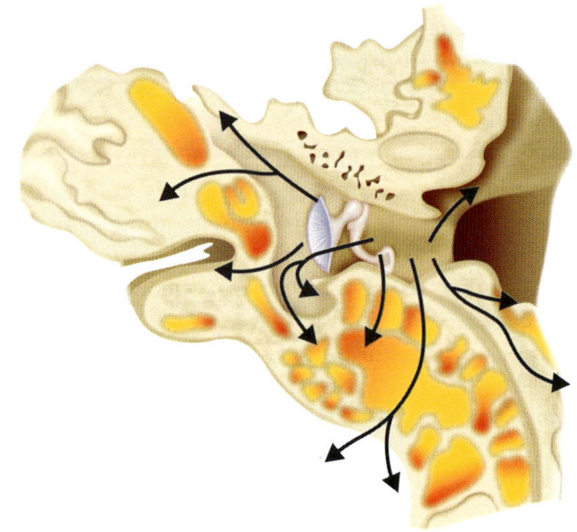

Fig. 3: Tumor spread

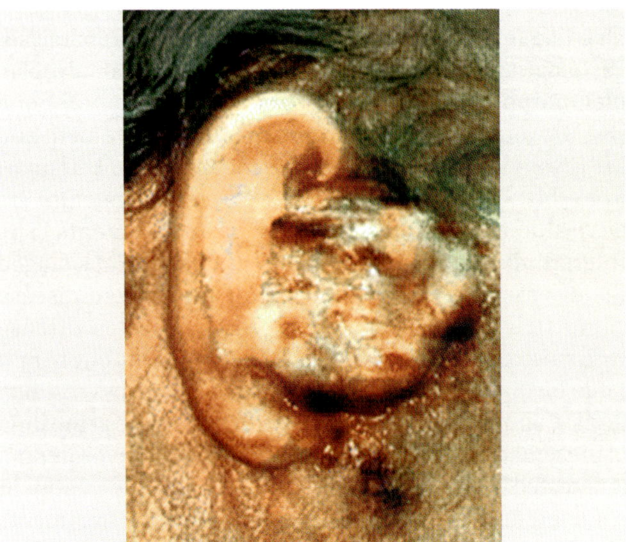

Fig. 2: Squamous cell carcinoma of temporal bone

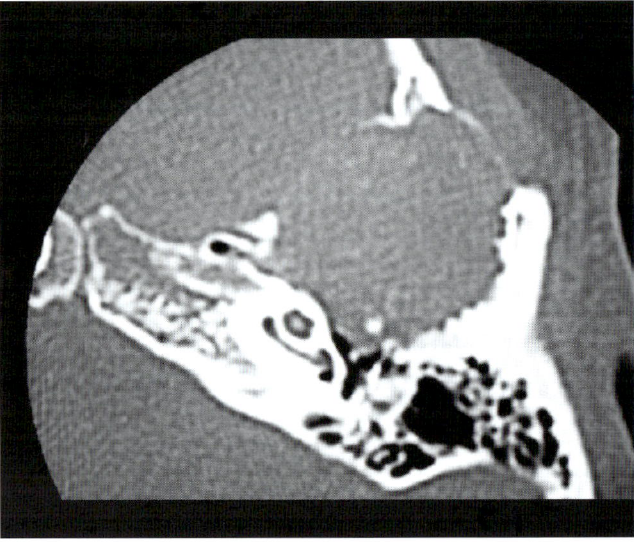

Fig. 4: CT scan of squamuous cell carcinoma of temporal bone

Table 3: Staging system

Stage	Description
T1	Tumor limited to external auditory canal without bony erosion or soft tissue extension
T2	Tumor with limited external auditory canal erosion or limited (0.05 cm) soft tissue extension
T3	Tumor eroding the osseous EAC (full thickness) with limited (0.05 cm) soft tissue involvement of middle ear or mastoid
T4	Tumor eroding the cochlear, petrous apex, medial wall of middle ear, carotid canal, jugular foramen, dura, facial nerve with extensive soft tissue involvement (>0.05 cm)

Lateral Temporal Bone Resection

For T1 and T2 lesions, lateral temporal bone resection would adequately remove the disease.

Important Steps

1. The pinna can be either excised or preserved according to the lateral extent of the disease and aesthetic requirement of the patient.
2. A cortical mastoidectomy with a posterior tympanotomy is performed delineating the facial nerve from the geniculate ganglion to the stylomastoid foramen.
3. Anterosuperiorly drilling is extended along the middle cranial fossa plate into the temporomandibular joint. The articular disc can be excised or the mandibular condyle is resected to achieve adequate tumor margin.
4. Inferiorly, the hypotympanum is drilled cutting the chorda tympani nerve.
5. The mastoid air cell system and the Eustachian tube are obliterated.
6. If possible, the tumor is removed en bloc with superficial lobe of parotid and neck dissection.

Extended (Total) Temporal Bone Resection

This is done for tumor that extends beyond the boundaries of external auditory canal, i.e. the T3 and T4 lesions.

Important Steps

1. Pinna has to be completely removed along with margins from adjacent scalp and skin.
2. 3 cm of bone above the middle cranial fossa tegmen plate and behind the sigmoid sinus is removed creating posterior and middle craniotomy.
3. The sigmoid sinus and the jugular bulb are delineated and dissection is made medially preserving the cortex

and proceeding medially to remove the labyrinth and transpetrous to expose the internal carotid artery petrous part.

4. The middle cranial fossa dura is retracted and looked for any intracranial involvement.
5. Inferiorly the sternocleidomastoid is freed from the mastoid tip and sigmoid sinus is ligated. The IX, X, XI cranial nerves are preserved only if not involved clinically and on gross examination.
6. The masseter is removed from the mandible and the ramus of the mandible is removed. The vertical ramus, coronoid process and condyle are removed along with the specimen.
7. The parotid gland is also resected anteriorly.
8. The entire specimen along with the entire structures lateral to the petrous internal carotid artery is removed en bloc. The petrous bone medial to the internal carotid artery can be removed separately, if required for margin.
9. The defect is reconstructed by various methods like temporalis flap, pectoralis major myocutaneous flap, latissimus dorsi flap, trapezius or free tissue transfer.

Radiotherapy has limited role in the bone covered area and is only given postoperatively or in inoperable cases. Osteoradionecrosis and perichondritis of the pinna are dose limiting complications. Chemotherapy has not much role.

VASCULAR TUMORS

Glomus Tumors

Glomus tumors are benign vascular tumors arising from the temporal bone. They arise in relation to the jugular bulb or the promontory. They arise from specialized neural crest elements called the paraganglion cells. Accordingly, they are divided into Glomus jugulare, Glomus tympanicum and Glomus jugulotympanicum. They are also called paraganglioma or chemodectoma. But all these terms are misnomers. Temporal bone Glomus bodies are ovoid, lobulated structures which derive supply from inferior tympanic branch of ascending pharyngeal artery. They are in close relation with the Jacobson's nerve and Arnold's nerve.

Histopathology

The paraganglioma consist of chief cells and the sustentacular cells. The chief cells produce neuropeptides and catecholamines which serve as hormones, para hormones, neurohormones and neurotransmitters, etc. However, only 1–3% of paraganglioma are found to be functional. Functional tumors produce many paraneoplastic syndromes and carcinoid syndromes according to the substance they release. Sustentacular cells are supporting cells. The tendency towards malignant degeneration is determined by the ratio of chief cells to sustentacular cells.

Staging

Glasscock-Jackson has provided separate staging system for Glomus jugulare and Glomus tympanicum.

For Glomus tympanicum
Type 1 is small tumor limited to promontory.
Type 2 is tumor completely filling middle ear space.
Type 3 is tumor filling middle ear and extending into mastoid process.
Type 4 is tumor filling middle ear, extending into external auditory canal, or anterior to internal carotid artery.

For Glomus jugulare
Type 1 is tumor involving jugular bulb, middle ear and mastoid process.
Type 2 is tumor extending into the internal auditory canal, may have intracranial extension.
Type 3 is tumor extending into the petrous apex, may have intracranial extension.
Type 4 is tumor extending beyond petrous apex into the clivus and infratemporal fossa, may have intracranial extension.

Clinical Features

The patient usually presents with pulsatile tinnitus and hearing loss. The degree of sensory neural hearing loss is determined by the degree of involvement of the labyrinth. Erosion of the tympanic membrane can cause bleeding from ear. In advanced skull base erosion, symptoms of cranial nerve involvement can set in like facial nerve palsy, dysphagia, hoarseness, aspiration, tongue paralysis and shoulder drooping. On examination, the most consistent finding is a reddish mass behind the tympanic membrane (Fig. 5). The typical Browns sign of blanching on siegalization is seen in only about 30% cases. If the margins are visible all around, Glomus tympanicum is the possibility because in Glomus jugulare the inferior margin is absent. But this has to be differentiated from other differentials of reddish mesotympanic mass like high jugular bulb, facial neuroma, aberrant internal carotid artery and meningioma. Biopsy should not be attempted due to risk of bleeding.

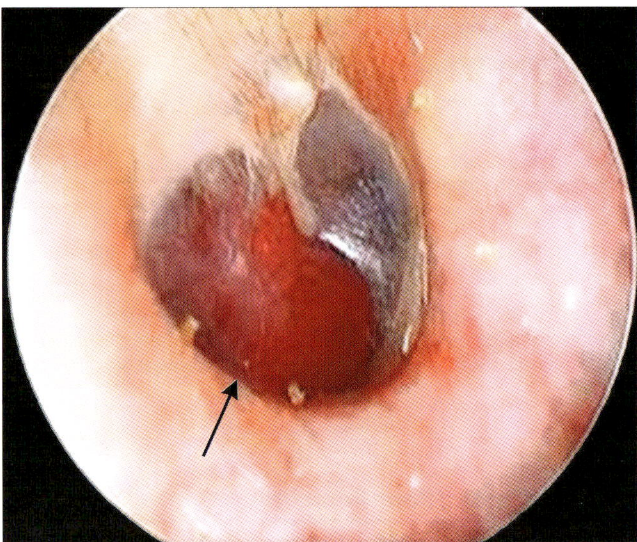

Fig. 5: Otoscopy finding in glomus jugulare

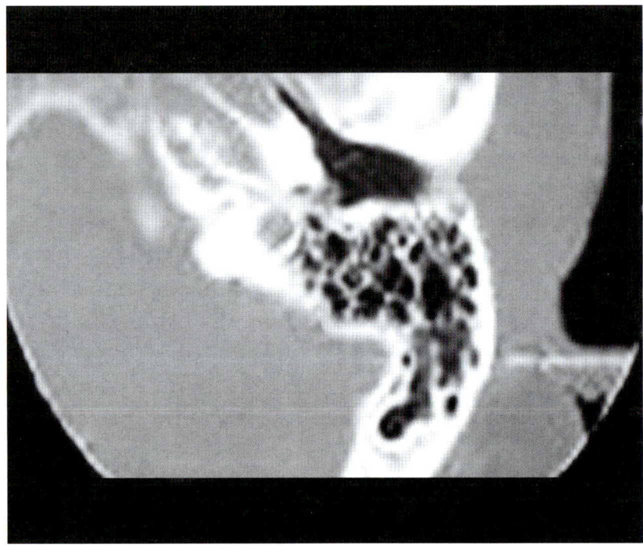

Fig. 6: CT picture of glomus tympanicum

Investigations

High resolution computerized tomography in axial and coronal planes is the best investigation. This would help to assess the extent of tumor and more importantly differentiate between Glomus tympanicum (Fig. 6) and jugulare (Fig. 7). If Glomus tympanicum is diagnosed usually no further investigation is required except when functional features are seen. If Glomus jugulare is detected, then for extensive lesions MRI (Fig. 8) is advised for assessing intracranial and soft tissue extension and to assess for multicentricity. Carotid angiography can be

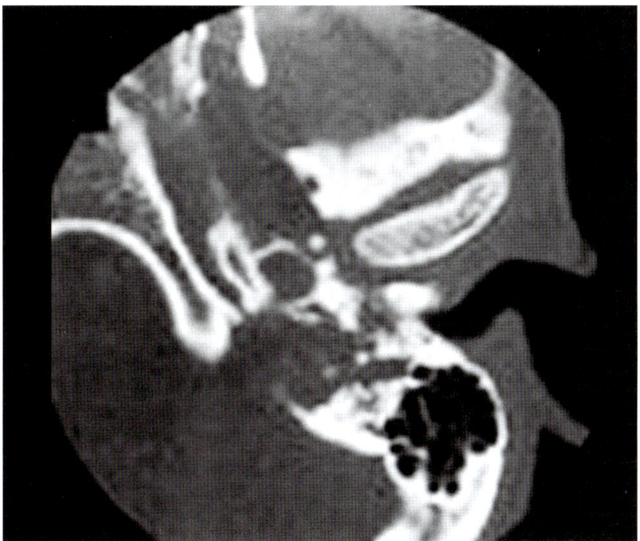

Fig. 7: CT with glomus jugulare

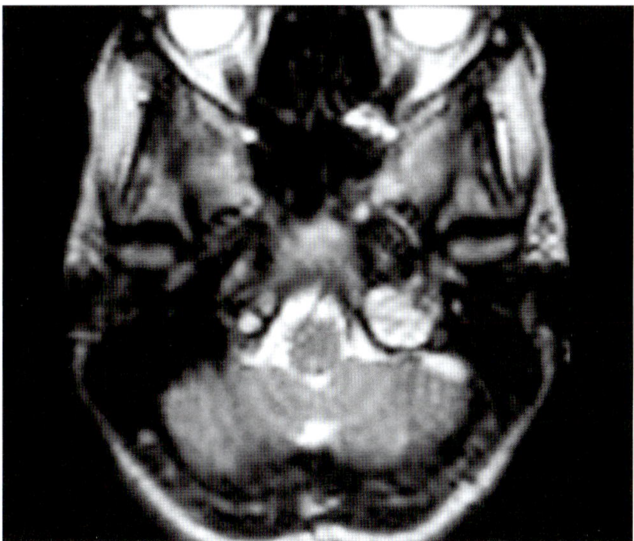

Fig. 8: MRI of glomus tympanicum

done to assess the involvement of the carotid artery and for embolization. Once embolised, the tumor has to be excised within 72 hours. For familial cases and those having neuroendocrine symptoms, a catecholamines assay has to be done and pheochromocytoma has to be ruled out.

Treatment

Glomus tumors are very slow growing tumors and hence there are situations where the surgical morbidity is more than the disease itself. A wait and observe policy is adopted when in the natural course of the patient's life span, the paraganglioma is not expected to cause excessive mortality and morbidity. Annual imaging is done to assess the behavior.

The definitive treatment of paraganglioma is surgery which is curative and radiotherapy which is palliative.[7]

Surgical Treatment

The major challenges during the surgery are to access the whole margins of the tumor, to access intracranial extensions and to expose and control the major vessels and cranial nerve.

Glomus Tympanicum

For type 1 tumor where the tumor is visualized circumferentially, a transcanal removal can be performed. When the tumor margins are indistinct as in type 2–4, a transmastoid approach is done. A posterior tympanotomy approach or an extended facial recess approach is performed. By this, the tumor can be visualized and its relationship with the internal carotid artery and the

ossicles can be assessed. When this is done the inferior tympanic branch of the ascending pharyngeal artery which is the pedicle of the tumor is cauterized and the tumor is delivered. In case of ossicular damage, a conventional ossiculoplasty is done. A canal wall down procedure can be performed if there is any need for further exposure.

Glomus Jugulare

For type 1 and 2 tumors which basically involve only the tympanic segment of the internal carotid artery, a hearing conservation method should be adopted.

1. A postauricular incision is made which provides access to both the mastoid and the neck.
2. The internal carotid artery, the internal jugular vein, cranial nerves of the skull base and the extratemporal portion of facial nerve is delineated and secured with vascular loops.
3. The internal jugular vein is ligated and the sigmoid sinus is occluded.
4. Mastoidectomy is performed and extended facial recess approach is adopted. The anteroinferior wall of the external auditory canal is skeletonized exposing the tympanic part of internal carotid artery.
5. Short mobilization of the facial nerve is done, mobilizing it from the second genu drilling the stylomastoid foramen area.
6. Proximal control of the sigmoid sinus is made by surgical packing. The tumor is dissected off from the internal carotid artery and the nerves of the jugular foramen.
7. The tumor is delivered and the oozing from the inferior petrosal sinus can be dealt by surgical packing.

For Type 3 and 4 Glomus tumors, i.e. when it goes into the petrous internal carotid artery or into the infratemporal fossa, extended infratemporal fossa approaches as described by Ugo Fisch, have to be adopted.

Steps

1. Incision is similar to the previous situation.
2. The external auditory canal is cut at the level of the bony cartilaginous junction and oversewn as a blind pouch. The external auditory canal, tympanic membrane and ossicles lateral to the stapes are resected.
3. The anteromedial ligaments of the temporomandibular joint are cut and the mandible is dislocated antero inferiorly.
4. The facial nerve undergoes long mobilization, i.e. from the first genu.
5. Further steps to access the inratemporal fossa like segmental mandibulectomy, TM joint resection, resection of zygoma, detachment of temporalis muscle and inferior reflection can be performed only when wider exposure is required.
6. The Eustachian tube is resected and the content of foramen spinosum is sacrificed. This exposes the internal carotid artery at the precavernous and pterygoid region.
7. Any intracranial extension is dealt by middle cranial fossa dural plate drilling.
8. The tumor is delivered in similar fashion by carefully dissecting it off from the internal carotid artery and the cranial nerves.
9. Defect reconstruction is done according to the defect. A vascularized temporoparietal fascia based on superficial temporal artery, sternocleidomastoid musculoskeletal facial flap, free abdominal fat graft, lower trapezius flap,and rectus abdominis flap have been mentioned.

NEURAL TUMORS

Vestibular Schwannoma

Vestibular schwannoma is a benign tumor arising from the Schwann cells of the vestibular portion of the vestibule cochlear nerve (Fig. 9).

Histopathologically , they comprise of two types of cells. The Antony A type of cells are densely packed cells with small spindle-shaped nuclei which are deeply stained. This appearance is also called the Verocay body. The Antony B cells are loosely arranged and scattered.

The etiology of vestibular shwannoma is not known. However, mutation of the long arm of chromosome 22 is to be responsible for unilateral or bilateral schwannoma made as in neurofibromatosis 2. The tumor grows slowly

and fills the internal auditory meatus protruding through medial porus end. The tumor only compresses the nerves rather than invading it. There is active bone resorption by increased vascularization, fibrosis and adhesion. Bone erosion can extend superiorly into the middle cranial fossa and inferiorly to the cochlear aqueduct. Once outside the porus, the tumor grows slowly into the pontine cistern causing compression of the 7th and 8th nerves and the anterior inferior cerebellar artery. They can further grow and compress the cerebellum, trigeminal nerve and abducent nerve. The internal auditory meatus is gradually widened. Further progression can compress the brain stem and fourth ventricle causing hydrocephalus.

At the Consensus Meeting on Reporting systems on Vestibular Schwannoma at Tokyo, 2001 a classification scheme was proposed as shown in Table 4.[8]

Symptoms of vestibular schwannoma depend on the disease extent. Initially, when the vestibular nerve is involved the patient experiences vertigo. Sooner when the 8th nerve is involved, the hearing is also affected along with tinnitus. A high-frequency sensory neural hearing loss with poor speech discrimination is the usual finding. Later, the imbalance worsens further when the cerebellum and its peduncles are compressed. Midfacial and corneal anesthesia is seen when the trigeminal nerve is affected. Voice change, nasal regurgitation and dysphagia are seen when the lower cranial nerves are affected. Weakness of the limbs, headache and visual loss are seen when the brain

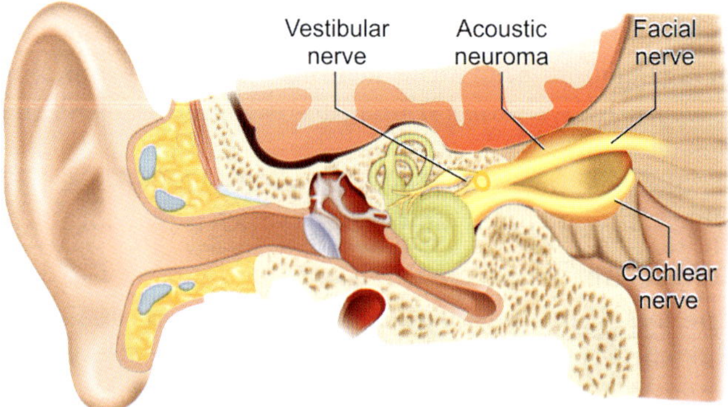

Fig. 9: Anatomy of vestibular schwannoma

Table 4: Classification scheme on vestibular schwannoma

Intrameatal tumor	Extrameatal size	mm
Grade 1	Small	1–10
Grade 2	Medium	11–20
Grade 3	Moderately large	21–30
Grade 4	Large	31–40
Grade 5	Giant	>40

stem is compressed and hydrocephalus develops. There are two variants of vestibular schwannoma. The medial vestibular schwannoma is a pure medial location of tumor, without intrameatal component. The internal auditory meatus is of normal size and is filled with yellow cerebro spinal fluid of high protein content. A cystic vestibular schwannoma is a cystic degeneration of the Antoni A cells of vestibular schwannoma.

Both high-resolution computerized tomography (Fig. 10) and gadolinium-enhanced magnetic resonance imaging (Fig. 11) are required for assessement of the tumor. Computerized tomography will give good details about the intracanalicular part and the amount of bony destruction and erosion. The magnetic resonance imaging is necessary to assess the intracranial part of the tumor.

Surgery is the treatment of choice for these tumors. However, in elderly patients, a wait and imaging protocol can be adopted as they are very slow growing and the surgical morbidity may be more than the disease morbidity. There are three approaches to remove these tumors, each having their pros and cons. A translabyrinthine approach avoids cerebellar retraction and postoperative ataxia, destroying residual hearing in the patient. The middle cranial fossa approach protects the residual hearing, but needs brain retraction and facial nerve injury. The retrosigmoid approach needs cerebellar retraction and has poor visualization of the fundus.

Facial Nerve Schwannoma

Facial nerve schwannoma though rare is the most common tumor of facial nerve. They are benign and very slow growing and as a result are detected late. As the name suggests they arise from the Schwann cells of the nerve sheath. They grow eccentrically from the nerve sheath and cause compression of the nerve. They mostly arise from the geniculate ganglion followed by the labyrinthine portion. They can present in any age and do not show any sex predeliction.

Histopathologically, they are composed of two types of cells, Antoni A cells which are compact interwoven bundles of cells with pallisading appearance of nuclei and the Antoni B cells which are scattered loosely arranged cells. Gradually, progressing facial palsy is the most common presenting symptom. Patients may have premonitory features like facial tingling, muscle fasciculations or hemifacial spasm. Sudden onset facial palsy has also been reported. The patient may also present with recurrent facial palsy with gradual progression of the weakness.[9] Other symptoms include hearing loss, which may be conductive, sensory neural or mixed according to the segment of nerve affected and pathway of spread. Rare presentations include otalgia, otorrhea and loss of taste sensation. High-resolution magnetic resonance imaging with gadolinium enhancement is the investigation of choice as it can detect even very small tumors of millimeters of size. Once the diagnosis is made, a HRCT can provide details regarding the extent of bony destruction and spread. Other investigations may include pure tone audiogram for assessment of hearing and electroneuronography to assess the percentage of nerve fibers involved by the tumor. Topodiagnostic tests, though not useful after the advent of radiology can be used to identify the site of lesion. Biopsy should never be attempted as they can lead to facial palsy. Even though surgery is the main stay of treatment, the merits

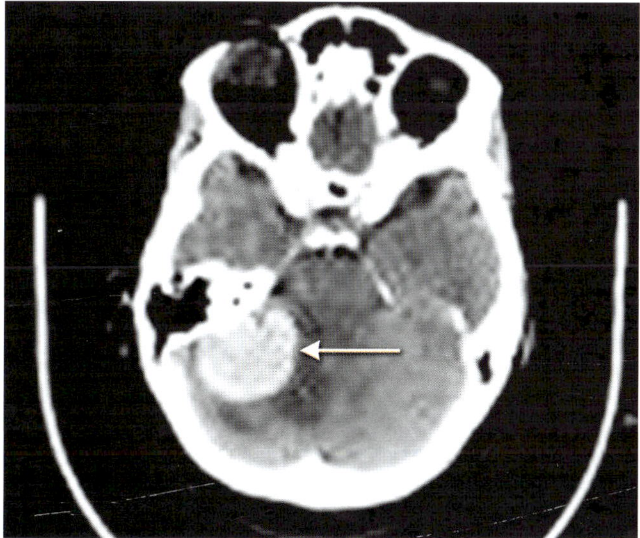

Fig. 10: CT with vestibular schwannoma

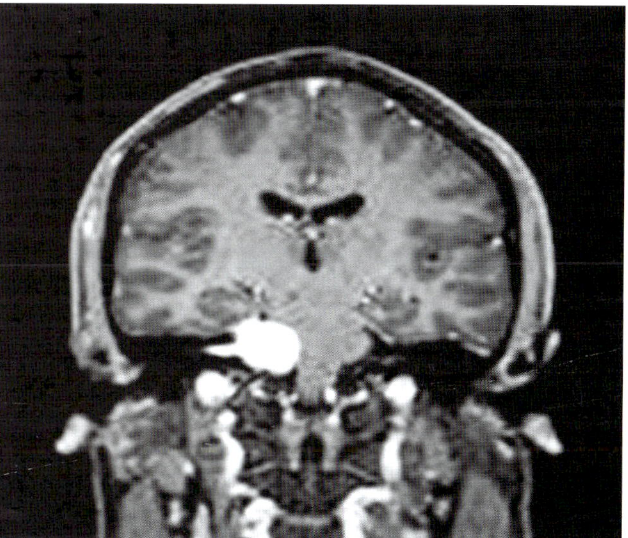

Fig. 11: MRI with vestibular schwannoma

of the surgery have to be weighed against the morbidities. A young patient with a small schwannoma and normal functioning facial nerve has to be counseled regarding the merits and demerits of surgery versus observation. Similarly, a small tumor in an elderly patient can also be managed by observation.

Surgery is the mainstay of treatment and the route and approach are determined by the site and extent of lesion. A small tumor of 2–3 mm size involving the geniculate ganglion and internal auditory meatus can be accessed by a middle cranial fossa approach. This would provide less morbidity in terms of hearing preservation. If the tumor is larger and involves the horizontal segment of the facial nerve with intracranial extension, a translabyrinthine approach can be adopted. For tumor involving the vertical portion of the facial nerve, a transmastoid approach would suffice. All the three approaches can be combined according to the extent of tumor. After the removal of the tumor and frozen section from the cut ends to ensure complete tumor removal, the gap is either covered by end-to-end anastomosis or interposition nerve grafting using greater auricular nerve or sural nerve.

In patients with normal or near normal facial nerve function a partial debulking or stripping of the tumor from the facial nerve has been also mentioned to avoid surgical morbidity. Gamma knife and linear accelerator radiosurgery has also been mentioned as alternatives to surgery.

REFERENCES

1. Wetli CV, Pardo V, Millard M, Gerston K. Tumors of ceruminous glands. Cancer. 1972;29:1169-78.
2. Gaffey MJ, Mills SE, Fechner RE, Intmann SR, Wick MR. Aggressive papillary middle ear tumor. A clinicopathologic entity distinct from middle ear adenoma. American Journal of Clinical Pathology. 1988;12:790-7.
3. Wiatrak, BJ and Pensak ML. Rhabdomyosarcoma of the ear and temporal bone. The Laryngoscope. 1989;99:1188-92.
4. Moffat DA, Grey P, Ballagh RH, Hardy DG. Extended Temoral bone resection for squamous cell carcinoma. Otolaryngology and Head and Neck Surgery.1997;116:617-23.
5. Leonetti JP, Smith PG, Kletzker GR, Izquiredo R. Invasion patterns of advanced temporal bone malignancies. American Journal of Otology.1996;17:438-42.
6. Arriaga M, Curtin H, Hirsch BE, Takahashi H, and Kamerer DB. "Staging proposal for external auditory meatus carcinoma based on preoperative clinical examination and computed tomography findings". Annals of Otology, Rhinology and Laryngology, vol. 99, no. 9, pp. 714–721, 1990
7. Semaan MT, Megerian CA. Current assessment and management of glomus tumors. Curr Opin Otolaryngol Head Neck Surg. 2008;16(5):420-6.
8. Kanzaki J, Tos M, Sanna M, Moffat DA. New and Modified reporting systems from the consenses meeting on reporting results in vestibular schwannoma. Otology and Neurotology. 2003;24:642-8.
9. Chung JW, Ahn JH, Kim JH, Nam SY, Kim CJ, Lee KS. Facial nerve schwannomas: different manifestations and outcomes. Surg Neurol. 2004;62(3):245-52.

Radiology of EAR

Chaturbhuj L Rajak

EXTERNAL EAR

Normal anatomy

The external ear has a lateral fibrocartilaginous part (length about 8 mm) and a medial bony part (length about 16 mm). The medial boundary of external auditory canal [EAC] is tympanic membrane.

Common External Ear Diseases/Conditions

- Congenital Anomalies
  - Atresia and Hypoplasia
- Inflammatory diseases
  - Malignant otitis externa
  - Keratosis obturans
- Benign neoplasms
  - Hemangioma, vascular malformations, ceruminomas, etc.
- Malignant neoplasms
  - Squamous cell carcinoma.

Atresia and Hypoplasia

Congenital anomalies of external ear are commoner than middle ear and include total atresia, webs, hypoplasia, stenosis of the EAC, microtia (a small auricle of the ear). [1]

In Microtia, there is bony stenosis of the EAC. In major microtia, there are also associated anomalies of middle ear (reduced pneumatization of the middle ear including mastoid) and inner ear (usually lateral semicircular canal hypoplasia).

In minor microtia also there are coexistent middle ear abnormality, viz. dysplastic malleus-incus complex, abnormalities of stapes (Fig. 1).

Malignant Otitis Externa

A severe inflammatory condition due to pseudomonas infection of EAC (usually at junction of bony and cartilaginous part) in elderly diabetic or HIV infected patients. [2]

CT Findings

- Soft tissue lesion in EAC
- Erosion of bony wall of EAC
- Sclerosis of the skull base.

MRI Findings

- Soft tissue edema of external ear
- Obliteration of parapharyngeal fat
- Obliteration of fat planes around carotid sheath
- Signal alteration of skull base with enhancement of bone.

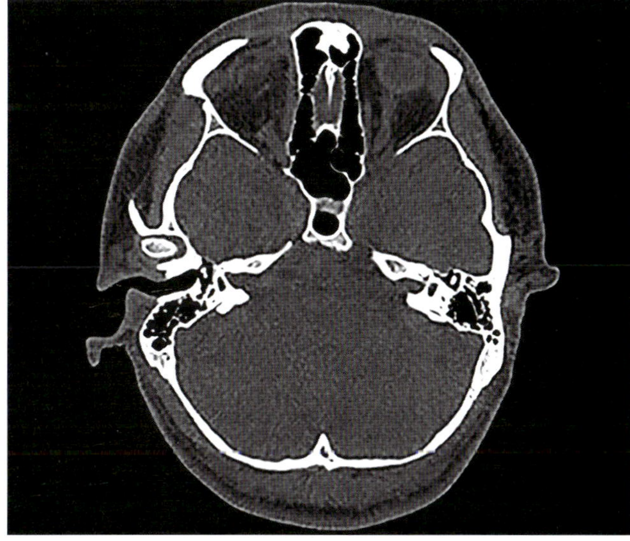

Fig. 1: Microtia—Axial computed tomography image showing bony stenosis and nonvisualization of the left external auditory canal. The middle ossicle is also dysplastic

Table 1: Differentiating points between KO and CC

KO	CC
Middle age	Old age
Very painful	Dull pain
Bilateral	Unilateral
Bone erosion is limited to external ear	More bone erosion and extends from middle ear to external ear

Keratosis Obturans

Keratosis obturans (KO) gives rise to a soft tissue lesion in EAC which is due to plugs of keratin.[3] These may be difficult to distinguish from congenital cholesteatoma (CC) if it infiltrate the EAC from middle ear. The differentiating points between the two are given in the table 1.

EAC Masses

EAC masses may be benign (Hemangioma, vascular malformations, polyps, minor salivary gland tumors, adenoma of ceruminous glands—ceruminomas) or malignant (squamous cell carcinoma).

Benign masses usually expand the EAC and cause bony scalloping. Malignant masses cause bone destruction and extension to middle ear, inner ear or temporomandibular joints.

MIDDLE EAR

Normal Anatomy

The middle ear cavity or tympanic cavity has three parts:
1. Epitympanic recess or attic—superior part.
2. Mesotympanum—the portion of the middle ear directly behind the tympanic membrane.
3. Hypotympanum—inferior to mesotympanum.

Tympanic membrane forms the lateral boundary of the middle ear. The handle of malleus attaches to the tympanic membrane at umbo.

The tympanic membrane is attached superiorly at scutum, which is a bony spur at superomedial margin of the EAC. The scutum is best seen in coronal images (Figs 2 and 3).

Malleus, incus and stapes are the three middle ear ossicles. Malleus has a head, neck, anterior process, lateral process and manubrium. Incus has body, short and long processes. Stapes has head, anterior crus, posterior crus and footplate.

The head of malleus articulates with the short process of the incus and gives rise to "icecream cone" appearance.

The long process (lenticular process) of incus articulates with the head of stapes. The footplate of stapes covers the oval window.

Tensor tympani muscle attaches to manubrium and neck of malleus. Stapedius muscle attaches to head of stapes.

Facial nerve traverses through middle ear after exiting from the internal auditory canal. Facial nerve lies in the anterosuperior part of the internal auditory canal which is separated by crista falciformis into superior and inferior parts. The labyrinthine part of the facial nerve courses anterosuperiorly and laterally from the internal auditory canal to geniculate ganglion. The geniculate ganglion lies above the cochlea, where the facial nerve forms its first genu. The horizontal (tympanic) part of the facial nerve courses posteroinferiorly and laterally from the geniculate ganglia on the undersurface of the lateral semicircular canal up to the facial nerve recess in the posteroinferior wall of the tympanic cavity. The facial nerve then makes its second genu. The descending (intramastoid) part of the facial nerve then courses inferiorly through the mastoid bone and emerges out at the stylomastoid foramen.

Common Middle Ear Disease/Conditions

Epidermoids (Congenital Cholesteatoma)

The most common site for skull base congenital epidermoid is temporal bone and the typical common locations for these lesions are the petrous apex, Koerner's septum (petrosquamosal suture) and mastoid air cells. [4]

CT/MRI Findings

- In MRI, epidermoids are hypointense in T1-weighted images, hyperintense in T2-weighted images and are brighter than CSF on FLAIR (fluid attenuated inversion recovery) and diffusion-weighted images
- On CT scan, these usually appear as a well-circumscribed hypodense lesion in temporal bone which causes bone erosion and scalloping. The scutum is usually intact
- Epidermoids may be solid or cystic and do not enhance while acquired cholesteatoma sometimes show peripheral enhancement. Patients with acquired cholesteatoma also have concomitant perforation of tympanic membrane, ear infections or previous ear surgeries.

Otitis Media

Otitis media is the inflammation of the tympanic cavity which is common in children.[5,6]

CT/ MRI Findings

- Opacification of epitympanic recess
- Fluid density in CT scan and fluid intensity in MR scan are seen filling the middle ear cavity (Figs 4 and 5).
- Thickening of tympanic membrane

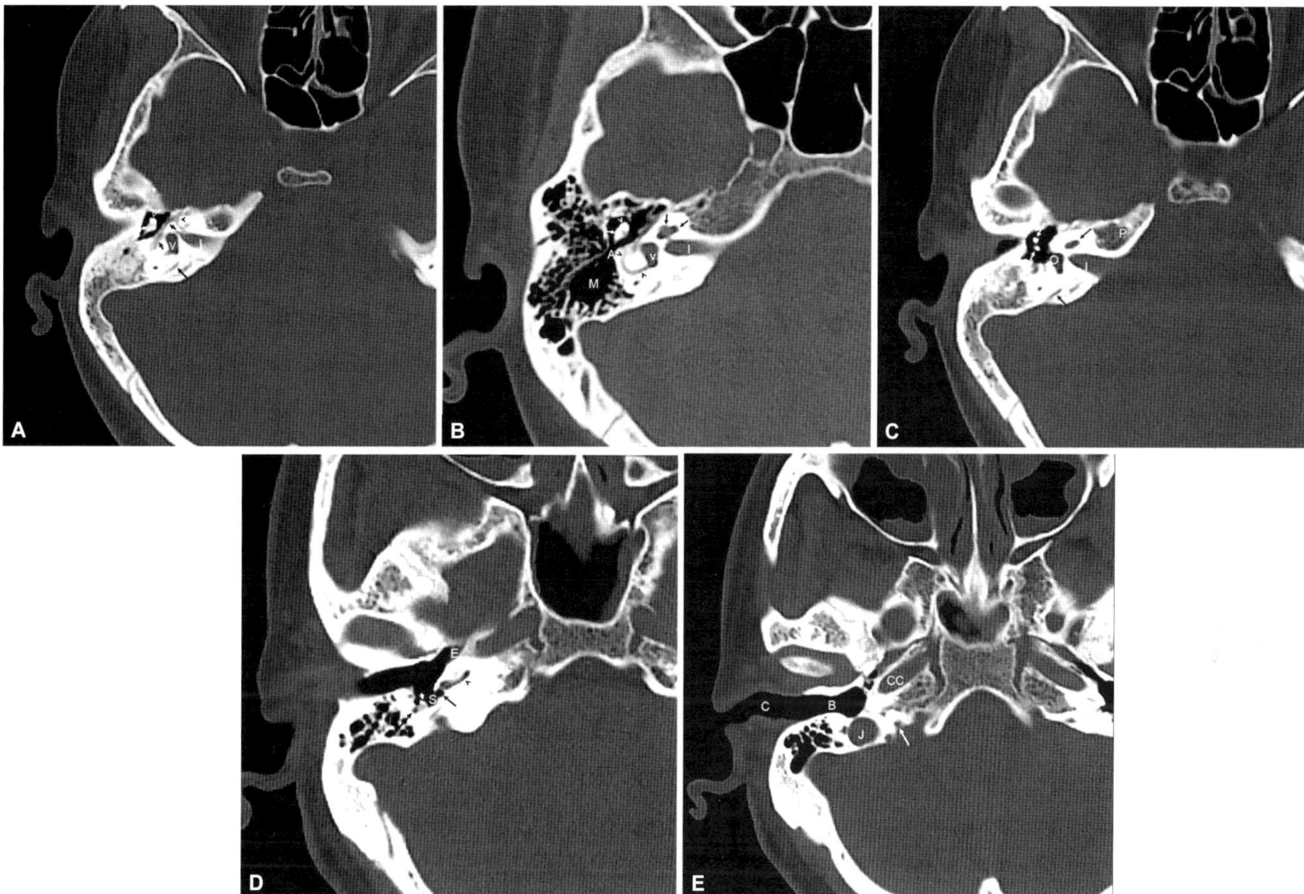

Figs 2A to E: Axial computed tomography of normal anatomy of the middle ear from cranial to caudal region. (A) Labyrinthine part of the facial nerve (black arrowhead), horizontal segment of the facial nerve (small black arrows), head of malleus (short white arrow), short process of incus (long white arrow), vestibule, internal auditory canal, vestibular aqueduct (long black arrow); (B) Head of malleus (short white arrow), short process of incus (long white arrow), aditus ad antrum, mastoid antrum, vestibule, lateral semicircular canal (black arrowheads), apical turn of cochlea (short black arrow), middle turn of cochlea (long black arrow), internal auditory canal; (C) Neck of malleus (short white arrow), long process of incus (long white arrow), oval window, vestibular aqueduct (short black arrow), basal turn of cochlea (long black arrow), internal auditory canal, petrous apex; (D) Cranial aspect of the Eustachian tube, tensor tympani tendon, apical turn of cochlea (black arrowhead), basal turn of cochlea (short black arrow), round window niche (long black arrow), sinus tympani, pyramidal eminence (short white arrow), facial nerve recess (long white arrow); (E) Cartilaginous and bony part of external auditory canal, jugular bulb, carotid canal, cochlear aqueduct (white arrow).
Abbreviations: V, vestibule; I, internal auditory canal; A, aditus adantrum; M, mastoid antrum; P, petrous apex; O, oval window; E, Eustachian tube; S, sinus tympani; C, cartilaginous; B, bony; J, jugular bulb; CC, carotid canal

- Obstruction of Eustachian tube
- Increased density and sclerosis of the mastoid seen in chronic otits media (Fig. 6)
- Ossicular erosions, seen in chronic infection, are rare and usually affect the long process of incus—ossicular erosion is usually a marker of acquired cholesteatoma
- In CT scan, the ossicular erosion appears as small lytic punched out lesion in ossicle
- Presence of air in inner ear in middle ear infection suggests a labyrinthine fistula

- Ossicular disruption may be seen in chronic infection but are usually caused by trauma
- A gap of 1 mm between the long process of incus and head of stapes is diagnostic of disruption
- May be seen in axial as well as coronal section
- Inflammatory processes cause erosion of the long process of incus and fibrosis causing disruption
- Incudostapedial joint is most commonly affected by trauma, hence dislocation and subluxation are common between incus and stapes

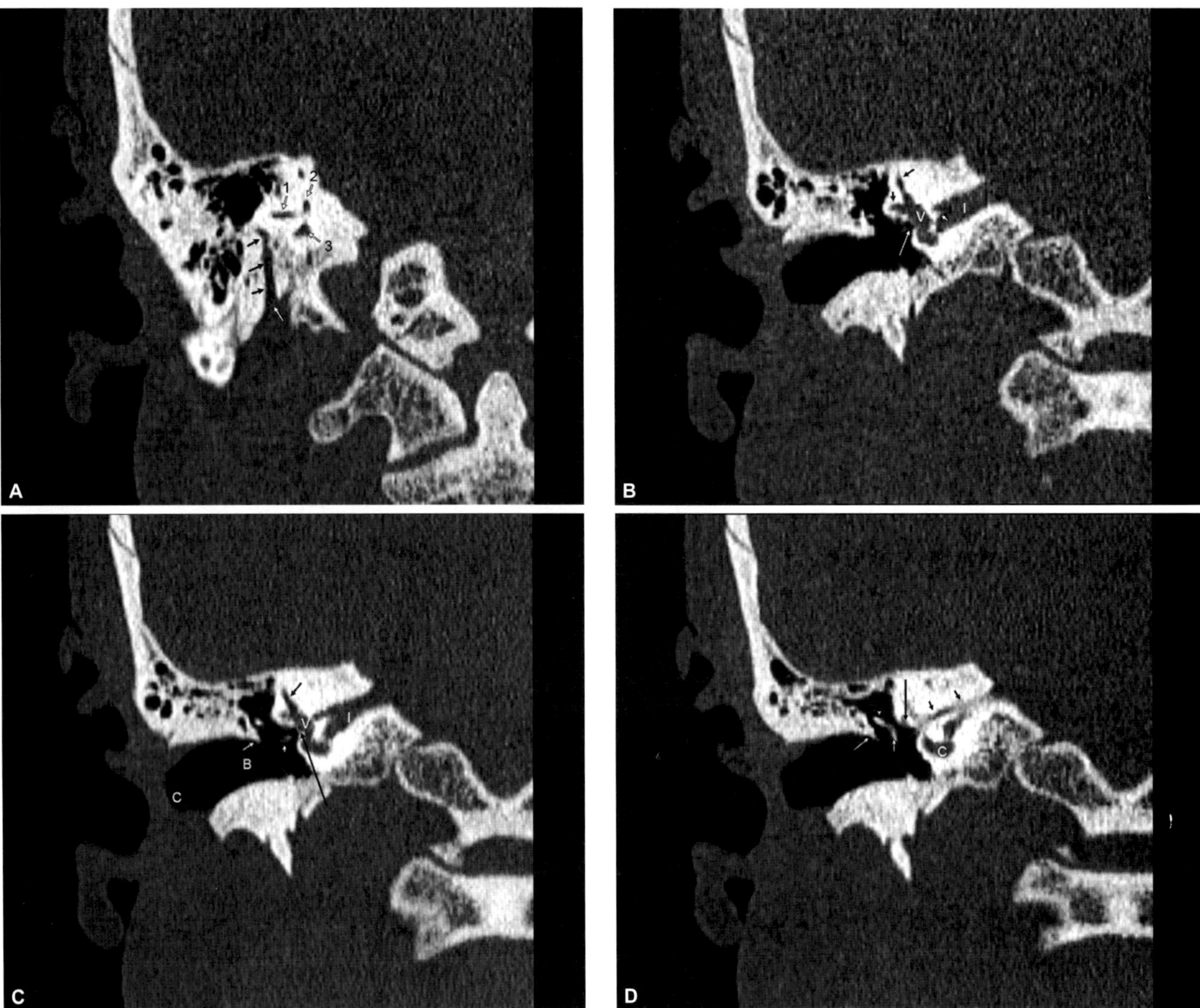

Figs 3A to D: Coronal computed tomography of the normal anatomy of the middle ear from anterior to posterior aspect. (A) Descending part of the facial nerve (black arrows), stylomastoid foramen (white arrow), lateral (arrow 1) and superior (arrow 2) semicircular canal, vestibule (arrow 3); (B) Scutum (long white arrow), head and neck of malleus (white arrowhead), incus (short white arrow), tympanic segment of the facial nerve (long black arrow), cochlea, facial nerve over cochlea (short black arrows); (C) Cartilaginous and bony part of external auditory canal, scutum (long white arrow), stapes (short white arrow), oval window (long black arrow), vestibule, superior semicircular canal (short black arrow), internal auditory canal; (D) Oval window (long white arrow), vestibule, lateral (short black arrow) and superior (long black arrow) semicircular canals, crista falciformis (short white arrow) of the internal auditory canal.
Abbreviations: V, vestibule; C, cochlea; C, cartilaginous; B, bony; I, internal auditory canal

- Complication of chronic otitis media:
  - Ossicular fixation
  - Tympanosclerosis—calcification around ossicles or ossicular ligaments.

Mastoiditis

Mastoiditis is the inflammation of the mastoid cells, which is usually due to spread of infection from middle ear via aditus ad antrum.[5,6]

CT/MR Findings

- Opacification of mastoid air cells
- Very bright on T2-weighted images (Figs 5A and B)
- Air-fluid levels (Fig. 7)
- Bone destruction
- Middle ear/petrous apex opacification
- Complications: Sigmoid sinus thrombosis, Epidural abscess, Meningitis, Subperiosteal abscess and Bezold's abscess. Bezold abscess is the spread of infection from

mastoid bone to the adjacent soft tissue and appears as inflammatory fluid collection inferior to tip of mastoid.

Acquired Cholesteatomas

Chronic infection of middle ear and mastoid leads to formation of cholesteatoma. It is due to ingrowth of stratified squamous epithelium through a perforated tympanic membrane or retraction pocket forming a collection of keratinous debris—cholesteatoma.[7]

CT/MRI Findings

- Cholesteatoma causes mass effect, expansion and bony erosion, which is the key point in differentiating them from otitis media without cholesteatoma

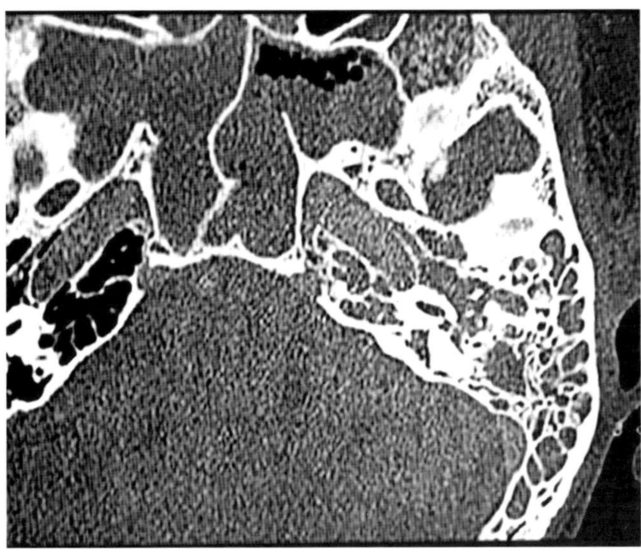

Fig. 4: Acute otitis media and mastoiditid—Axial computed tomography image showing soft tissue density in the middle ear cavity and masoid air cells. The trabecular pattern of the mastoid is maintained with no evidence of sclerosis, a finding seen in chronic mastoiditis

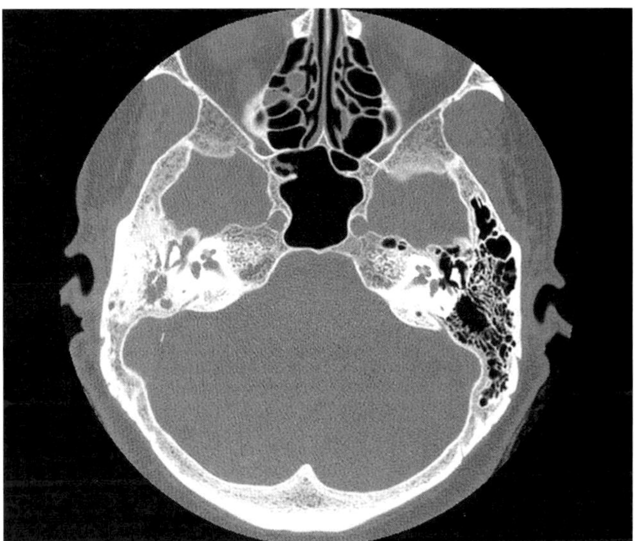

Fig. 6: Chronic suppurative otitis media and mastoiditis—Axial computed tomography image showing soft tissue density in the right tympanic cavity. Absence of body erosion and normal ossicle in this case rules out presence of cholesteatoma. The right mastoid is also sclerotic with paucity of mastoid air cells

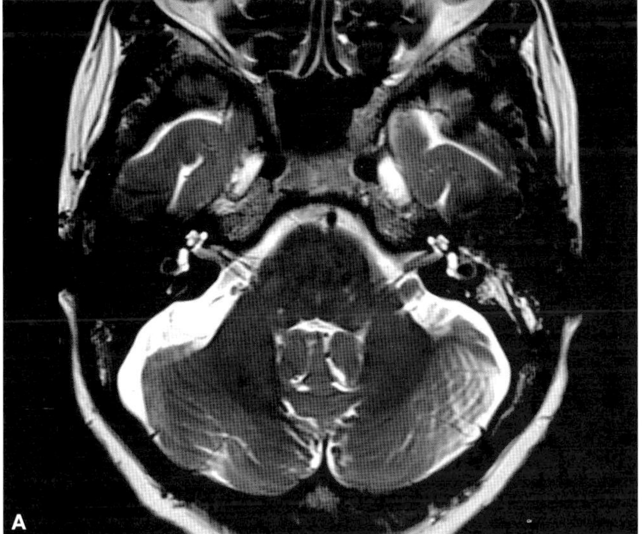

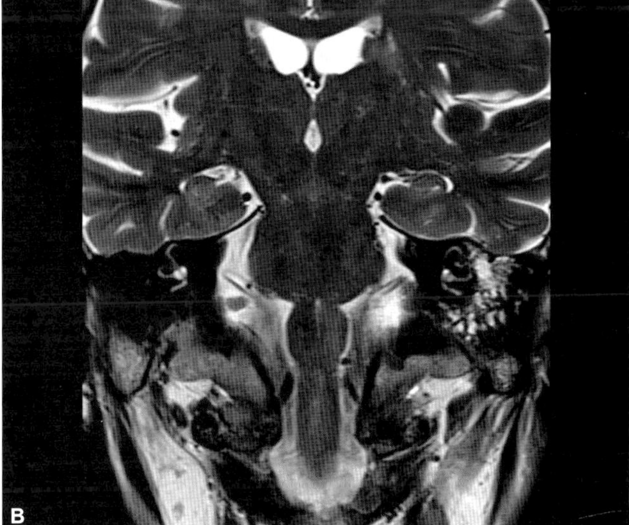

Figs 5A and B: Acute otitis media and mastoiditis—Axial (A) and Coronal (B) MRI showing high-signal intensity consistent with fluid collection and secretary changes in the middle ear cavity and mastoid air cells on left side

- Soft tissue mass in middle ear—involvement of epitympanic space, Prussak's space, middle ear cavity, hypotympanum, etc.
- Erosion of scutum (Fig. 8)
- Displacement or erosion of ossicles
- Medial displacement of malleus and incus are common
- Head of malleus and body of the incus are most vulnerable areas for erosion by pars flaccida cholesteatoma

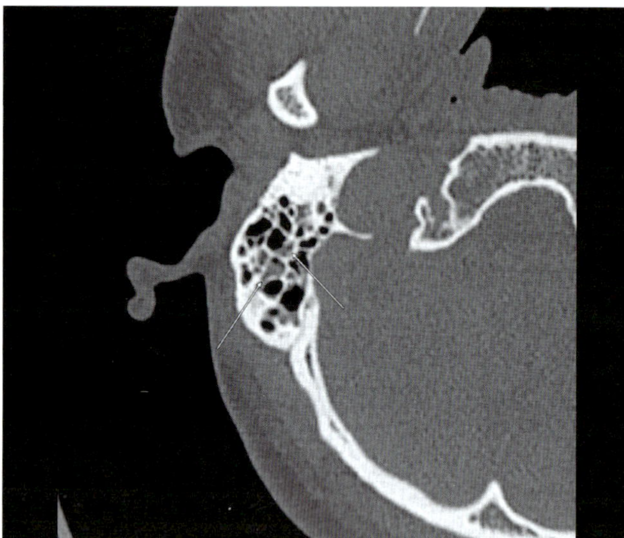

Fig. 7: Acute mastoiditis—Axial computed tomography image showing opacification of the mastoid air cells with fluid levels (arrow)

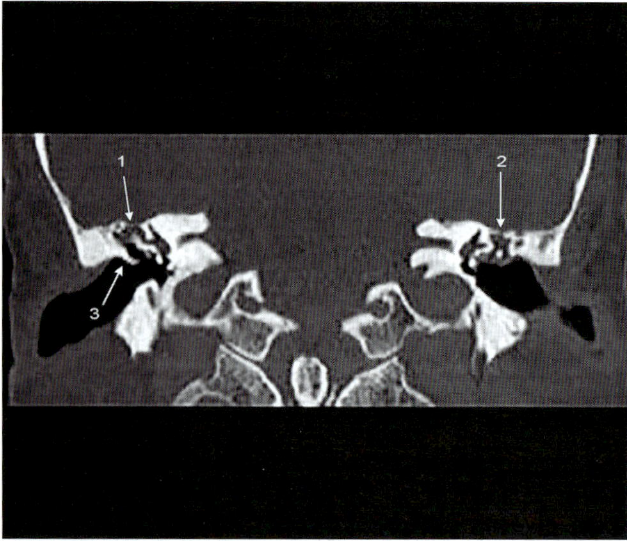

Fig. 8: Atticoantral cholesteatoma—Coronal computed tomography image showing soft tissue mass lesions in bilateral epitympanum causing ossicular disruption (arrow 2). Erosion of the tegmen tympani (roof of epitympanic space) is also seen in right side (arrow 1) and erosion of the scutum is seen in left side. A normal scutum is seen on right side (arrow 3)

- Perforations of the pars tensa of tympanic membrane associated with cholesteatoma are rare and cholesteatoma in these patients extends directly into the central part of the middle ear
- On MRI, cholesteatoma appears hypointense in T1-weighted images and has intermediate signal in T2-weighted images
- Cholesteatoma does not enhance unlike granulation tissue (postoperative) which enhances
- Complications
  - Erosion of bony labyrinth causing lateral semicircular canal fistula—presence of soft tissue mass in the region of oval window or lateral margin of lateral semicircular canal causing dehiscence of the bony labyrinth
  - Erosion of tegmen tympani—roof of the epitympanic space (Fig. 8)
  - Erosion of lateral or inferior wall of the tympanic part of the facial nerve canal (Figs 9A and B).

Benign Neoplasms

Glomus Tympanicum

It is a paraganglioma located at lateral aspect of cochlea in the middle ear—most classical location is at cochlear promontory.[8]

CT/ MR Findings

A strongly enhancing small soft tissue mass in middle ear (Figs 10A and B).

They engulf the adjacent middle ear ossicle as opposed to cholesteatoma which erodes them.

Glomus Jugulare

They are the paragangliomas which arises from glomus body around the jugular vein in the jugular foramen.

Thus, glomus jugulare are soft tissue masses extending from skull base superiorly into the middle ear cavity, and when large enough may simulate a localized glomus tympanicum, when it is called a glomus-jugulotympanicum.

CT/MRI Findings

- Soft tissue mass at base of skull eroding the jugular foramen (Fig. 11)
- A typical salt-and-pepper appearance is seen in contrast-enhanced T1-weighted MR images because of internal flow voids in the enhancing soft tissue mass (Figs 12A and B)
- A high asymmetric large jugular bulb may have dehiscent wall and may mimic a mass lesion but bone erosion or soft tissue destruction is essential to label it a glomus tumor.

INNER EAR

Inner ear comprises:
- Osseous labyrinth (otic capsule)
- Vestibule—the common chamber in which semicircular canals join Semicircular canals—Lateral/Superior/Posterior

- Cochlea—It has two and half turns. Cochlea has a base and an apex (cupola). It is divided by a bony central canal called the modiolus.

Membranous labyrinth (Figs 13A to D)
- Perilymph—within the cochlea, scala vestibuli and scala tympani
- Endolymph—within semicircular canals, cochlear duct and vestibular aqueduct.

Congenital Anomalies

The salient features and radiological findings of common congenital anomalies of the inner ear are as follows:[9]

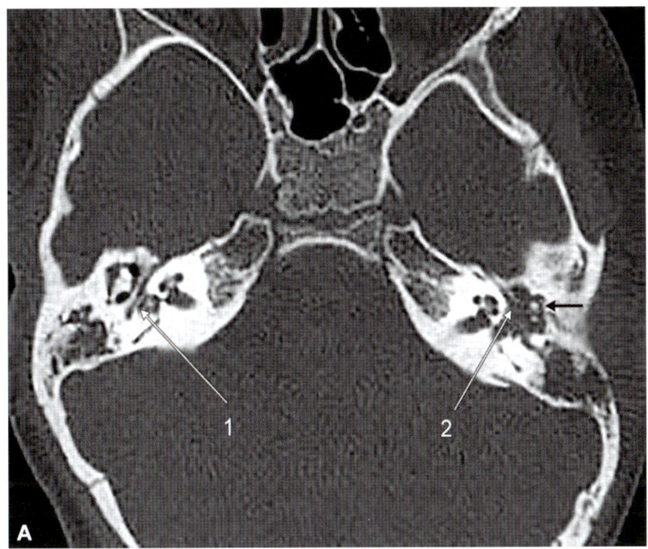

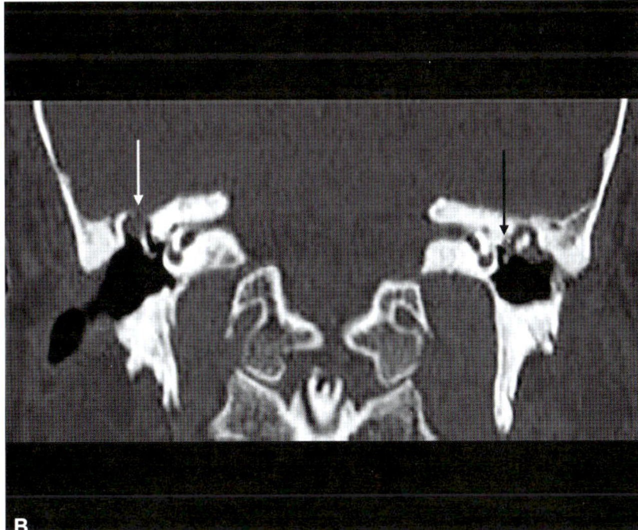

Figs 9A and B: Bilateral cholesteatoma—(A) Axial computed tomography image showing sclerosis of bilateral mastoids with soft tissue lesions in middle ear cavity and mastoid antrum with lytic destruction of antrum on both sides. There is also ossicular destruction (black arrow) and erosion of the lateral wall of the tympanic portion of the facial nerve (arrow 2) in left side. The horizontal facial nerve canal is normal on right side (arrow 1); (B) Coronal image showing erosion of the inferolateral wall of the facial nerve in left side (black arrow) and erosion of the tegmen tympani (white arrow) on left side

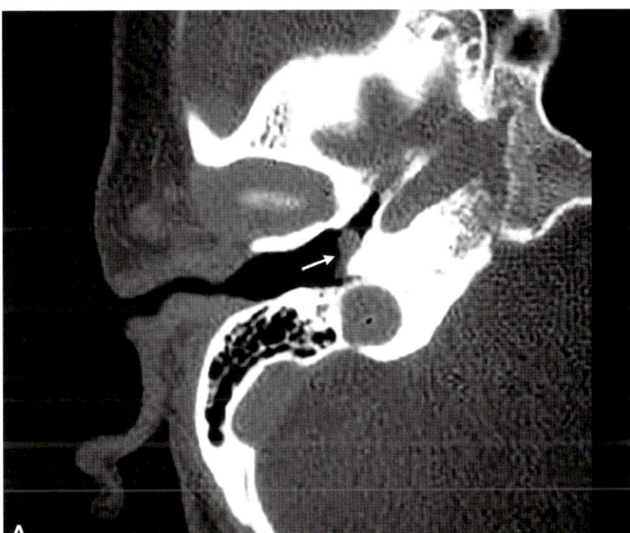

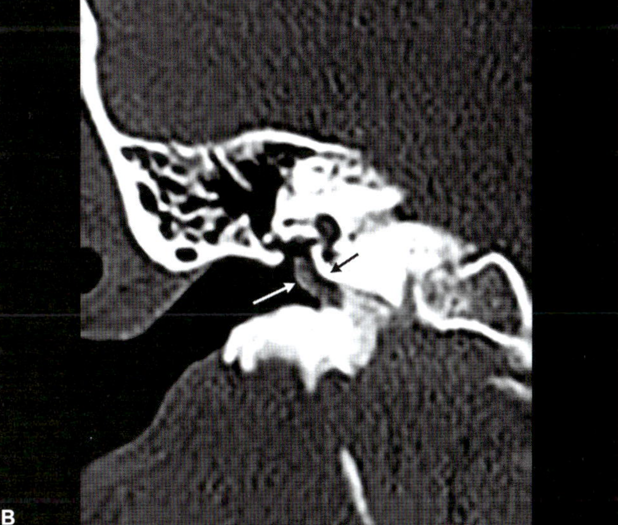

Figs 10A and B: Glomus tympanicum—Axial (A) and coronal (B) CT images showing a small soft tissue mass (white arrow) located over cochlear promontory (black arrow)

Mondini's Deformity

- Most common cochlear malformation
- Incomplete development of two and half turns of the cochlea (Figs 14A and B)
- Basal turn is relatively well-formed
- Middle and apical turns are poorly formed and balloon into a cyst

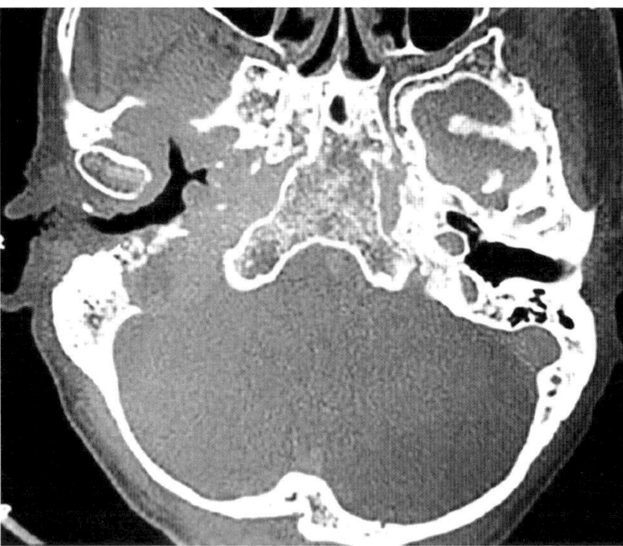

Fig. 11: Glomus jugulare—Axial computed tomography image showing a soft tissue mass (white arrows) at right base of skull enlarging and eroding the right jugular foramen and extending into the middle ear. There is also erosion of the right carotid canal by the mass. A normal carotid canal is seen on left side (black arrow)

- Associated abnormality seen in Mondini's deformity—enlargement of endolymphatic sac, large vestibular aqueduct.

Cock's Deformity (Michel's Dysplasia or Common Cystic Cavity)

- Second most common cochlear malformation
- A common cystic cavity comprising the vestibule and the cochlea (Figs 15A and B)
- Absent modiolus of the cochlea

Michel's Aplasia

- It is complete labyrinthine aplasia
- Total absence of inner ear structure
- Absence of stapes and oval window
- Bilateral in 50%
- Narrow or aplastic IAC
- Association: Platybasia, Abnormal course of facial nerve, Jugular vein anomalies.

Enlargement of Cochlear Aqueduct

- Usually, cochlear aqueduct narrows from medial to lateral
- A cochlear aqueduct size of >1.5 mms in medial part or >1.2 mms in mid-part is diagnostic.

Semicircular Canal (SC) Abnormalities

- Superior SC is first to develop followed by posterior SC and lateral SC is last to develop

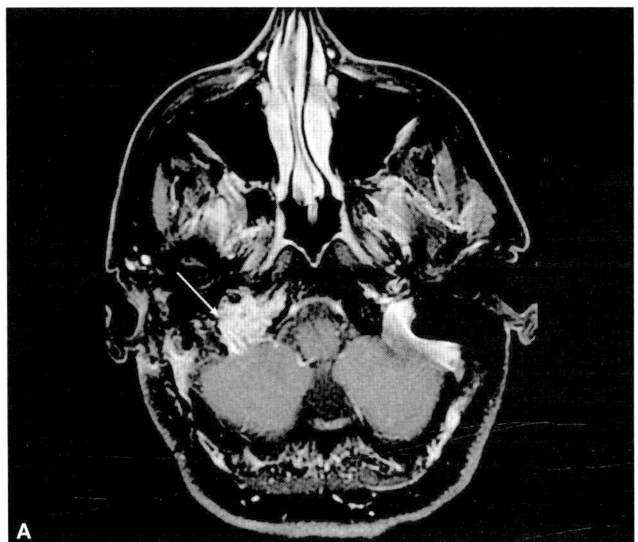

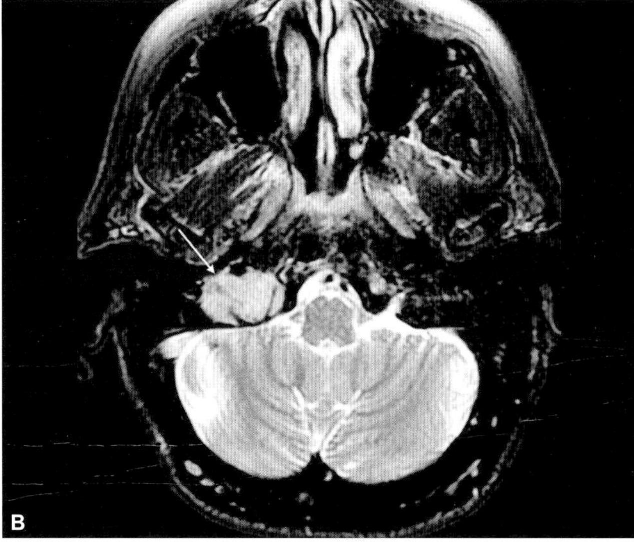

Figs 12A and B: Glomus jugulare—(A) Axial T2-weighted MR scan showing a predominantly hyperintense mass (arrow) in right jugular fossa with internal hypointensities due to flow voids (salt and pepper sign); (B) Postcontrast T1-weighted axial MR image showing diffuse enhancement of the mass (arrow) with salt and pepper appearance

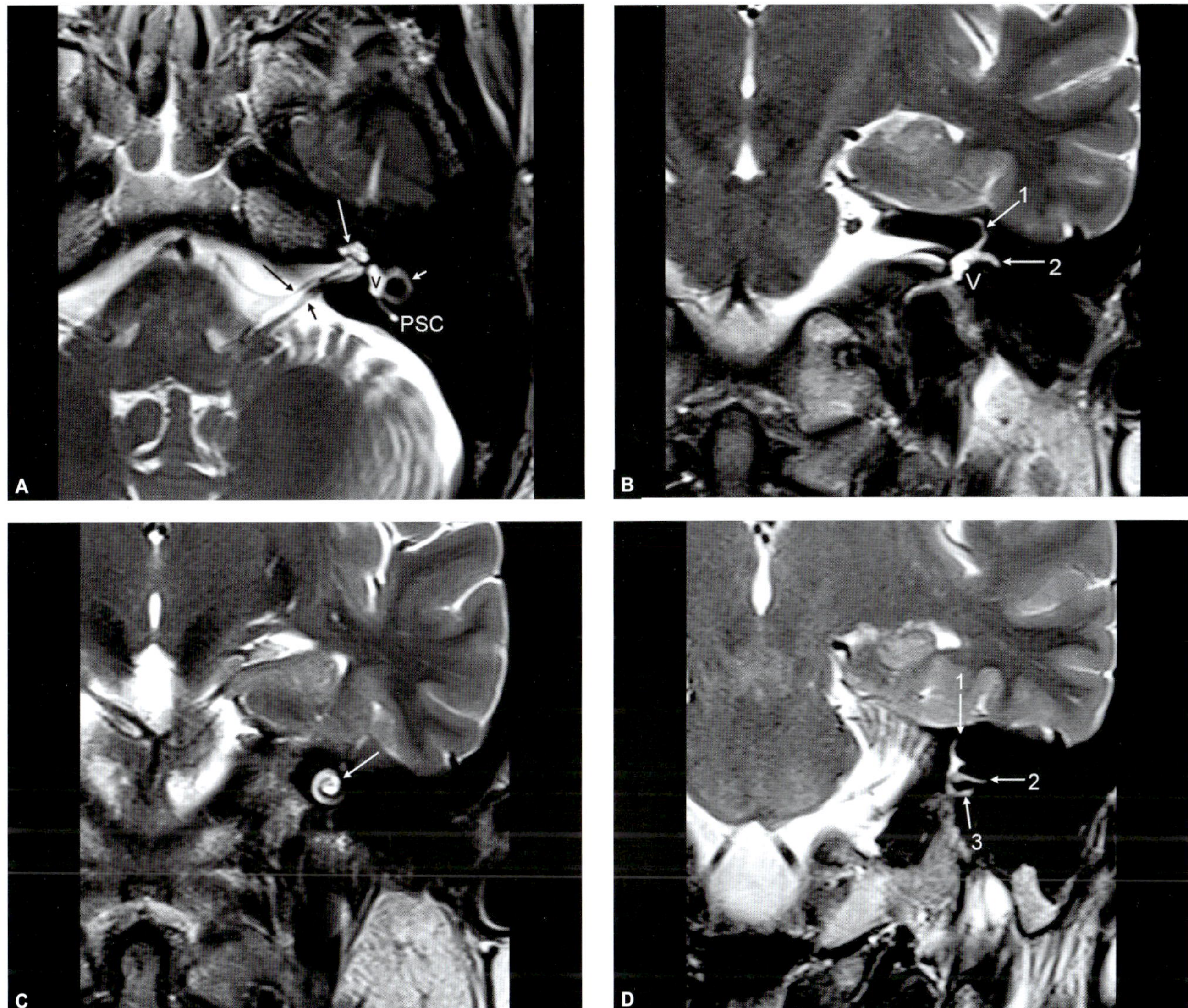

Figs 13A to D: (A) Axial T2-weighted MR image showing basal and apical turn of cochlea (long white arrow), vestibule, lateral semicircular canal (small white arrow), portion of posterior semicircular canal, facial (long black arrow) and vestibulocochlear (short black arrow) nerves; (B) Coronal T2-weighted MR image showing cochlea; (C) Coronal T2-weighted MR image showing vestibule, superior (arrow 1) and lateral (arrow 2) semicircular canals; (D) Coronal T2-weighted images showing superior (arrow 1), lateral (arrow 2) and posterior (arrow 3) semicircular canals
Abbreviations: V, vestibule; PSC, posterior semicircular canal

- Lateral SC hypoplasia is most common
- Lateral SC hypoplasia is also associated in superior/posterior SC hypoplasia
- Hearing loss
- There is compensatory enlargement of vestibule in semicircular canal hypoplasia
- Aplasia of semicircular canals is seen in CHARGE syndrome.

Enlargement of Vestibular aqueduct

- Enlarged vestibular aqueduct is the most common cause of congenital sensory neural hearing loss
- Normal duct is <1.5 mm in diameter at mid point and is about the same size as adjacent semicircular canal
- Enlarged when >1.5–2 mms
- MRI—Dilated endolymphatic sac is seen as hyperintense (than CSF) tubular structure in T1-weighted images due to high protein, hyperosmolar fluid.

Inflammatory Lesions of Inner Ear

Labyrinthine Ossification

It is a condition of bony replacement of labyrinthine portion of the inner ear.[10]

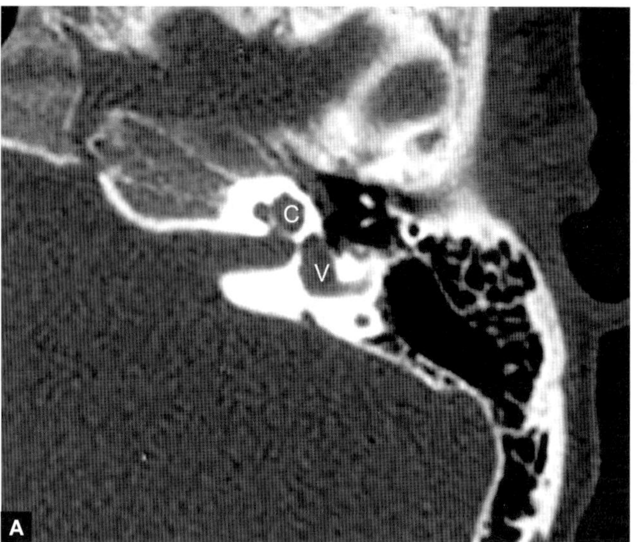
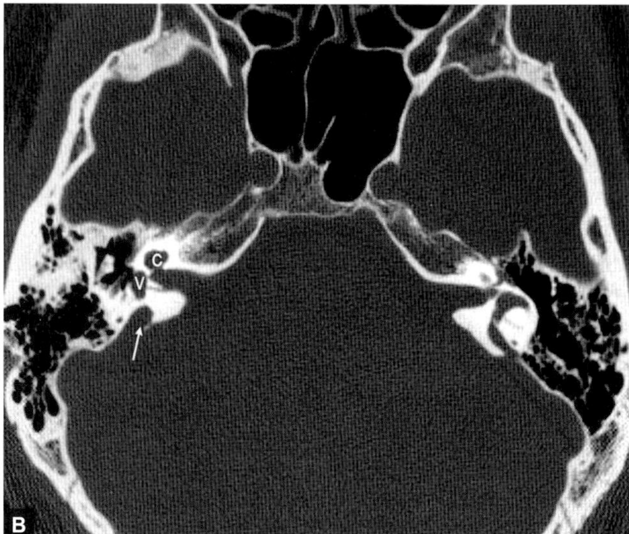

Figs 14A and B: Mondini's deformity—Axial computed tomography (A) showing malformed cochlea and dilated deformed vestibule on left side. Axial computed tomography (B) showing deformed right cochlea, and dilated vestibular aqueduct (white arrow) but normal vestibule
Abbreviations: V, vestibule; C, cochlea

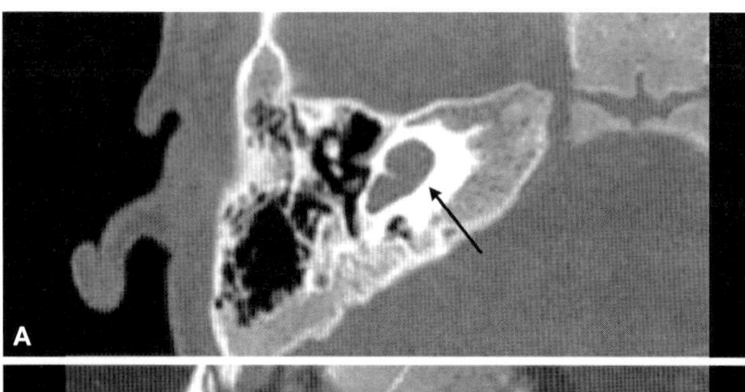
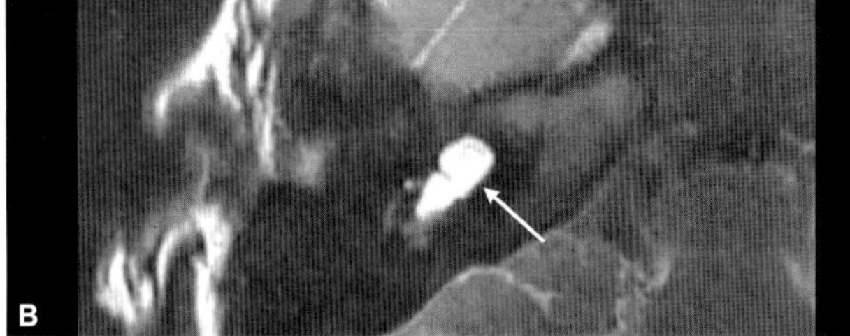

Figs 15A and B: Michel's dysplasia—Axial computed tomography (A) and axial T2-weighted MR scan (B) showing a common cystic cavity (arrow) replacing cochlea and vestibule

CT/MRI Findings

- CT—Dense sclerosis of cochlea, vestibule and semicircular canal as well as round window niche.
- MRI—Fibro-ossific change of cochlea are better seen in T2-weighted images MRI as fibrous obliteration of cochlea may not be seen on CT.

Causes

- Postoperative
- Trauma/hemorrhage
- Chronic otitis media
- Chronic labyrinthitis
- Paget's disease
- Otospongiosis.

Otospongiosis

Otospongiosis is an uncommon cause of sensorineural hearing loss where there is replacement of endochondral bone by spongy bone. It is usually (80%) bilateral and is seen in young/middle-aged female.[11]

CT Findings

- CT—lytic radiolucent erosion of the labyrinthine margin of the oval window, round window niche or the cochlea
- Depending on the involvement of the osseous labyrinth it is classified into cochlear and retrocochlear/fenestral otospongiosis.

Cochlear Otospongiosis

- Middle and basal turns of cochlea are involved showing areas of demineralization
- A double ring (lucent) sign is seen at basal turn of cochlea (Fig. 16)
- In late stage of otospongiosis, sclerosis develops which gives rise to increased bone density.

Fenestral Otospongiosis

- More common than cochlear otospongiosis
- It involves anterior margin of oval window (80–90%) and round window niche (30–50%)

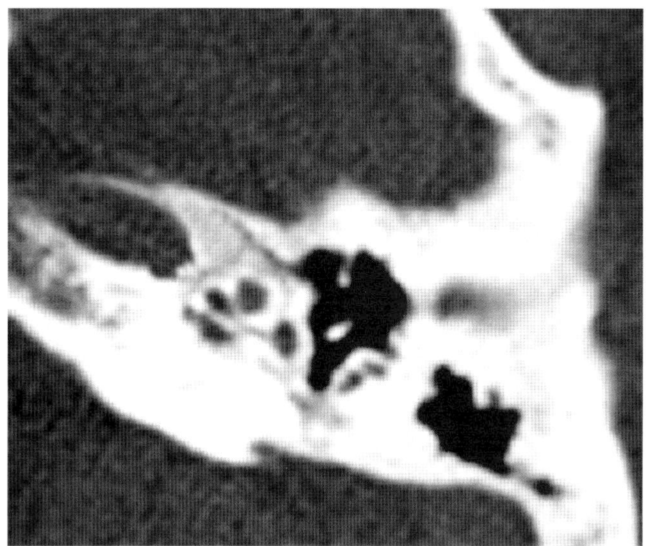

Fig. 16: Cochlear otospongiosis—Axial computed tomography showing area of demineralization around the cochlea (black arrow)

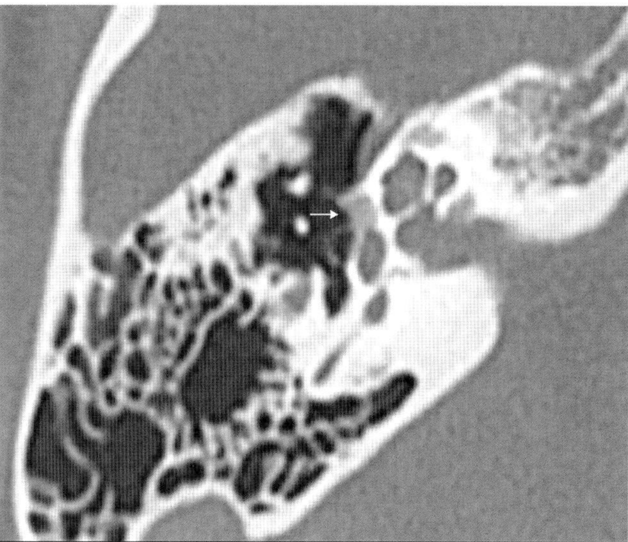

Fig. 17: Fenestral otospongiosis—Axial computed tomography showing a lytic bony mass (arrow) at anterior margin of the oval window

- Stapes gets adherent to oval window
- Oval window niche is narrowed with plaque of new bone anteriorly (Fig. 17).

Paget's Disease

Paget's disease is a bone forming disease of the inner ear. It may cause either sensorineural or conductive deafness.

CT Findings

- In early phase of disease, a diffuse lytic lesion is seen involving bony labyrinth
- In late stage of disease, increased density is seen in labyrinth
- D/D with cochlear otosclerosis
- Paget's disease begins at periphery and spreads centrally while cochlear otosclerosis starts centrally and extends outwards.

Petrous Apicitis

Petrous apicitis is the inflammation of the pneumatized petrous apex. The pneumatization of petrous apex is seen in about one-third of the population which may develop petrous apicitis.[12]

CT/MRI Findings

- Opacification of petrous apex
- High signal intensity in T2-weighted and low signal intensity in T1-weighted images
- In chronic infection, due to accumulation of high viscosities and high protein content in the fluid the signal intensity changes appearing hyperintense in T1-weighted images and hypointense in T2-weighted images
- The dura near the Gasserian ganglian (Meckel's cave) may show enhancement on MR.

Cholesterol Granuloma

Cholesterol granuloma is a benign tumor of the petrous apex.[12]

CT/MRI Findings

- Seen at apex of temporal bone
- Appear as a lytic lesion within petrous apex filled with soft tissue
- They have high signal intensity in all MRI pulse sequences because of the hemorrhagic product and cholesterol debris (D/D: Acquired cholesteatoma are dark in T1-weighted images) (Fig. 18)
- Both petrous apex fat and cholesterol granuloma will have high signal in T1-weighted images. Fat suppressed sequence and bone expansion (seen in cholesterol granuloma) helps distinguish between the two.

Acoustic (VIII Nerve) Schwannoma

Acoustic schwannoma usually presents as a cerebellopontine angle mass lesion extending into internal auditory canal (Figs 19A to D). Intralabyrinthine schwannoma is a rare tumor and are usually diagnosed in contrast-enhanced MRI (Figs 20A to D).[13]

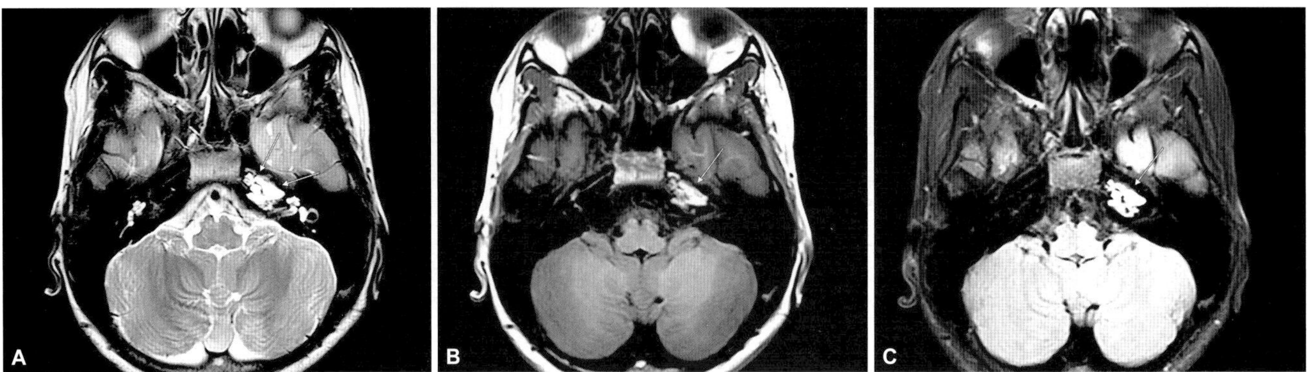

Figs 18A to D: Cholesterol granuloma—(A) Axial T2-weighted image showing a lobulated well-defined hyperintense mass (arrow) at left petrous apex; (B) Lesion is bright in T1-weighted image; (C) Lesion in also bright in this fat saturated FLAIR image

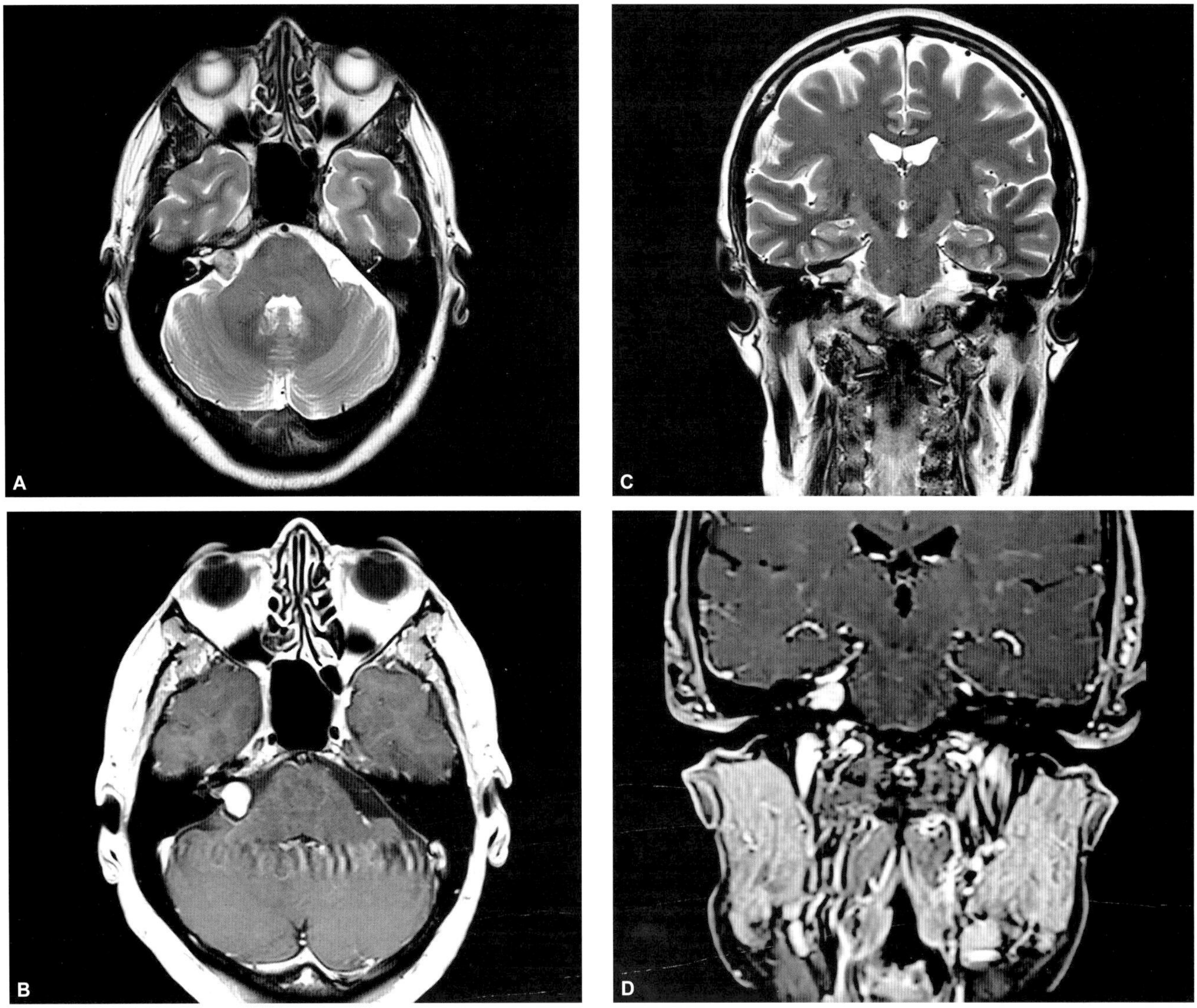

Figs 19A to D: Axial (A) and coronal (B) T2-weighted MR images showing right cerebellopontine angle mass extending into internal auditory canal consistent with acoustic schwannoma. Postcontrast T1-weighted axial (C) and coronal (D) MR images showing marked homogeneous enhancement of the mass

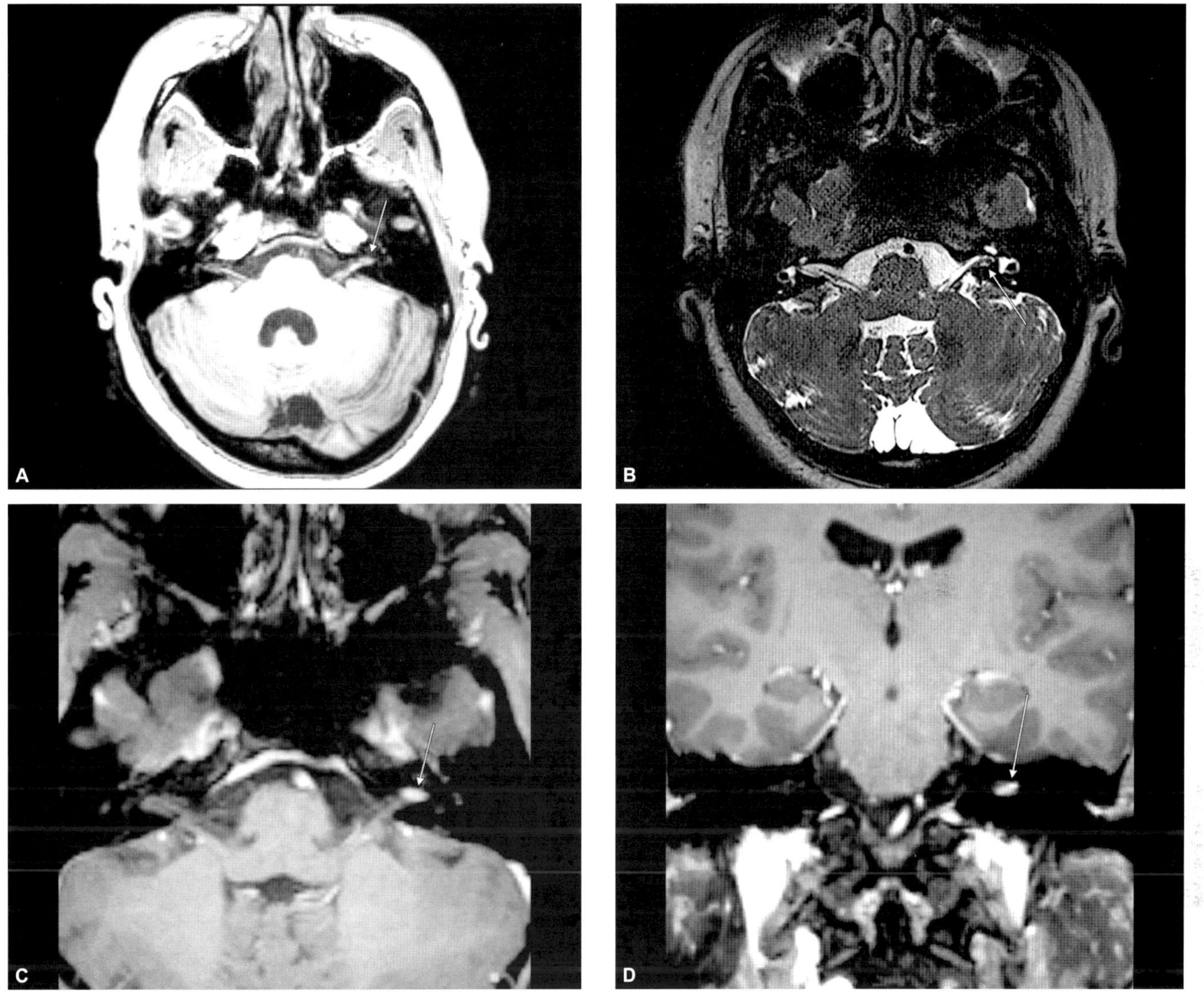

Figs 20A to D: Left intracanalicular Acoustic Schwannoma—(A) Axial T1-weighted image showing isointense nodular lesion (arrow) in left IAC inseparable from left seventh-eighth nerve complex; (B) Axial T2-weighted image also shows nodular hypointense lesion; (C and D) Axial and coronal postcontrast T1-weighted images shows enhancement of the mass

MRI Findings

- Typical acoustic schwannomas arise from cochlear branch of VIIIth cranial nerve
- An extra-axial mass in cerebellopontine angle cistern extending into internal auditory canal giving it an icecream cone appearance
- Intralabyrinthine schwannoma are usually situated close to round window niche or within scala tympani of basal and second turn of cochlea
- Enhances markedly on MR.

Enhancement of VII Cranial Nerve

Intracanalicular facial nerve enhancement is always abnormal. The usual causes of enhancement of the facial nerve are:[14]

- Schwannoma
- Lymphoma
- Bell's palsy
- Viral neuritis
- Ramsay Hunt syndrome

- Guillain-Barre syndrome
- Perineural tumor spread.

Usual site of enhancement of VII cranial nerve in Bell's palsy are enhancement of distal intrameatal segment or labyrinthine segment proximal to geniculate ganglion.

Trauma

Traumatic fracture of temporal bone may be vertical (transverse), horizontal (longitudinal) or complex (mixed or oblique) depending on the orientation of the fracture line to the petrous ridge.[15]

Vertical Fracture

- The fracture line traverses in a superoinferior orientation (Fig. 21)
- Less common than horizontal fracture
- Higher incidence (40%) of facial nerve injury
- Two types:
    - Lateral—which involves cochlea or vestibule
    - Medial—which involves IAC and petrous pyramid.

Horizontal Fracture

- Fracture line runs along the plane of temporal bone (Figs 22A to C)
- Beginning from EAC, through the middle ear and extends toward the sphenoid bone
- Common (70–90%) than vertical fracture

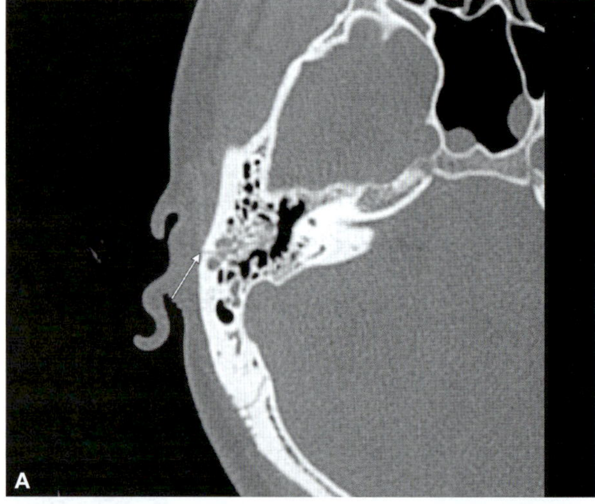

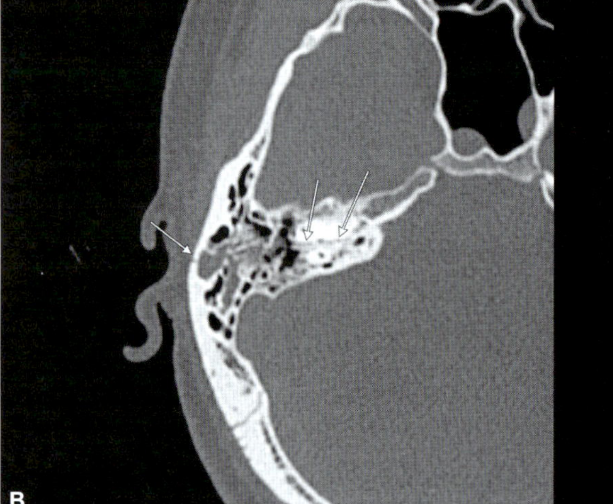

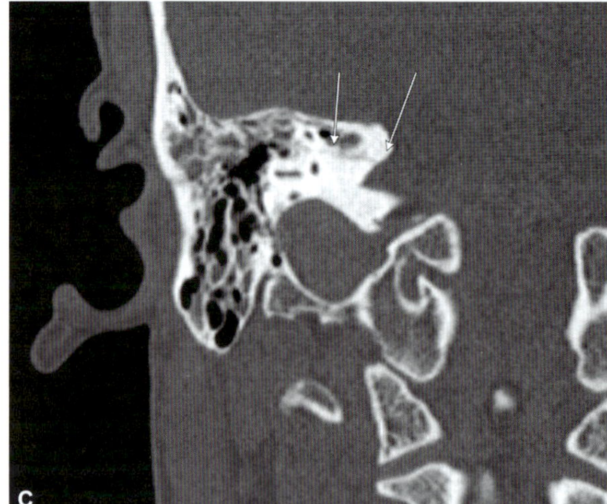

Figs 22A to C: Horizontal temporal bone fracture—(A) Axial computed tomography image showing thin fracture line (arrow) extending from mastoid to middle ear; (B) Extension of the fracture line (arrow) into labyrinth; (C) Coronal image also demonstrating the labyrinthine extension of the fracture

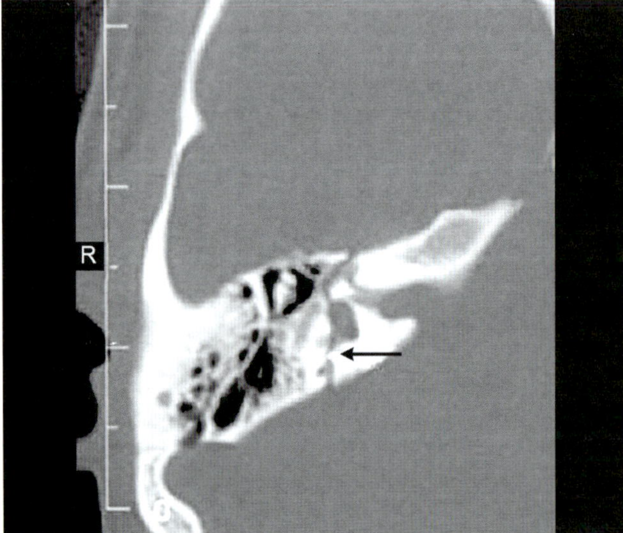

Fig. 21: Vertical temporal bone fracture—Axial computed tomography showing a fracture line in a superiorinferior orientation traversing the facial nerve canal, vestibule and lateral semicircular canal

- Ossicular dislocation:
    - Incudostapedial joint dislocation is most common, and the weakest ossicular articulation
    - Fracture of long process of incus with separation of more than 1 mm from stapes head at posterolateral aspect is diagnostic.
- Hemotympanum
- Injury of facial nerve
- Involvement of labyrinth is rare
- Involvement of EAC and glenoid fossa of temporo-mandibular joint is common.

REFERENCES

1. Mayer TE, Brueckmann H, Siegert R, Witt A, Weerda H. High-Resolution CT of the Temporal Bone in Dysplasia of the Auricle and External Auditory Canal. AJNR Am J Neuroradiol. 1997;18:53-65.
2. Curtin HD, Wolfe P, May M. Malignant external otitis: CT evaluation. Radiology. 1982;145(2):383-8.
3. Chakeres DW, Kapila A, LaMasters D. Soft-tissue abnormalities of the external auditory canal: subject review of CT findings. Radiology. 1985;156(1):105-9.
4. Robert Y, Carcasset S, Rocourt N, Hennequin C, Dubrulle F, Lemaitre L. Congenital Cholesteatoma of the Temporal Bone: MR Findings and Comparison with CT. AJNR Am J Neuroradiol. 1995;16:755-61.
5. Mafee MF, Singleton EL, Valvassori GE, Espinosa GA, Kumar A, Aimi K. Acute otomastoiditis and its complications: role of CT. Radiology. 1985;155(2):391-7.
6. Mafee MF, Aimi K, Kahen HL, Valvassori GE, Capek V. Chronic otomastoiditis: a conceptual understanding of CT findings. Radiology. 1986;160(1):193-200.
7. Swartz JD. Cholesteatomas of the middle ear. Diagnosis, etiology, and complications. Radiol Clin North Am. 1984;22(1):15-35.
8. Jackson CG. Glomus tympanicum and glomus jugulare tumors. Otolaryngol Clin North Am. 2001;34:941-70.
9. Urman SM, Talbot JM. Otic capsule dysplasia: clinical and CT findings. Radiographics. 1990;10(5):823-38.
10. Swartz JD, Mandell DM, Faerber EN, Popky GL, Ardito JM, Steinberg SB, et al. Labyrinthine ossification: etiologies and CT findings. Radiology. 1985;157(2):395-8.
11. Valvassori, GE. Imaging of otosclerosis. Otolaryngol Clin North Am. 1993;26:359-71.
12. Connor SE, Leung R, Natas S. Imaging of the petrous apex: a pictorial review. Br J Radiol. 2008;81(965):427-35.
13. Karen L, Salzmana H, Davidsona HC, Harnsbergera HR, Glastonburya CM, Wigginsa RH, et al. Dumbbell Schwannomas of the Internal Auditory Canal. AJNR. 2001;22:1368-76.
14. Saremi F, Helmy M, Farzin S, Zee CS, Go JL. MRI of Cranial Nerve Enhancement. AJR Am J Roentgenol. 2005;185(6):1485-97.
15. Wiet RJ, Valvassori GE, Kotsanis CA, Parahy C. Temporal bone fractures. State of the art review. Am J Otol. 1985;6(3):207-15.

Cochlear Implant

KK Handa, Arpit Sharma

INTRODUCTION

Cochlear implant is a device that helps in restoring useful hearing in severely to profoundly deaf people when the organ of hearing situated in the inner ear has not developed or is destroyed by disease or injury. Normally, sound is transmitted down the ear canal, through the middle ear, to the inner ear. The sense organ of hearing in the inner ear consists of hair cells which protrude into a gelatinous membrane. These cells move with sound and their vibrations produce electric current and stimulate the auditory nerve. Auditory nerves send the signals to higher brain centers which are interpreted as sound.

In partially damaged hair cells, hearing aid helps by amplification but with severe to profound loss no amplification helps and thus cochlear implant is required. Cochlear implant directly stimulates the nerve and bypasses the inner ear. However, hearing from cochlear implant is different from normal hearing and takes time to learn with the help of speech therapist.

HISTORY

Alessandro Volta was the first to stimulate the auditory system electrically, by connecting a battery of 30 or 40 'couples' (approximately 50V) to two metal rods that were inserted into his ears. When the circuits were completed, he received the sensation of boom within the head, followed by a sound similar to that of boiling of thick soup. Duchenne of Boulogne, in 1855, stimulated the ear with an alternating current and felt a sound that resembled, 'the beating of a fly's wings between a pane of glass and a curtain'. In 1868, Brenner found that hearing was better with an electrical stimulus that created a negative polarity in the ear, and that correct placement of the electrodes could reduce the unpleasant side effects. In 1957, Djourno and Eyries provided the first detailed description of the effects of directly stimulating the auditory nerve in deafness. The clinical applications of electrical stimulation of the auditory nerve were refined by House (1976) and Michelson (1971) through scala tympani implantation of electrodes driven by implantable receiver-stimulators.

In 1972, a speech processor was developed to interface with the House 3M single-electrode implant and was the first to be commercially marketed. More than 1,000 of these devices were implanted between 1972 and the mid 1980s. In 1980, the age criteria for use of this device was lowered from 18 to 2 years. The FDA formally approved the marketing of the 3M/ House cochlear implant in November 1984. Later, introduction of multiple channel devices enhanced the spectral perception and speech recognition capabilities compared to the single-channel device.

COMPONENTS

Cochlear implant has external (outside) parts and internal (surgically implanted) parts.[1]

External Parts (Fig. 1)

The external parts include a microphone, a speech processor, and a transmitter. The **microphone** looks like a behind-the-ear hearing aid. It picks up sounds just like a microphone of the hearing aid and sends them to the speech processor.

The speech processor may be housed behind the ear with the microphone, or it may be worn on a belt or pocket. The **speech processor** analyzes and digitizes the sound signals and sends them to a transmitter worn on the head just behind the ear.

The **transmitter** sends the coded signals to an implanted receiver just under the skin.

Internal Parts (Fig. 2)

The internal (implanted) parts include a receiver-stimulating system and electrodes. The receiver is surgically fixed to the skull bone behind the ear. The **receiver** takes the coded electrical signals from the transmitter and delivers them to the array of electrodes that have been inserted in the cochlea during surgery. The **electrodes** stimulate the fibers of the auditory nerve to send information to the brain where it is interpreted as meaningful sound and thus the implanted person starts learning language and speech communication skills.

Types of Cochlear Implants

1. Digisonic Neurelac France
2. Advanced Bionics, United States
3. MED-EL, Austria
4. Cochlear Corporation, Australia

Types of Electrodes

- Straight
- Contour
  - Split array
  - Compressed array.

PREOPERATIVE SELECTION

Cochlear implants are FDA approved for adults 18 years and older (no upper age limit). Initially, implants were only approved for adults who were postlingually deaf and had no improvement with high-powered hearing aids. This group of people has consistently been shown to be benefited by implantation. As more was learned about the

benefits of cochlear implantation, the criteria were relaxed. Now, adult criteria include bilateral severe-to-profound sensorineural hearing loss with 70 dB pure tone average, little or no benefit from hearing aids (must attempt binaural high-powered hearing aids for at least 6 months), and psychological suitability. Audiological examination should show word discrimination scores less than 40% in the best-aided condition. The patient should have no anatomical deformity that would preclude implantation success. Finally, the patient should have no physical condition that would preclude a general anesthetic.

Pediatric implantation is indicated in children 12 months or older with bilateral severe-to-profound sensorineural hearing loss with pure tone averages of 90 dB or greater in the better ear. The child must have had no appreciable benefit with hearing aids (evaluated with parental survey when younger than 5 and 30% or less on sentence recognition tests under best-aided conditions when 5 years old or older). Children must tolerate wearing hearing aids for a period (as all cochlear implants have external components), and show some aided communication ability. Children must be enrolled in educational programs that support aural/oral learning and have no medical contraindications. Parents must be highly motivated and have reasonable expectations.[2]

IMPORTANCE OF NEURAL PLASTICITY

The main factor which influences the candidacy is neural plasticity. Neural plasticity is the ability of the central nervous system to be programmed to learn a task. The mechanism of learning to articulate is initiated at a very early age by babbling and normally hearing persons learn to articulate most of the sounds they will require

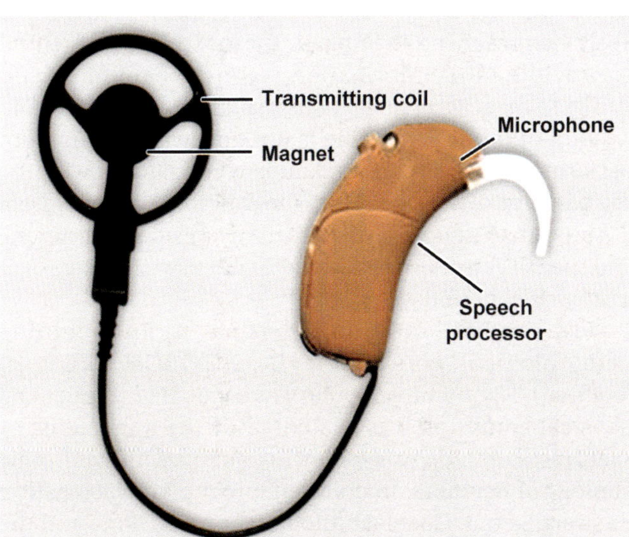

Fig. 1: External parts of cochlear implants

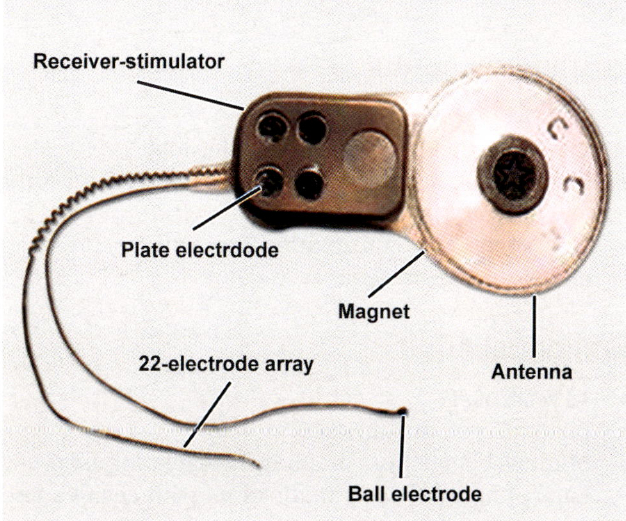

Fig. 2: Internal parts of cochlear implants

before uttering any meaningful words. Neural plasticity of speech articulation is more severe than that of listening. If a person has never utilized the auditory mechanism, the neural plasticity needed to learn to listen probably fades between the age of 6 and 8 years. Speech articulation can only be accomplished if speech sounds are learnt before the age of 2–3 years, and this justifies the early diagnosis and management of congenital deafness.

ChIP (Children's Implant Profile)

It is used as a means of determining which children may except to receive benefit from a cochlear implant. Eleven factors are assessed: chronological age, duration of deafness, medical/radiological findings, multiple handicapping conditions, functional hearing level, speech-language abilities, family structure and support, parent-child expectations, education environment, availability of support services and cognitive learning style.

GENERAL CRITERIA FOR COCHLEAR IMPLANT SURGERY

Prelingual and Postlingual Children (AAO HNS Criteria)

- Bilateral severe-to-profound hearing loss (only profound hearing loss in children < 2 years old)
- Lack of auditory development with a proper binaural hearing aid trial as documented by objective testing or a parental questionnaire (for very young children)
- Properly aided open-set work recognition scores <20–30% in children capable of testing
- Suitable auditory developmental education plan
- Lack of medical contraindication.

Postlingual Adults

- 18 years of age
- Bilateral severe-to-profound hearing loss
- Properly aided sentence (HINT) recognition scores <40%
- Lack of medical contraindication, with cochlea and auditory nerve present.

Prelingual Adults

- 18 years of age
- Bilateral profound deafness
- Minimal benefit from properly fitted hearing aid
- Lack of medical contraindication, with cochlea and auditory nerve present

Factors Generally Associated with Better Outcomes in Cochlear Implantation

Adults and Children

- Shorter duration of deafness
- Better preoperative word or sentence recognition (or both)
- Lip-reading ability
- Higher intelligence quotient (I.Q.)
- Better preoperative residual hearing
- Optimized implant technology and processing strategy
- Cause of deafness (e.g. meningitis associated with poor outcomes)
- Intact, nonossified cochlea.

Additional Factors in Children

- Younger age at implantation
- Motivated family assistance
- Oral preoperative education
- Oral education rehabilitation program as opposed to total communication.

PREOPERATIVE COUNSELING

The importance of counseling was always acknowledged and each candidate and family members were counseled explaining the anatomy and physiology of hearing, cochlear pathology responsible for his/her deafness, surgical procedure, the types of implants, the working procedure, switch on, mapping, possible complications and the importance of postoperative auditory verbal therapy. The patient's intelligence quotient, speech, language and auditory skills were assessed. It is very important that candidate and family understand exactly what gain is likely after receiving an implant. The most effective method of providing this information is for the candidate and family to meet someone who is using a cochlear implant. It is important that meeting is not only with star implant performers but with an implantee who matches with the age and type of hearing loss of the candidate. For children, it is important that family realize the acquisition of listening and speech can only be gained after intensive tutorage over a prolonged period.

Prior to implantation, a basic workup including hematological, chest X-ray, ECG, TORCH screen (if required), TB immunoglobulin was conducted. The general physical condition was evaluated by the anesthetist. A specialist's opinion was sought in patients with syndromic etiology of deafness. In children, preimplant vaccination was carried out. Cochlear implantation was done and the response of electrodes was confirmed using neural response telemetry (NRT) and effectiveness was assessed especially in children. Facial nerve monitoring was done whenever necessary.[3]

CANDIDANCY CATEGORIES

a. **Postlingual:** Onset of deafness has occurred after completion of speech development.
b. **Perilingual:** Onset of deafness has occurred while speech development was occurring.
c. **Prelingual:** Onset of deafness occurred prior to any development of speech.
   - Primary candidate—have not acquired language by any other means of communication
   - Secondary candidate—have used other mode of communication (usually sign) to develop language
   - Change-over candidate—have developed auditory skills using a hearing aid.

IDEAL CANDIDATE FOR COCHLEAR IMPLANT

There are number of factors that determine the degree of success to expect from the operation and the device itself. Cochlear implant centers determine implant candidacy on an individual basis and take into account a person's hearing history, cause of hearing loss, amount of residual hearing, speech recognition ability, health status, and family commitment to aural habilitation/rehabilitation.

A prime candidate is described as:
- Having severe to profound sensorineural hearing impairment in both ears
- Having a functioning auditory nerve
- Having lived a short amount of time without hearing
- Having good speech, language, and communication skills, or in the case of infants and young children, having a family willing to work toward speech and language skills with therapy
- Not being benefited by other kinds of hearing aids
- Having no medical reason to avoid surgery
- Living in or desiring to live in the "hearing world"
- Having realistic expectations about results
- Having the support of family and friends
- Having appropriate services set up for postcochlear implant aural rehabilitation (through a speech language pathologist, deaf educator, or auditory verbal therapist).

Contraindications for Cochlear Implantation

Not all patients with sensorineural hearing loss are good candidates for cochlear implantation. For example, patients with pure tone thresholds greater than 90 dB with residual hearing through 2000 Hz often do better with hearing aids than with implantation. Computed tomography findings may also preclude implantation. The absence of the cochlea (Michel deformity), and a small internal auditory canal (associated with cochlear nerve atresia) are contraindications to implantation on that side. However, when implantation of a dysplastic cochlea is to be undertaken, informed consent is especially important. Cochlear implants in these patients are associated with increased risk of poor result, CSF leak, and meningitis.

The presence of active middle ear disease is a contraindication to surgery. This process should be treated and resolved before implantation. Patients with a history of canal wall down mastoidectomy may need surgery to reconstruct the posterior canal wall or close off the canal before implantation.

Meningitis may lead to hearing loss and ossification of the cochlea. Labyrinthitis ossificans is usually identifiable on CT scan (brightly lit cochlea with obliteration of the basal cochlear duct) and is a relative contraindication when there is a patent contralateral basal turn. MRI is often better at delineating patency of the cochlea and should be pursued if there is any question. Very young children with hearing loss after meningitis should be followed with CT/MRI until they reach implantable age. Early implantation may be indicated if evidence of ossification is noted. Adults and children with acute meningitis should be treated with steroids to avoid hearing loss. Those who sustain hearing loss secondary to meningitis should be observed for 6 months before implantation due to the substantial number of patients that will regain their hearing in at least one ear. Advanced otosclerosis can also cause ossification of the basal turn of the cochlea. This finding is most often noted on CT scan. This is not a contraindication as long as the surgeon is prepared to perform a drill out or pursue implantation into the scala vestibuli. Patients with otosclerosis can achieve excellent results from implantation.

A diagnosis of neurofibromatosis II (history of progressive hearing loss and suggestive MRI findings), mental retardation, psychosis, organic brain dysfunction, and unrealistic expectations may also be contraindications.[4]

SURGICAL TECHNIQUE

Most commonly and widely practiced technique is the classical technique where the electrode is inserted via the facial recess approach.[5]

Classical Technique

A C-shaped incision was first used for the 3M single-electrode implant that had only a coil, but no electronics placed behind the ear but gave inadequate exposure to multiple electrodes implant. Other disadvantages of this incision were compromise in blood supply of flap and management of mastoid emissary vein. For this reason an inverted J–shaped incision was developed which although cut the posterior branches of the superficial temporal artery, there was a good arterial supply from below from the occipital artery as well as musculocutaneous vessels and excellent dependent venous drainage. A modification of this incision by Lehnhardt has replaced the upward postauricular limb of the inverted J with an incision in the external auditory canal. Before making the incision, its site is determined after a dummy package is positioned over the skin, taking into consideration the age of the child, the head shape, and the extent of the mastoid air cells as seen on X-rays. Space of 2 cm is left behind the ear for the placement of a microphone and behind-the-ear speech processor unit. A flap of skin and subcutaneous fascia followed by a separate anteriorly based flap of deep fascia and periosteum is raised. A limited mastoidectomy is carried out exposing the mastoid antrum, the lateral semicircular canal, and the short process of the incus. The removal of bone should be sufficient to carry out the posterior tympanotomy. Posterior tympanotomy is the surgical approach to the middle ear to expose the round window through the mastoid air cells via a triangular space between the facial nerve, chorda tympani, and the floor of the fossa incudis. A bed is made in the skull bone to place the container for the receiver-stimulator electronics, so that it will not move or protrude as a swelling. Access to the scala tympani can be gained either through the round window membrane or more usually a fenestration anteroinferior to it (cochleostomy). After accessing scala tympani by any of the aforementioned technique, electrode arrays are inserted and both array and receiver-stimulator is fixed. After the skin is sutured and the bandage applied, a transorbital X-ray should be taken while the patient is still under the anesthetic to check the electrode position.

The alternative methods are Veria technique, Suprameatal approach and the middle fossa approach.[6]

Veria Technique (Fig. 3)

The surgical procedure begins after the patient receives a general anesthesia. The patient's head is shaved over the postauricular area. The extent of hair removal depends on the incision to be used—generally four fingerbreadths above and behind the ear is sufficient. The patient is then prepped and draped in a fashion similar to other otologic procedures. A dummy receiver is placed over the skin and positioned approximately 1 cm posterior to the auricle. A postauricular incision is made 1–2 cm posterior to the implant. Several incisions have been proposed and include a large C-shaped incision, a 4–5 cm superior elliptical extension of the routine postauricular incision, a small 4–5 cm straight incision posterior and an incision posterior-superior to the auricle (Fig. 4).

The superficial layer (skin and subcutaneous tissue) is elevated first followed by the deep layer of muscle and periosteum (Wurzburg flap). Tympanomeatal flap is elevated and round window niche identified. Posterior canal wall is straightened by drill work. A suprameatal hollow is made measuring 5 mm × 5 mm × 5 mm posterosuperior to the bony canal. Through the anterosuperior portion of hollow, a tunnel is drilled in the posterior canal wall by 1.6 mm burr with a guard (TRIFON PERFORATOR)(Fig. 5). Tunnel is widened to about 3 mm. The distance between guard and burr is 0.6 mm. Drilling is done towards the round window. Tunnel is drilled, patency is confirmed and smoothened. Mucosa over the promontory is incised and elevated in anteroinferior direction to round window. Cochleostomy is done in above area. Irrigation is done inside the cochlea to remove bone dust and filled with gel foam. Tympanomastoid portion of temporal bone is drilled to make the implant bed using the template. Tunnels are made above the bed and sutures passed through these tunnels and over the implant for anchoring and fixing the implant. Implant is secured in position by nonabsorbable

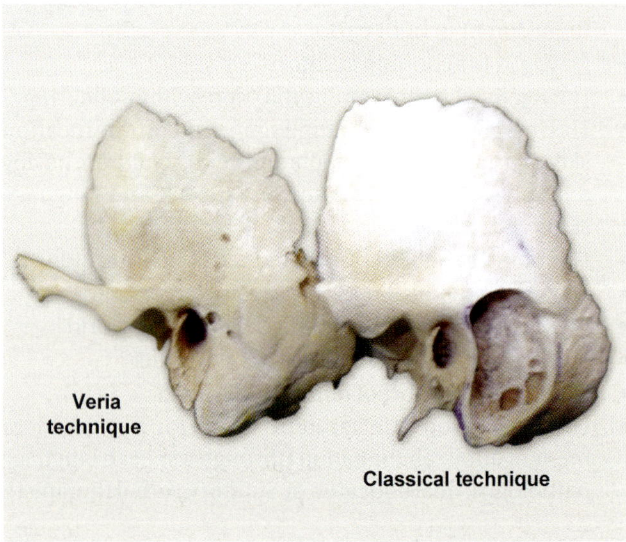

Fig. 3: Veria technique (minimal invasive) and classical technique (mastoidectomy)

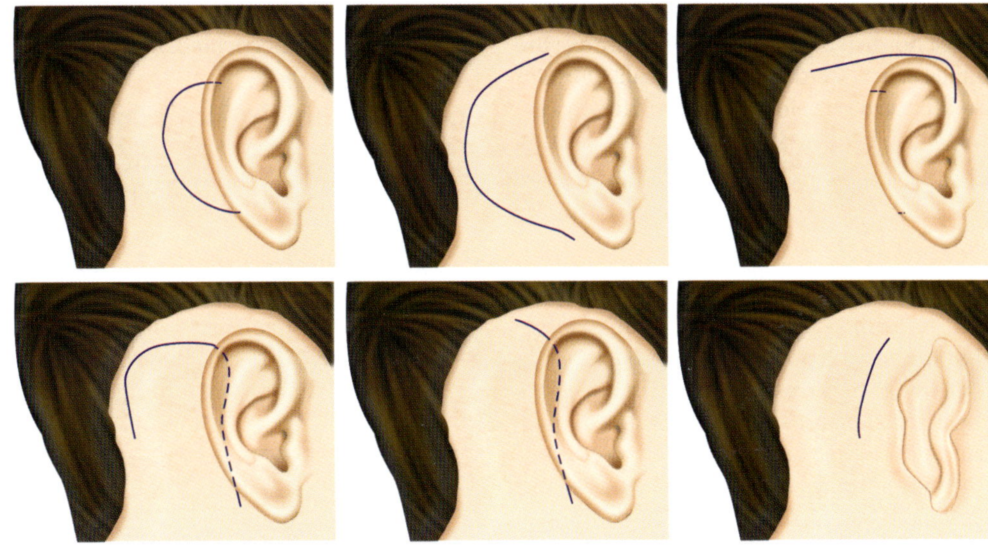

Fig. 4: Different type of skin incisions in cochlear implant surgery

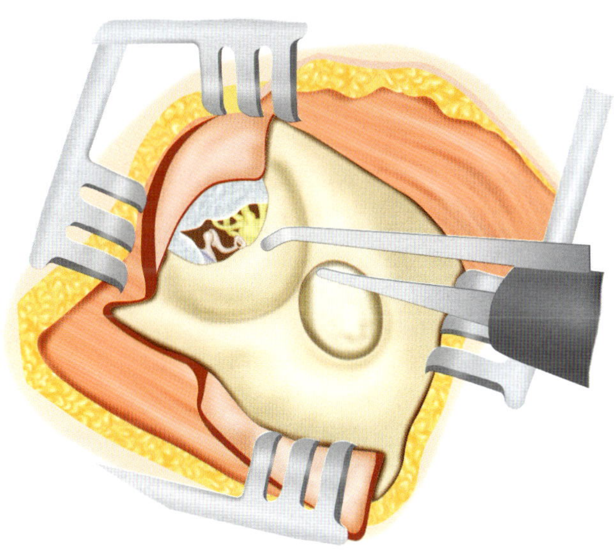

Fig. 5: Trifon's perforator

"double suture". Rest of implant inserted between bone and periosteum. A groove is drilled from implant site towards the suprameatal hollow where in the end a tunnel is made connecting the hollow with the drilled groove. Electrode is passed through the tunnel, then through the suprameatal hollow in the posterosuperior tunnel, through the middle ear finally into the cochlea. The rest of the electrode array is placed like a loop in the suprameatal hollow and partly covered with bone dust. Mucosa is repositioned. Cochleotomy covered with temporalis fascia. Tympanomeatal flap is repositioned. Working of implant is

confirmed with diagnostic interface box (DIB). Telemetry is done. Wurzburg flap and subcutaneous tissue is closed by interrupted absorbable sutures. Skin is closed by continuous nonabsorbable sutures. Antibiotic impregnated wick kept in the external auditory canal.

The advantages of this technique are:
- Less traumatic, because no mastoidectomy and posterior tympanotomy is needed
- Better approach to the cochlea ensures proper opening and prevents malpositioning of the electrode array
- The second turn and the apex of the cochlea can be easily opened in cases of obliteration or ossification
- It is suitable for very young children, where the mastoid has not yet been sufficiently developed[7]
- It is suitable for revision cases and makes cochlear implantation simple and safe for the hands of the average ear surgeon.

Suprameatal Approach

Kronenberg J (2001) introduces a new approach for cochlear implantation by means of which mastoidectomy is avoided and the duration of the operation is decreased. This is the so-called suprameatal approach. This technique eliminates the need for mastoidectomy and posterior tympanotomy. The middle ear is entered through a retroauricular tympanotomy flap, and the electrode is introduced into the cochlea via a tunnel drilled in the suprameatal region superior to Henle's spine. The average length of the drilled tunnel in children is 7 mm and in adults 12 mm. The suprameatal approach is simple and safe technique that does not endanger the facial nerve and the chorda tympani. A wide exposure of the promontory enables exact determination of scala tympani and smooth introduction of the electrodes into the cochlea. This technique may also be used in malformed or ossified cochlea.

The Middle Cranial Fossa Approach

Colletti V et al. (1998) proposed the placement of cochlear implant to be performed through the middle cranial fossa. The anatomy of petrous bone makes the approach to the cochlea through middle cranial fossa possible. The cochlea is in contact with the anterior petrous wall in its anterosuperior region. The basal and middle turns are reachable in the angle between the labyrinthine portion of facial nerve and N. petrosus superficialis major. The surgical technique is as follows: A temporal craniotomy measuring 3 × 3 cm is performed. The lower bony margin should lie maximally close to the floor of middle cranial fossa. The bone flap is removed plastically. The dura is elevated from the middle cranial fossa floor towards foramen spinosum. A. meningea media is visualized. N. petrosus superficialis major is identified and followed to ganglion geniculi. The elevation of dura continues medially till the location of eminentia arcuata. The bone is drilled in a triangular area limited by N. petrosus superficialis major and the projection of the labyrinthine portion of facial nerve. The basal turn of the cochlea is easily identified by its bluish color. A cochleostomy of about 1.5 mm is performed in its highest part. The method makes possible the stimulation of middle and apical turn of the cochlea, where the number of functioning ganglion cells is usually greater, compared to the basal turn.

Transepitympanic Approach

This approach utilizes a transepitympanic pathway for electrode array and an endomeatal approach for cochleostomy. This transepitympanic approach avoids mastoidectomy and posterior tympanotomy. The electrode array is guided into the middle ear via a lateral epitympanotomy between the superior posterior wall of the outer ear canal and the posterior process of incus. Cochleostomy is done via an endomeatal approach following elevation of tympanomeatal flap.

Advantages of transepitympanic approach includes—safer, less invasive, landmark surgery (surgical steps under visualization of superior wall of outer ear canal, incus, bony labyrinth, chorda tympani nerve, tympanic segment of facial nerve) and a routine approach for ear surgeon.

Advantages of transcanal cochleostomy includes—wide overview on promontory, clear visualization of landmarks

for positioning of cochleostomy, facilitates identification of the site and angle of cochleostomy.[8]

Cochlear Implant Surgical Steps

- Incision (Fig. 6)
- Raising of Posteriorly Based Flap (Fig. 7)
- Implant (Fig. 8)
- Fixing the Receiver stimulator (Fig. 9)
- Cochleostomy with the Implant (Fig. 10)
- Postoperative telemetry (Fig. 11)
- Postoperative X-ray to check the Implant (Fig. 12)
- Important radiological findings (Figs 13 and 14)

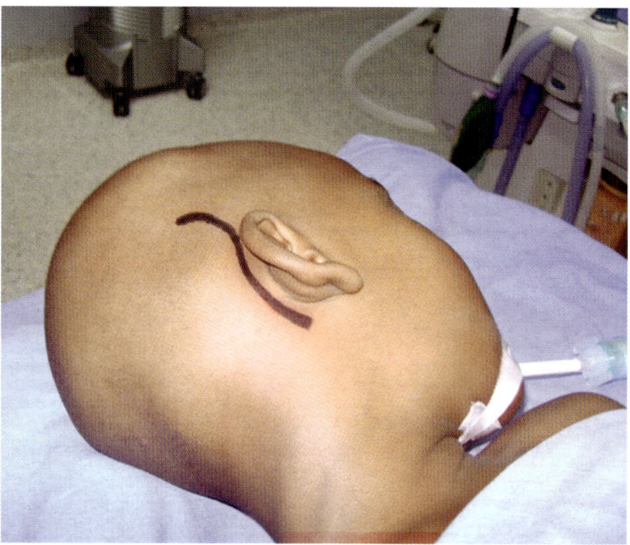

Fig. 6: Incision for cochlear implant surgery

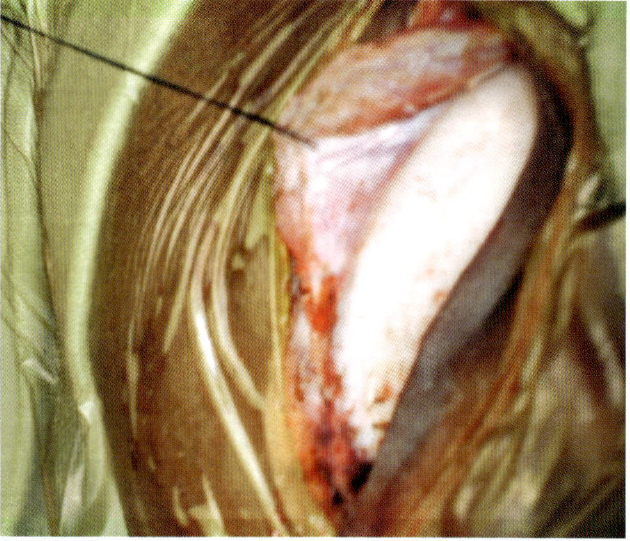

Fig. 7: Raising of posteriorly based flap

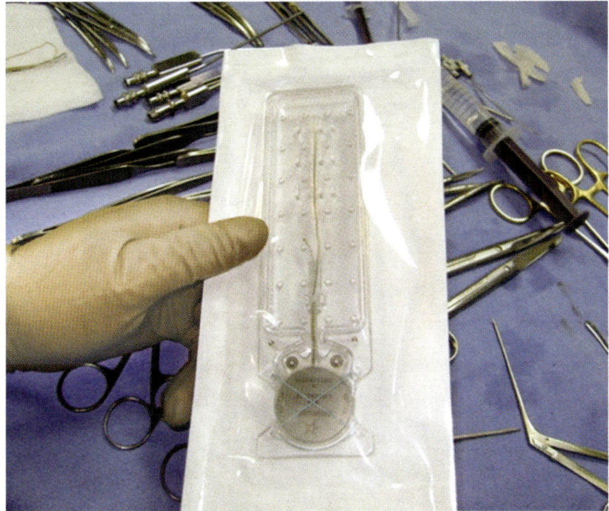

Fig. 8: Implant

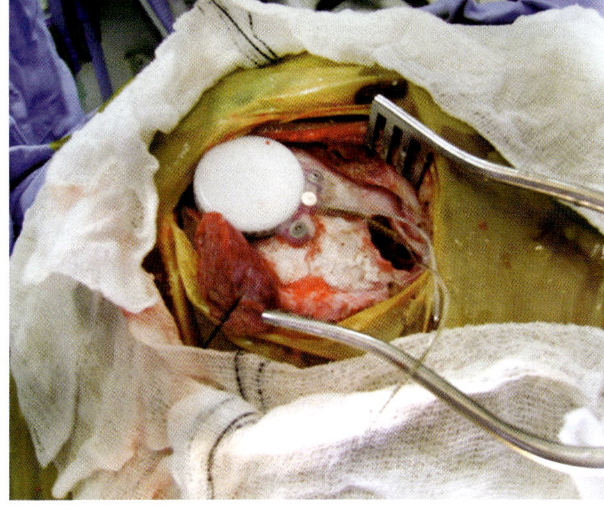

Fig. 10: Cochleostomy with the implant

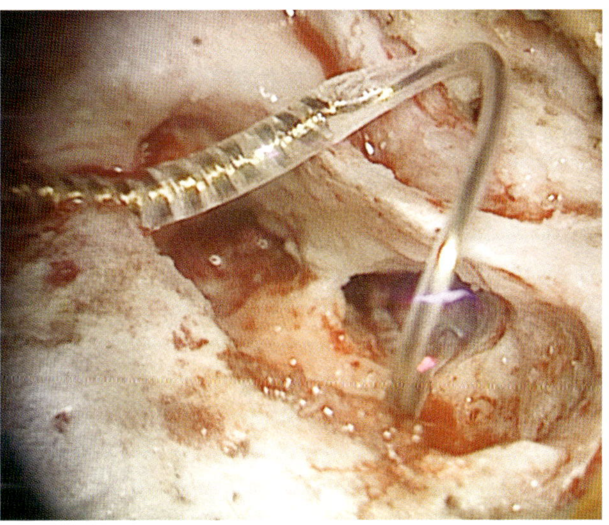

Fig. 9: Fixing the receiver stimulator

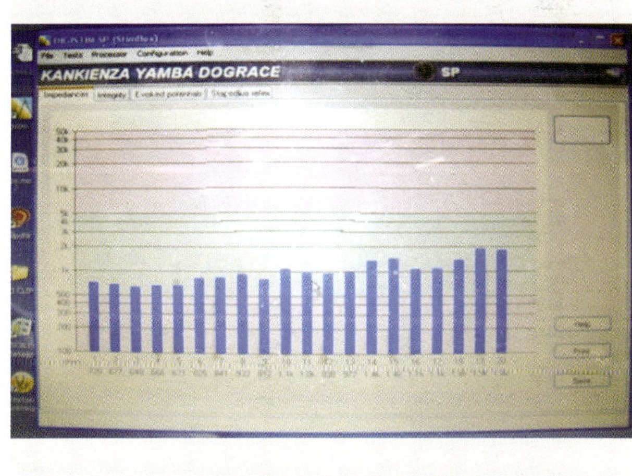

Fig. 11: Postoperative telemetry

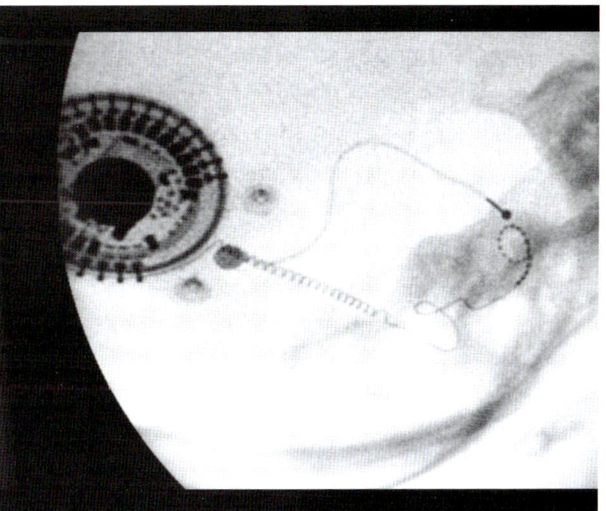

Fig. 12: Postoperative X-ray to check the implant

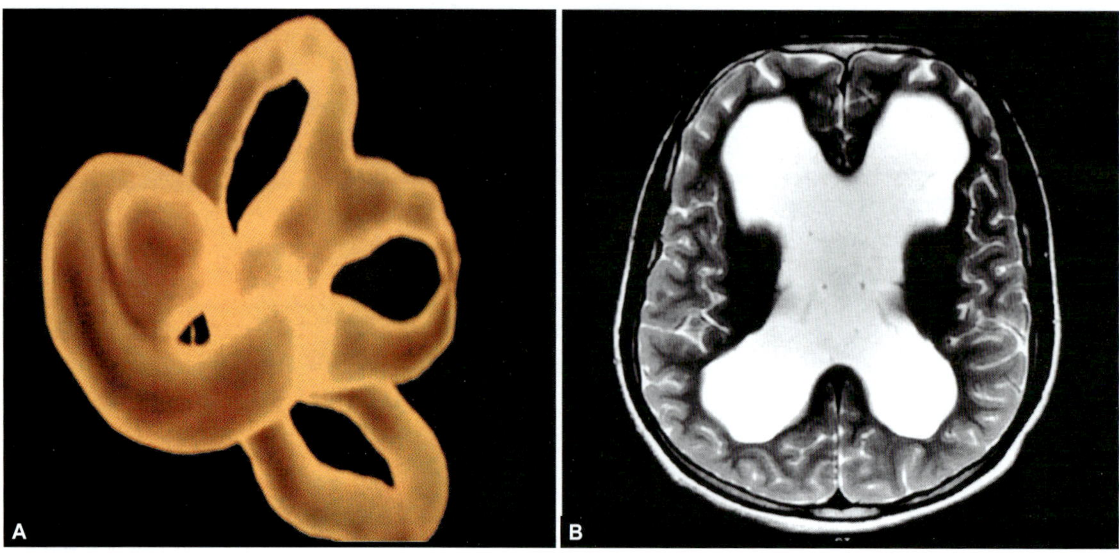

Figs 13A and B: (A) Normal 3-D reconstruction of cochlea; (B) Postmeningitic hydrocephalous

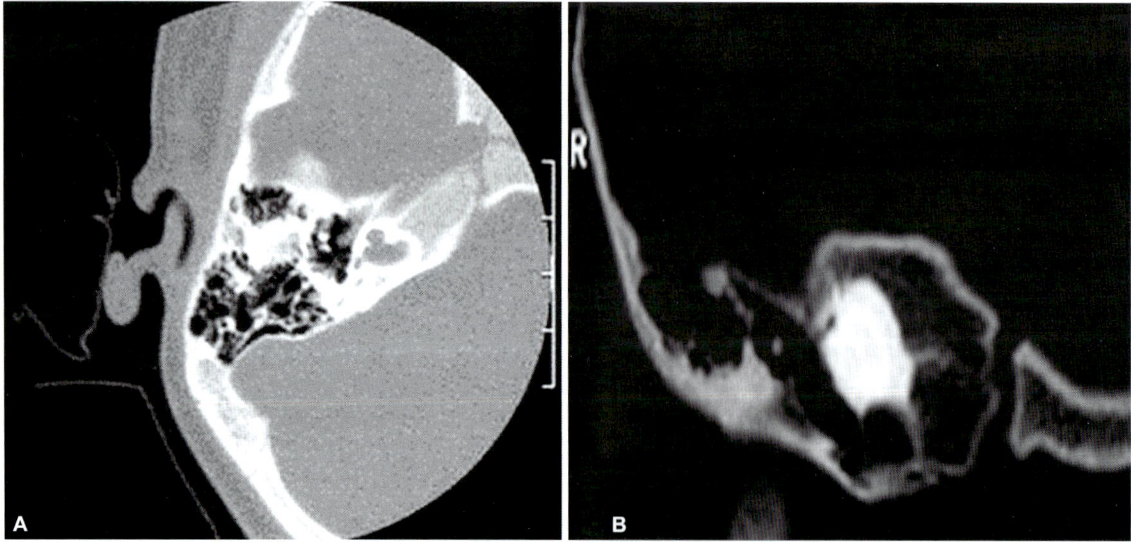

Figs 14A and B: (A) Mondini's dysplasia (common cavity cochlea); (B) Postmeningitic labirynthitis ossificans

COMPLICATIONS

The surgical complication rate after cochlear implantation is estimated to be only 5%. The most common problems are wound infection and wound breakdown. Rarely, extrusion of the device, facial nerve injury, bleeding, CSF leaks and meningitis can occur. Device-related complications include intracochlear damage, slippage of the array, breakage of the implant, and improper or inadequate insertion.

Recent reports of increased incidence of meningitis in cochlear implant recipients have prompted the CDC to recommend vaccination of implanted or soon to be implanted patients. Children less than 2 years old who have implants should receive pneumococcal conjugate vaccine (Prevnar). Children with implants 2 years and older who have completed the conjugate series should receive one dose of the pneumococcal polysaccharide vaccine (Pneumovax 23 or Pnu-Imune 23). Children with implants between 24 and 59 months who have never received vaccination should receive two doses of pneumococcal conjugate vaccine 2 months apart and then one dose of pneumococcal polysaccharide vaccine at least 2 months later. Finally, persons age 5 years and older with cochlear implants should receive one dose of pneumococcal polysaccharide vaccine.

Flap complications can be avoided by using an incision that does not compromise the blood supply to the postauricular region. Seroma formation may be avoided by use of a mastoid compressive dressing for at least 2 days. If a seroma develops, it can be evacuated using an 18-gauge or larger needle using sterile technique. A mastoid dressing should be reapplied for 2 days. Initially, raising a supraperiosteal flap and then raising a subperiosteal and pericranial flap based in opposite directions results in complete coverage of the internal receiver with fascia, which creates a secure closure that minimizes postoperative complications.

Promptly treat minor infections with oral and topical antibiotics. Intravenous antibiotics and, if necessary, flap revision can save an otherwise extruding device secondary to major infection. Implant migration can be avoided by securing the device deep within the bony well with secure tie-down sutures. Electrode migration is minimized by packing the cochleostomy with tissue, such as temporalis fascia or muscle. Facial stimulation usually can be managed by deactivating certain offending electrodes.

A CSF/perilymph gusher via the round window is common in patients with cochlear anomalies, such as enlarged vestibular aqueduct syndrome, common cavity, and wide internal auditory canal syndrome. These complications are best managed by packing the round window with fascia after implant insertion. Dizziness after surgery typically is short-lived and usually resolves with observation. When device failure is believed to have occurred, perform telemetry and consider consultation with the manufacturer before explantation and reimplantation.[9]

Classification of Complication

Short-term Complications

- Facial paralysis
- Wound infection
- Skin/flap necrosis
- Misplacement of electrode array
- Short-term increase in tinnitus.

Long-term Complicatons

- Gradual hearing deterioration
- Device failure
- Extrusion of electrode array
- Extrusion of implant through the scalp
- Facial nerve twitching following stimulation

- Progressive partial facial nerve paralysis
- Long-term balance disturbances
- Long-term increased tinnitus
- Numbness of scalp
- Taste disturbances
- Nonusers.

POSTOPERATIVE REHABILITATION

Unless intensive postoperative rehabilitation is undertaken, cochlear implantation is likely to provide little benefit. Each patient's need for rehabilitation is different based on preoperative auditory experience. For the prelingually deaf patient, auditory and speech training are imperative if they are to improve their communication abilities. Postlingually deaf patients often need training in more complex listening skills. Cochlear implants in children are successful when the implantation is followed by a intensive treatment by a multidiscipline rehabilitation team. The goal of a pediatric rehabilitation team is to enable the hearing-impaired child to be able to learn passively from his environment. The rehabilitation must address both receptive language skills as well as expressive language abilities. A structured program with dedicated team members is integral to a successful cochlear implant program.

REFERENCES

1. Graeme Clark. Cochlear implants. Fundamentals and applications. Publisher Springer: 2003.
2. Clark GM. The university of Melbourne/Cochlear Corporation (Nucleus) programme. Otolaryngological Clinics of North America. 1986;19:329-54.
3. Clark GM and Hallworth RJ. A multielectrode array for a cochlear implant. Journal of Laryngology and Otology. 1976;90:623-7.
4. Cochlear Corporation. Surgical procedure manual: Nucleus 22 channel cochlear implant system, Issue 5. Englewood, CO: Cochlear Corp; 1987.
5. Nomura Y. Otological significance of the round window. Advances in Otorhinolaryngology. 1984;33:27-37.
6. Shambaugh G. Surgery of the ear. Philadelphia: WB Saunders; 1959.
7. Luxford W and House W. Cochlear implants in children. Ear and Hearing. 1977;6:205-35.
8. Clark GM. A surgical approach for a cochlear implant. An anatomical study. Journal of Laryngology and Otology. 1975;89:9-15.
9. Dowell RC, Blamey PJ and Clark GM. Potential and limitations of cochlear implantation in children. Annals of Otology, Rhinology and Laryngology. 1995;104 (sup 166):324-7.

Hearing Aids, Implants and Assistive Listening Devices

Indranil Chatterjee

INTRODUCTION

A hearing aid is an electroacoustic device which is designed to amplify and modulate sound that will enable a user to use his/her remaining hearing effectively. Earlier devices, known as ear trumpets or ear horns, were passive funnel-like amplification cones designed to gather sound energy and direct it into the ear canal.[1] Hearing aids partially overcome the deficits associated with hearing loss. For a sensorineural hearing loss, there are several deficits to overcome. Some sounds are inaudible. Other sounds can be detected because part of their spectra (typically the high-frequency) remains inaudible. The range of levels between the weakest sound that can be heard and the most intense sound that can be tolerated is less for a person with sensorineural hearing loss than for a normal hearing person. To compensate for this, a hearing aid has to amplify weak sounds more than it amplifies for intense sounds.[2]

COMPONENTS OF HEARING AID

A modern electronic hearing aid, however, is an amplifier whose function is to increase intensity of the sound and amplify voice and speech, effectively so that the person has a better sense of what is being said and to deliver it to the ear with as little distortion as possible. Since the acoustic energy of sound cannot be amplified directly, it is necessary to convert it to an electrical signal; this signal is amplified and then changed back to acoustical energy. For this process to happen, the hearing aid should contain these basic components:
- Microphone
- Amplifier
- Receiver
- Power supply
- Tone control
- Volume control
- Ear mold/tubing
- Compression/AGC systems.

The basic components of hearing aid include microphone, amplifier and receiver in analog, digital and programmable hearing aids. However, the circuits differ in programmable and digital hearing aids compared to analog hearing aids.

TYPES OF HEARING AIDS

Hearing aids by manner of placement—placement in the ear.

Body Worn Aids (Fig. 1)

This was the first type of hearing aid invented by Harvey Fletcher while working at Bell Laboratories. Body aids consist of a case and an earmould, attached by a wire. The case contains the electronic amplifier components, controls and battery while the earmould typically contains a miniature loudspeaker. The case is typically about the size of a pack of playing cards and is carried in a pocket or on a belt. Without the size constraints of smaller hearing devices, body worn aid designs can provide large amplification and long battery life at a lower cost.

Behind the Ear (Fig. 2)

The body of the instrument is worn behind the ear (BTE). It 'hooks' over the pinna. It is attached via plastic tubing to an earmould, which holds it in place in the ear. BTEs can be used for mild to profound hearing loss. As the electrical components are located outside the ear, the chance of moisture and earwax damaging the components is reduced, which can increase the durability of the instrument. A new type of BTE aid called the mini BTE (or "on-the-ear") aid.

It also fits behind/on the ear, but is smaller. A very thin, almost invisible tube is used to connect the aid to the ear canal. Mini BTEs may have a comfortable ear piece for insertion ("open fit"), but may also use a traditional earmould. Mini BTEs allow not only reduced occlusion or "plugged-up" sensations in the ear canal, but also increase comfort, reduce feedback and address cosmetic concerns for many users.

In the Ear (Fig. 3)

The complete hearing aid is in the ear (ITE) or ear canal. The hearing aid is housed in a hard plastic shell which is often custom made by taking an ear impression. ITC aids are smaller, filling only the bottom half of the external ear. CICs are usually not recommended for people with good low-frequency hearing, as the occlusion effect is much more noticeable. In-the-ear hearing aids are typically more expensive than behind-the-ear counterparts of equal functionality, because they are custom-fitted to the patient's ear.

Spectacle Hearing Aid (Fig. 4)

During the late 1950s through 1970s, before in-the-ear aids became common (and in an era when thick-rimmed eyeglasses were popular), people who wore both glasses and hearing aids frequently chose a type of hearing aid that was built into the temple pieces of the spectacles. However, the combination of glasses and hearing aids was inflexible—the range of frame styles was limited, and the user had to wear both hearing aids and glasses at once or wear nothing.

Special function hearing aid/noninvasive special function hearing aid (Hearing aid for unilateral hearing loss) are discussed further.

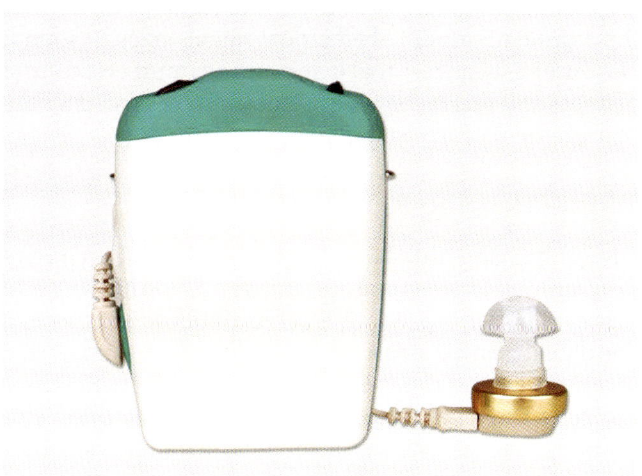

Fig. 1: Body worn hearing aid

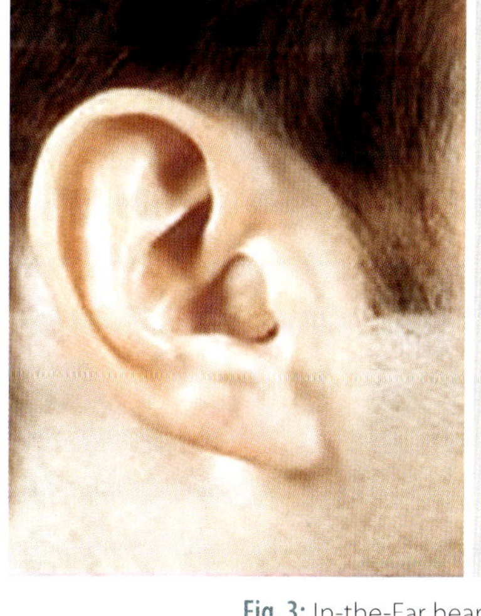

Fig. 3: In-the-Ear hearing aid

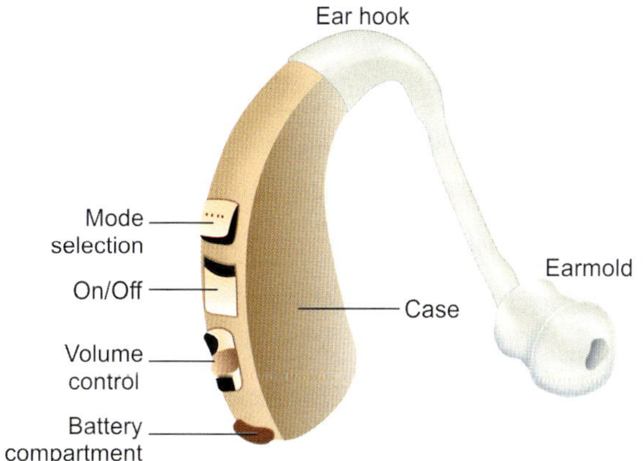

Fig. 2: Behind the ear hearing aid

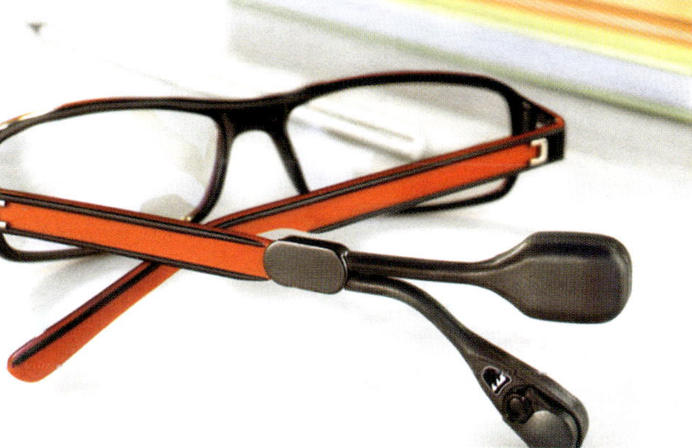

Fig. 4: Spectacle hearing aid

Contralateral Routing of Offside Signals (Fig. 5)

Contralateral routing of offside signal (CROS) is a type of hearing aid that is used to treat unilateral hearing loss. It takes sound from the ear with poorer hearing and transmits to the ear with better hearing. Systems can involve two behind-the-ear units connected either by wire or by wireless transmission. There are also systems incorporated into eyeglasses. A CROS (Contralateral Routing of Signal) aid is made up of two instruments—a microphone (transmitter) and a hearing aid (receiver). Patients wear the transmitter on the deaf ear and the receiver on the hearing ear. Sound is transmitted via a wire connecting each unit, infrared or radiofrequency. Almost all CROS aids fitted in this country use a wire to transmit sound. As with a BAHA device, the time delay associated with the transmission gives the user the necessary temporal cues to help determine from which side the sound originated. If a person has a degree of hearing loss on the hearing side as well, amplification can be added to the receiver side as well as the transmitter, creating what is known as a "BICROS" aid.

Hearing Aid by Signal Processing Approaches

- Analog hearing aid
- Digital hearing aid.

Invasive Special Function Hearing Aid

- Bone-anchored hearing aid
- Middle ear implant
- Cochlear implant
- Brainstem implant
- Electroacoustic stimulation.

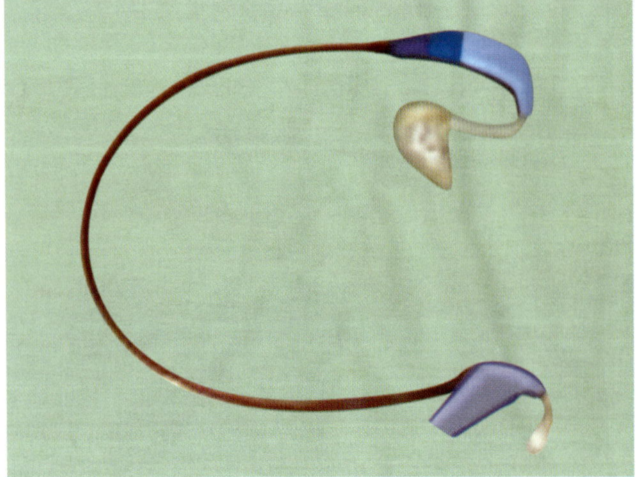

Fig. 5: CROS Hearing aid

Hearing Aid by Mode of Presentation

- Air conduction/Bone conduction
- Monoaural/Binaural.

Hearing Aid by Mode of Operation

- Single channel versus multichannel hearing aid
- Nonadaptive versus adaptive hearing aids.

Analog Hearing Aids

Analog hearing aids allow for the representation of a continuously changing physical variable (i.e. sound) by another physical variable (i.e. electrical current). The first block encountered by an acoustic signal is a microphone, which converts sound into electricity. The small signals produced by microphones are made more powerful by the hearing aid amplifier. The sound that is amplified is delivered by the receiver to the ear. The receiver is a miniature headphone that use electromagnetism to convert the amplified, modified electrical signals back to sound. The disadvantages are that it does not allow precise control of filters and that technology is becoming outdated for the management of acoustic signal.

Digital Hearing Aids

Digital hearing aids have all the features of analogue programmable aids, but they convert sound waves into digital signals and produce an exact duplication of sound. The digital hearing aids allow for more complex processing of sound during the amplification process, which may improve their performance in certain situations (for example, background noise and whistle reduction). They also have greater flexibility in hearing aid programming so that the sound they transmit can be matched to the needs for a specific pattern of hearing loss. Digital hearing aids also provide multiple program memories.

Table 1 explains about the feature of three different types of hearing aid, i.e. Analog, Programmable and Digital hearing aids. Programmable hearing aid can be analog and digital also and manipulations are possible in programmable hearing aids as per requirements. Digital hearing aids converts the analog into digital signal.

Linear and Nonlinear Amplification

Linear amplification (Fig. 6) means that the relationship between input and output is proportional, so that, low-intensity sounds are amplified to the same extent as high-intensity sounds.[3] A problem with this type of linear amplification is that it doesn't address the nonlinearity of

Table 1: Analog Vs Programmable Vs Digital Hearing Aids

Feature	Analog	Programmable	Digital
Signal processing	Continuously varying amplitude over time	Manipulation of acoustic parameters as per requirements	Sampling technique, changing signals into varying discrete voltages
Output	Replica of input	Varied over memories and programs	Analog to digital converted signal
Amplifiers	Class A or B Analog Vs Programmable Vs Digital Hearing Aids	Class D	Class D in combination with Class H
S/N Ratio	Poor	Better	Improved
Additional Features	Absent	WDRC	AGC
Best Suited for	Flat hearing loss	Sloping hearing loss	Reduced speech scores in noise

Fig. 6: Linear amplification

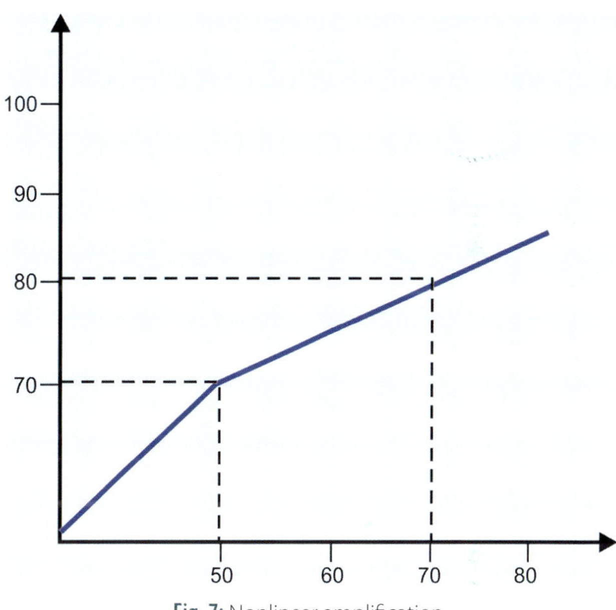

Fig. 7: Nonlinear amplification

loudness growth that occurs with sensorineural hearing impairment. A linear device amplifies both soft and loud sounds identically. As a result, if a low-intensity sound is made loud enough to be audible, a high-intensity sound is likely to be made too loud for the listener.

Nonlinear amplification (Fig. 7) means that the relationship between input and output is not proportional, so that, for example, low-intensity sounds are amplified to a greater extent than high-intensity sounds.[3] Nonlinear amplification is achieved with something called compression circuitry. Compression is a term that is used to describe how the amplification of a signal is reduced as a function of its intensity. Compression techniques are used both to limit the maximum output of a hearing aid and to provide nonlinear amplification across a wide range of inputs.

Techniques of Nonlinear Amplification

Nonlinear prescription can be viewed as specifying the gain frequency response for several input levels for both the average gain and the shape of the frequency response will vary with input level. Alternatively, the prescription can be viewed as specifying an input-output (I-O) curve for several frequencies. It is necessary to specify the I-O curve for at least as many frequencies as there are channels in a multichannel hearing aid. There are several various techniques for nonlinear amplification, they are:

- Loudness growth in half-octave bands (LGOB)
- Independent hearing aid fitting forum (IHAFF)
- Madsen aurical method
- Scaladapt
- FIG6
- DSL[i/o]
- NAL-NL1.

ELECTROACOUSTICS CHARACTERISTICS

The performance characteristics of a hearing aid, that is the changes affected in a signal as it is transduced from acoustic to electric to acoustic energy are known as the electroacoustic characteristics. One ear simulator with four cavities is known as the Knowles DB100 ear simulator. Another ear simulator in common use is the BRUEL and KJAER 4138 ear simulator. It operates on the same principles, except that it has two simulators, have a very similar variation of impedance with frequency. But unfortunately, the standard 2-cc coupler is larger than the average adult ear canal with a hearing aid in place, so the hearing aid generates lower SPL in the coupler than in the average ear. This difference is called real ear to coupler difference (RECD). An ear simulator or artificial ear is a far more sophisticated device for the calibration of an ear phone. Like the acoustic coupler, it contains a calibrated microphone for the measurement of the sound pressure developed within a cavity. Several standards published by the ANSI and International electroacoustical commission (IEC) specify how hearing aids should be tested. ANSI S3.22 specifies that hearing aids be measured in a 2-cc coupler; whereas IEC 118-0 specifies that hearing aids be measured in an ear simulator. The ITE and ITC hearing aids usually connected directly to a coupler or ear simulator. BTE and body aids, however, connect to the real ear via an earmold, so an earmold simulator is added between the coupler or the ear simulator and the hearing aid. In addition, BTE hearing aids use tubing when connecting to the real ear, so they also require tubing when connecting to the coupler or simulator. ANSI S3.3 describes a 2-cc coupler as being used in several different applications.

Common Electroacoustic Characteristics

Gain: The gain is the amount in decibels, by which the sound pressure level developed by the hearing aid in the coupler exceeds the sound pressure level in the sound field at the hearing aid microphone. Simply, gain equals output minus input.

Frequency response: The frequency range of a hearing aid refers to the useful range of the frequency response. It is expressed by two numbers first, low-frequency limit of the amplification and high-frequency limit of amplification. The relation between frequency and gain constitutes one area of interest in specifying electroacoustic behavior of hearing aid.

Saturation sound pressure level: The saturation sound pressure level (SSPL) value represents the maximum root mean square (RMS) sound pressure level obtainable in the coupler as generated by the receiver of the hearing aid.

Measurement of OSPL Frequency Response

The purpose of this test is to determine the sound pressure level obtained in the HA-2 coupler while giving an input 90 dB SPL and the hearing aid gain control in the full on position as a function of frequency.

It is important to know at what level a hearing aid limits its output when it receives a high-level input signal. The maximum possible level should not exceed the threshold of discomfort for a user.

Measuring on Full on Acoustic Gain Frequency Response

Acoustic gain is defined as the output SPL in an earphone coupler and the input SPL. It is a measure of how much the input signal is amplified. Acoustic gain is a function of frequency and the user gain control setting as well as other factors. When the gain control is set to its maximum position, i.e. full-on, and the input SPL is adjusted to a suitable value that will not overload the hearing aid, the full-on gain may be measured and recorded as a function of frequency.

The purpose of this test is to determine the full-on acoustic gain obtainable with the hearing instrument. The output sound pressure level in the HA-2 coupler is measured at full-on gain control setting with an input below the hearing instrument's saturation sound pressure level (Normally 60 dB SPL).

Measurement of Basic Frequency Response

The purpose of this test is to measure the frequency response of a hearing aid without acoustic (feedback) or mechanical (vibration problems). If one compares the shape of the full-on acoustic gain frequency response to the basic frequency response, then acoustic or mechanical problems can be identified. The more similar the shapes of the curves are, the more stable is the hearing aid.

Frequency Range

To provide a general idea of the range of frequencies over which a hearing aid might be considered effective, a standardized method of determination has been adopted. The method is based on the frequency response curve. A horizontal line is drawn at a specific location. The frequency range is defined by the intersections (f1 and f2) of the response curve and the horizontal line. The location of the horizontal line is 20 dB downward from the average value of points R1, R2 and R3 at 1000, 1600 and 2500 Hz, respectively.

Nonlinear Distortions

The purpose of this test is to determine the degree of the amplitude nonlinearity in the sound output under specified conditions.

The ability of a hearing aid to deliver a clean signal at the required output level is indicated by measuring its nonlinear distortion characteristics.

The total harmonic distortion is a measure of nonlinearity.

The amplitude nonlinearity can be described in terms of harmonic distortion and intermodulation distortion.

Harmonic distortion: When the input is a sine wave, the distortion products occur at frequencies that are harmonics (i.e. integer multiples) of the input frequency. Consequently, the process is called harmonic distortion.

Intermodulation distortion: When a more complex signal is peak-clipped, the distortion products occur at frequencies that are harmonics of all the frequencies in the input signal, and at frequencies that are combination of all the harmonics. If two tones, with frequencies f1 and f2 are input, for e.g. distortion component will occur at 2f1, 3f1, 4f1, 2f2, 3f2, 4f2, f2-f1, 2f2-f1, 2f1-f2, 3f1-f2, to name but a few frequencies. Although the mechanism causing the distortion is exactly the same as for harmonic distortion (peak clipping is the most common cause), the result is called **intermodulation distortion.**

Total Harmonic distortion: The power of all the distortion products is summed and expressed relative to the power of the wanted output signal component; this ratio is referred to as total harmonic distortion.

The gain control is adjusted to the reference test position and the input sound pressure level increased to 70 dB SPL. The total harmonic distortion is measured an input level of 70 dB at 500, 800 and 65 dB at 1600 Hz. In the event, the specified frequency response curves rises 12 dB or more between any distortions test frequency and its second harmonic, distortion tests at that frequency may be omitted.

Equivalent input noise level: The quantity is not too important because the internal noise levels of normally operating modern hearing aid electronics are low compared to ambient noise levels typically encountered. The space to carry out this test must be extremely quiet to avoid false readings due to ambience noise when making the test for this quantity.

Measurement of Battery Current

The purpose of this test is to determine the current consumption of the H/A in operation.

Test procedure: With the gain control in the reference test gain position, measure the battery current at the reference test frequency with an input sound pressure level of 60 dB SPL and at the reference test frequency. A 1000-Hz tone is introduced into the free field at an intensity of 65 dB SPL

and battery current drain is measured. When other than a standard hearing aid battery is used as a power source, the internal impedance of the power source is to be stated. The tolerance for battery current drain is such that it shall not exceed the value specified by the manufacturer for that model of hearing aid.

Coupler SPL with Induction coil: The sensitivity of a telecoil is measured with the aid set to the 'T' mode and oriented to produce the greatest coupler SPL. The aid is placed in a strong magnetic field created with a "Telecoil Magnetic field simulator" and the gain control set to the reference test position. A frequency response (sound pressure level for an inductive telephone simulator or SPLITS) curve can be made between 200 and 5000 Hz. A high-frequency average of the SPLITS curve (HFA-SPLITS) or a special purpose average (SPA-SPLITS) can be calculated as described for acoustic gain. Also available are simulated telephone sensitivity (STS) HFA-SPLITS (HFA-SPLITS-Reference test gain + 60 dB of merit for how much the volume control will have to be rotated when switching from microphone position to telephone position, or STS SPA-SPLITS (SPA-SPLITS-reference test gain + 60 dB).

I/O Characteristics

Automatic gain Control (AGC) Aids: It is important to know how output SPL varies with as a function of input SPL from 50 to 90 dB in 5 dB steps, measured at one of the following frequencies; 250, 500, 1000, 2000, or 4000 Hz. The curves are drawn on a grid with output SPL as the ordinate and input SPL as the abscissa.

Dynamic AGC Characteristics

The AGC function takes time. The "Dynamic AGC characteristics" is a method to determine the attack and release times for the AGC function. With the aids gain control set to the reference-test position, a 2000 Hz input tone is abruptly alternated between 55 and 90 dB SPL.

The attack time is defined as the time between the abrupt increase and the point where the output level has stabilized to ±3 dB of the steady-state value for the 90 dB input.

The release time is defined as the time between the abrupt drop and the point where the hearing aid output stabilized to ±4 dB of the steady state 55 dB input SPL. Times are stated in milliseconds.

HEARING AID CARE

- Avoid high temperatures
- Don't leave the hearing aid in the direct sunlight, in a hot car, on a heater, or on any other piece of equipment that generates heat. Heat can damage the hearing aid

amplifier and can cause batteries to deteriorate. Avoid Moisture—Keep the hearing aid dry. Even perspiration can cause damage to the hearing aid. Protect the aid from hard knocks—Avoid dropping the hearing aid or bumping it against hard objects. Removing the aid—Get into the habit of turning the switch to the "OFF" position before you take off the aid. When the switch is in the "ON" position, the battery is discharging whether the child is wearing the hearing aid or not. If the aid doesn't have an "OFF" switch, open the battery compartment so that the battery is not touching the battery contacts. Repairs—Do not attempt to repair the hearing aid. If the aid is not functioning properly, ask the audiologist or hearing aid dealer for assistance. Many times a loaner aid can be supplied by a hearing aid dispenser while the aid is being repaired. Tubing and Cords—If the child has a behind-the-ear or eyeglass type of hearing aid, the tubing should be replaced when it becomes dry, brittle, and yellow. If the child has a body aid, the cord will eventually wear out or develop a short and need to be replaced. Avoid twisting the cord, and do not use safety pins to position the cord since the pin could inadvertently pierce the cord.

BONE-ANCHORED HEARING AIDS

Introduction (Fig. 8)

Most patients with hearing loss can be successfully fitted with a conventional hearing aid which involves the placement of an occlusive earmold in the external ear canal. For some hearing impaired persons, however, the fitting of a conventional hearing aid is problematic in spite of favorable audiological criteria. For example, in patients

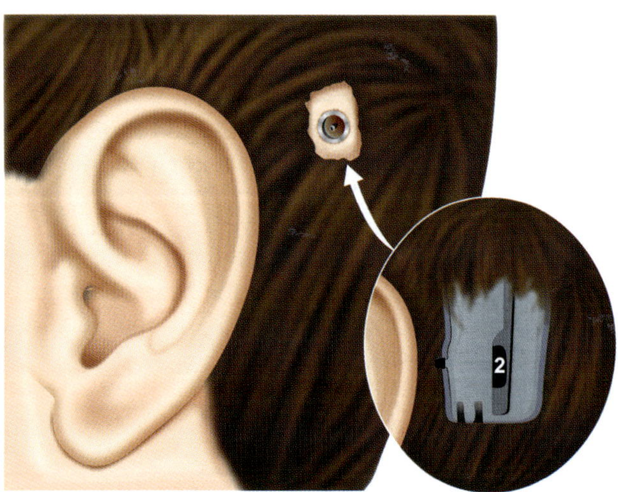

Fig. 8: Bone-anchored hearing aid

with stenosis of the external ear canal due to congenital middle ear malformation or agenesis, an earmold cannot be placed.[4] Hearing impaired persons with chronic suppurative otitis media (CSOM) suffer from ear discharge that often exacerbates when an occlusive earmold is placed. Another group of patients for whom a conventional hearing aid is often problematic are those with a canal wall down mastoidectomy cavity. They have a wide external ear canal and acoustic feedback frequently occurs. In some otological conditions, thus, the occlusive earmold of the conventional hearing aid is the major bottleneck in restoring hearing. For these patients, a bone-anchored hearing aid (BAHA) does not imply occlusion of the external ear canal and offers a valid alternative to conventional hearing aids. More recently, the indications for a BAHA have been extended to include unilateral deafness. For these patients, the BAHA is implanted at the deaf side, and bone conduction routes sound to the functional cochlea. Compared to a conventional contralateral routing of sound (CROS) hearing aid, patients report high satisfaction with the BAHA.

Principles

The BAHA stimulates the cochlea through bone conduction, in a similar way as a tuning fork does. Because the external and middle ear are bypassed, pathological conditions of these structures do not interfere with hearing as they would do with a conventional hearing aid. Bone conduction stimulation of the cochlea results from several physical phenomena.[5]

- Sound transmission in the external ear canal (predominantly at high-frequencies)
- Inertia of the tympano-ossicular chain and the inner ear fluids (predominantly at low-frequencies)
- Compression of the inner ear spaces (predominantly at mid frequencies).

For bone-anchored hearing aids, the latter two phenomenas are quantitatively most important and hearing gain will eventually be limited by the amount of sensorineural hearing loss. Sound radiation in the ear canal does occur with a BAHA, but this sound energy reaches the inner ear strongly attenuated due to the pathologic state of the middle ear that indicates the use of the BAHA. As sound waves propagate through the bones of the skull, the contralateral cochlea is stimulated as well, which is a second benefit of the BAHA, as will be discussed forthwith. By using a percutaneous titanium bone-integrated fixture, the BAHA overcomes the limitation of transcutaneous devices, such as a bone conduction hearing aid incorporated in a headset or spectacles. Most interestingly, acoustic feedback or Larsen's effect does not occur with the BAHA.

INDICATIONS AND PATIENT SELECTION CRITERIA

Audiological Indications

- For the BAHA Compact, the average bone conduction threshold should be better than or equal to 45 dB HL (measured at 500 Hz, 1 kHz, 2 kHz and 3 kHz). Recently, a BAHA with digital sound processing, the BAHA Divino, has been released. Its maximal amplification is identical to the BAHA Compact, but it has automatic gain control (AGC) capability and two microphones: an omnidirectional microphone and a directional front-facing microphone. The BAHA Cordelle II is a body worn device and has the more powerful K-amp amplifier, which yields an output that is on average 13 dB stronger than the BAHA Classic
- A maximum speech discrimination score should be better than 60% in the poorer ear[7,8]
- The pure tone average of air conduction threshold of the normal hearing ear should be better than or equal to 20–25 dB HL (measured at 500 Hz, 1 kHz, 2 kHz and 3 kHz in the audiometric test frequencies)
- Using a test band or rod, the candidate can evaluate the sound quality and possible gain of the BAHA device prior to implantation. Pure tone and speech audiometry can be carried out and thus expectations are obtained.

Otological Indications

- Congenital malformations with agenesis or atresia of the middle or external ear. In cases of microtia or a completely absent pinna, an epithesis can be provided with two additional fixation points
- Chronically, draining ears do not allow use of an air conduction hearing aid, such as mastoidectomy cases with poor sound transmission and recurrent problems of humidity, discharge or infection in case of occlusion by a hearing aid or recurrent external otitis
- Patients with unilateral conductive hearing loss (and not appropriate for or refusing surgical correction) or unable to be aided by conventional air conduction hearing devices[3]
- Congenital or acquired unilateral total deafness,[8-10] e.g. after acoustic neuroma surgery where preservation of hearing was not possible.

Contraindications

- An average bone conduction threshold worse than 60 dB HL (measured at 500 Hz, 1 kHz, 2 kHz and 3 kHz)
- Mentally retarded or uncooperative patients; drug addicts, very small children (<2 years). In USA, the lower age limit is 5 years.

SURGERY

Since Anders Tjellström performed the first three screw implantations in 1977, the surgical procedure and the equipment have evolved significantly. The operation nowadays usually consists of a one-stage procedure, carried out under general or local anesthesia in the outpatient clinic. Currently, two types of incisions and surgical approaches are used, though the details of the actual implantation are identical in both procedures.[8]

The first approach uses a horseshoe-shaped skin flap that is mobilized somewhat posterosuperior to the pinna. The flap is elevated and thinned as much as possible before closure. When available, a dermatome can be used for thinning the skin. No subcutaneous fat tissue or hair follicles may remain. The second approach uses a single, straight incision through which the surrounding skin is undermined and thinned. The actual drilling site has to be chosen carefully, especially in small children or in postradiotherapy cases. Detailed spiral CT studies can be helpful in these particular cases, where sometimes a two-stage procedure is preferred. There are two types of self-tapping fixation screws: their lengths are 3 and 4 mm, respectively. After drilling a 3 mm deep hole, the presence of solid bone is assessed. If there is solid bone, then the drilling continues to a depth of 4 mm and the 4 mm fixture is used. This is usually the case. During the second stage, after osseointegration of the screw, the skin is again incised and thinned and, subsequently, the abutment is screwed onto the fixation screw. The so-called osseointegration takes about 3–4 months in healthy individuals, but in most centers, the fixture screw is loaded for the first time approximately 2 months after surgery. In cases of very thin bone or after radiotherapy, a longer waiting time is warranted.

EFFICACY

When reporting the outcome of a BAHA, several issues have to be considered—implantation success, skin tolerance, audiometric performance, and finally, overall patient satisfaction. Most studies report high success rate of osseointegration (>90%). As to complications, they are rare and generally limited to skin reactions. Loss of the fixture is reported to happen sporadically. Previously irradiated bone, bone disease and very thin cortical bone are negative prognostic factors, but not a contraindication.[11,12] Several clinical studies comparing the audiometric performance of the Bone-anchored hearing aid to those of air conduction hearing aids have been carried out. Especially, patients with a pure conductive hearing loss and a limited sensorineural loss up to 45 dB (0.5–3 kHz) are very satisfied, although sensorineural losses up to 60 dB (0.5–3 kHz) can be fitted using a body-worn device connected to the transducer (Cordelle II).

All studies on BAHA almost unanimously agree on a number of facts:

1. Neither conventional air conduction hearing aids, nor bone-anchored hearing aids rehabilitate hearing impaired patients to the level of normal hearing people. Although this might seem an obvious observation, it is important to convey this message to the patient prior to implantation to ensure they have realistic expectations.[13]
2. Both air conduction hearing aids and bone-anchored hearing aids yield very similar audiometric performances. Both were effective in improving aided free field hearing thresholds. The best improvement in hearing was observed between 1 and 2 kHz. In tests of temporal acuity, the BAHA scored slightly better, though not statistically significant.[14]
3. In terms of subjective improvement using validated questionnaires, the BAHA scored better. Almost all patients preferred their BAHA to the air conduction device they used beforehand. Of course, one has to take into account the problems these patients had with their conventional hearing aids encompass the indication for switching to BAHA.[14,15]
4. 99% of all patients confirmed reduced occurrence of ear discharge and discomfort.
5. In cases of single-sided deafness, studies demonstrate strongly positive patient reactions to the BAHA system. Although source localization was not improved, subjective benefit (quality of life) was reported consistently. Also, an objective improvement in speech recognition in noise was reported (except for the condition where the talker is at the side of the hearing ear). This suggests that reducing the head shadow by use of a BAHA has overall positive effects on hearing, compared to unilateral hearing. The results with BAHA were also consistently better than those with conventional CROS devices.[16] One recent review, however, comments on the validity of these studies, since they invariably consist of small numbers of patients, who have not always tried CROS devices for a long enough period according to the authors.[17]
6. Bilateral fitting of BAHA has been carried out on a limited scale. The results show that sound localization, speech recognition in quiet and in noise is significantly better compared to the monaural BAHA group.[18-20]

Conclusion

The Bone-anchored hearing aid is a valuable solution for a selected group of patients who cannot be satisfactorily helped by either functional surgery or a conventional hearing aid. Level A scientific evidence is at hand illustrating the effectiveness and safety of the procedure, as well as a significant improvement of speech discrimination and quality of life. Although an elegant and minimally invasive procedure, an operation is nonetheless required. Belgian social security reimburses the costs of the operation and the titanium implants. Furthermore, a partial reimbursement of the sound processor is provided, similar to a classic bone conduction hearing aid. The gain in quality of life significantly outweighs the inconveniences associated with this type of hearing.

MIDDLE EAR VIBRANT BRIDGE

The middle ear vibrant bridge (Fig. 9) is a new category of implantable middle ear hearing device. The implant directly vibrates the small bones in the middle ear. The vibrant bridge is indicated for use in adults, 18 years or older, with a moderate to severe sensorineural hearing loss and no interest in conventional hearing aids. The vibrant bridge is the first FDA-approved implantable middle ear hearing device to treat sensorineural hearing loss. A proven, safe and effective treatment that leaves the ear canal completely open, the vibrant bridge features a 94% improvement in patient satisfaction, with thousands of patients worldwide. The vibrant bridge is intended for use in adults (18 years or older) who have moderate-to-severe sensorineural hearing loss and desire an alternative to an acoustic hearing aid. The Vibrant bridge utilizes a hearing technology that directly

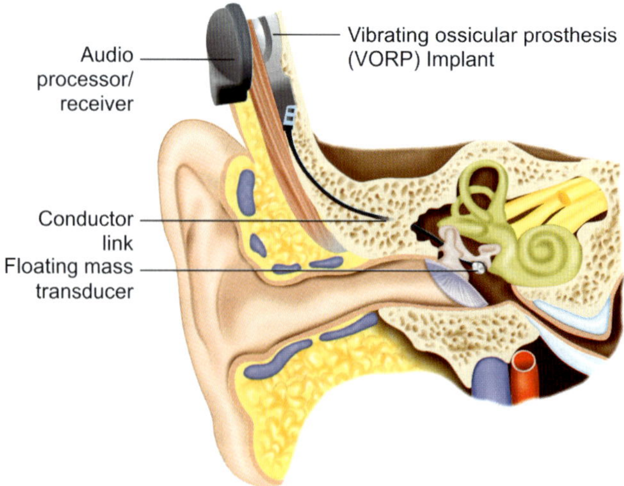

Fig. 9: Middle ear vibrant bridge

drives the ossicular chain (middle ear bones), bypassing the ear canal and tympanic membrane. It consists of two major components: Internal receiver and the tiny floating mass transducer.

1. The implant, called the Vibrating Ossicular Prosthesis™ (VORPTM), and,
2. The externally-worn receiver, called the Audio Processor™ (approximately the size of a quarter).

The vibrant bridge is a direct drive device which mechanically vibrates the bones in the middle ear without surgically altering the structures of the middle ear.

The tiny Floating Mass Transducer™, attached to the incus bone in the middle ear, is approximately the size of a grain of rice. It is 100% digital and is programmed by an Audiologist 8 weeks after the implant procedure to fit the user's specific hearing loss. The Vibrant bridge converts sound into mechanical energy which is directly transmitted to the auditory ossicles.

The external audio processor picks up the sound from the environment and transmits it across the skin to the receiver of the VORP. The signal is then transmitted to the floating mass transducer (FMT) causing it to vibrate. The FMT mechanically stimulates the ossicles, mimicking the natural process of hearing. The VORP is surgically implanted under the skin behind the ear. The FMT is attached to the long process of the incus bone during the surgical process. The ossicular motion creates a movement in the cochlea, stimulating the hair cells. The hair cells provide stimuli to the auditory nerve, which is interpreted as sound by the brain.

Efficacy of Vibrant Bridge

The efficacy of implantation of the vibrant bridge on residual hearing was evaluated by several different clinical measures. A shift in pure-tone averages (PTAs) of less than 10 dB at 3 months after activation was seen in 96% of study participants. The mean shift in PTA was 2.7 dB for all of the subjects. The vibrant bridge yielded a mean improvement in functional gain at all frequencies and greater than 10 dB at 2000, 4000 and 6000 Hz. Additionally, the number of subjects who reported improvement was significant across all seven subscales compared with the presurgery aided condition (familiar talkers, ease of communication, reverberation, reduced cues, background noise, aversiveness of sounds, and distortion of sounds).

Difference Between Cochlear Implant and Vibrant Bridge

The vibrant bridge is not a cochlear implant and it is not currently approved for conductive hearing loss. Cochlear implants are for the estimated 10% of the hearing-impaired population who suffer from severe to profound hearing loss. They are implanted directly in the inner ear, or cochlea, where they electronically stimulate the nerves through a series of electrodes. In contrast, the vibrant bridge is implanted in the middle ear and is for the 60% of hearing-impaired people with moderate-to-severe sensorineural hearing loss. Hearing aids, which are worn in the ear canal, amplify sound acoustically in order to increase the movement of the eardrum and indirectly vibrate the middle ear bones. In contrast, the vibrant bridge provides an enhanced signal to the inner ear by directly vibrating the middle ear bones while leaving the ear canal open and the eardrum undisturbed. Patients generally wear the device all day (as long as sixteen hours) and generally report a "more natural sound," better speech understanding and like the device much better than hearing aids. For many patients who cannot wear hearing aids due to medical necessity, a middle ear implant like the vibrant bridge is the only available alternative.

Candidacy for the Vibrant Bridge

With nothing in the ear canal, the vibrant bridge is a particularly good treatment option for current hearing aid wearers who suffer from occlusion or feedback, and those who are looking for better sound quality or improved cosmetics. Occlusion is the sensation of hearing distorted, muffled sounds experienced when an object blocks the ear canal. It is a common complaint among hearing aid users, who often find that the presence of the hearing aid, or hearing aid earmold, in their ear canal distorts not only outside sounds but also the sound of their own voice. People who experience a hearing loss due to disease or trauma to the middle ear are not candidates for the device. To be a candidate for this procedure, patients should meet the following criteria:

- Moderate-to-severe sensorineural hearing loss
- Normal middle ear function
- 50% minimum speech recognition score at the implant ear under headphones
- Realistic expectations and highly motivated
- Stable hearing loss.

Surgery

The procedure to implant the vibrant bridge is done on an outpatient basis and it takes approximately 1.5–2 hours. Implant patients are exposed to the normal risks of middle ear surgery and general anesthesia. The surgery is performed under general anesthesia. There is minimal postopertive pain. An incision is made being the ear and a bed is made for the internal receiver. The mastoid bone is opened and the middle ear is then entered through the mastoid and the floating mass transducer is placed on the incus. The internal receiver is sutured to the skull and the skin is closed. A dressing is worn for one day. Sutures are self-dissolving and the patient can resume most activities the next day. The external processor is fitted 3 weeks after surgery. At activation, the device is connected to the Siemens programming software and programmed for the individual's hearing loss.

The Vibrant Bridge for Conductive and Mixed Hearing Loss

The vibrant bridge is now being investigated by Dr Maw for the treatment of conductive and mixed hearing losses, which can occur in patients with chronic disease of the middle ear. It can be placed at the opening to the inner ear, the round window, bypassing the middle ear bones which may be absent or diseased, and therefore, eliminates the conductive, or mechanical hearing loss of the ear. It can also amplify sound to overcome a sensorineural, or nerve hearing loss, if also present. After surgery, the device is programmed to compensate for the loss of sensitivity of the inner ear. In the current study, the vibrant bridge is being evaluated for patients who have middle ear problems that cannot be resolved with other surgical procedures, or in patients who have persisting mechanical middle ear problems after previous ear surgery. This is a clinical scenario that is frequently encountered by ear surgeons, and is often caused by poor function of the Eustachian tube, the tube which connects the middle ear to the back of the nose.

AUDITORY BRAINSTEM IMPLANTS

The successful employment of a cochlear implant demands the presence of an intact cochlear nerve and an implantable cochlea. There are a number of conditions in which the cochlear nerves are absent or the cochlea is so dysplastic that a cochlear implant cannot be inserted. In these cases, electrical stimulation of the auditory pathways may be considered at a more central site. The ABI was developed to deal with this situation, originally for the condition of Neurofibromatosis Type 2 (NF2). The hallmark of this condition is the presence of bilateral vestibular schwannomas (acoustic neuromas), benign tumors that arise on the audiovestibular nerves. As a result of the tumors themselves and/or the surgery to remove them, the majority of these patients end up totally deaf, and nearly always without functioning auditory nerves. The ABI stimulates the auditory pathway at the level of the cochlear nucleus

complex, which is located in the pons in the lateral recess of the fourth ventricle. The device has a modified electrode with a carrier paddle with 21 disc electrodes. Technically, insertion of the electrode is not easy, as surgical landmarks are not always obvious. Following the removal of the vestibular schwannoma either via the translabyrinthine or retrosigmoid route, the opening of the lateral recess of the fourth ventricle is explored, the so-called foramen of Luschka. This is found at the pontomedullary junction by following the stump of the auditory nerve inferiorly and the glossopharyngeal nerve superiorly. The choroid plexus will usually be seen coming out of the foramen of Luschka and cerebrospinal fluid will be seen to emerge from it, especially if the anesthetist raises the intracranial pressure. Arachnoid adhesions may have to be broken down in order to gain access to the foramen, and it is usual to have to deal with a plexus of veins or even to have to move an arterial loop in order to do so. The walls of the lateral recess are recognized by their smooth white appearance. The electrode paddle is slipped into the lateral recess with the electrode discs pointing upwards to make contact with the dorsal cochlear nucleus. The correct position of the implant is verified by eliciting the electrically evoked auditory brainstem response (EABR). Adjacent cranial nerves (facial, glossopharyngeal, accessory and trigeminal) are monitored to minimize the risk of nonauditory stimulation. From the point of view of neuroanatomy, there is a major problem with the frequency maps, or tonotopicity, of the cochlear nucleus compared with the cochlea. A surface electrode will function most effectively if the frequency map is distributed across the surface of the nucleus. In the cochlear nucleus, the map is disposed obliquely through the depths of the nucleus, and to take advantage of this arrangement a penetrating electrode has been developed, though it has not been used in clinical trials. Relatively, few ABIs have been performed worldwide, but most users have environmental awareness and assistance with lipreading. A realistic comparison is with the performance that one used to see with single-channel cochlear implants. Other possible indications for the ABI are a congenital absence of the cochlear nerve and total obstruction of the cochlea.[21] It is too early yet to state with confidence if these children will be able to use their implants to gain access to speech.[22] There is a real possibility that a nontumor patient who receives an ABI should do better than one whose cochlear nucleus has been damaged by pressure from a large tumor and surgical attempts to remove it.

Surgical Technique

The ventral cochlear nucleus is the main target for placement of the ABI. The correct placement is confirmed using electrophysiological recordings. Electrically evoked auditory brainstem responses elicited by stimulation of the nucleus are recorded from electrodes placed on the scalp, and the position of the ABI electrode is optimized using information derived from the recording.

Candidacy

The patients with NF2 and bilateral acoustic schwannoma can be the ABI candidate.

In NF2 patients, the goal is to restore some auditory function in order for these individuals to continue to be a part of the hearing world and to improve their quality of life.

The ABI is placed during removal of their first tumor even if they have hearing on other side. This approach allows patients to become familiar with the use of other device and prepares them for the loss of hearing on the other side, when they will experience hearing loss in both ears.[23,24]

Processor Fitting and Programming

The threshold level and maximum comfortable levels of each electrode were first assessed to select the optimal electrode configuration. The monopolar mode was initially utilized to identify the electrodes that elicit auditory sensations. Electrodes that induce unpleasant sounds or nonauditory effects were excluded for future use.

To determine an ABI recipient's perception of pitch and define the appropriate tonotopic order of the electrodes, the place-pitch scaling and ranking results were obtained. On average, for the first 6 months from activation, the SPEAK encoder strategy was applied in all patients using the investigational protocol for the clinical trial of the Multichannel Auditory Brainstem Implants. When the patients reach an auditory performance level without any improvement for 3 months, i.e. a 'plateau phase', the ACE strategy is utilized. ACE processor have higher stimulation rates, which allows better spectral and temporal resolution of speech signals and improvement in open-set speech recognition scores within a short-period of time.

Benefits of ABI

Most ABI recipients benefit from the device through increased sound awareness. Because few ABI recipients are able to understand speech without lipreading, the level of performance achieved with the ABI is poorer than that obtained by people with a cochlear implant (CI). However, the environmental and speech sounds that patients receive through the ABI help significantly to improve their communication and quality of life. ABI sound always is most beneficial when it can be combined with lipreading cues.

ELECTRIC ACOUSTIC STIMULATION (FIG. 10)

Inclusion criteria for electric stimulation of the auditory nerve via cochlear implantation have significantly broadened over the years. Encouraged by promising results in traditional cochlear implant (CI) patients, the application of cochlear implantation has been used in patients with increasing amounts of residual hearing. Most of these patients are able to achieve considerably good speech reception after cochlear implantation, and in some cases residual hearing could even be preserved.

Combined electric acoustic stimulation (EAS) of the auditory system is the concept of using CI technology and acoustic amplification in the same ear and is a relatively new treatment for patients with a considerable amount of residual hearing in the low-frequency range. In EAS, the aim is to preserve low-frequency hearing after cochlear implantation which can be used for acoustic amplification, while a CI provides electric stimulation to the auditory system in the high-frequency range to compensate for the hearing loss in the high frequencies.

In 1999, von Ilberg et al.[25] first discussed the possibility of using electric and acoustic stimulation simultaneously in patients without losing functional residual hearing in the low frequencies. Evidence in animal experiments demonstrated the possibility of using electric and acoustic stimulation of the central auditory system simultaneously without interferences and the first patient

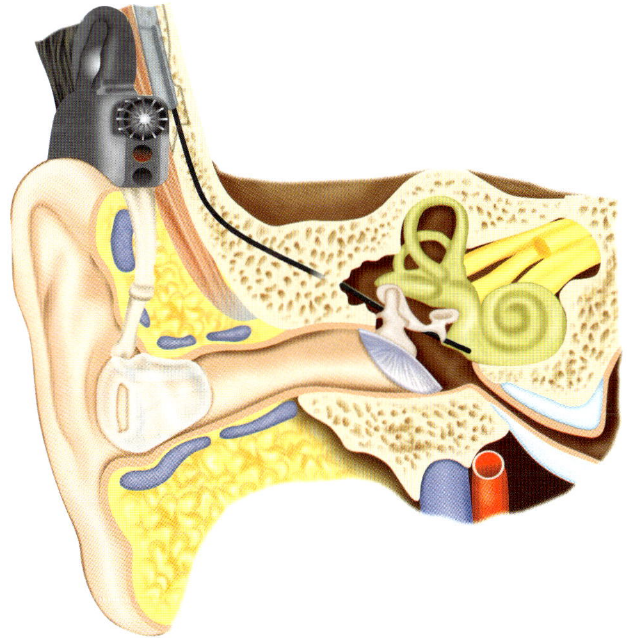

Fig. 10: Electroacoustic stimulation

with a considerable amount of residual low-frequency hearing was implanted for EAS. Long-term experience with EAS shows that preserved residual hearing after cochlear implantation remains stable over time in most patients, and encouraging results in speech reception are reported with the use of combined electric and acoustic stimulation.[26-28]

Indications and Criteria for Electric Acoustic Stimulation

Electric acoustic stimulation (EAS) is a prosthetic hearing rehabilitative treatment used in patients with normal hearing or mild to moderate hearing loss in the low-frequencies up to approximately 1 kHz, sloping to a severe-to-profound sensorineural hearing loss in the high frequencies. These patients do not benefit much from conventional hearing aids (HAs), as HAs are efficient for mild-to-moderate hearing loss, while severe hearing loss in the high-frequency range (>1 kHz) is difficult to compensate for with an HA. However, traditionally cochlear implantation is not considered as a treatment for these patients with a considerable amount of residual hearing either. Maximum-aided speech understanding of monosyllables should be 60% or lower. Along with the audiogram and speech reception results, there are certain criteria for EAS candidacy—there should not be any progressive hearing loss, an autoimmune disease or hearing loss as a result of meningitis or otosclerosis or ossification of the cochlea and there should be no malformation of the cochlea. The maximum air-bone gap is 15 dB. There should also be no contraindications to use amplification devices in the EAS ear. The detection of dead regions in the cochlea could also be helpful when selecting EAS patients.

Hearing Preservation and Electrode Design

The success of EAS depends on the preservation of residual hearing. In order to preserve residual hearing after cochlear implantation, several EAS soft surgery techniques have been developed. The round window approach [27] and cochleostomy are most commonly used in EAS surgery. These specific surgery techniques are based on the concept of soft surgery [29] and are designed to induce as little acoustic and mechanical trauma as possible to the inner ear in order to preserve residual hearing. Special measures are taken to reduce the risk of infection and inflammation to a minimum—antibiotics are given intravenously before implant surgery, and applied locally during surgery before electrode insertion. The use of steroids diminishes inflammatory or apoptotic reactions. The operating field is also cleaned just before insertion of the electrode of

array into the cochlea. Although partial consensus on hearing preservation surgery is achieved, the effect and importance of some issues remain a topic of debate. For a large part, a minimal invasion into the cochlea is considered to be responsible for hearing preservation. Studies in temporal bones show a significantly higher risk of cochlear trauma with deep electrode insertions of more than 360°.[30-32] When using a thinner and more flexible electrode, less force is needed when inserting the electrode into the cochlea.[33] Electrodes have been designed to be more atraumatic to the cochlea to ensure hearing preservation.

Electric Acoustic Stimulation Fitting

The majority of the patients implanted for EAS use the combination of HA and CI after cochlear implantation. The acceptance of the combined use of HA and CI seems to depend on the postoperative hearing thresholds. Correct fitting of the CI and HA are important to achieve the best possible speech reception results using EAS. Research has shown that CI and HA should be fitted according to the patient's residual hearing, with a small amount of overlap between the frequency range of the HA and CI.[34] The HA should be fitted to provide an appropriate amount of amplification in the low frequencies. The half-gain rule can be used for fitting of the HA. However, often more gain is needed in the low frequencies than is recommended by the fitting software. No amplification needs to be provided in the high frequencies as the patient has no functional residual hearing in the high-frequency range. Other factors that influence HA fitting are power of the HA and the amount of venting in the earmold. Electric stimulation for frequencies with hearing loss of more than 80 dB HL seems to provide the highest speech reception at least when testing is acute.

Outcomes Using Electric Acoustic Stimulation

Several studies show good results using EAS in patients with profound hearing loss in the high-frequency range. Patients using EAS have better speech reception results than traditional CI patients. Rubenstein et al. [35] also found that people with more residual hearing preoperatively tend to have better speech reception results after cochlear implantation. Even when using CI on its own, speech reception results are generally better than those of regular CI patients. The combination of CI and HA can also result in an additive or synergistic effect, providing better speech reception than with either device used alone.[36] Better speech reception in quiet and in noise might be due to better preserved hair cells and spiral ganglion. Compared to CI users, LAS users also perform better on music perception testing. LAS users' scores were not significantly lower than the scores of normal-hearing listeners. The successful outcomes of LAS in adults have led to an extended use of LAS in children.[37]

Counseling

Patients with severe sloping high-frequency hearing loss are not deaf, but often do not fit in the hearing world either. They have great difficulties with speech perception, even when fitted with HA. With low-frequency hearing and the additional help of lipreading these patients are able to get by. Often these patients have tried several HAs with limited success. Still many patients are wary of LAS surgery because they fear losing their residual hearing and becoming deaf after implantation. It is important that the risk of losing residual hearing is explained and that patients are aware that rehabilitation will take time. With reports of initial declines of speech perception after cochlear implantation preoperative counseling is important.[38]

Electric Acoustic Stimulation in the Future

The rate of hearing preservation continues to increase due to improved surgical techniques as well as new developments in electrode design. An important opportunity to prevent hearing loss after EAS surgery may be in intracochlear drug treatment to protect the organ of Corti against apoptotic physiopathological pathways.

ASSISTIVE LISTENING DEVICES

An assistive listening device (ALD) is any type of device that can help you function better in your day-to-day communication situations. An ALD can be used with or without hearing aids to overcome the negative effects of distance, background noise, or poor room acoustics. So even though you have a hearing aid, ALDs can offer greater ease of hearing (and therefore reduce stress and fatigue) in many day-to-day communication situations.

According to **National Association of the Deaf**, assistive listening devices (ALDs), essentially are amplifiers that bring sound directly into the ear. They separate the sounds, particularly speech, that a person wants to hear from background noise. They improve the "speech to noise ratio". Research indicates that people who are hard to hearing require increasing the signal to noise ratio of about 15–25 dB in order to achieve the same level of understanding as people with normal hearing. An ALD allows them to achieve this gain for themselves without making it too loud for everyone else.

FM Devices

There are two types of FM devices:
- Large Area System
- Personal System.

The underlying mechanism involves frequency modulated radio waves transmit a signal from the talker or sound source to listener. FM transmitters work as a miniaturized radio station. The FM transmitter and receiver must be tuned to each other. This transmission happens on reserved radio spectrum 216–217 MHz. In 1982, the Federal Communications Commission authorized the use of frequencies within the 72–76 MHz band as the designated radiofrequencies that could be used by people with hearing loss. ALS manufacturers differ in how they allocate this band.

FM System (Fig. 11)

FM or frequency modulation systems, the sound is transmitted on a specific frequency or channel similar to a radio. The Federal Communications Commission (FCC) has designated specific frequencies for these types of systems. FM systems can be used for whole rooms or by individuals. Large areas can be set up with single or multiple speakers depending on the size of the room. These systems can be permanently installed in a given location or there are also several versions that are portable. Individual systems typically have a receiver that looks like a Walkman or MP3 player and uses different styles of earphones or headsets and may be useful for 1-1 communication, car rides, and watching TV. With miniaturization, there are now small receivers than can be connected directly to a person's hearing aids through direct audio input (DAI). Any time an

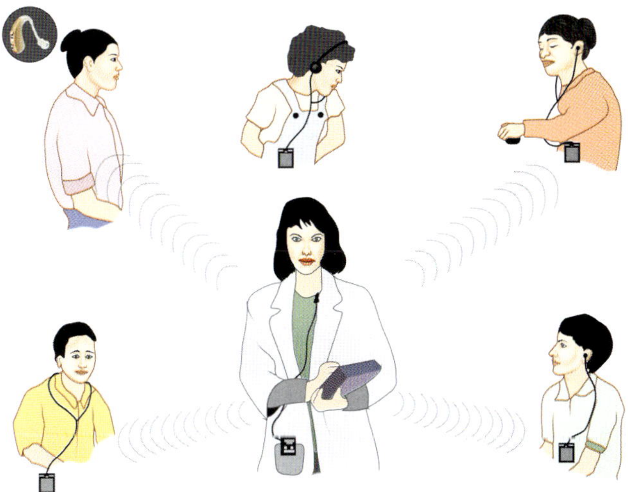

Fig. 11: FM system

FM system is coupled to a hearing aid, special settings and connections are required from an audiologist. Sometimes when several FM-based systems are used in the same building, there can be problems with cross-over between rooms and channels. Real-time captioning—provides a typewritten account of all verbal information presented within a lecture, meeting, discussion or presentation. All of these systems require the skills of a trained captionist and specialized software or equipment, such as a computer. They typically vary based on the amount of information represented within the visual display of information ranging from summaries to word for word transcription. CART (Communication Access Real-Time Captioning)— provides a word-for-word transcription (similar to a court reporter) using a stenotype machine, laptop computer and real-time software. C-Print—Developed as a speech to text communication access system at the National Technical Institute for the Deaf (NTID), a college of Rochester Institute of Technology (RIT). This system condenses information using a meaning-for-meaning translation (not verbatim). Remote Captioning—Rather than having a captionist physically present, the user can listen using a phone, cell phone, or computer microphone which allows the captionist to transmit the text back to the consumer using a modem, internet or some other data connection. The purpose of an earmold is to seal amplified sound inside the ear. An earmold that does not have a proper seal will permit sound to escape, resulting in acoustic feedback. To avoid this, an accurate ear impression must be obtained.

REFERENCES

1. Sandlin RE. Textbook of hearing aid amplification, 2nd ed. San Diego: Singular Publishing Group; 2000.
2. Dillon H. Hearing Aids. Sydney: Boomerang Press; 2001.
3. Stach BA. Clinical Audiology. An Introduction. San Diego: United States of America: Delmar Singular Publishing Group Inc. 1998;135-48.
4. Snik AF, Mylanus EA, Cremers CW. The bone-anchored hearing aid- a solution for previously unresolved otologic problems. Otolaryngol Clin North Am. 2001;34:365-72.
5. Stenfelt S, Goode RL. Bone-conducted sound- physiological and clinical aspects. Otol Neurotol. 2005;26:1245-61.
6. Snik AF, Mylanus EA, Cremers CW. The bone-anchored hearing aid in patients with a unilateral air-bone gap. Otol Neurotol. 2002;23:61-6.
7. Niparko JK, Cox KM, Lustig LR. Comparison of the bone-anchored hearing aid implantable hearing device with contralateral routing of offside signal amplification in the rehabilitation of unilateral deafness. Otol Neurotol. 2003;24:73-8.
8. Hol MK, Bosman AJ, Snik AF, Mylanus EA, Cremers CW. Bone anchored hearing aids in unilateral inner ear deafness- an evaluation of audiometric and patient outcome measurements. Otol Neurotol. 2005;26:999-1006.
9. Vaneecloo FM, Ruzza I, Hanson JN, et al. The monaural pseudo-stereophonic hearing aid (BAHA) in unilateral total deafness- a study of 29 patients [in French]. Rev Laryngol Otol Rhinol. 2001;122:343-50.
10. Bosman AJ, Hol MK, Snik AF, Mylanus EA, Cremers CW. Bone-anchored hearing aids in unilateral inner ear deafness. Acta Otolaryngol. 2003;123:258-60.
11. Mylanus EA, Cremers CW. A onestage surgical procedure for placement of percutaneous implants for the bone-anchored hearing aid. J Laryngol Otol. 1994;108:1031-5.
12. Holgers KM, Tjellström A, Bjursten LM, Erlandsson BE. Soft tissue reactions around percutaneous implants- a clinical study of soft tissue conditions around skin-penetrating titanium implants for bone-anchored hearing aids. Am J Otol. 1988;9:56-9.
13. Bance M, Abel SM, Papsin BC, Wade P, Vendramini J. A comparison of the audiometric performance of bone anchored hearing aids and air conduction hearing aids. Otol Neurotol. 2002;23:912-9.
14. Mylanus EA, Van der Pouw KC, Snik AF, Cremers CW. Intraindividual comparison of the bone-anchored hearing aid and air-conduction hearing aids. Arch Otolaryngol Head Neck Surg. 1998;124:271-6.
15. Wazen JJ, Caruso M, Tjellström A. Long-term results with the titanium bone-anchored hearing aid- the U.S. experience. Am J Otol. 1998;19:737-41.
16. Lin LM, Bowditch S, Anderson MJ, May B, Cox KM, Niparko JK. Amplification in the rehabilitation of unilateral deafness- speech in noise and directional hearing effects with bone-anchored hearing and contralateral routing of signal amplification. Otol Neurotol. 2006;27:172-82.
17. Baguley DM, Bird J, Humphriss RL, Prevost AT. The evidence base for the application of contralateral bone anchored hearing aids in acquired unilateral sensorineural hearing loss in adults. Clin Otolaryngol. 2006;31:6-14.
18. Dutt SN, McDermott AL, Burrell SP, Cooper HR, Reid AP, Proops DW. Patient satisfaction with bilateral bone-anchored hearing aids- the Birmingham experience. J Laryngol Otol Suppl. 2002;28:37-46.
19. Snik AF, Beynon AJ, Mylanus EA, van der Pouw CT, Cremers CW. Binaural application of the bone anchored hearing aid. Ann Otol Rhinol Laryngol. 1998;107:187-93.
20. van der Pouw KT, Snik AF, Cremers CW. Audiometric results of bilateral bone-anchored hearing aid application in patients with bilateral congenital aural atresia. Laryngoscope. 1998;108:548-53.
21. Colletti V, Carner M, Miorelli V, Guida M, Colletti L, Fiorino FG. Cochlear implantation at under 12 months- Report on 10 patients. Laryngoscope. 2005;115:445-9.
22. Grayeli AB, Escoubet B, Bichara M, Julien N, Silve C, Friedlander G, et al. Increased activity of the diastrophic dysplasia sulfate transporter in otosclerosis and its inhibition by sodium fluoride. Otol Neurotol. 2003;24(6):854-62.
23. Otto SR, Brackmann DE, Hitselberger WE, Shannon RV, Kuchta J. Multichannel auditory brainstem implant- Update on performance in 61 patients. Journal of Neurosurgery. 2002;96(6):1063-71.
24. Nevison B, Laszig R, Sollmann WP, Lenarz T, Sterkers O, Ramsden R, et al. Results from a European clinical investigation of the Nucleus multichannel Auditory Brain implant. Ear and Hearing. 2002;23:170-83.

25. Von Ilberg C, Kiefer LTAlein I, Piconingdorf T, Hartmann R, Stuntbeeher E, Klinke It. Eleciro-acoustic stimulation of the auditory system. OBI. 1999;61:334-40.

26. Gantt BI, Turner C, Gfeller KE, Lowder MW. Preservation of hearing in cochlear implant surgery- advantages of combined electrical and acoustical speech processing. Laryngoscope. 2005;115:796-802.

27. Skarzynski H, Iorens A, Ihotrowska A, Anderson I. Preservation of low frequency hearing in partial dealness cochlear implantation (PDCI) using the round window surgical approach. A< ta Otolaryngol. 2007;127:41-8.

28. Gstoenner WK, Van De fleyning O'Connor AF, Ntorera C, Sainz M, Vet Moire K, McDonald S, et al. Electric acoustic stimulation of the auditory system- results of a moth-centre Investigation. Acta Otolaryngol. 1999;119:229-33.

29. Kiefer I, Gstettner W, Baumgartner W, 10 Pok S, Tillem I, Ye Q, et al. Conservation of low frequency hearing in cochlear implantation. Acta Otolaryngol. 2004;124:272-80.

30. Gstocitner W, Franz P, Plea H, Baum-II, Armor Czerny C. Intracochlear position of cochlear implant electrodes. Acta Otolarptgol. 1999;119:229-33.

31. Adunka OF, Unkelbach MH, Mack MG, Radeloff A, Gstoettner WG. Predicting basal cochlear length for electric-acoustic stimulation. Otolaryngol Head Neck Surg. 2005;131:488-92.

32. Adunka OF, Kiefer J. Impact of electrode insertion depth on intracochlear trauma. Otolaryngol Head Neck Surg. 2006;135: 374-82.

33. Adunka OF, Kiefer J, Unkelbach MH, Leh nert T, Gstoettner W- Development and evaluation of an improved cochlear implant electrode design for electric acoustic stimulation. Laryngoscope. 2004;114:1237-41.

34. Vermeire K, Anderson I, Flynn M, Van de Ileyning P. The influence of different speech processor and hearing aid settings in electric acoustic stimulation patrons. Ear and Hearing. 2038-29-76-36.

35. Rubinstein IT, Parkinson WS, Tyler RS, Gant BI. Residual speech recognition and cochlear implantation criteria. Am I Otol. 1999;20:445-52.

36. Kiefer Pok M, Adunka OF, Sturzbecher E, Baumgartner W, Schmidt M, Tilkin I, et al. Combined eke- hie and acoustic stimulation of the auditory system-results of clinical study. Audiol Neurotol. 2005;10:134-44.

37. Skarayfiski H, Lorens A, Piotrowska A, Anderson I. Partial deafness cochlear implantation in children. Int I Nihau Otorhinolaryngol. 2007;71:1407-13.

38. Adunka OF, Buss E, Clark MS, Pillsbury IK, Buchman CA. Effect of preoperative residual hearing on speech perception after cochlear implantation. Laryngoscope. 2008;118:2044-9.

Biofilms in Otology

Dev Roy

INTRODUCTION

A biofilm is a structured community of bacteria embedded in a self-producing slime like extracellular matrix composed of proteins, polysaccharides, nucleic acids known as extracellular polymeric substances (EPS), which is attached to an inert or living surface.[1] Only 1% of bacteria exist in a free-floating or planktonic form while the remaining 99% exist as biofilms.[2] A mature biofilm undergoes through the following stages: 1. Seeding, 2. Attachment to inert or living surface, 3. Colonization, 4. Growth phase, 5. Seeding again, thus completing a cycle (Fig. 1). The unique feature of biofilms is shedding of isolated bacteria from its surface, which seeds infection to distant parts of the body similar to septic emboli. This planktonic shedding of bacteria is a continuous process, which appears to increase during conditions of physiological stress and starvation.[3] These bacteria then get attached to an inert or living structure. The bacterial community then secretes extracellular matrix in which colonization of the bacteria takes place. As more bacteria and other multicellular organisms like algae, parasites and protozoa get attached and colonize, the biofilms grows in size. This increase in growth results in formation of a matured biofilm. These matured biofilms then start shedding bacteria which seeds infection in distant parts, thus completing a life cycle.[4] Planktonic shedding and seeding of bacteria are key to biofilm survival (Fig. 2).

Most of the bacteria are susceptible to antimicrobials. But when the bacteria are enclosed in a biofilm, their behaviour is different and complex and has a unique feature of resistance to antimicrobials.[5] There is variety of defense mechanisms against immune system of the host, which results in resistance against the antimicrobials. The free floating bacteria are susceptible to antimicrobials, but once they are in a biofilm, the behavior changes and they exhibit a spectacular defense mechanism against the immune system of their host and antimicrobial agents. The bacterial colonies show a highly organized growth involving complicated intercellular communicating systems, which help them to protect themselves against the host and the hostile environment. [6]There is also a division of work among bacteria of different species as well as with fungi, algae and protozoa. There is an organized handling of wastes and nutrients in such a manner that when antimicrobial agents are added, they are depleted to suboptimal levels in the bulk fluid before they reach the biofilm. The colony of bacteria responds to changing environment by intercellular signaling between individual members within the biofilm. Through the process of quorum sensing, pathogenic bacteria can coordinate their virulence to evade immune capture and successfully infect their host.[6,7]

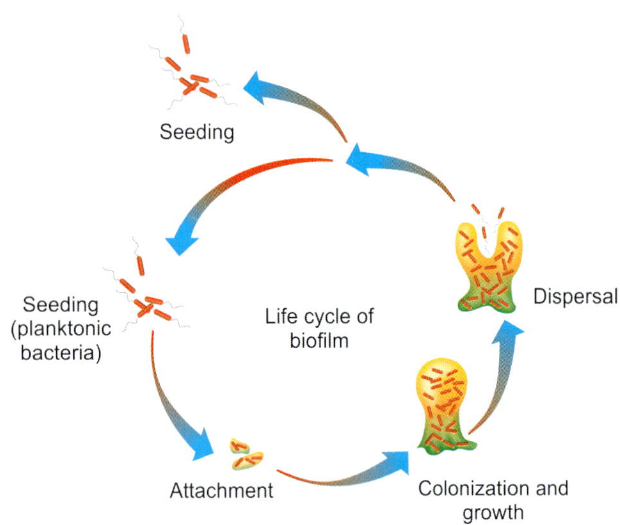

Fig. 1: Life cycle of Biofilm

The unique feature of biofilms is resistance to antibiotics. Bacteria in a biofilm are up to 1000 times more resistant to action of antibiotics than their planktonic counterparts.[8] The causes of antibiotic resistance are as follows:

- Poor antimicrobial penetration
- Decreased oxygen and nutrient requirements
- Increased expression of resistance genes (e.g., beta-lactamase)
- Reduced permeability to topical and intravenous antibiotics
- Slower growth rate
- Oxygen depleted microenvironment
- Quorum sensing involves intercellular transmission of molecules and genetic information which permits coordinated behavior and reaction to local environment.[6-8]

DIAGNOSIS

Various animal models have been used to culture biofilms. The most common culture is using Chinchilla animal. In Chinchilla, *S. pneumonia* can be inoculated into the middle ear, giving rise to otitis media. The advantage of using chinchilla model is bacteria can be inoculated in the middle ear and induce otitis media; it does not spread outside the middle ear and is easily accessible for culture.[9,10] The bacterial biofilms can be identified by scanning electron microscopy (SEM) and confocal laser microscopy (CFLM). There are newer and more sophisticated methods like fluorescent in situ hybridization (FISH), lectin-binding and immunohistochemical techniques.[11-14] In vivo studies of middle ear biofilms in humans are difficult since adequate samples from the middle ear are needed to carry out the tests. Moreover, study of adenoid biofilms is only possible after adenoidectomy. Hence, to carry out in vivo studies animal model of chinchilla is used. In the quest for noninvasive in vivo detection of middle ear biofilms, there is a new tool called Optical coherence tomography (OCT). This is based on ultrasound like near infrared laser waves, which produce 3D images. It can be used in children, causes no tissue injury and there is no radiation exposure. The OCT has recently been used to detect in vivo biofilm in patients with otitis media.[15] In a follow-up study, in similar adult population acoustic parameters of the tympanic membrane from the ear have been evaluated. These in vivo studies have limited application since the sample size is small. But still, OCT remains a highly promising noninvasive method of detecting biofilms which may play a major role in biofilm related diseases in middle ear. Despite new technology, the prohibitive costs of the above tests limit their practical role in routine clinical situations for identifications of biofilms.

ROLE IN OTITIS MEDIA WITH EFFUSION

In otitis media with effusion (OME), it is difficult to culture bacteria. The recent discovery of mRNA and DNA in the culture media suggests that OME may be a biofilm disease.[12,14,16] There are various explanations for development of recurrent otitis media. Initially, there is exposure of nasopharynx to known middle ear infection followed by colonization and subsequent formation of biofilm by these bacteria. Eustachian tube dysfunction creates a negative pressure and allows planktonically shed bacteria from nasopharynx to enter the middle ear cavity. It is followed by colonization and subsequent biofilm formation in the middle ear, which results in development of recurrent acute otitis media.[8] With antibiotic treatment, there is a good response, leading to sterile middle ear effusion. Initially, there is a partial response to antibiotic treatment; however this treatment may result in chronicity. The adenoid in the nasopharynx contains biofilm; they shed planktonic bacteria to reinfect the middle ear, resulting in recurrence of the middle ear infection.[17] Based on the above evidence, the practice of "watchful waiting" may promote biofilm formation. Treatment by insertion of grommets helps in draining the middle ear fluid and has a drying effect. Grommets alter middle ear flora by providing ventilation and increased oxygen tension.[13,18] Some patients after grommet insertion develop chronic otorrhea. As a foreign body, grommets may promote biofilm growth.[19] Biofilms have been cultured from grommets removed from affected children. Thus, biofilm has been implicated as a cause of chronic postgrommet insertion otorrhea.

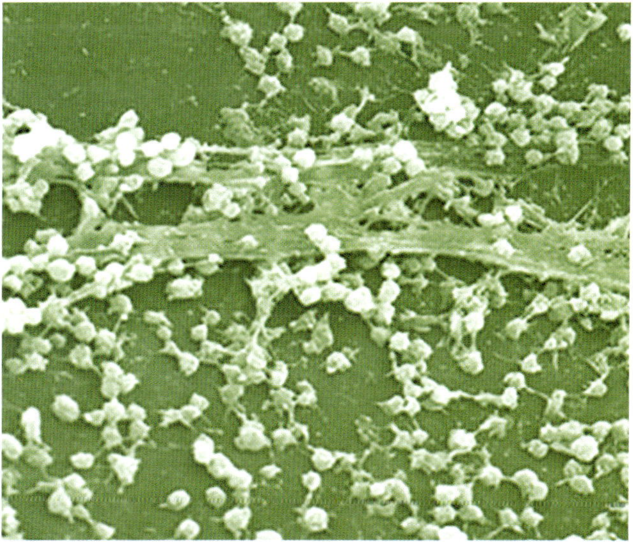

Fig. 2: Mature Biofilms showing *Staph aureus*

A number of studies have been carried out to identify surface adherence properties of grommets and have shown a reduction to biofilm formation. There are several studies that show protective effect of coated grommets. MRSA is inhibited by vancomycin-coated tubes, *P. aeruginosa* biofilms are inhibited by polyvinylpyrrolidone (PVP) and piperacillin–tazobactam coated tubes.[20,21] In cases of chronic otorrhea or recurrent and persistent otorrhea, removal of grommets and treatment with antimicrobials are effective. In addition to grommet insertion, removal of the adenoids by curettage or diathermy results in better resolution of middle ear effusion, possibly due to removal of biofilms from the nasopharynx.[17]

ROLE IN CHOLESTEATOMA

Cholesteatoma is a chronic disease with resistance to medical therapy. The culture of cholesteatoma has shown colonies of *pseudomonas aeruginosa* and *staphylococcus aureus*. These form biofilms and have a role in the pathogenesis of this condition. Matrix samples of cholesteatoma were induced in gerbils. The cholesteatoma produced contain gram-positive, gram-negative bacteria and acellular polysaccharide matrix similar to biofilms. Based on this finding, recurrent infection in cholesteatoma may be related to biofilm formation.[22] Recurrent active otorrhea is due to release of planktonic bacteria, which respond to antimicrobial treatment, since planktonic bacteria are more susceptible to antibiotic therapy as compared to bacteria in biofilms. Unfortunately, the resistant biofilm remains within the cholesteatoma and releases further bacteria and thus ensures the chronicity of the condition. Bacterial endotoxins release and binding of sessile bacteria to epithelial cells are thought to lead to regulation of signals that contribute to increased epithelial turnover and keratin production. The definitive treatment of cholesteatoma includes mastoid surgery with microsurgical removal of the cholesteatoma matrix and associated biofilm. It is important to remove the hypertrophic granulation tissue from the normal tissue. There are many reasons for failure after the operation. If the tissue with the potential to harbor biofilms, such as granulation tissue, cannot be removed, residual biofilm may be one reason for surgical failure.[23]

In presence of cholesteatoma, the use of patient's own ossicles for reconstruction after removal of the cholesteatoma matrix is not appropriate. One can argue that there is a risk of cholesteatoma matrix remaining on the ossicles. But studies have show that presence of biofilms is significantly higher in middle ear as compared to mastoid and ossicles. In addition, biofilm formation is less on the ossicles, probably because they remain suspended in the middle ear.[24]

Chronic suppurative otitis media, infected mastoid cavity and chronic otitis externa—in these conditions, the moist, warm environment of the middle ear, Eustachian tube and mastoid cavity provides a safe haven for chronic infection, fungal overgrowth and suspected biofilm formation. Control of discharge is a problem. The use of aural toilet, saline irrigations and adjunctive use of topical antibiotics helps in these conditions. The topical regimen that involves the physical agitation, disruption or removal of the biofilms by active irrigation or debridement with microdrill might improve the efficacy of treatment.[24]

COCHLEAR IMPLANT INFECTION

A cochlear implant was removed from a pediatric patient due to chronic otorrhea despite antibiotic treatment. Scanning EM revealed presence of fungal candida biofilm in the cochlear implant receiver and the electrode array. The child received 6-week course of liposomal amphotericin. Cochlear replantation was done in the same ear, 8 months after the first implant was removed.[25] Whenever there is recurrent and chronic infection not responding to antibiotics, removal of the implant with the embedded biofilm on its surface will help in greater antibiotic penetration and faster resolution of the infection.

TREATMENT

Cases of chronic infection apparently resistant to antibiotic treatment, particularly in the presence of implantable devices or foreign body must raise concern of biofilms. The most important step in treating biofilm infection is first to have a high index of suspicion. The mainstay of treatment includes antiseptic techniques, removal of infected foreign bodies, and provision of meticulous debridement. However, with the understanding of the biofilms and how bacteria interact to form biofilms newer methods can be developed in the future. Specific enzymes are known to be capable of digesting the biofilms' protective mucoid extracellular polysaccharide (EPS) coat. With pseudomonas, the EPS is alginate, which can be treated with alginase and simultaneous antibiotic treatment. The alginase dissolves the biofilm intercellular matrix and allows greater penetration of the antibiotic and has higher curative rates.[26] Some chemicals like N-acyl homoserine lactone group are involved in bacterial intercellular signaling; furanones are similar to N-acyl homoserine. These furanones can be used to disrupt intercellular signaling and making the biofilms more susceptible to antimicrobials. In case of tracheoesophageal valve colonization, probiotic biofilms are developed to combat pathogenic biofilms.[27] Some bacteria produce biosurfactants which release bacteria from the biofilms, damage the biofilm matrix and make them susceptible to host immune system and antimicrobial agents.[28]

CONCLUSION

A biofilm is a complex matrix of multicellular colonies, which have the capability to exploit the environment and protect themselves from the host and antimicrobial treatment. Standard tests are unreliable in identifying biofilms and conclusive tests are expensive. Conventional antibiotic sensitivity may be misleading, since they test sensitivity of free-floating bacteria and not the bacteria embedded in the biofilms. An index of suspicion of the presence of biofilms is important in chronic and resistant diseases. The mainstay of treatment remains manual irrigation, removal of the implanted foreign body and debridement. Understanding the biofilms will enable us to develop novel therapeutics in the treatment of biofilms.

REFERENCES

1. Costerton JW, Stewart PS, Greenberg EP. Bacterial biofilms: a common cause of persistent infections. Science. 1999;284:1318-22.
2. Fergie N, Bayston R, Pearson JP, Birchall JP. Is otitis media with effusion a biofilm infection? Clin Otolaryngol. 2004;29:38-46.
3. Costerton JW, Geesey GG, ChengKJ. How bacteria stick. Sci Am. 1978;238:86-95.
4. Kolter R, Losick R. One for all and all for one. Science. 1998;280:226-7.
5. Hall-Stoodley L, Stoodley P. Evolving concepts in biofilm infections. Cell Microbiol. 2009;11(7):1034-43.
6. Stewart PS, Costerton JW. Antibiotic resistance in biofilms. Lancet. 2001;358(9276):135-8.
7. Mah TF, O'Toole GA. Mechanism of biofilm resistance to antimicrobial agents. Trends microbiol. 2001;9(1):34-9.
8. Coticchia JM, Chen M, Sachdeva L, Mutchnick S. New paradigms in pathogenesis of otitis media in children. Paed Otolaryngol. 2013;1:1-7.
9. Giebink GS. Otitis media: The chinchilla model. Microb drug Resist. 1999;5(1):57-72.
10. Watanabe N, DeMaria TF, Lewis DM, Mogi G, Lim DJ. Experimental otitis media in chinchillas. II. Comparison of middle ear immune responses to S pneumonia type 3 and 23. Ann Otol Rhinol laryngol Suppl. 1982;93:9-16.
11. Post JC. Direct evidence of bacterial biofilms in otitis media. Laryngoscope. 2001;111(12):2083-94.
12. Hall Stoodley L. Hu FZ, Gieseke A, Nistico L, Nguyen D, Hayes J, et al. Direct detection of bacterial biofilm on the middle ear mucosa of children with chronic otitis media. JAMA. 2006;296(2):2002-11.
13. Barakate M, Beckenham E, Curotta J, da Cruz M. Bacterial biofilms adherence to middle ear ventilation tubes: scanning electron micrograph and literature review. J Otolaryngol Otol. 2007;121(10):993-7.
14. Bakaletz LO. Bacterial biofilms in the upper airway-evidence for role in pathology and implication for treatment of otitis media. Paediatr Respir Rev. 2012;13(3):154-9.
15. Nguyen CT, Robinson SR, Jung W, Novak MA, Boppart SA, Allen JB. Investigation of bacterial biofilm in the human middle ear using optical coherence tomography and acoustic measurements. Hear Res. 2013;301:193-200.
16. Rayner MG, Zhang Y, Gorry MC, Post JC, Chen Y, Ehrlich GD. Evidence of bacterial metabolic activity in culture negative otitis media with effusion. JAMA. 1998;279:296-9.
17. Nistico L, Kreft R, Gieseke A, Cottichia JM, Burrows A, Kampang P, et al. Adenoid reservoir for pathogenic biofilm bacteria. J Clin Microbiol. 2011;49(4):1411-20.
18. Jang CH, Cho YB, Choi CH. Structural features of tympanostomy tube biofilms formation in ciprofloxacin resistant Pseudomonas otorrhea. Int J Paediatr Otorhinolaryngol. 2007;71:591-5.
19. Vlastarakos PV, Nikolopoulos TP, Korres S, Tavoulari E, Tzagaroulakis A, Ferekidis E. Grommets in otitis media with effusion: the most frequent operation in children. But is it associated with significant complications? Eur J Paediatr. 2007;166:385-91.
20. Jang CH, Park H, Cho YB, Choi CH, Park IY. The use of piperacillin-tazobactam coated tympanostomy tubes against ciprofloxacin resistant Pseudomonas biofilm formation: an in vitro study. Int J Paediatr otorhinolaryngol. 2009;73(2):295-9.
21. Ojano-Dirain CP, Silva RC, Antonelli PJ. Biofilm formation on coated silicone tympanostomy tubes. Int J Paediatr Otorhinolaryngol. 2013;77(2):223-7.
22. Chole RA, Faddis BT. Evidence for microbiofilms in cholesteatoma. Arch Otolaryngol Head Neck Surg. 2002;128:1129-33.
23. Lampikoski H, Jero J, Kinnari TJ. "Mastoid biofilm in chronic otitis media". Otology and Neurology. 2012;5:785-8.
24. K Ercan, Dag I, Incesulu, Gurbuz MK, Acar M, Birdanc L. Investigation of presence of biofilms in chronic Suppurative otitis media, nonsuppurative otitis media, and chronic otitis media with cholesteatoma by scanning electron microscopy. The Scientific World Journal. 2013;1-6.
25. Cristobal R, Edmiston CE Jr, Runge Samuelsson CL, et al. Fungal biofilm formation on cochlear implant hardware after antibiotic induced fungal growth within the middle ear. Paediatr Infect Dis J. 2004;23:774-8.
26. Bayer AS, Park S, Ramos MC, et al. Effects of alginase on the natural history and antibiotic therapy of experimental endocarditis caused by mucoid Pseudomonas aeruginosa. Infect Immun. 1992;49:713-8.
27. van der Mei HC, Free RH, Elving GJ, et al. Effect of probiotic bacteria on prevalence of yeasts in oropharyngeal biofilms on silicone rubber voice prosthesis in vitro. J Med Microbiol. 2000;60:3979-85.
28. van Hoogmoed CG, Der Kuijl-Booij, Der Mei HC, Busscher HJ. Inhibition of streptococcus mutants NS adhesion to glass with and without a salivary conditioning film by biosurfactant releasing Streptococcus mitis strains. Appl Environ Microbiol. 2000;66:659-63.

Anesthesia for Ear Surgery

Enakshi Saha

Ear is a very complex and delicate structure serving two very important functions:

1. Auditory function
2. Vestibular function.

Ear is divided into external, middle and inner ear.

Middle ear harbors the delicate ossicles that conduct the sound waves to the inner ear. Besides that, it is in very close proximity to the following anatomical structures:

- Superiorly—temporal lobe of brain
- Inferiorly—jugular vein, internal carotid artery
- Facial canal containing the facial nerve
- Chorda tympani nerve.

Inner ear serves the following functions:

- Transduction of sound pressure into neurochemical impulses in the auditory nerve
- Maintaining optic fixation to help to maintain upright posture.

Therefore, the need for high degree of precision during surgical manipulation in ear cannot be overemphasized. Skilful anesthesia service goes a long way in providing optimal environment to carry out such high precision surgery.

Commonly Performed Otologic Procedures

- Tympanoplasty/tympanotomy
- Myringotomy/Grommet insertion
- Mastoidectomy
- Ossiculoplasty
- Stapedectomy/stapedotomy
- Insertion of cochlear implant
- Facial nerve decompression/repair/grafting
- Otoplasty.

Options for Anesthesia in Ear Surgery

- Local anesthesia
- General anesthesia

Patient's consent is taken for operation to be done under local/general anesthesia or monitored anesthesia care (MAC)

LOCAL ANESTHESIA

Prerequisite for successful local anesthesia (LA) is adequate patient cooperation. Patient has to keep his head still as long as the surgery is being carried out. Hence, it is unsuitable for very long procedures.

Procedure for Local Anesthesia

To allow optimum effect of the local anesthetic agent, infiltration should be done 10–15 minutes before the start of surgery. A sedative premedication (midazolam, diazepam) is desirable before local anesthetic injection. Monitoring the vital signs (ECG, O_2 saturation, BP) is mandatory before starting the procedure.

When retroauricular incision is indicated, about 10 mL of local anesthetic solution is infiltrated along the incision line near the retroauricular fold. From the same region, the needle is advanced anteriorly and a few mL of anesthetic solution is injected beneath the skin of the external auditory canal. Anesthetic solution is then injected subperiosteally through the external auditory canal from four different points—anteriorly, superiorly, posterosuperiorly and posteroinferiorly. About 0.3 mL of anesthetic solution is injected in each point. When a transcanal approach is indicated, the injection is made only in the canal.

The solution most commonly used for local infiltration is 2% lignocaine with adrenaline (1:100000) or bupivacaine 0.25% (Fig. 1).

Advantages of Local Anesthesia

- Cost-effective
- Saves operating room time/pollution

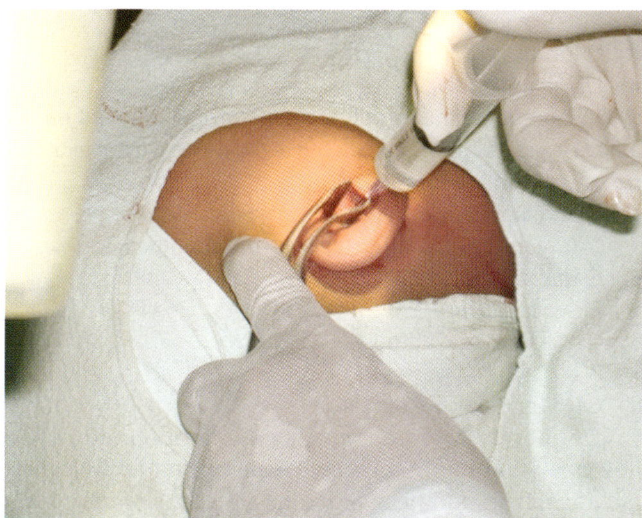

Fig. 1: Four quadrant local anesthesia using 2% xylocaine with 1:100000 adrenaline being infiltrated

- Bleeding reduced to minimum as adrenaline is added
- Intraoperative assessment of hearing and/or facial nerve function is possible.

Risks of Local Anesthesia

- Anaphylaxis
- Neurogenic shock
- Hypertension, tachycardia, cardiac arrhythmia due to absorption of adrenaline.

Local anesthesia is unsuitable in the following situations:

- Pediatric population
- Uncooperative adults
- Procedures of long duration
- Claustrophobia
- Hypersensitivity to local anesthetic agents.

GENERAL ANESTHESIA

General anesthesia (GA) with endotracheal intubation and muscle relaxation provides the most optimum situation to carry out the delicate and high precision procedures inside the ear. General anesthesia with laryngeal mask air way (LMA) insertion, instead of endotracheal intubation, is helpful as it is not that invasive. Special issues during conduct of general anesthesia for ear surgery are discussed below:

Use of Nitrous Oxide

Nitrous oxide (N_2O) is 34 times more soluble than nitrogen. It freely diffuses into air containing spaces. During ear surgery it quickly diffuses into middle ear cavity. Since middle ear cavity is a closed noncompliant space, the pressure inside the cavity rises due to diffusion of nitrous oxide.

Middle ear pressure changes during nitrous oxide anesthesia can impede hearing, influence surgical outcome, increase postoperative nausea and vomiting, and occasionally cause facial nerve injury.[1] The main factors influencing middle ear pressure changes during N_2O anesthesia are duration of anesthesia, the concentration of N_2O, and the patency of the Eustachian tube, which functions like a relief valve.

There is a definite threat to disruption of tympanic membrane and worsening deafness due to intraoperative rise in middle ear pressure. Tympanic membrane grafts tend to get disrupted due to rise in middle ear pressure. Hence, it is recommended that nitrous oxide should be put off at least 15 minutes prior to tympanic graft placement. It would be best if oxygen, air together with volatile agents could be used instead of oxygen and nitrous oxide anesthesia.

Studies have confirmed that elimination of nitrous oxide during middle ear surgery definitely prevents this unwanted rise in middle ear cavity pressure and thereby, the adverse effects.[2]

Use of Neuromuscular Blocking Agents

Facial nerve paralysis represents the most outward and noticeable cranial neuropathy. It causes an obvious facial deformity and has an emotional impact that leads to social isolation and reduced self-esteem.

Due to intimate association of the middle ear with the course of the facial nerve, there is considerable chance of iatrogenic injury to the motor component of the facial nerve during middle ear surgery. Various studies have estimated the incidence of such unfortunate event to be as low as 0.65 to as high as 33.3%.[3-5]

Facial nerve monitoring can go a long way in minimizing such complications and avoiding litigations. The absence of mechanically evoked responses during facial nerve stimulation allows safe dissection. Monitoring can help to locate the facial nerve, guide the dissection and drilling, and confirm its integrity, thereby allowing more definitive surgical treatment while preserving neural function.[6]

The facial EMG monitoring needs a functional and intact facial neuromuscular junction to enable facial muscles responsive to nerve stimulation. Neuromuscular blocking agents, as an important ingredient for maintaining general anesthesia, act directly on the nerve muscle junction and block the signal transmission. It leads to patient's paralysis and immobilization as required in general anesthesia, but at the same time, it may interfere the facial nerve monitoring during the surgery. Hence, muscle relaxation has to be kept to minimum to facilitate facial nerve monitoring. Neuromuscular monitoring with a peripheral nerve stimulator should be employed to assess the depth of muscle paralysis. Studies has shown that 50% neuromuscular block provides optimum balance for facial nerve monitoring and ensuring immobilization during surgery.[7-9] Use of muscle relaxants can be minimized by making judicious use of volatile and intravenous anesthetic agents and opioids.

Degree of Head Rotation

Optimum head rotation is essential to bring the operative field into clear view during microsurgery of middle ear. Usually, this is not of much concern in patients without any cervical spine pathology.

However, when the cervical spine is diseased (subluxation, osteoarthritis, rheumatoid arthritis, vertebral artery insufficiency) inappropriate head and neck rotation may cause grave neurological injury.

Optimum venous drainage from brain may be hindered by twisting and kinking of draining vessels during head and neck rotation. This promotes brain swelling and rise in intracranial tension. It can cause enhanced brain damage in patients with intracranial pathology.

It is a wise practice to assess the safe range of head and neck rotation preoperatively in a patient with preexisting head and neck pathology.

Deliberate Hypotension

In middle ear surgery, even minor bleeding impairs the surgeon's ability to operate under an optical microscope. For this reason, arterial blood pressure must be decreased to achieve a bloodless cavity in the middle ear. The cochlear microcirculation is a crucial factor in the maintenance of the normal homeostatic environment of the inner ear, and studies have shown the deleterious effect of hypotension in the pathogenesis of sudden hearing loss.[9,10]

The inner ear or the cochlea is supplied by labyrinthine artery, an end artery, which is a branch of anterior inferior cerebellar artery or may directly arise from basilar or vertebral artery. It is presumable that the blood flow regulation to the inner ear is closely related to that of the brain. However, different animal and human studies have failed to decisively conclude about direct correlation between cerebral blood flow and cochlear microcirculation.

Laser Doppler flowmetry in animal studies has shown that acceptably consistent inner ear blood flow is maintained in arterial blood pressure range of 50–10 mm of Hg.[11] It is safe not to reduce mean arterial pressure below the lower limit of cerebral autoregulation.

Vital organ hypoperfusion is a very important complication of deliberate hypotension. Patient should be closely monitored for avoidance of such complications. Recommended monitoring includes the following:

- Electrocardiogram (ECG)
- Invasive blood pressure is a must so that beat-to-beat variation of arterial blood pressure can be measured

- Pulse oxymetry
- Capnometry
- Urine output.

Various pharmacological agents are employed either alone or in combination to achieve the desired level of blood pressure. Some of them are:

- Volatile anesthetic agents
- Intravenous anesthetic agents and opioids
- Ganglion blockers
- Directly acting vasodilators
- α-2 adrenergic agonists
- β-blockers
- Calcium channel blockers.

Deliberate hypotension is contraindicated in the absence of optimum technical expertise and monitoring facilities. It should be avoided in patients suffering from significant cardiac, pulmonary, renal or hepatic disease, ischemic cerebrovascular disease, severe anemia, severe systemic hypertension and in extremes of age.

Reactionary hemorrhage and hematoma formation may be a problem in the postoperative period when the blood pressure is restored to normal levels. Return of blood pressure to normal level before the operation ends is important, so that the surgeon can check any bleeding. Besides that, some grave complications can result from this technique such as:

- Myocardial infarction
- Cerebral artery thrombosis
- Acute tubular necrosis
- Hepatic necrosis
- Pulmonary infarction
- Central retinal artery thrombosis
- Ischemic optic neuropathy
- Sudden hearing loss, as mentioned above.

Monitored Anesthesia care (MAC): Operation is done under local anesthesia with the Anesthetist taking care of patient's sedation, analgesia, existing comorbid diseases and possibility of complications.

Common Complications Following Ear Surgery

Postoperative Nausea and Vomiting

Middle ear surgery performed under local or general anesthesia has a significantly high incidence of postoperative nausea and vomiting. It is highly distressing to the patients and detrimental to their postoperative recovery. Nausea and vomiting can significantly delay hospital discharge and thereby increase costs.

- A multimodal strategy should be adopted to minimize this unpleasant complication following ear surgery:

- Nitrous oxide should be avoided during general anesthesia to prevent changes in middle ear pressure
- Optimum pain management must be done in the postoperative period
- Use of opioids must be kept to minimum
- Sudden changes in posture must be avoided as the vestibular apparatus is sensitive in the postoperative period
- Hydration must be adequate
- Gastric distention should not be allowed to occur
- Pharmacologic prophylaxis must be provided either alone or in combination.

Different groups of drugs are effective against postoperative nausea and vomiting. These are:

- Antihistamines—diphenhydramine
- Phenothiazines—promethazine, prochlorperazine
- Benzamides—metoclopromide
- Anticholinergics—scopolamine, hyoscine
- 5 HT$_3$ receptor antagonists—ondansetron, granisetron, dolasetron
- Steroids—dexamethasone.

Postoperative Vertigo

Postoperative vertigo is encountered mainly after stapes surgery. Slight postoperative symptoms of vertigo are very common following stapedotomy. Persistent vertigo and balance disorders are rare. This may occur if the piston of the stapes prosthesis is too long or there is a perilymph fistula.

Postoperative Deafness

Postoperative deafness is a devastating complication following ear surgery. This can occur as a result of intraoperative injury to cochlear structures. Risk of deafness exists after both middle ear and inner ear surgery. Extensive drilling during middle ear surgery can cause noise-induced hearing loss. During resection of extensive cholesteatoma, damage to the inner ear can occur in the form of stapes subluxation or semicircular canal fistula. This may exacerbate preexisting tinnitus or may cause new onset tinnitus in the postoperative period.

Facial Nerve Paralysis

Facial paralysis or paresis (partial paralysis) following ear surgery is a possibility as the facial nerve courses its way through the middle ear to supply the muscles of the face. However, the incidence is very less. It can be related to one of several things:

1. The administration of local anesthetic can cause a temporary paralysis, lasting for several hours after the procedure.

2. The thorough removal of all diseased tissue in middle ear and mastoid surgery can sometimes necessitate exposing a segment of the facial nerve in its bony canal. This exposure can result in temporary nerve inflammation which can lead to transient facial nerve paralysis. This type of injury generally recovers over weeks to months, unless transection or dehiscence been taken place.

3. It is possible to inadvertently nick, bruise, or divide the facial nerve during middle ear and mastoid surgery. This is characterized by immediate, complete paralysis that does not recover. If the injury was not recognized during the operation, sometimes re-exploration for assessment of the extent of injury, and possible decompression, repair, or grafting with segment of great auricular nerve/sural nerve is warranted.

REFERENCES

1. Hohlrieder M, Keller C, Brimacombe J, Eschertzhuber S, Luckner G, Abraham I, von Goedecke A. Middle ear pressure changes during anesthesia with or without nitrous oxide are similar among airway devices. Anesth Analg. 2006;102:319-21.
2. Karabiyik L, Bozkirli F, Çelebi H, Göksu N. Effect of nitrous oxide on middle ear pressure: a comparison between inhalational anesthesia with nitrous oxide and TIVA. European Journal of Anaesthesiology. 1996;13(1):27-32.
3. Schuring AG. Latrogenic facial nerve injury. Am J Otol. 1988:9; 432-3.
4. Wiet RJ. Latrogenic facial paralysis. Otolaryngol Clin North Am. 1982:15;773-80.
5. Lin JC, Ho KY, Kuo WR, Wang LF, Chai CY, Tsai SM. Incidence of dehiscence of the facial nerve at surgery for middle ear cholesteatoma. Otolaryngol Head Neck Surg. 2004;131(4):452-6.
6. Lennon RL, Hosking MP, Daube JR, Welna JO. Effect of partial neuromuscular blockade on intraoperative electromyography in patients undergoing resection of acoustic neuromas. Anesth Analg. 1992;75:729-33.
7. Kizilay A, Aladag I, Cokkeser Y, Miman MC, Ozturan O, Gulhas N. Effects of partial neuromuscular blockade on facial nerve monitorization in otologic surgery. Acta Otolaryngol. 2003;123:321-4.
8. Yi-rong C, Jing XU, Lian-hua C, Fang-lu C. Electromyographic monitoring of facial nerve under different levels of neuromuscular blockade during middle ear microsurgery. Chinese Medical Journal. 2009;122(3):311-4.
9. Imamura SI, Nozawa I, Imamura M, Murakami Y. Clinical observations on acute low-tone sensorineural hearing loss. Ann Otol Rhino Laryngol. 1997;106:746-50.
10. Pirodda A, Saggese D, Ferri GG, et al. The role of hypotension in the pathogenesis of sudden hearing loss. Audiology. 1997;36:98-108.
11. Kawakami K, Makimoto K, Fukuse S, Takahashi H. Autoregulation of cochlear blood flow: a comparison of cerebral blood flow with muscular blood flow. Eur Arch Oto Rhino Laryngol. 1991;248:471-4.

Superior Canal Dehiscence Syndrome: Diagnosis and Management

Dev Roy, Anirvan Banerjee

INTRODUCTION

Vertigo is a common symptom, presenting to the ENT surgeon. There are numerous differential diagnoses for vertigo; superior semicircular canal dehiscence (SSCD) syndrome is a new entity.[1] The dense otic capsule normally has two mobile windows namely oval and round, but an acquired dehiscence in the superior, posterior or lateral semicircular canal results in a third mobile window. The bone conducted sounds and intracranial pressure changes are transmitted across this third mobile window giving rise to abnormal vestibular function. The symptoms include sound- or pressure-induced rotatory vertigo, conductive deafness with normal middle ear function and amplification of certain internal body sounds like heart beat and eye ball movement.[2] The etiology is probably due to thinning of the bone over the semicircular canal during development. CT scan studies of cadaveric temporal bones have found a 0.4- 0.5% dehiscence in the bone overlying the superior canal.[3]

Symptoms of SSCD include:

- Dizziness/vertigo/ unsteadiness
- Autophony—person's own speech
- Tullio phenomenon
- Oscillopsia
- Hyperacusis—the over-sensitivity to sound
- Deafness—Low-frequency conductive
- A feeling of fullness in the affected ear
- Pulsatile tinnitus
- Headache/migraine.

Clinicophysiological Symptoms and Signs

- **Vertigo and balance disorders**—In the normal ear, movement of stapes does not cause any change of pressure at the two ends of semicircular canal. However, in SSCDS the bony dehiscence acts as a 'third window' to the inner ear in addition to oval and round window. The mobility of this third window results in deflection of superior canal ampulla. The direction of the vertical and rotational nystagmus depends on the effect of these stimuli on the superior canal ampulla. Change in pressure in the middle ear or intracranial pressure results in vertigo and ocillopsia. The activities like blowing of nose, cough, lifting heavy objects, pressing on the tragus or significant pressure during bowel movements can trigger the symptoms[4,5]
- **Tullio phenomenon**—Vertigo or unsteadiness is induced by loud noises; volume is not necessarily a factor. It can also be triggered by normal everyday sounds. The presence of Tullio may also mean that involuntary eye movements (nystagmus), sometimes rotational, are set off by sound, giving the sufferer the impression that the world is going round, clockwise or anticlockwise, depending on the site of the dehiscence. A change of pressure within the middle ear (for example when flying or nose-blowing) may equally set off a bout of disequilibrium or nystagmus[6,7]
- **Autophony**—The patients report hearing their own voice as a disturbingly loud and distorted sound deep inside the head. Additionally, they may hear the creaking and cracking of joints, the sound of their footsteps when walking or running, their heartbeat and the sound of chewing and other digestive noises. Some are able to hear the sound of the eyeballs moving in their sockets (e.g. when reading in a quiet room) is almost exclusively associated with SSCDS[8]
- **Low-frequency conductive hearing loss**—It is present in many patients with SSCDS and is explained by the dehiscence acting as a "third window." Vibrations entering the ear canal and middle ear are then abnormally diverted through the superior semicircular

canal and up into the intracranial space where they become absorbed instead of being registered as sound in the hearing center, the cochlea. In some patients, there is true enhancement of low-frequency hearing via bone-conducted sound. A clinical sign of this phenomenon is the ability of the patient to hear (not feel) a tuning fork placed upon the anklebone. Due to the difference in resistance between the normal round window and the pathological dehiscence window, this hearing loss is more serious in the lower frequencies and may initially be mistaken for otosclerosis[9,10]

- **Pulsatile tinnitus** is caused by the gap in the dehiscent bone allowing the normal pulse-related pressure changes within the cranial cavity to enter the inner ear abnormally. This pressure changes, thus affect the sound of the tinnitus
- **Brain fog** and **fatigue** are caused by the brain having to spend an unusual amount of its energy on the simple act of keeping the body in a state of equilibrium when it is constantly receiving confusing signals from the dysfunctional semicircular canal
- **Headache** and **migraine** are also often mentioned by patients showing other symptoms of SCDS.

It is important to note that third window dehiscence may be present in other parts of the ear

Classification of third window lesions based on locations
- Superior canal dehiscence
- Posterior canal dehiscence
- Lateral canal dehiscence
- Large vestibular aqueduct syndrome
- DFN-3 (X-linked deafness with stapes gusher)
- Dehiscence between the cochlea and carotid canal
- Pagets disease of the temporal bone.

Clinical Findings

The main clinical finding is the presence of nystagmus in presence of sound or pressure stimuli. This can better visualized by Frenzels glasses since it eliminates visual suppression and magnifies the eye movements. Typically, the nystagmus has a vertical and torsional component. The direction of nystagmus can be predicted based on direction of endolymph flow within the superior canal (ampullifugal or ampullipetal) in response to valsalva maneuver or pressure in the external auditory canal.[11] Positive pressure within the external auditory canal (EAC), Valsalva maneuver against pinched nose, tragal compression and high intensity sounds will result in flow of endolymph from vestibule to the dehiscence. This ampullifugal flow of endolymph will result in vertical and rotational nystagmus, with a slow component pointing upwards and towards the opposite side of the affected ear. Similarly, negative pressure in the

EAC, Valsalva against closed glottis and jugular venous compression causing a raise in intracranial pressure. This will cause an inward bulging of the membrane at the dehiscence, resulting in an ampullipetal flow of the endolymph. The nystagmus will be in the opposite direction.[11-13]

Investigations

Tuning Fork Tests

Rhinne's test shows conductive hearing loss in the affected ear with low-frequency tuning fork 128, 256, 512 Hz. Weber is lateralized to the affected ear. Patients may also hear a low-frequency tuning fork (128 and 256 Hz) placed on the lateral malleoli of the foot.[14,15]

Audiometry and Tympanometry

Tonal audiometry shows "conductive hearing loss' with air bone gap of 5–10 dB in two or more frequencies especially in the lower and mid frequencies. The bone conduction thresholds are lower than 0 dB hearing level. Therefore, air-bone gap may exist even when air conduction thresholds are normal. The audiometry may mimic otosclerosis.[9-11] Some patients may have mild to moderate sensorineural loss. Tympanometry shows normal pressure. The speech discrimination and acoustic reflexes are normal.

Vestibular Function Test

Caloric test are normal. Electronystagmography shows no abnormal findings on sound and pressure stimuli, due to vertical and torsional nystagmus although patients complain of vertigo. The nystagmus is best documented by video-oculography or magnetic field scleral tests.[7]Patients with larger dehiscence (>0.5 mm) show reduced vestibular function on the affected side.

Vestibular-evoked Myogenic Potential testing (VEMP)

Vestibular-evoked myogenic potential responses have been a useful assessment technique for confirming suspected presence of SSCD. [14,16]

There are two types of VEMPs based on the position of electrodes. The ocular VEMPS, the surface electrode is placed below the eye and in cervical VEMP the electrodes are placed on the ipsilateral sternocleidomastoid muscle. These electrodes record excitatory responses to clicks or tone bursts. The patients with the syndrome have reduced threshold for VEMP response in the affected ear for both air and bone conduction and larger VEMP amplitudes with 80% specificity and sensitivity. VEMP testing is useful in testing whether a patient presenting with conductive hearing loss has ossicular fixation or true dehiscence. In dehiscence, the threshold is lowered while in ossicular fixation the VEMP responses are either absent or show elevated response.[14,16,17]

Radiology

CT Scan

High-resolution CT scan of temporal bone is the most important diagnostic criteria to demonstrate dehiscence of the bone in SSCD (Fig. 1).

The conventional CT scan of 1mm collimation when used for SSCD confirmation gave high number of false positive results.[18] Currently, multislice temporal bone CT scan is done with fine cuts of 0.5–0.6 mm collimation reformatted to the plane of superior semicircular canal such that images are parallel (Poshchl's view) and orthogonal (Stenver's view) to the plane. The temporal bone is scanned as a volume of tissue rather than multiple narrow slices. These factors allow extremely high-resolution of reconstructions in any desired plane produced from volume data. The positive predictive value of conventional 1mm CT scan in diagnosis of SSCD is 50% but improves to 93% by using multislice 0.5 mm helical CT scans of the temporal bone with oblique coronal reconstructions.[18]

Treatment

Conservative treatment for superior canal dehiscence best benefits patients with mild or no symptoms.[19] For most patients understanding the cause of symptoms, avoidance of the stimuli and reassurance is sufficient. In some patients, pressure-induced symptoms may dominant, these patients may benefit from grommet insertion, although its efficacy is variable.[20] But if the symptoms are debilitating then surgical

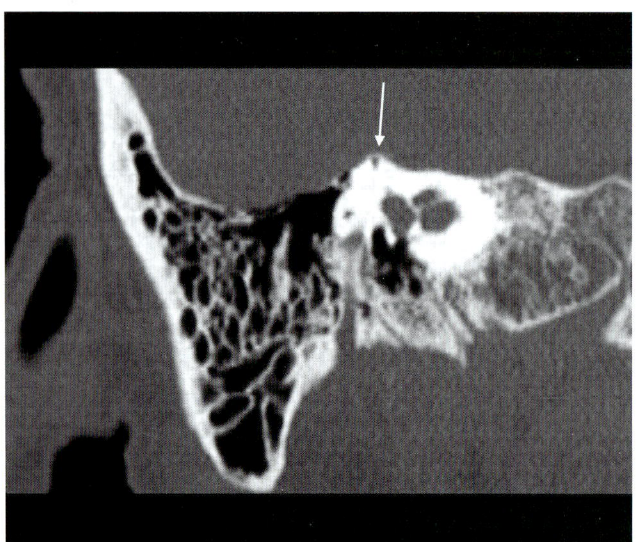

Fig. 1: Right temporal bone CT scan, arrow showing superior canal dehiscence

occlusion or resurfacing of the superior semicircular canal is beneficial.

Surgery

SSCD should be treated surgically, if there are clinical symptoms, which are debilitating.[21] The superior canal dehiscence can be approached via two methods—middle cranial fossa craniotomy and transmastoid approach.[19,22] Once the superior canal dehiscence is identified, there are two techniques—one is to plug or obliterate the canal and other is to resurface the canal. There are advantages and disadvantages of both the approaches and techniques used. Plugging the canal lumen with bone dust, bone wax or fascia stops the endolymph flow. Plugging can be done via transmastoid or middle cranial craniotomy approach. Resurfacing stops the communication between brain and inner ear. However, it can only be done via middle cranial approach.

Transmastoid Superior Canal Occlusion[19,22]

In this approach, a mastoidectomy is performed and the superior semicircular canal is identified near the ossicular heads. The superior semicircular canal is then ablated with a combination of bone dust, bone wax and fascia. Brantberg et al.[6] although this approach can be effective, the risk of sensorineural hearing loss increases with this procedure because of limited exposure versus middle fossa craniotomy.

Traditional Middle Fossa Craniotomy and Repair of Fistula[23]

In this procedure, a middle cranial fossa craniotomy is done on the affected side. The temporal lobe is gently retracted. Upon elevation of the dura, care is required to avoid stretching the greater superficial petrosal nerve, which could injure the facial nerve. The region of the superior semicircular canal is located with identification of the arcuate eminence. A dehiscence of the superior semicircular canal can be resurfaced with bone wax, bone cement, or fascia, or the canal can be ablated with wax or bone cement. The resurfacing can be done by five layered technique—fascia, bone paste, cartilage, bone paste and fascia or three layered cartilage fascia, cartilage, and bone paste. The disadvantage of middle cranial fossa approach is temporal lobe retraction increases the risk of epilepsy. Moreover, the surgery has to be done in cooperation with neurosurgeon.

Endoscopic Craniotomy Approach[24]

In this procedure, patients undergo a middle cranial fossa craniotomy through a small, limited-access craniotomy of

2 cm or less on the affected side. The temporal lobe is gently retracted. Upon elevation of the dura, a small endoscope is gently inserted, and the dehiscence is identified and resurfaced. This approach has an average hospital stay of 2 days and a smaller incision than the typical middle fossa approach originally described. There is improvement in 90% of the symptoms with no adverse outcomes. This approach allows visualization of the dehiscence without the need for a larger craniotomy.

Minimally Invasive Approach via Transcanal Oval and Round Window Reinforcement[25,26]

In this technique, reinforcing the other two natural windows can dampen the effects of a third window at the superior semicircular canal. By dampening the hyper compliance of the inner ear at the oval and round windows, rather than intracranial or transmastoid, the risks of craniotomy, which include death, stroke, cranial palsies, cerebrospinal fluid leaks and hearing loss, are avoided. This procedure can be performed under local anesthesia. A transcanal approach to the middle ear is performed with elevation of the tympanic membrane. Small amounts of fascia or tragal cartilage are used to reinforce both the oval and round windows. The risks of the procedure, performed on an outpatient basis, are extremely low.[25,26]

There are studies which measured the following symptoms, including autophony, sensitivity to bone conduction, pulsatile tinnitus, sensitivity to loud sounds, dizziness on straining, dizziness on increased middle ear pressure loss, aural fullness, and imbalance.[26] Most patients had improvement in their preoperative symptoms.

Combination Approach

In this technique, the superior canal defect is repaired via the middle fossa approach with concomitant reinforcement of the oval and round windows. The authors claim improved outcomes over middle fossa repair alone, reporting a resolution of vertigo.[27]

CONCLUSION

Since this is a recently described syndrome, most ENT surgeons are not aware of this diagnosis. It should be a part of differential diagnosis of vertigo and in cases of conductive hearing loss as a differential diagnosis of otosclerosis.[9] It is best diagnosed by multislice CT scan[18] and VEMP testing.[14,16] Mild cases should be treated conservatively while severe or debilitating symptoms are treated initially by minimally invasive procedure of reinforcing the oval and round window with fascia or tragal cartilage via trans canal approach.[25] The middle cranial fossa approach or transmastoid approach plugging or resurfacing should be reserved for the patients with persistent symptoms.[22,23]

REFERENCES

1. Minor LB, Solomon D, Zinreich JS, Zee DS. Sound- and pressure-induced vertigo due to bone dehiscence of the superior semicircular canal. Arch Otolaryngol Head Neck Surg. 1998;124:249-59.
2. Minor LB. Superior canal dehiscence syndrome. Am J Otol. Jan 2000;21(1):9-19.
3. Carey JP, Minor LB, Nager GT. Dehiscence or thinning of the overlying the superior semicircular canal in a temporal bone survey. Arch Otolaryngol Head Neck Surg. 2000;126:137-47.
4. Rosowski JJ, Songer JE, Nakajima HH, Brinsko KM, Merchant SN. Clinical, experimental, and theoretical investigations of the effect of superior semicircular canal dehiscence on hearing mechanism. Otol Neurotol. 2004;25(3):323-32.
5. Mong A, Loevner LA, Solomon D, Bigelow DC. Sound- and pressure-induced vertigo associated with dehiscenceof the roof of superior semicircular canal. AJNR AM J Neuroradiol. 1999;20:1973-5.
6. Tullio P. Das Ohr und die Entstehung der Sprache und Schrift Berlin. Urban & Schwarzenberg. 1929.
7. Ostrowski VB, Byskosh A, Hain TC. Tullio phenomenon with dehiscence of the superior semicircular canal. Otol Neurotol. 2001;22(1):61-5.
8. Albuquerque W, Bronstein AM. 'Doctor, I can hear my eyes': report of two cases with different mechanisms". Journal of Neurology, Neurosurgery, and Psychiatry. 2004;75(9):1363-4.
9. Merchant SN, Rosowski JJ, McKenna MJ. Superior semicircular canal dehiscence mimicking otosclerotic hearing loss. Adv Otorhinolaryngol. 2007;65:137-45.
10. Mikulec AA, McKenna MJ, Ramsey MJ, Rosowski JJ, Herrmann BS, Rauch SD. Superior semicircular canal dehiscence presenting as conductive hearing loss without vertigo. Otol Neurotol. 2004;25(2):121-9.
11. Minor LB, Carey JP, Cremer PD, Lustig LR, Streubel SO, Ruckenstein MJ. Dehiscence of bone overlying the superior canal as a cause of apparent conductive hearing loss. Otol Neurotol. 2003;24(2):270-8.
12. Cremer PD, Minor LB, Carey JP, Della Santina CC. Eye movements in patients with superior canal dehiscence syndrome align with the abnormal canal. Neurology. 2000;55:1833-41.
13. Banerjee A. Superior Canal dehiscence (SCD) Syndrome- A missed diagnosis. The Otolaryngologist. 2007;1(2):72-5.
14. Banerjee A, Whyte A, Atlas MD. Superior canal dehiscence: review of a new condition. Clin Otolaryngol. 2005;30(1):9-15.
15. Watson SRD, Halmagyi GM, Coltebach JG. Vestibular hypersensitivity to sound (Tullio phenomenon): structural and functional assessment. Neurology. 2000;54:722-8.
16. Brantberg K, Verrecchia L. Testing vestibular-evoked myogenic potentials with 90 dB clicks is effective in the diagnosis of superior canal dehiscence syndrome. Audiol Neuro Otol. 2009;14(1):54-8.

17. Streubel SO, Cremer PD, Carey JP, Weg N, Minor LB. Vestibular-evoked myogenic potentials in the diagnosis of superior canal dehiscence syndrome. Acta Otolaryngol Suppl. 2001;545:41-9.
18. Belden CJ, Weg N, Minor LB, Zeinveich SJ. CT evaluation of bone dehiscence of superior semicircular canal as a cause of sound- and/or pressure-induced vertigo. Radiology. 2003;226:337-43.
19. Amoodi HA, Makki FM, McNeil M, Bance M. Transmastoid resurfacing of superior canal dehiscence. Laryngoscope. 2011;121:1117-23.
20. Chien WW, Carey JP, Minor LB. Canal dehiscence. Curr Opin Neurol. 2011:24:25-31.
21. Minor LB. Clinical manifestations of superior semicircular canal dehiscence. Laryngoscope. 2005;15(10):1717-27.
22. Mikulec AA, Poe DS, McKenna MJ. Operative management of superior semicircular canal dehiscence. Laryngoscope. 2005;115(3):501-7.
23. Martin JE, Neal CJ, Monacci WT, Eisenman DJ. Superior semicircular canal dehiscence: a new indication for middle fossa craniotomy. Case report. J Neurosurg. 2004;100(1):125-7.
24. Shaia WT, Diaz RC. Evolution in surgical management of superior canal dehiscence syndrome. Curr Opin Otolaryngol Head Neck Surg. 2013;21(5):497-502.
25. Silverstein H, Kartush JM, Parnes LS, Poe DS, Babu SC, Levenson MJ. Round window reinforcement for superior semicircular canal dehiscence: A retrospective multi-center case series. Am J Otolaryngol. 2014;35(3):286-93.
26. Silverstein et al. Round Window Reinforcement for Superior Canal Dehiscence. Oto-HNS. 2012;147:93.
27. Gianoli GJ, Soileau JS. The dehiscent middle fossa: prevalence, manifestations, associated findings and results of 24 surgical explorations for superior semicircular canal dehiscence. Publication pending: presented as triologic thesis, 2005.

Middle Ear Surgery

Asok K Saha

Common topics in middle ear surgery presented in this chapter:
- Surgical approaches to middle ear and mastoid diseases
- Tympanoplasty
- Ossiculoplasty
- Mastoid surgery
- Endoscopic ear surgery.

SURGICAL APPROACHES TO MIDDLE EAR AND MASTOID DISEASES

Surgical approaches to middle ear and mastoid surgery are:
- Rosen's permeatal (transcanal) approach
- Lempert's endaural approach
- Wilde's postaural approach

Rosen's Permeatal (Transcanal) Approach

This approach is used when meatus is adequately wide and free of infection. It allows inspection of middle ear aseptically and provides separation of middle ear from the exterior after completion of surgery. Permeatal approach is used for[1]—
- Myringotomy in acute suppurative otitis media, hemotympanum and secretory otitis media along with grommet insertion
- Tympanic membrane reconstruction
- Ossicular chain examination and its reconstruction in tympanoplasty
- Stapedectomy or stapedotomy/Revision stapes surgery
- Labyrinthectomy in uncontrolled vertigo in nonhearing ear
- Tympanic neurectomy in recurrent sialoadenitis of parotid gland
- Singular neurectomy for uncontrolled BPPV of the posterior semicircular canal

- Excision of glomus tympanicum
- Reconstruction of round window following spontaneous rupture.

Contraindication

- Narrow EAC
- Otitis externa.

Anesthesia (Fig. 1)

- Premedication—Injection Phenergan 50 mg IM and morphine 0.1 mg/kg body weight are given 1 hour before surgery
- Usually, local anesthesia is used in adult patients
- Hypotensive general anesthesia with orotracheal intubation is used for children and apprehensive patients
- In local anesthesia, 1 mL of 2% xylocaine with 1:1,00,000 adrenaline is injected as follows:
  - 0.4 mL into posterior meatal wall just lateral to where the skin becomes closely adherence to the periosteum

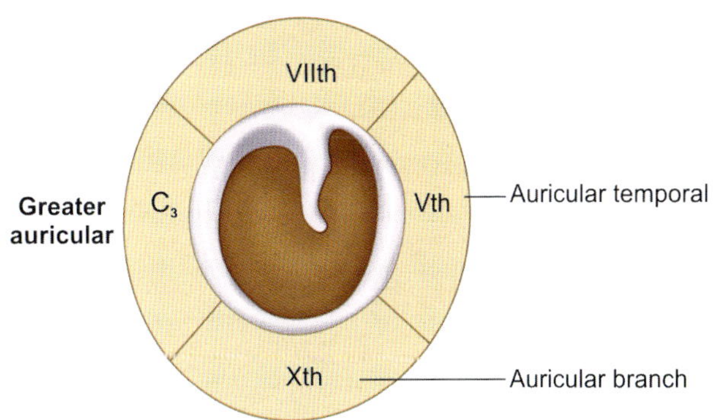

Fig. 1: Four quadrant anesthesia for ear surgery

- 0.2 mL into anterior meatal wall at same level
- 0.2 mL into superior meatal wall at same level
- 0.2 mL into inferior meatal wall at same level
- Some additional solution may be instilled into tympanic cavity.

Positioning of the Patient

- Patient is kept supine on the table and head is placed slightly lower down and rotated to the opposite side. Surgeon should be seated comfortably on a rolling chair
- A suitable size black ear speculum is inserted in the EAC under operating microscope with ×8 magnification.

Incision (Fig. 2)

Incision begins at 6 o' clock position on the inferior meatal wall close to the annulus. It then slopes outwards and upwards to a point of 6–8 mm from the annulus at 9 o' clock position. It ends at 12 o' clock position at about 2 mm above the lateral process of malleus.

Anterior Tympanotomy

The dissection should begin posterosuperiorly where the canal wall skin is thick. The posterior canal wall skin together with the periosteum is reflected anteriorly until the fibrous annulus is reached. Fibrous annulus is then reflected from the bony sulcus. Posterior canal wall skin and posterior half of pars tensa are then folded and placed over the anterior canal wall to expose the posterior part of mesotympanum.

Middle Ear Structures (Fig. 3)

- Chorda tympani lying immediately behind the tympanic membrane is reflected downwards to see the long process of incus, incudostapedial joint and oval window. Promontory is seen over the medial wall of middle ear. Oval window is situated above and behind the promontory; round window is situated below and behind the promontory. Transverse part of facial nerve canal is detected just above the oval window
- Posterosuperior bony overhang is curetted to see the stapedius tendon, pyramid, stapes and oval window clearly.

Reposition of TM flap (Fig. 4)

- Tympanomeatal flap is repositioned at the end of the procedure. Gelfoam soaked with antibiotic solution is then placed over the incision line. Gauze smeared with antibiotics is kept in the EAC.

Complications

- Tear of tympanic membrane during reflection of TM
- Loss of taste sensation due to injury of chorda tympani

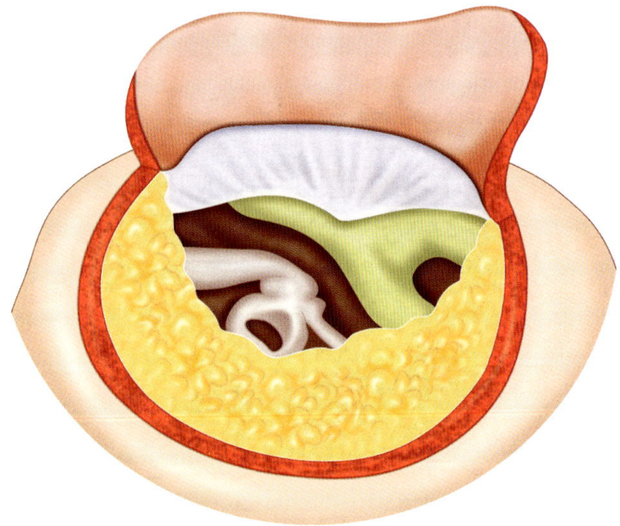

Fig. 3: Elevation of tympanomeatal flap

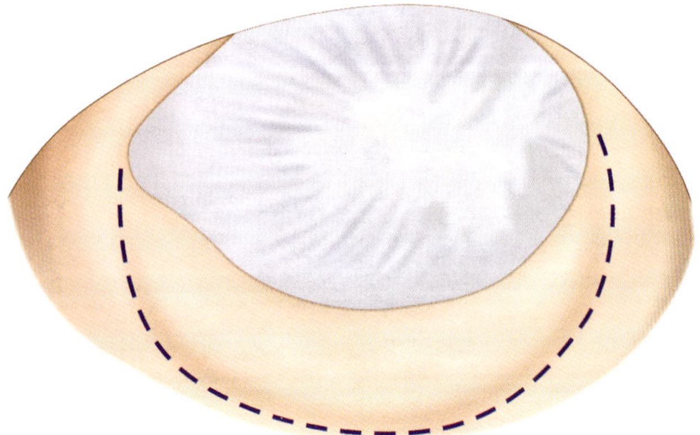

Fig. 2: Incision on posterior canal wall skin

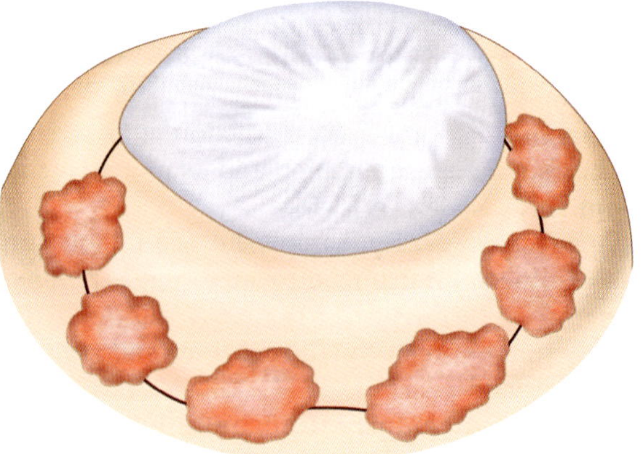

Fig. 4: Reposition of tympano-meatal flap

- Dead ear and persistent vertigo may happen following trauma to round window or oval window.

Lempert's Endaural Approach

This approach provides head-on access to mesotympanum, outer attic wall and antrum. Microscope can be rotated through a wide area of a circle to improve visibility of key area like facial recess and sinus tympani.

The endaural approach is used for[2]—

- Eradication of disease from epitympanum
- Correction of acquired meatal stenosis
- Modified radical mastoidectomy in a contracted acellular mastoid (inside out approach) while X-ray shows anteriorly placed sigmoid sinus and low lying dura
- Tympanoplasty in case of posteriorly situated central perforation
- Stapedectomy in a narrow EAC
- Fenestration of lateral semicircular canal.

Merits

- Meatal flap is easily constructed
- Tympanum is directly accessible
- Final cavity is small where antrum is free of disease
- No need for making meatoplasty separately
- Ideal for inside-out approach
- Lesser operating time compared to postaural approach.

Demerits

- Increased chances of perichondritis
- Increased chances of meatal stenosis
- Difficult to access mastoid tip cells
- Difficult to eradicate disease in a well-pneumatized mastoid.

Incision (Fig. 5)

There are two parts of the incision:
1. First part—Incision is made from 12 o' clock to 6 o' clock on the posterior canal wall at the junction of the cartilaginous with bony meatus.
2. Second part—Incision is made in the incisura terminalis and it joins the first incision at its superior end.

The incision extends vertically upwards in front of the auricle to a point halfway between the meatus and upper edge of the auricle.

Exposure of MacEwen's triangle (Suprameatal triangle)

The incision is deepened till meatal bone is felt. The periosteum is then separated upwards and backwards to expose the suprameatal spine, the suprameatal triangle and bony cortex of the mastoid process. The classic Lempert endaural retractor with blades of different sizes is used (Fig. 6). Small blade fits against the tragus whereas the wide blade retracts the posterior aspect of the incision thus exposing the mastoid cortex.

Mobilization of Meatal Skin

Meatal skin is separated from squamotympanic (anterosuperior) and tympanomastoid (posterior) sutures to expose epitympanum. Temporalis muscle is retracted upwards and meatal skin is mobilized posteriorly.

Exposure of Mastoid Antrum (Fig. 7)

- Antrum is entered through MacEwen's triangle by drilling with a cutting burr (6 mm). The direction of bone work is downward, forward and medially
- Continuous irrigation and suction is essential during the procedure.

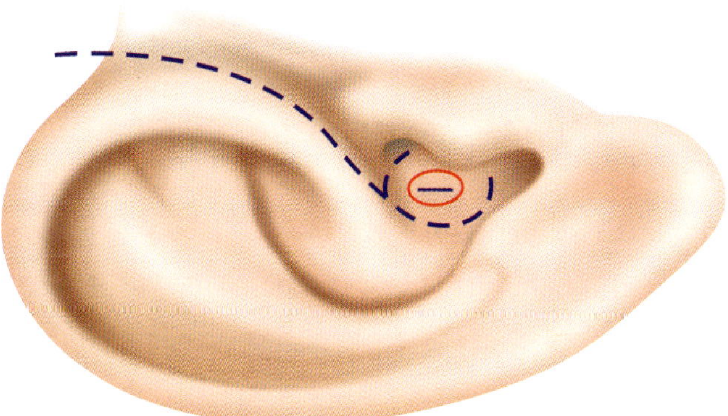

Fig. 5: Lempert's endaural incision

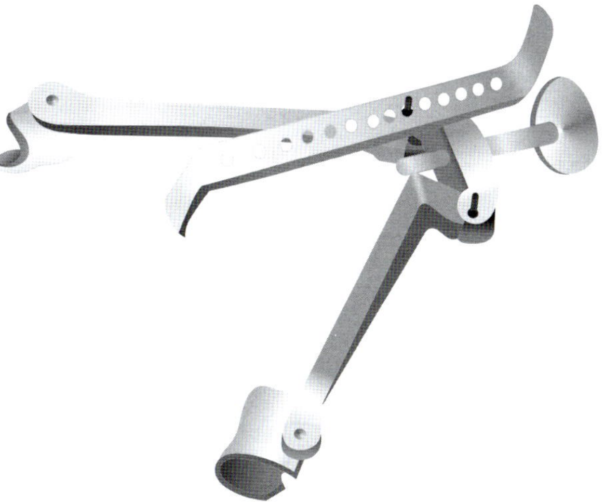

Fig. 6: Lempert endaural retractor

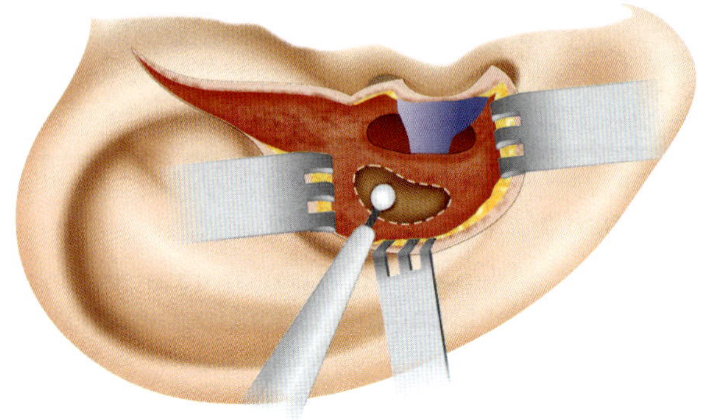

Fig. 7: Exposure of mastoid autrum

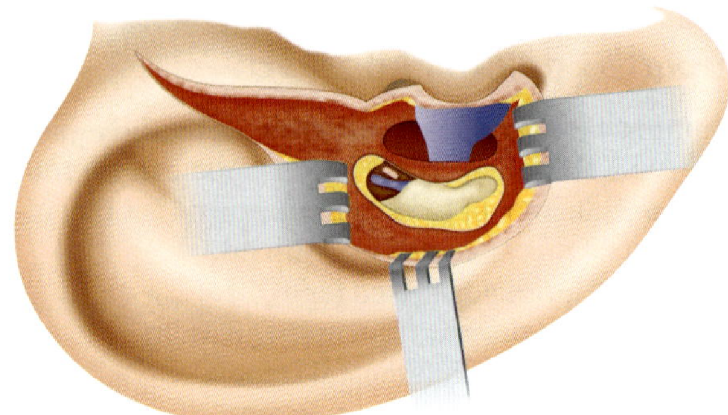

Fig. 8: Exposure of attic

Exposure of the Attic (Fig. 8)

This is made by drilling through the root of zygoma from antrum to expose the head of malleus and body of incus. Short process of incus is seen in fossa incudis and situated inferior to the aditus to antrum. After removal of incus, lateral semicircular canal which lies medial and posterior to the short process of incus is identified. Horizontal part of facial nerve lies below the anterior end of lateral SCC. Drilling of mastoid posteriorly exposes sinodural angle above, tip cells below and sinus plate behind.

Wound Closure (Fig. 9)

Gauze smeared with antibiotics is put in the EAC. Edge of the wound is closed with interrupted suture by 2.0chromic catgut. The skin is closed with interrupted silk suture. Then mastoid dressing is done.

Complications

- Facial nerve paralysis may happen on the operated side due to surgical trauma
- Perichondritis may develop from inferior cholesteatoma
- Vertigo and deaf ear are usually due to disease or surgical trauma
- Meatal stenosis is a late complication which may be prevented by careful closure of the wound and putting of the pack.

Wilde's Postauricular Approach

It provides wide exposure of entire mastoid, epitympanum, access to anterior recess of deep meatus and allows access to posterior fossa dura.

The postauricular approach is used for[3]

- Cortical Mastoidectomy and/or draining of subperiosteal abscess

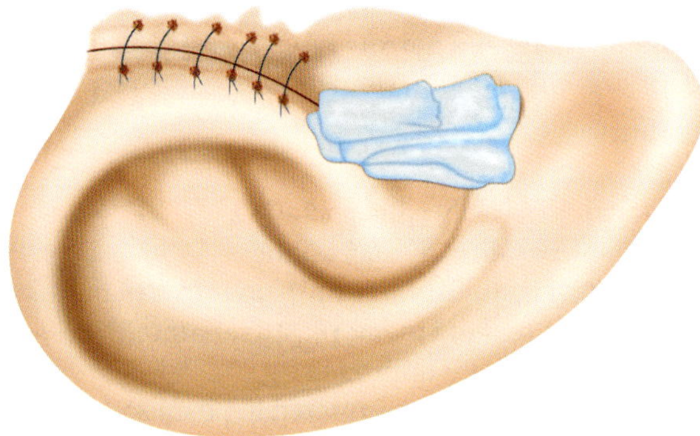

Fig. 9: Wound closure

- Cellular mastoid with large cholesteatoma cavity as evidenced by X-ray mastoid
- Canal wall up procedures (combined approach intact canal wall tympanoplasty with facial recess approach or tympanomastoid surgery)
- Canal wall down procedure (radical and modified radical Mastoidectomy and Bondy's procedure)
- In Meniere's disease, for exposure of endolymphatic sac and translabyrinthine vestibular neurectomy
- Facial nerve decompression or repair of this nerve in traumatic palsy
- Translabyrinthine removal of acoustic tumors confined to the porus acusticus
- Retrolabyrinthine approach to cranial nerves in CP angle
- Carcinoma of the middle ear
- Glomus jugulare
- Cochlear implant insertion.

Surgical Steps

- Incision—A curved incision is made three-eighth of an inch or 0.096 cm behind the postauricular sulcus from

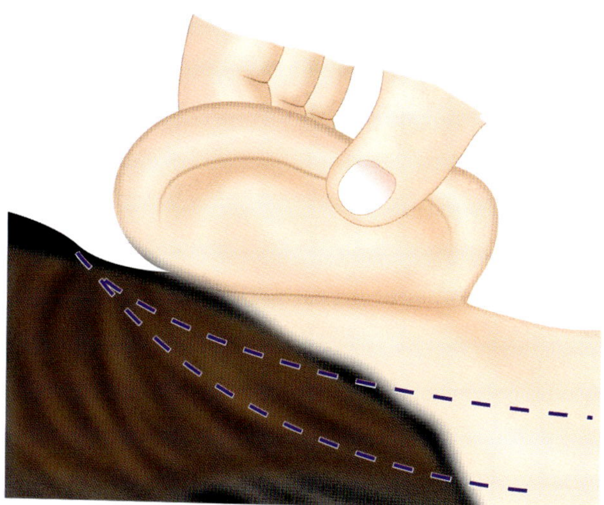

Fig. 10: Incision is made behind the postauricural sulcus

12 o' clock position to 6 o' clock position at the mastoid tip (Fig. 10)[4]

- In infants and young children, the incision is more horizontally placed to avoid injury to the facial nerve as the mastoid tip is not developed and the nerve is relatively more superficial
- The incision is deepened up to the periosteum by dividing the subcutaneus tissue and muscles of auricle with a cutting diathermy needle
- Separation of periosteal flap and mobilization of meatal skin—Periosteum is then divided by T-shaped incision. Vertical limb of T runs parallel to the posterior meatal opening and horizontal limb follows the temporal line. The periosteal flaps are then separated to expose the mastoid cortex, suprameatal triangle and spine and posterior canal margin. Posterior canal skin together with periosteum is reflected anteriorly from the underlying bone up to tympanic margin. The meatal skin is then mobilized superiorly and inferiorly
- Exploration of mastoid—Mastoid is explored as in endaural approach
- Wound closure—The periosteal margins are closed with interrupted catgut suture. The skin is closed with interrupted silk suture. Mastoid dressing is then applied.

Merits of Postauricular Approach

- The approach gives greater flexibility in holding the soft tissue and enables the surgeon to design flap to reduce the size of the cavity
- Greater exposure provides effective saucerization of the cavity.

Demerits of Postauricular Approach

- Increased incidence of meatoplasty closure
- Increased incidence of postaural fistula
- Postaural depression associated with dust collection
- Thick scarring
- Alteration of the angle of the pinna with the skull.

TYMPANOPLASTY

Definitions

- **Tympanoplasty** is the operation performed to eradicate the disease in middle ear and to reconstruct the hearing mechanism including tympanic membrane and ossicles with or without mastoid surgery. Tympanoplasty also includes canalplasty and meatoplasty for creation of a dry self-cleaning cavity.
  In 1965, the American Academy of Ophthalmology and Otolaryngology Subcommittee on Conservation of Hearing defined that tympanoplasty is the operation performed to eradicate the disease in middle ear and to reconstruct the hearing mechanism with mastoid surgery with or without tympanic membrane grafting
- **Myringoplasty** is the operation where reconstruction or repair of tympanic membrane is performed only assuming the middle ear mucosa is normal and ossicular chain is intact
- **Canalplasty** is the operation of widening the external auditory canal and is an integral part of tympanoplasty. It provides appropriate surgical access for grafting anterior perforation of tympanic membrane and facilitates cleansing and second stage Ossiculoplasty
- **Ossiculoplasty** is the procedure to restore the sound transformer mechanism from TM to oval window
- **Conchomeatoplasty** is used to enlarge the opening of EAC with removal of cartilage so that widening of cartilaginous EAC is in proportion to bony meatus.

Aims of surgery are:
- To create intact tympanic membrane
- To eradicate disease from middle ear and mastoid
- To create air containing middle ear space
- To restore hearing by securing connection between TM and cochlea.

Pre-requisites for tympanoplasty are:
- Hearing with AC<BC (with tuning fork tests)
- Adequate cochlear reserve; BC 30 dB or greater than AC
- Patent Eustachian tube
- Functional state of ossicular chain/labyrinthine windows should be assessed
- Tympanic mucus membrane should be healthy
- Regular follow-up postoperatively.

Wullstein's Classification (1956)

This classification relates to the pathology of the middle ear conductive mechanism and predicts the level of postoperative hearing improvement.

Types of Tympanoplasty (Fig. 11)

Wullstein described five types of tympanoplasty:
- Type I tympanoplasty—Ossicular chain is intact and mobile; only reconstruction of the TM is required
- Type II tympanoplasty—Malleus handle is absent; reconstruction of tympanic membrane is done over malleus remnant and long process of incus
- Type III tympanoplasty—Malleus and incus are absent; stapes superstructure is intact; reconstruction of tympanic membrane is done over an intact and mobile stapes (myringostapediopexy or columella tympanoplasty)
- Type IV tympanoplasty—Stapes superstructure is absent; tympanic membrane is reconstructed as a round window baffle. A narrow middle ear is then formed to create an air pocket around the round window (cavum minor)
- Type V tympanoplasty—Stapes is fixed; fenestration is made on LSCC covered by a graft.

Indications for Tympanoplasty[5]

- Conductive hearing loss resulting from TM perforation or ossicular dysfunction
- Progressive hearing loss due to COM
- Perforation or hearing loss persisting for more than 3 months following infection, trauma or surgery.

Contraindications for Tympanoplasty[6]

- Malignant tumors of external or middle ear
- Extensive and uncontrolled cholesteatoma
- Invasive life-threatening pseudomonas infection in diabetes
- Intracranial complications of COM
- Eustachian tube dysfunction
- Functionally dead ear unless patient participates in water sports
- Only hearing ear to avoid risk of SNHL.

Preoperative evaluation

In addition to usual investigations like audiometry/tympanometry/X-ray mastoid and paranasal sinuses/CT temporal bone, examination under microscope and Gelfoam patch test are helpful.

Otomicroscopy includes examination of ear canal and tympanic membrane for—
- Size and location of perforation
- Retraction pockets, granulation or cholesteatoma
- Status of middle ear through perforation

The Gelfoam patch test is as follows—

- Perforation is closed with moist Gelfoam. Audiogram is repeated following closure of perforation. If audiogram shows improvement in hearing, it indicates ossicular chain continuity. If the test shows no improvement of hearing indicating possibility of stapes fixation that needs 2nd stage stapes surgery
- In bilateral COM with mucosal disease, patch test determines the side of surgery. If patch test shows no improvement on one side, it is better to operate on the other side where there is increased improvement of hearing with Gelfoam in position
- In severe bilateral mixed hearing loss, adequate masking is to be done. Increased hearing on better side by patch test provides better masking efficiency with exact evaluation of cochlear reserve in the worse ear.[7]

Choice of Surgical Approaches[8] for Myringoplasty

- Transcanal approach is used for wide meatus permitting total visualization of perforation. This approach is mostly used for repairing anterior traumatic perforation
- Endaural approach is used for posterior perforation
- Postauricular approach is selected for anterior perforation where margins cannot be seen through EAC.

Graft Materials

- Full thickness skin graft (FTSG)—Berthold (1878) who coined the term 'myringoplasty' first applied FTSG
- Split thickness skin graft (STSG)—Wullstein and Zollner (1950) first used STSG over de-epithelialized TM. Initial result is good but subsequent desquamation and infection cause high failing rate

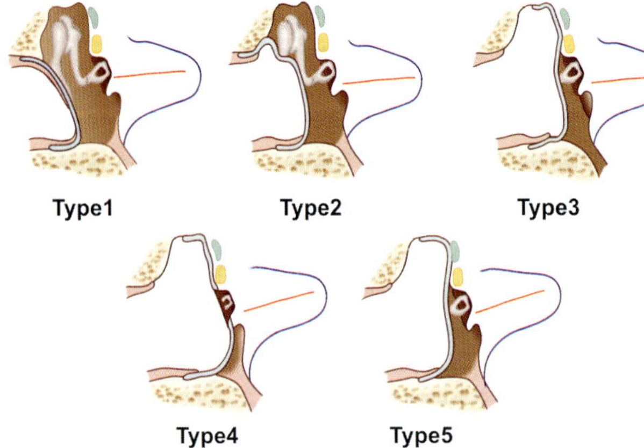

Fig. 11: Types of tympanoplasty

- Vein graft—Shea (1957) first performed medial grafting with vein patch that may atrophy resulting in graft failure
- Temporalis fascia—Heermann (1960) and Storrs (1961) introduced the use of Temporalis fascia graft (TFG). Harvesting of TFG needs no separate incision. It has low metabolic rate. It is sturdy and obtained in large quantity
- Homograft TM—It has excellent success similar to TFG. But there is risk for transmission of infectious disease (AIDS, HepB)
- Tragal perichondrium—It is used in revision surgery and has excellent results
- Cartilage—Salen and Jansen (1963) first reported the use of cartilage for reconstruction of TM. It is excellent for prevention of recurrent retraction pockets and most successful when it is placed posterosuperiorly and on pars flaccida. It is recommended by Vrabec (2002) to be placed over TORP or PORP to prevent extrusion. Hearing results are comparable to TFG [Gerber (2000) and Dornhoffer (1997)].

Grafting Technique

Reconstruction of TM is commonly done using temporalis fascia by
- Onlay technique (lateral grafting)
- Underlay technique (medial grafting)
- Interlay technique (inlay grafting).

Onlay/lateral Grafting

The graft is placed lateral to the fibrous layer of the denuded drum remnant (Fig. 12)
Advantages of onlay grafting are:
- Excellent exposure
- High graft take rate
- Applicable to all cases
- Middle ear volume is not reduced.

Disadvantages of onlay grafting:
- Longer healing time
- Possibility of blunting
- Lateralization or epithelial pearls
- Meticulous precision is required.

Underlay/medial Grafting

The graft is placed medial to tympanic annulus. The procedure involves opening of middle ear to see the ossicular status and middle ear structure. This technique is mostly used by the surgeon (Fig. 13).
Advantages of underlay grafting are:
- As the integrity of anterior tympanomeatal angle is maintained, blunting does not occur
- As the graft is placed under malleus lateralization doesn't occur
- Graft take rate is high and technique is simple.

Disadvantages of underlay grafting are:
- Residual perforation—In case of large perforation where anterior drum remnant of TM is less than 4 mm and blood supply is not adequate anteriorly, small window is made about 2 mm lateral to the annulus at 3 o' clock position to pull through the graft.[9] Otherwise residual perforation remains
- Medialization of graft with adhesions with the promontory
- Chronic myringitis—As the squamous epithelium grows inwards around the edge of perforation endothelium grows outwards around the edge and on the outer surface of the fascia resulting in myringitis.
- There is reduction of middle ear space.

Interlay Technique

Graft is placed between the fibrous and mucous layers of tympanic membrane. This technique is not usually used by the surgeons (Fig. 14).

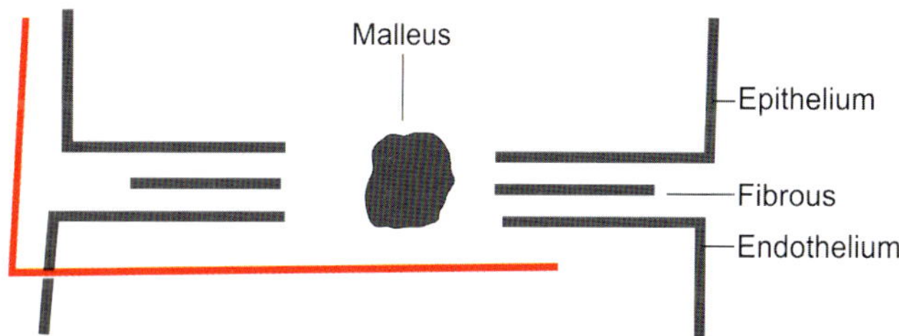

Fig. 13: Underlay technique

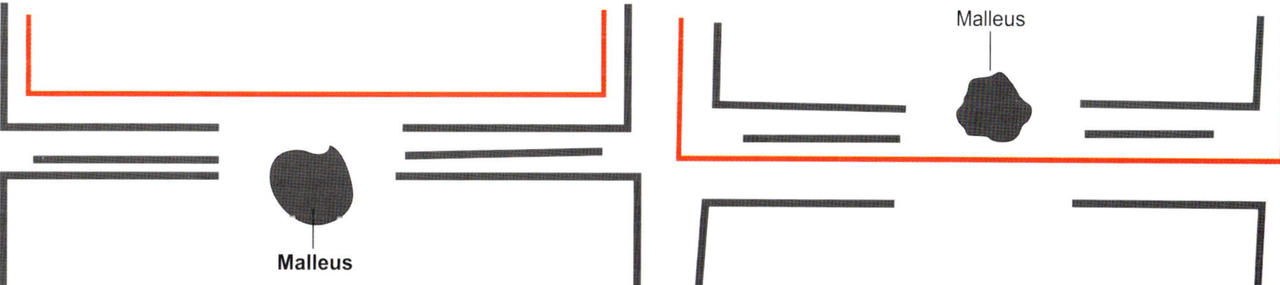

Fig. 12: Onlay technique

Fig. 14: Interlay technique

Advantages of interlay technique are:
- No lateralization, no medialization or epithelial pearl formation.

Disadvantages of interlay technique are:
- Meticulous precision is required.

Causes of Graft Failure

- Infection
- Technical error
- Insufficient tubal function
- Poor patient preparation.

Ugo Fisch[10] advocated terms "overlay" and "underlay" in different sense than usual, referring placement of graft in relation to bone and not in relation to TM. "Overlay" refers to placement of graft over the bony tympanic sulcus or over a bony ledge newly made in the bone where bony tympanic sulcus is absent.

"Underlay" means placement of graft under tympanic membrane and surrounding bone.

Usually, anteriorly the graft is placed under the anterior remnant of tympanic membrane and under the lateral wall of protympanum. Posteriorly, the graft is placed over the posterior tympanic sulcus and under the remnant of TM. The graft lies medial to the handle of malleus. This is a combination of anterior underlay and posterior overlay technique (Fig. 15).

Total Overlay (Fig. 16)

In case of perforation with no remnant of TM—A new bony sulcus is made by drilling to support the graft at the lateral opening of tympanic cavity. The graft is placed over the anterior and posterior tympanic sulcus and medial

to the handle of malleus. Edges of graft are covered by meatal skin.

Grafting of Anteroinferior Perforation (Fig. 17)

Inferior tympanomeatal flap is elevated up to the edge of perforation (4'o clock). Epithelium covering the tip of malleus is elevated to the underlying bone but elevation of TM from lateral surface of malleus is carefully avoided. The graft is then placed—
- Over the anteroinferior tympanic sulcus
- Medial to the malleus
- Over the posterior tympanic sulcus.

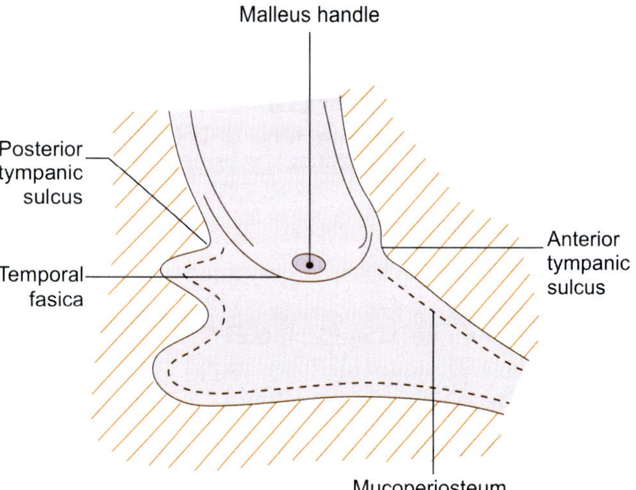

Fig. 16: Total overlay technique (after U Fisch 1994)

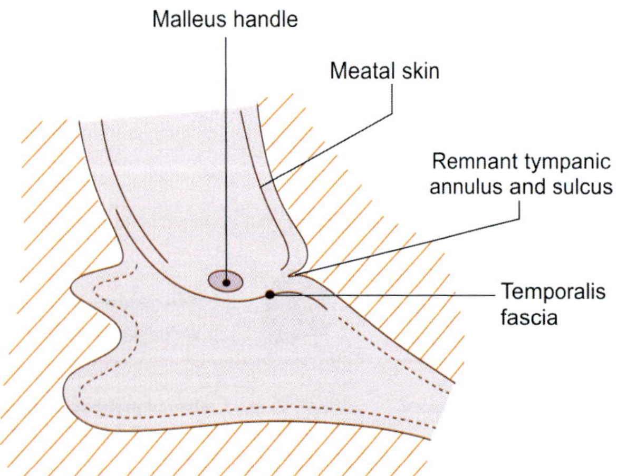

Fig. 15: Anterior underlay and posterior overlay technique (after U Fisch 1994)

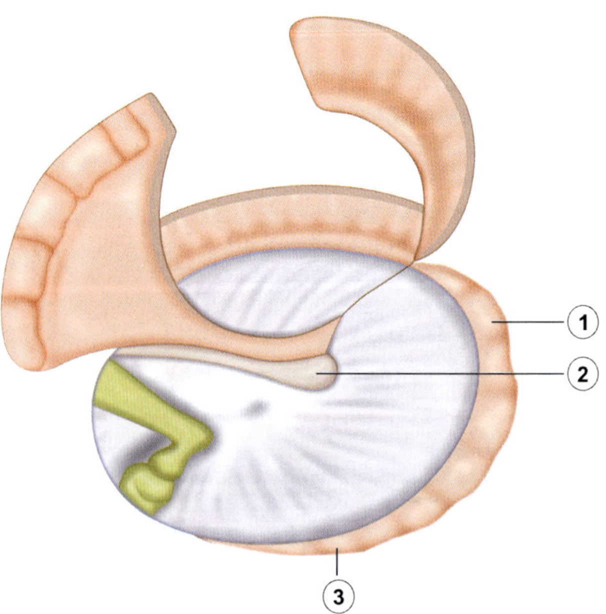

Fig. 17: Grafting of anteroinferior perforation[10]: (1) anteroinferior tympanic sulcus, (2) handle of mallelus, (3) posterior tympanic sulcus

Support of the intratympanic gelfoam is not needed as it may cause obstruction of Eustachian tube.

Grafting of Anterosuperior Perforation (Fig. 18)

Perforation of anterosuperior quadrant of pars tensa needs anterior support.

Gelfoam soaked in Ringer's solution is put in the tympanic cavity to support the graft against undersurface of remnant of TM. The posterior sulcus is extended to the oval window. Graft is then placed on—

- Inferior tympanic sulcus
- Medial to tip of handle of malleus
- On the posterior tympanic sulcus
- Anteriorly undersurface of tympanic membrane and surrounding bone.

Alternatively, tympanic annulus is detached from the sulcus from 1'o to 2'o clock for right side or 10'o to 11'o clock for left side and graft is pulled through window thus made between the annulus and sulcus (Fig. 19). The graft is then placed—

- On the inferior tympanic sulcus
- Medial to handle of malleus
- On the posterior tympanic sulcus
- Between anterosuperior tympanic annulus and sulcus.

OSSICULOPLASTY

Definition

Ossiculoplasty is a surgical procedure designed to repair the damaged ossicles of the middle ear with autograft/ homograft or nonbiological prosthesis to restore sound transmission from TM to inner ear.

Belluci's Classification of Tympanoplasty

This relates to the prognosis for obtaining an ear free of infection after surgery. Grouping is made accordingly to the following criteria:

- H/o of onset of ear infection
- Unilateral/bilateral
- Relationship between ear and nose infection
- Tests of Eustachian tube function
- Pathology of TM and middle ear mucosa
- Character of ear discharge and type of organism
- Radiology.

Group I: Good prognosis
- One episode of infection or trauma; no recurrence; dry ear.

Group II: Fair prognosis
- Recurrent AOM associated with URTI; alternating periods of quiescence with acute middle ear infection.

Group III: Poor prognosis
- Persistent discharge (COM); no periods of quiescence; mastoiditis.

Group IV: Very poor prognosis
- Chronic discharge (COM) associated with naso-pharyngeal malformation (cleft palate and chronic adhesion).

Cholesteatoma may be present in all four groups.

Illustrations of surgical steps of Type I tympanoplasty-underlay grafting are shown in Figures 20A to H.

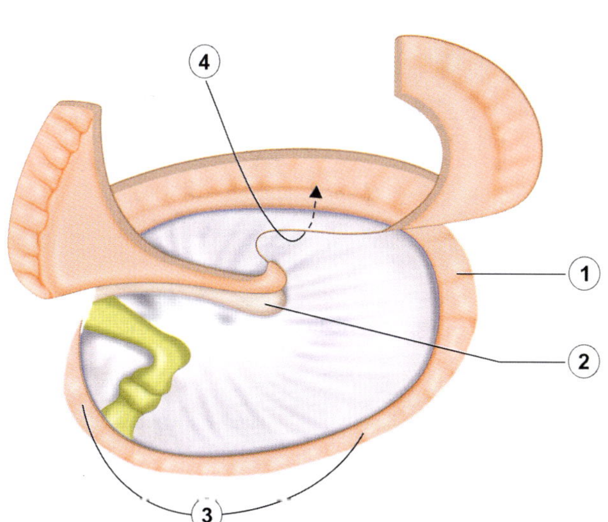

Fig. 18: Grafting of anterosuperior perforation: (1) inferior tympanic sulcus, (2) middle tympanic sulcus, (3) posterior tympanic sulcus, (4) anterior under surface of tympanic membrane and adjacent bone

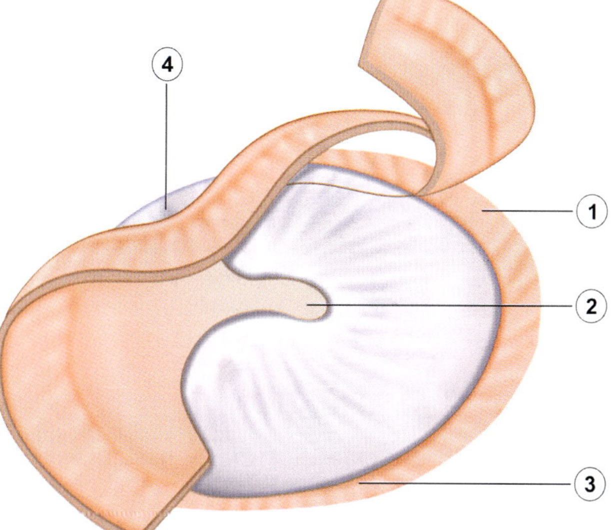

Fig. 19: Alternate technique of grafting for anterosuperior perforation: (1) inferior tympanic sulcus, (2) middle tympanic sulcus, (3) posterior tympanic sulcus, (4) anterior superior tympanic anulus and sulcus

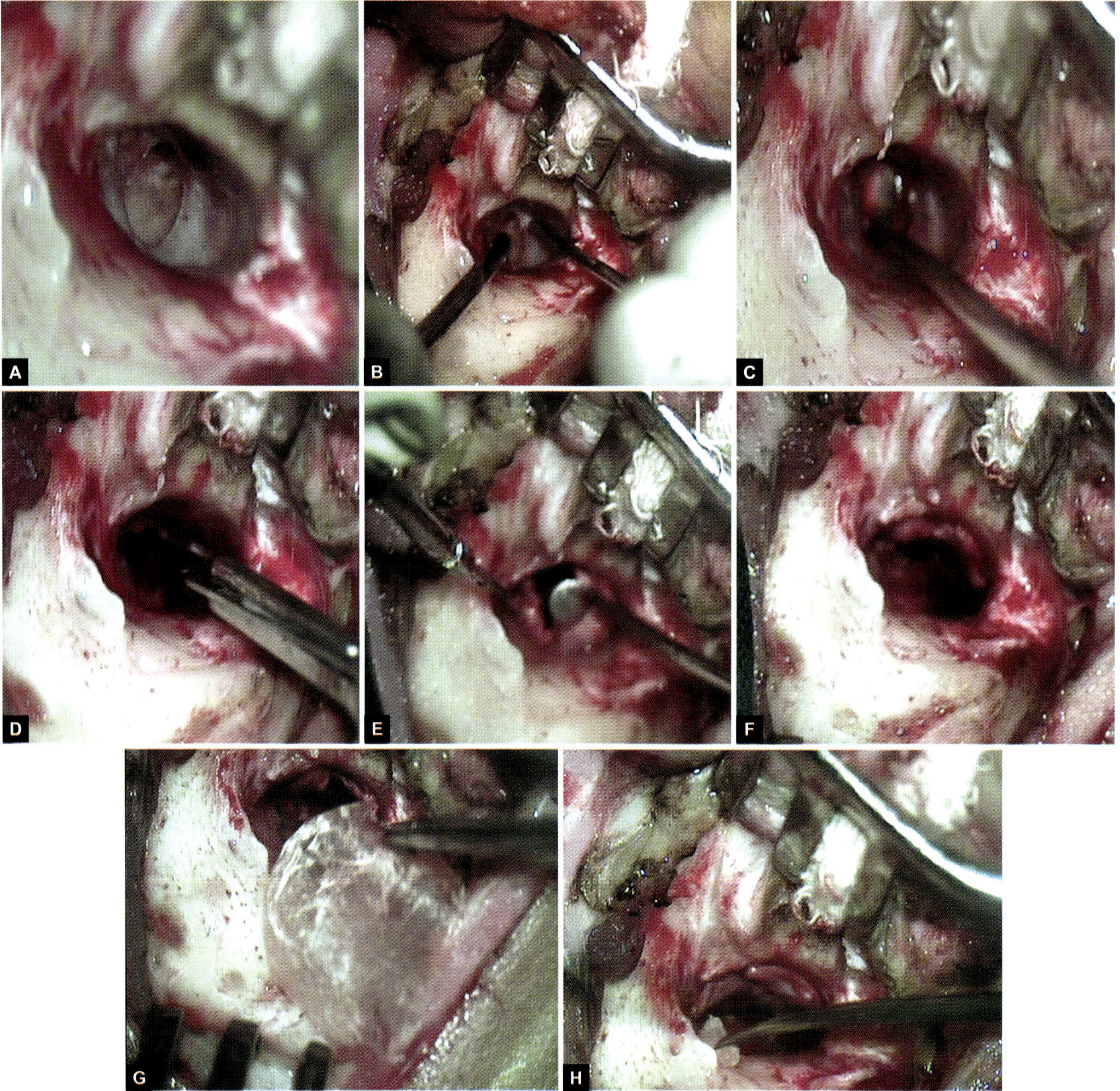

Figs 20A to H: Surgical steps of Type I Tympanoplasty—(A) Central perforation under microscope (postauricular approach); (B) Freshening of margin of perforation; (C) Desquamation of undersurface of remnant of TM; (D) Incision made at 12'0 clock position in EAC; (E) Elevation of TM flap; (F) TM flap is placed over the anterior wall; (G) Placement of temporal's facia graft (TFG); (H) Placement of gelfoam over the TFG

AUSTIN'S CLASSIFICATION[10]

This relates to the classification of ossicular chain defects. Incus is presumed to be absent in all cases. TM reconstruction is done in all cases (Table 1).

Group A—Requires reconstruction of tympanic membrane (ROTM) and reconstruction of ossicular chain from handle of malleus to stapes head.

Table 1: Austin's classification

		Malleus Handle	
		Present	Absent
Stapes superstructure	Present	M^+S^+	M^-S^+
		A	B
	Absent	C	D
		M+S-	M-S-

Abbreviations: M, Malleus; S, Stapes

Group B—Requires ROTM and malleus and incus.

Group C—Requires ROTM, ossicular chain from malleus handle to the stapes footplate.

Group D—Requires ROTM, malleus and stapes arch.

Kartush added three more classes as a modification to this scheme

- O – Intact ossicular chain
- E – Ossicular head fixation
- F – Stapes fixation

Middle ear risk index (MERI) is used to stratify patient groups and to predict the success rate of surgery. For accurate prediction of the results of ossiculoplasty, status of middle ear and its ossicles is to be ascertained (Table 2).

Reconstruction of ossicular chain is done by:

i. Autograft ossicular bone: This was first performed by Hall and Rytzner (1975). It involves two techniques—

- Interposition technique—Patient's own sculptured ossicles (incus) is used to serve continuity between malleus and stapes (Portman 1963/Sheehy 1965). Use of autogenous ossicular bone graft was not supported by Jankees (1957). Occult osteitis in the ossicles might cause failure of control of infection in CSOM as evidenced from histological confirmation of infection present in ossicles (Grippando 1958)[9,10]

- Transposition technique—Incus remnants and/or malleus are partially mobilized from the normal anatomical positions and placed onto the stapes head or footplate. When long process of incus is missing, the incus is removed and malleus attached to TM by umbo is transposed onto the stapes head, called tympanomalleostapediopexy by Bell (1958).[11]

ii. Allograft ossiculoplasty—Incus acquired from healthy middle ear is preserved in 70% ethyl alcohol and ossiculoplasty is performed as allograft incus interposition technique (House et al. 1966). Donor should be free from malignant disease, hepatitis, syphilis or CSOM. No difference in microscopic or histological appearance between autografts and allografts is found. Austin (1971) observed limited osteoblastic activity and/or mass absorptive erosion representing a rejection phenomenon in alcohol preserved incus allografts.

Hildyard (1967)[12] used cadaver acquired ossicular bone after autoclaving (autoclaved allogenic ossicular bone) as a TM-to-footplate interposition.

- Loose interposition technique—Also called TM to stapes head interposition or TM to footplate interposition may encounter problems, such as displacement of graft, lateral retraction of stapes head or footplate and fibrous and bony ankylosis between graft and posterior bony annulus, facial canal and promontory

- Stable ossicular interposition techniques—Malleus stapes assembly (MSA) or malleus footplate assembly (MFA) which is stable and produces better postoperative hearing gain than tympanic membrane to stapes head or tympanic membrane to footplate interposition (Figs 21A and B).

Table 2: Middle ear risk index	
Risk Factors	**Risk Value**
Ear discharge (Bellucci)	
Dry	0
Occasionally wet	1
Persistently wet	2
Wet, cleft palate	3
Perforation	
Absent	0
Present	1
Cholesteatoma	
Absent	0
Present	1
Ossicular status (Austin/Kartush)	
O M+I+S+	0
A M+S+	1
B M+S-	2
C M-S+	3
D M-S-	4
E Ossicular head fixed	2
F Stapes fixed	3
Middle ear granulation and effusion	
No	0
Yes	1
Previous surgery done	
None	0
Staged	1
Revision	2
Total	
MERI-0	: Normal
MERI-1 to 3	: Mild disease
MERI-4 to 6	: Moderate disease
MERI-7 to 12	: Severe disease

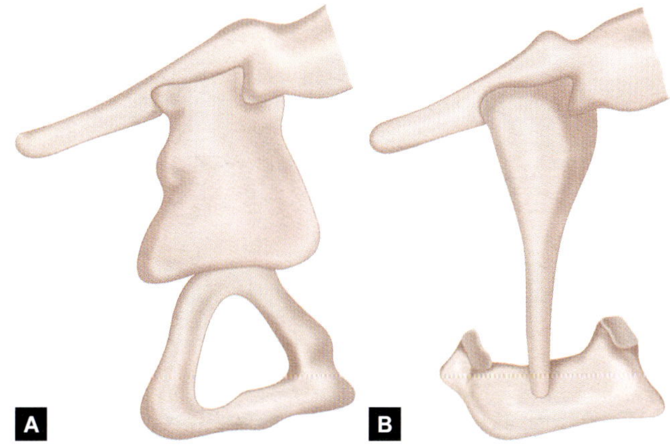

Figs 21A and B: (A) Malleus/stapes assembly (MSA); (B) Malleus/foot plate assembly (MFA)

For MSA, a notch is made into incus short process to accommodate malleus neck or handle and incus body is drilled to fit the stapes head.

For MFA, incus short process is drilled to fit the malleus neck or handle and long process is placed on the stapes footplate. This technique was described by Austin in 1971 (Fig. 22).

Functional results are comparable if the ossicles is placed horizontal position as it is placed in vertical position.

Incus interposition with autograft ossicle may be—

- Incus interposition with intact malleus (including malleus head)
- Incus interposition with handle only (malleus head removed)
- Retention or elimination of malleus head does not alter the functional result
- In both open and close cavity, presence of tensor tympani tendon prevents anterior migration of malleus handle and is essential for good functional result
- Interposed incus should tightly fit between stapes head and malleus handle
- Articulation to malleus is made in such a way that the incus body is higher than the malleus handle to provide stability of interposed incus and better contact with intersurface of TM.

Functional results of ossicular defects following ossiculoplasty—

- In presence of a mobile intact stapes, malleus handle and an intact anterior TM (Incus is missing) ossicular reconstruction provides a closure of air-bone gap to within 10 dB
- In presence of malleus and mobile footplate (incus and stapes superstructure absent) ossicular reconstruction results in a closure of air-bone gap within 20 dB.

In presence of mobile stapes, mobile footplate and fixed stapes with close cavity or open cavity average air-bone gap following ossiculoplasty is 30 dB.

iii. Tympanomeatal and tympano-ossicular allografts—Glasscock and Sheehy used alcohol preserved composite allograft with enbloc TM and ossicles for ear surgery in case of absent TM, malleus, incus with or without stapes superstructure. But result was very poor. Subsequently, Marquet preserved the cadaver acquired de-epithelialized TM to repair perforation and reported successful myringoplasty.

iv. Autologous and allogenic cortical bone grafts—Autologous cortical bone grafts are obtained from mastoid cortex, external auditory meatus and spine of Henle and used it in TM to stapes head, TM to footplate interposition, malleus to stapes and malleus to footplate assemblies. Hearing gains are same for ossicular and cortical bone graft in TM to stapes head interposition and malleus to stapes assembly. Autogenic cortical bone graft has limited use in tympanoplasty.

v. Autologous and allogenic cartilage grafts—Autologous cartilage graft is usually obtained from tragal cartilage and conchal cartilage. Allogenic cartilage graft is obtained from nasal septal cartilage. It is used for TM to stapes head interposition (short columella) and TM to footplate interposition (long columella).

Disadvantage includes—Creeping resorption of cartilage columella.

For satisfactory hearing, gain materials used for ossiculoplasty must have certain physical and structural characteristics—

- Reconstructive ossicular chain should be rigid enough to transmit high frequencies
- Materials should not be too firm to sublaxate in the vestibule when subjected to inward pressure
- Ossicle or prosthesis used should be at right angle to the stapes footplate
- A wide surface area should be presented at fascial graft-prosthesis interface
- Material should have good dampening properties to avoid unwanted vibration transmitted to footplate.

Tragal cartilage with perichondrium on both sides satisfying these characteristics is commonly used. Perichondrium retained on both sides of tragal cartilage prevents late resorption.

Cartilage techniques used in ossiculoplasty[7] are—

- If the malleus is present, a Y-shaped cartilage is preferred to be placed between malleus to footplate (Fig. 23)

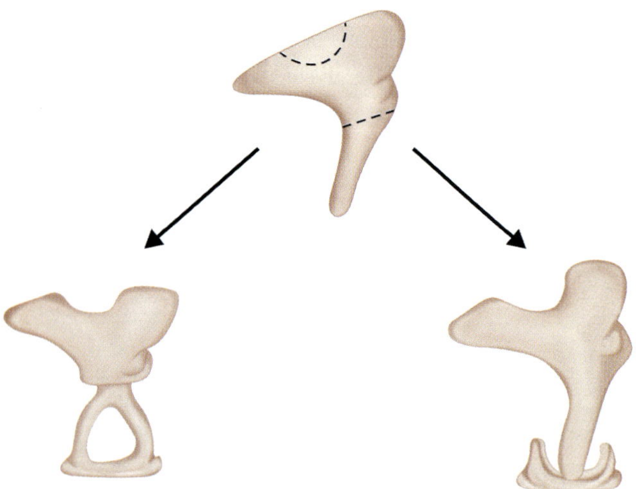

Fig. 22: Notched incus with short process to fit between malleus neck and stapes head, notched incus with long process to fit between malleus neck and stapes footplate (after Wahrs)

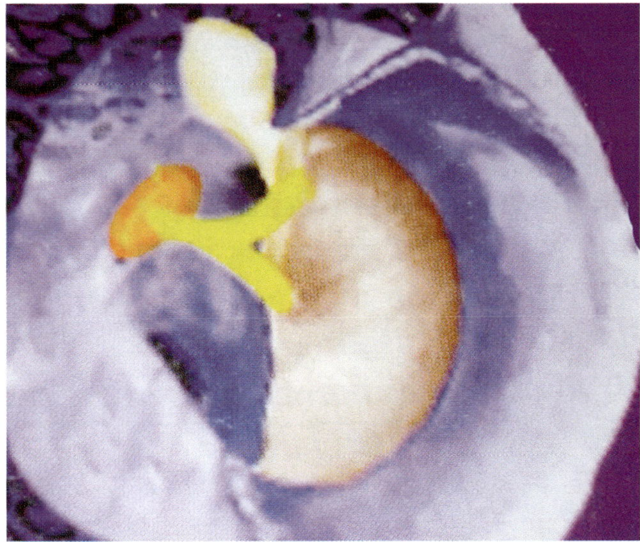

Fig. 23: Y-shaped cartilage tympanoplasty

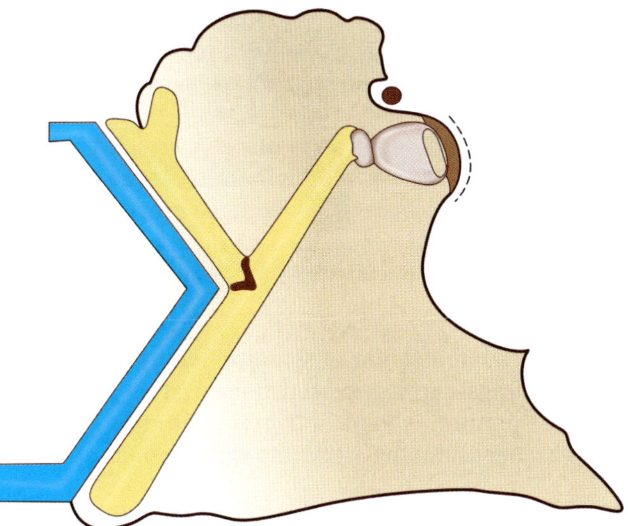

Fig. 24: Two cartilage technique

- If the malleus is absent, the two cartilage technique is used to reconstruct the ossicular chain for better stabilization and single stage procedure (Fig. 24).

The first cartilage extends from a notch made in the inferior annulus to stapes head or to the footplate. The second cartilage is placed in the superior annulus to a notch made in the first cartilage for pressure contact.

Advantages of cartilage ossiculoplasty—

- Chances of extrusion are minimal unlike allopastic materials [partial ossicular replacement prosthesis (PORP) or total ossicular replacement prosthesis (TORP)] which are foreign body and may extrude
- Ankylosis with raw area does not happen as is seen with autograft ossicles or PORP/TORP
- Footplate sublaxation into oval window resulting in SNHL never occurs as cartilage is elastic and not a solid connection like TORP/PORP
- Hearing gain is maintained in long-term as less chances of loss of contact with drum or footplate if drum is retracted outwards.

vi. Glues and adhesives—Marquet and Portman (1982) have used Fibrin glue or Tissucol. It forms a stable adhesive by combining human fibrinogen, Factor XIII and aprotinin with thrombin and calcium chloride. It is used in stabilizing ossicular bone assemblies without inducing an inflammatory response in middle ear.

Biomaterial[13] used as grafts in tympanoplasty—

- Metallic—Stainless steel, gold, platinum and titanium
- Nonmetallic plastics (solid)—polyethylene, Teflon, silastic
- Plastics (porous)—proplast$_1$, proplast$_2$, plastipore (high density polyethylene) and polycele (ultra high mol. wt. polyethylene)

- Ceramics-bioinert (aluminium oxide ceramics), bioactive (calcium silicate glass ceramics) and biodegradable (hydroxyaptite-tricalcium phosphate ceramics)

Spandrel II and Fisch Titanium Total (FTT) Prosthesis[14]

The Spandrel prosthesis is now used with good results in ossicular reconstruction. It has derived from the idea of Shea's total ossicular replacement prosthesis (TORP).

In spandrel prosthesis, diameter is reduced to 0.6 mm and head of the prosthesis is shaped into L- form. A stainless –steel wire is introduced in the shaft for increase its stability and in the head for improved sound transmission. A shoe is also attached to the stem for better holding of the prosthesis over stapes footplate. This design of prosthesis is called spandrel I. The term spandrel means shape of a triangular space lying beneath the string of a stair. Spandrel I is now modified to Spandrel II (Fig. 25) which also consists of head with shaft and shoe; metal plat form is moved to the centre of the head, wire core is 0.12 mm in diameter and thickness of head is reduced to 0.1 mm. Polycel casing of head and shaft stablilizes the sound transmitting wire core. The shoe of the prosthesis is perforated (0.3 mm) to allow entry of the wire core to protrude a fraction of millimeter (0.5) beyond its base to act as an anchoring spike that keeps the prosthesis firmly in position at the oval window (Fig. 26).

Length of the spandrel is determined by the distance between the TM and stapes footplate with a malleable measuring rod. The prosthesis is placed on the stapes footplate in two ways—

- By placing the foot without spike in stapes footplate or
- By fixing the foot with spike through a small fenestrum (0.2 mm) made on the stapes footplate depending on the patient's acceptance of associated risk.

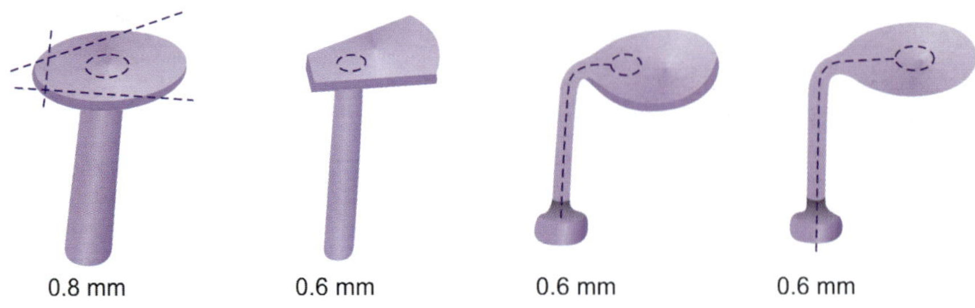

Fig. 25: Spandrel II

Further stabilization of spandrel foot is done by few pieces of tragal cartilage placed in the oval window niche.

The spandrel is kept in contact with the handle of malleus. Repositioning of TM flap is then done.

Fisch Titanium Total (FTT) Prosthesis (Fig. 27)

Like the Spandrel II FTT comprises
- Head with shaft
- Shoe with spike

Head diameter = 5 mm
Head thickness = 0.1 mm
Shaft diameter = 0.6 mm
Length of shaft = 10 mm
Shoe or foot diameter = 1.0 mm
Length of the shoe = 1.5 mm

Perforation in shoe is up to 1.0 mm with diameter of 0.6 mm

Through perforation shaft is introduced 1.0 mm into the shoe.

Spike length = 0.3 mm
Spike diameter = 0.1 mm

Total length of the assembled FTT is 0.5 mm longer than shaft. Prosthesis stem may be cut to the desire length. Prosthesis head may be trimmed to the desire size and shape. Each ring of prosthesis head = 1 mm. Therefore, removal of both rings may reduce head diameter by 2 mm. Functional result does not alter with different prosthesis diameters indicating fixation of the prosthesis is more beneficial than the size of the prosthesis (Fig. 28).

Fixation of FTT onto the stapes footplate is obtained by—
- Inserting the spike of prosthesis shoe into the perforated stapes footplate. Perforation is made by using Erbium YAG laser or coupling the shaft without shoe on the center of the footplate with a cartilage disk.

Once the shoe is placed on the stapes footplate, prosthesis head is placed under the center of the TM by rotating the head of prosthesis with a hook (1.5 mm, 45°), placed in one of the multiple holes of the prosthesis head and another hook (2.5 mm, 45°) holding in the left hand kept under intact portion of TM. Then TM flap is repositioned.

The Spandrel II provides closure of air-bone gap of about 25 dB and it helps specially the patient with bilateral hearing loss. It yields better hearing gain than type III tympanoplasty.

The FTT prosthesis is preferred over the spandrel II prosthesis for ossicular reconstruction as it has good sound transmission properties and titanium is superior biocompatible alloplast.

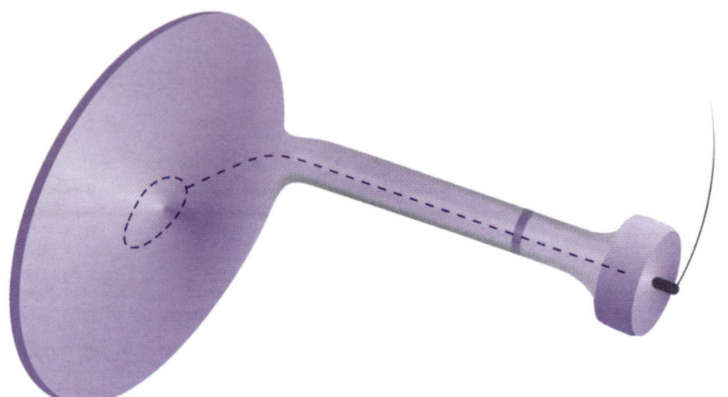

Fig. 26: Spandrel with spike

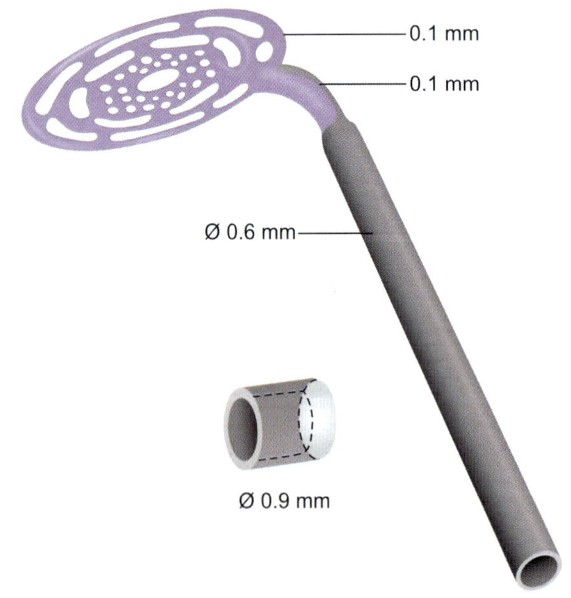

Fig. 27: Fisch titanium total prosthesis with shoe

MASTOID SURGERY

Middle ear infection when extends to the mastoid and does not resolve with appropriate antibiotics requires surgery involving mastoid. Mastoidectomy is the surgical procedure done to remove mastoid air cells.

Indications are—

- Mastoiditis
- COM with subtotal or total perforation
- COM with posterior marginal perforation with retraction of remnant of TM
- COM with cholesteatoma.

Mastoidectomy is also performed as a part of other procedure, such as cochlear implant/access to middle ear and facial nerve/access to internal acoustic meatus.

Types of Mastoidectomy

Cortical or Simple Mastoidectomy (Schwartze Procedure)

The principle of the procedure involves the removal of mastoid cells without affecting the middle ear as well as identifying of the aditus ad antrum.

Indications

- Acute mastoiditis
  - When the signs and symptoms have not been adequately controlled by an adequate course of an appropriate antibiotics (>48 hours)
  - When patient presents with following complications, such as intracranial complications, subperiosteal/subcutaneous abscess in the postauricular region, Bezold's or citelli's abscess in the neck and Labyrinthitis.
- Secretory otitis media and idiopathic hemotympanum
  - When this is persistant and accompanied by marked hearing loss which continues to recur despite frequent insertion of grommets.
- Tubercular mastoiditis
- Acute viral mastoiditis with vertigo and SNHL requiring mastoidectomy with atticotomy and posterior tympanotomy to achieve drainage of the round and oval window niche to avoid inner ear injury
- Decompression of facial nerve
- Endolymphatic shunt insertion and ultrasonic Labyrinthectomy in Meniere's disease.

Surgical Procedure

Surgical procedure is performed through postauricular approach under local anesthesia or general anesthesia in case of children or apprehensive patients.

- Mastoid antrum is entered through MacEwen's triangle. Disease polypoid mucosa along with diseased ear cells

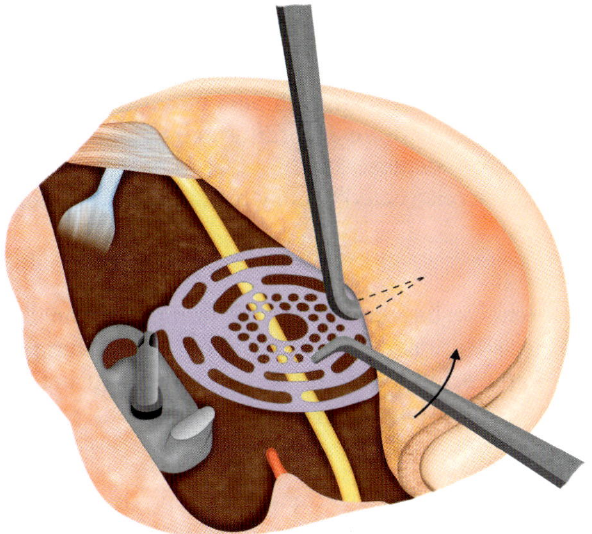

Fig. 28: Fisch titanium total head is rotated under temporal fascia

are removed superiorly up to middle fossa dural plate, posteriorly to the level of sinus plate, inferiorly to the tip cells and anteriorly to the zygomatic cells until the appearance of normal looking cells. Aditus ad antrum if blocked due to thickened mucosa is removed and airway patency is established.

Intact Canal Wall or Closed Cavity Tympanomastoidectomy

The principle of this procedure is the removal of cholesteatoma matrix from attic, antrum and middle ear with preservation of posterior wall of EAC. Combined transcanal and transmastoid approach helps to remove cholesteatoma from tympanic cavity and mastoid on both sides of preserved bony canal. Choice of close method is taken if Eustachian tube is functioning, good pneumatization of tympanomastoid cleft, and limited extent of cholesteatoma (Fig. 29).

Procedure involved following steps—A simple mastoidectomy with removal of polypoid mucosa, disease mastoid air cell and cholesteatoma with sac from the antrum.

Tympanomeatal flap is elevated. Extent of cholesteatoma in middle ear is assessed. Transcanal atticotomy and canalplasty to widen the bony canal are performed. Particular attention is given to work in the attic.

Complete clearance of cholesteatoma and granulation tissue from attic, antrum and middle ear including facial recess with removal of the diseased ossicles is performed.

Cholesteatoma in sinus tympani and Eustachian tube area is difficult to remove because of limited visibility of these areas.

Posterior tympanotomy or facial recess approach is taken for better clearance of disease which is discussed later. Reconstruction of lateral attic wall is performed with a concheal cartilage with perichondrium. Ossicular reconstruction is done according to ossicular defect as described in ossiculoplasty.

TM is reconstructed usually by autologus temporalis fascia graft.

Advantages

- The ear can be reconstructed at normal position
- No cavity problem during swimming and bathing
- Better hearing gain compared to open cavity method
- Fitting a hearing aid is easier if required.

Disadvantages

- Higher reccurence rate compared to open method (36%)
- Excessive thinning of posterosuperior wall may result in bone resorption and posterosuperior retraction pocket
- Posterior tympanotomy may result in retraction pocket when cavity is large[15]
- Patient will return for regular follow-up since second look operation is frequently necessary within 6–18 months of primary operation.

Contraindication

Intact canal wall or close cavity procedure is contraindicated in presence of only hearing ear.

- Labyrinthine fistula
- Extention of cholesteatoma into inaccessible area
- Cholesteatoma destroyed 1/3rd of posterior canal wall. Due to disappointing recurrences shift of opinion in recent ear has occurred towards canal wall down procedure.

Posterior Tympanotomy (Approach Through the Facial Recess) (Fig. 30)

It basically combines a complete simple mastoidectomy and tympanoplasty with preservation of the posterior wall of the EAC. The middle ear is exposed through the lateral tympanic or facial recess. It is an intact canal wall procedure. Opening the facial recess from behind through a triangular area of bone is called antrum threshold angle (Fig. 31) which is bounded by facial nerve medially, the chorda tympani nerve laterally and the fossa incudis superiorly. Through the posterior tympanotomy, the structures visualized are—

- Stapedius tendon exiting the pyramidal process
- Long process of incus
- Incudostapedial joint
- Stapes superstructures
- Round window niche
- Promontory
- Horizontal segment of facial nerve coursing anteriorly superior to stapes
- Chochleariform process—anchoring the tensor tympani medially as it courses towards the neck of the malleus.

Eustachian tube opening in the middle ear can be visualized through the facial recess medial to the neck of malleus.

Indications for posterior tympanotomy

- Patient with cholesteatoma involving the mastoid, attic and upper portion of middle ear. There should not be evidence of cholesteatoma extending into the hypotympanum
- Middle ear should have good aeration/Eustachian tube function

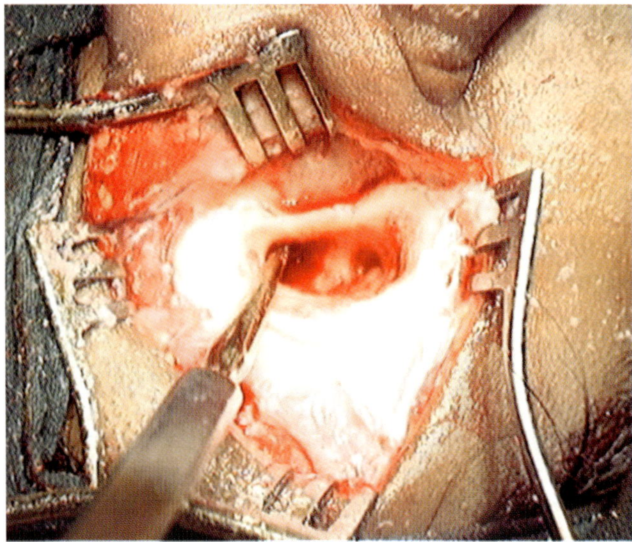

Fig. 29: Intact canal wall or closed cavity tympanomastoidectomy

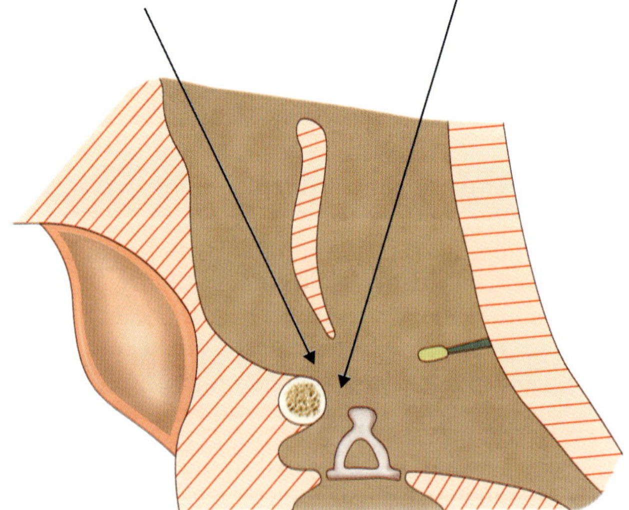

Fig. 30: Combined approach of transcanal and transmastoid technique with posterior tympanotomy

- Mastoid is well pneumatized with pneumatization extending into the root of zygoma
- Pure tone audiometry shows good bone conduction thresholds.

Contraindication

- Only hearing ear
- Labyrinthine fistula
- Poor Eustachian tube function.

Canal Wall Down or Open Method

The principle of this procedure includes complete mastoidectomy and removal of postosuperior canal wall at the level of facial canal. The tympanic membrane is left in place or tympanic membrane is reconstructed with or without ossiculoplasty to separate mucosal-lined middle ear space from mastoid cavity and ear canal (modified radical mastoidectomy). The aims of this surgical technique are—

- Radical exenteration of tympanomastoid cell tract
- Adequate exteriorization of both mastoid and epitympanum (attic).

For adequate exteriorization open cavity is shaped as an inverted truncated cone with the lateral diameter twice the size of the medial diameter so that lateral removal of bone reduces the volume of the open cavity (Fig. 32).[16]

This procedure is indicated in—

- Invasive cholesteatoma involving mastoid, epitympanum and middle ear
- Discharging mastoid cavity following previous surgery
- Recurrent and residual disease following close cavity tympanomastoidectomy
- Scelerotic mastoid with extensive disease
- Anteriorly placed lateral sinus with low lying dura.

Open cavity with tympanoplasty procedure involves following steps:

- Wide removal of bone is done over the root of zygoma with skeletonization of middle fossa dura, sinodural angle, sigmoid sinus, digastric ridge and stylomastoid foramen
- Removal of posterior bony wall and bridge over the aditus
- Identification of tympanic and mastoid segments of facial canal and lowering of the inferior buttress and facial ridge. Lowering of facial ridge is done with diamond burrs. Constant suction irrigation during surgery is important to maintain clear operating field by washing away bone dust and blood and to avoid thermal injury of underlying facial nerve.

The level of mastoid segment of facial canal is assessed by a line drawn from tympanic segment of facial nerve to the stylomastoid foramen.

- The inferior edge of posterior semicircular canal (PSCC)
- Pyramidal segment of facial nerve lies 2 mm anterolateral to the inferior edge of PSCC.

- Posterior buttress is left higher if disease is absent to preserve a mesotympanic space
- Anterior buttress of the canal bridge is preserved to maintain mesotympanic space anteriorly. Extended canalplasty is performed by
  - Removal of anterior buttress to the level of attic
  - Removal of bone over the root of zygomatic cell tract
  - Lowering inferior tympanic ring to the level of stylomastoid foramen.

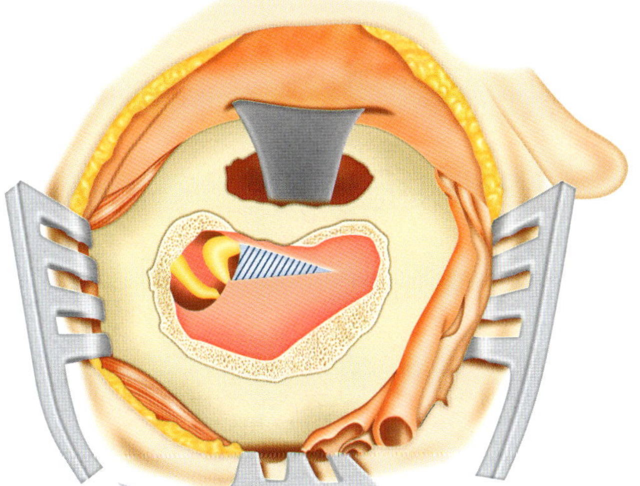

Fig. 31: Antrum threshold angle

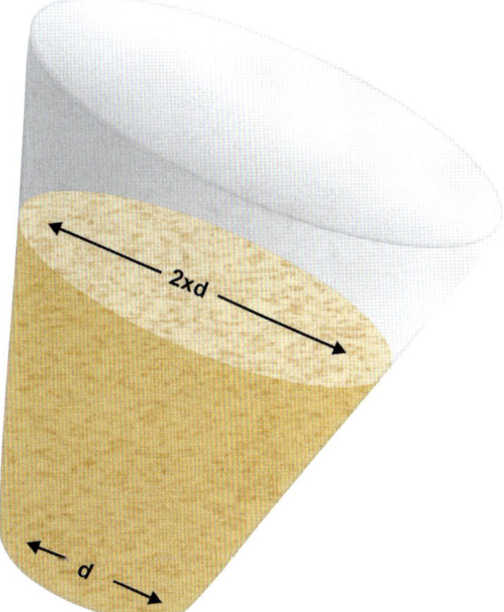

Fig. 32: Open cavity showing reduction in volume by lateral removal of bone

Facial bridge—It is a bony bridge that connects the posterior bony canal with the anterior bony canal at anterior buttress and overlies the ossicles and tympanic segment of facial canal.

Anterior buttress—It is the bony buttress where the superior bony canal meets the tegmen.

Posterior buttress—It is the bone where the posterior canal wall meets the floor of EAC lateral to the mastoid segment of facial canal.[17]

- Removal of cholesteatoma from oval window and round window—Cholesteatoma matrix is removed at the anterior edge of the footplate with fisch footplate elevator. Oval window is covered with a piece of pressed tragal perichondrium. Cholesteatoma matrix is removed completely from the round window without rupture of round window membrane with a diamond drill
- Anteroinferior canalplasty is done followed by formation of tympanic sulcus (Fig. 33)
- The ossicular reconstruction is performed according to the ossicular deficit
- The mastoid tip is removed before grafting
- Temporalis fascia graft is placed by underlay technique. If the disease mucosa is removed from promontory silastic sheeting should be used to prevent the graft from adhering to the raw areas of bone with thin silastic (0.005 inch) or thick silastic (0.01 inch). The piece of silastic sheet should be shaped so as to extend into the Eustachian tube orifice as well as to cover the bony promontory up to the round window. The silastic sheet is used only when second stage surgery is planned. In one stage surgery gelfilm is used

- Gelfoam pieces soaked in antibiotic ear drop are put to keep the temporalis fascia graft and meatal skin in place
- A wide conchomeatoplasty (Fisch) is performed by making superior and inferior meatal flaps from conchomeatal skin flap with removal of adequate amount of conchal cartilage and the suturing the meatal flaps and conchal skin (Fig. 34)
- Widened meatus and exteriorized cavity is packed with 1.25 cm width ribbon gauge smeared with antibiotic ointment to keep the meatal skin in contact with bony cavity
- Postauricular incision is closed by interrupted suture with 3.0 silk.

Bondy's Modified Radical Mastoidectomy

Gustave Bondy (1910) developed the technique of modification of radical mastoid surgery for COM with attic cholesteatoma in patient having chronic ear discharge and pars flaccida perforation with intact pars tensa and normal hearing.

Technique

It is a canal wall down procedure which is performed like MRM without disturbing intact pars tensa, tympanic cavity and ossicles. A potential candidate for Bondy's MRM having following desirable features are as follows:

- Good hearing
- A small scelerotic mastoid
- Good Eustachian tube function
- Intact tympanic membrane except pars flaccida perforation and cholesteatoma matrix limited lateral to the ossicular chain
- Aerated middle ear space.

Procedure

- Posterior canal is lowered to the posterior annulus and vertical facial nerve level

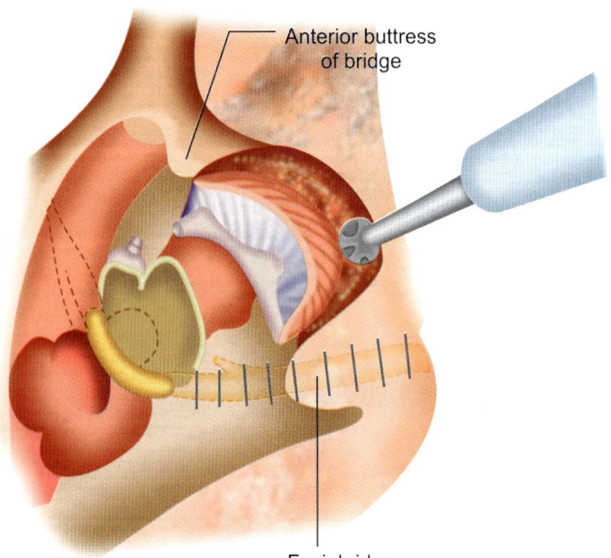

Fig. 33: Extended canalplasty

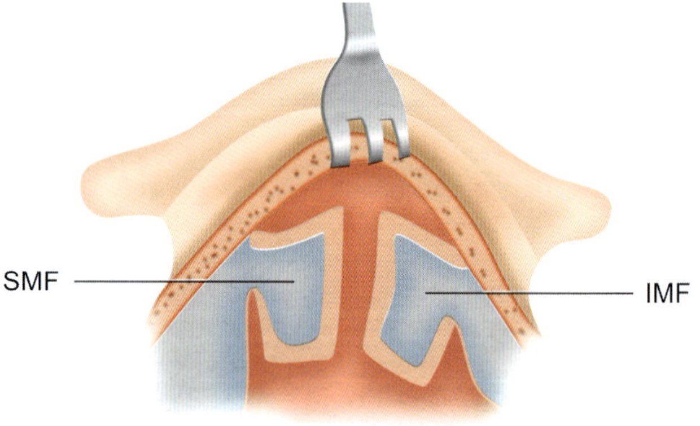

Fig. 34: Wide conchomeatoplasty is performed by making SMF and IMF from conchomeatal skin

Abbreviations: SMF, superior meatal flap; IMF, inferior meatal flap

- Floor of mastoid cavity and EAC are same level for dependent drainage
- Scutum is removed and any cholesteatoma in attic is exteriorized. Cholesteatoma is then marsupialized and enucleated
- Cholesteatoma matrix in the mastoid is removed
- Cholesteatoma matrix is preserved over the ossicular chain and labyrinth if a fistula is suspected
- Once the ear is healed, the cholesteatoma matrix will resemble normal squamous epithelium
- Aims of the surgery are—safe and dry ear without disturbing hearing mechanism.

Radical Mastoidectomy (Open Cavity without Tympanoplasty)

The principle of the procedure is (Figs 36A to N)—
- The eradication of cholesteatoma or chronic granulation from middle ear and mastoid
- Creation or conversion of antrum, mastoid air cells, aditus, attic and middle ear into one cavity
- Exteriorization of cavity to the external auditory meatus
- Removal of remnants of TM, malleus and incus except stapes and obliteration of Eustachian tube to reduce the risk of chronic otorrhea
- No tympanoplasty is performed.

A graft can be placed in the middle ear to reduce mucosalization. A classic radical mastoidectomy includes removal of posterosuperior bony canal wall at the level of facial ridge with eradication of disease from tympanic mastoid region.

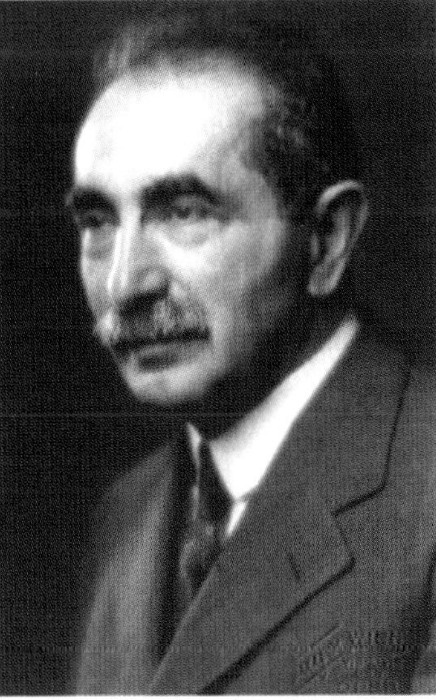

Fig. 35: Gustave Bondy (1870-1954) popularized for the modified radical mastoidectomy with preservation of middle ear structure

Exteriorization of the middle ear and mastoid cavity with wide meatoplasty is performed. Tympanic membrane and ossicles are not reconstructed.

Indications

- Unresectable cholesteatoma extending into the Eustachian tube
- Cochlear fistula over promontory due to cholesteatoma
- Chronic perilabyrinthine osteitis/cholesteatoma
- Malignancy of middle ear
- Destruction of entire middle ear mucosa with severe SNHL or dead ear
- Cholesteatoma that cannot be removed and must be cleaned and inspected periodically
- As a definite revision of operation to eliminate chronic infection resulting from incomplete previous surgeries
- COM (squamosal) with intracranial complication where reconstruction is not advisable.

Basic Steps of Operation

- Complete mastoidectomy is performed by postaural route (outside in). Inside out approach may also be used
- All the ossicles and mucous membrane from middle ear space except stapes superstructures and mucosa around the oval window are removed
- Facial nerve is delineated on its lateral/anterior surfaces
- Eustachian tube is obliterated using bone dust, fat or cartilage
- Tensor tympani tendon is severed and muscle extracted after fracturing the bony process away from the facial canal
- Completed radical mastoidectomy converts the middle ear, hypotympanum, epitympanum and mastoid into one large cavity
- Healing occurs by in growth of skin from the ear canal and the concha
- A large external auditory meatus may be created by removal of an elliptical segment of concheal cartilage
- If disease removal is completed temporalis fascia grafting is placed to the middle ear and the mastoid cavity for quick healing of the cavity
- If entire disease clearance is not possible then cavity is kept uncovered.

Disadvantage

Recurrent infection of the middle ear space through the perforated tympanic membrane needs closure of perforation by tympanoplasty.

Contraindications for Open Cavity Procedure

- Benign type of chronic mucoid otorrhea with central perforation without cholesteatoma

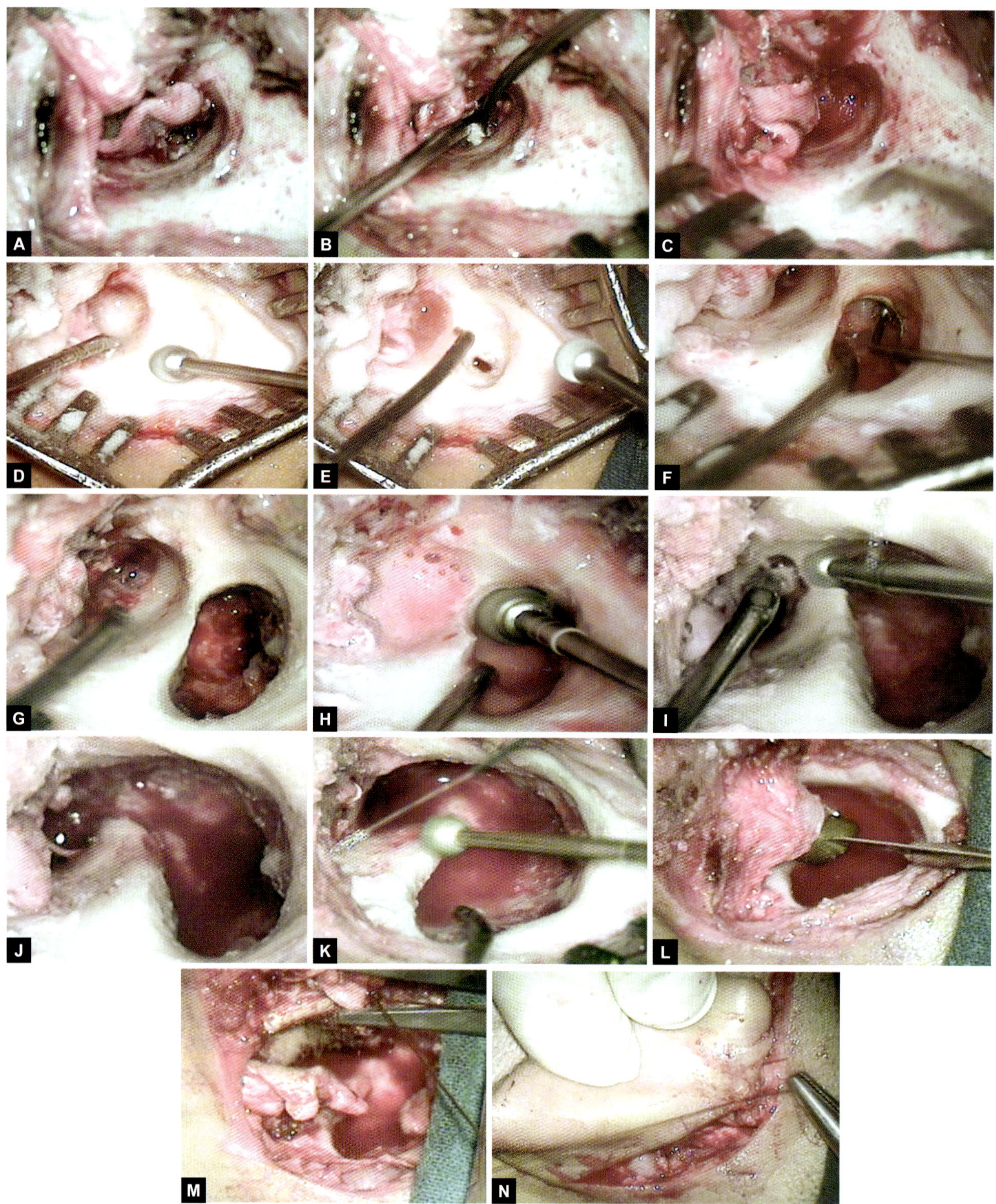

Figs 36A to N: Tympanomastoid surgery in active squamosal disease/radical mastoidectomy in COM with cholesteatoma. (A) Elevation of TM flap; (B) Cholesteatoma in mesotympanum; (C) Mesotympanum following removal of cholesteatoma; (D) Entering antrum through MacEwen's triangle; (E) Antrum is entered; (F) Widening of the antrum; (G) Both mesotympanum and mastoid cavity are seen; (H) Removal of the bridge 1; (I) Removal of the bridge 2; (J) Removal of the bridge 3; (K) Lowering of ridge; (L) Incision for wide conchomeatoplasty; (M) Conchomeatoplasty is on progress; (N) Closure of postauricular incision

- Acute otitis media with coalescent mastoiditis
- Persistent secretory otitis media
- Chronic allergic otitis media
- Tubercular otitis media.

Age is not a contraindication for this operation since it can be done quite well under local anesthesia.

Key Consideration

Successful and safe mastoid surgery requires routine identification of key anatomic structures in addition to tagmen, sigmoid sinus and facial nerve.

Inside Out Technique (Fig. 37)

- Opening of the cavity from front to back. It means first attic then aditus and finally antrum following the course taken by cholesteatoma
- It is usually helpful for limited attic cholesteatoma or postero superior cholesteatoma. All the diseased areas are widely opened and cleared away following removal of diseased cells and their mucosa in toto
- Facial ridge is lowered to make a hemispherical cavity for aeration and supervision
- With time cavity will be healed by newly formed squamous epithelium. Aim of surgery is to make a cavity which is well aerated to remain biological stable. It follows the principle Va/S ratio where Va = volume of air circulating from outside, S = surface area of the cavity essential for aeration
- Ideally, the ratio Va/S is 1. If S is large then Va should be large for correctly furnished mastoidectomy
- In open cavity Va can be increased by wide meatoplasty and lowering of the facial ridge and S can be decreased by obliteration of the cavity with muscleplasty.[18]

Advantages of this Procedure

- Small cavity—The size depending upon the extent of cholesteatoma
- The approach is rational as the disease is followed according to course of cholesteatoma.

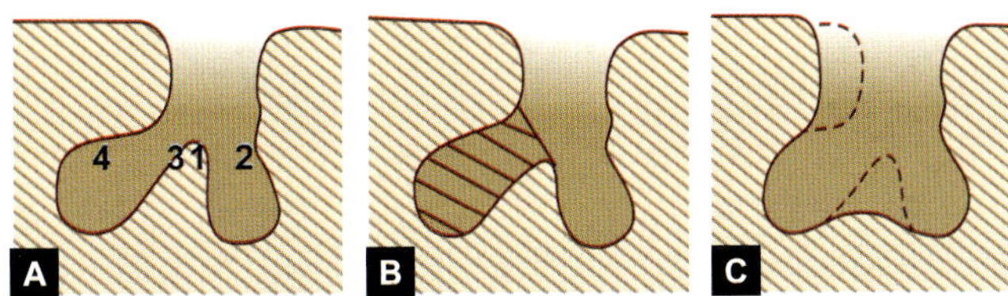

Figs 37A to C: (A) Incorrectly finished mastoid cavity where V/s ratio is very small. (1) EAC (2) Middle ear cavity (3) Facial ridge (4) Mastoid cavity; (B) Same Mastoid cavity after obliteration reducing surface area of the cavity; (C) Same Mastoid cavity after revision surgery. Meatoplasty and removal of facial ridge are performed to increase V for ventilation

Flexible Otologic Surgery[19]

The flexible technique provides a conservative sequential method of eradication of disease that is individualized to the patient's needs. Pathogenesis of chronic otitis media is influenced by pathological and anatomical obstructive sites along middle ear cleft—pathological obstructions, such as tympanosclerosis, granulation tissue and or cholesteatoma or anatomical obstruction along Eustachian tube, middle ear and mastoid may lead to generalized or localized pathologic conditions. Thus, a procedure is required that allows enough flexibility to expose and eradicate the diseases as it is followed through various anatomic location within the air. Various sites of obstruction are—

- Soft Eustachian tube
- Hard Eustachian tube (protympanum)
- Mesotympanum
- Attic
- Additus and antrum
- Mastoid air cell systems.

Obstruction of Eustachian tube may cause generalized pathologic condition in the middle ear and the mastoid.

Obstruction of aditus and antrum may result in localized pathologic condition of the mastoid.

Selective obstruction of mastoid air cell may lead to localized pathologic condition in mastoid region, such as cholesterol granuloma.

Main steps involved in flexible approach are—

- Incision—Endaural standard lempert I, II and rarely III (carried inferiorly to expose mastoid tip) are used.
  A Körner flap (skin flap from posterior canal connected to concha) can be fashioned
- Canalplasty—A posterior flap is elevated. Osseous canal is exposed from annulus laterally. Canal is drilled lateral to annulus so as to allow better exposure of the annulus and associated mesotympanum. A laterally based anterior flap is elevated and anterior canal is drilled to expose anterior aspect of mesotympanum
- Exploratory tympanoplasty—Middle ear is entered posteriorly after elevating the fibrous annulus. Width and depth of middle ear space is increased by cutting tensor tympani and lateralizing malleus. Site of possible obstruction are cleared of the disease. Silastic sheet is routinely placed over the promontory between the Eustachian tube and round window niche. Ventilation tube is then inserted
- Atticotomy—Posterosuperior part of bony canal is removed for better exposure of the ossicles or to follow the disease of mesotympanum extending backward to the mastoid via aditus adantrum
- Mastoidotomy—Mastoidotomy is done:
  - Where mastoid pathology is unsure otherwise surgeon proceeds directly to mastoidectomy

– Where good pneumatisation of mastoid is identified
– Better understanding of pathology in antrum and check the patency of aditus ad antrum.

Mastoidectomy and tympanoplasty:

- Close cavity tympanomastoidectomy is done in patient with pneumatic mastoid
- Open cavity or intact bridge mastoidectomy is done in diploic or sclerotic mastoid associated with COM
- Tympanic membrane repair and ossicular reconstruction may be done.

Therefore, it is the stepwise surgical procedure and flexible approach for surgeon to allow the sequential steps of surgery according to individual patient's need for providing satisfactory functional outcome.

Surgical steps of cartilage tympanoplasty are shown in Figures 38A to F.

Mastoid Cavity Obliteration

Open cavity technique for treating COM with cholesteatoma results in formation of a mastoid cavity which is not always free from any problems. Large mastoid cavity following mastoidectomy may results in following problems:

- Chronic discharge from the cavity
- Dizziness due to direct caloric stimulation of exposed semicircular canal by air/water entering the cavity
- Regular supervision for cleaning the cavity
- Difficulty in using the hearing aid.

The idea of mastoid obliteration was first introduced by Mosher (1911)[20] who used superiorly based postauricular soft tissue flap for cavity obliteration. The mastoid obliteration may be performed as a primary procedure in the same sitting as canal wall down mastoidectomy or open technique but it may be done as a secondary revision procedure. Leaving smaller surface for epithelization helps to promote healing of the cavity and reduces the above problems.

Indications for the Mastoid Obliteration

- Dead ear (no auditory function)
- Severe mental retardation preventing postoperative care of the cavity
- Dural hernia with or without CSF leak
- Temporal bone resection for malignancy.

Contraindication for Cavity Obliteration

- Possibility of residual cholesteatoma
- Presence of osteonecrosis
- Metabolic disorder like diabetes mellitus

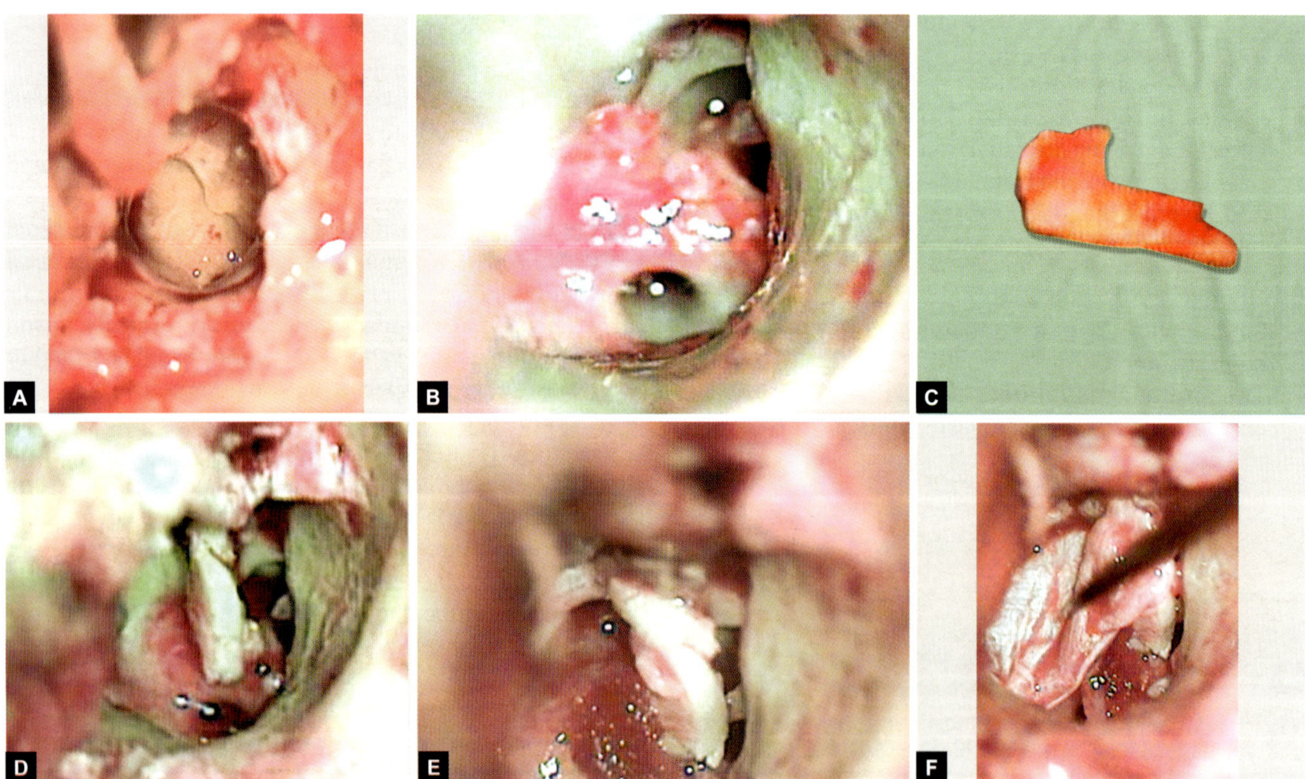

Figs 38A to F: Cartilage Tympanoplasty: (A) Large central perforation; (B) Long process of incus is eroded; (C) Cartilage is prepared for ossicular repair; (D) Placement of cartilage over stapes Superstructure; (E) Cartilage is secured by gelfoam; (F) Placement of temporalis fascia graft (TFG) and tympano meatal (TM) flap on cartilage

- Materials used for obliteration are biological materials—bone chips, bone dust/patte, conchal cartilage, free abdominal flap graft and local flaps
- Nonbiological materials are—hydroxyapatite crystals and ceramic
- Local flaps—pedicled flaps resurface the cavity and cover the raw surfaces that interfere with re-epithalization.

Types of flap commonly used include:

- Palva's flap—Meatally based musculoperiosteal flap. A laterally based postauricular musculoperiosteal flap is rotated into the mastoid cavity. Palva (1950) used bone paste and chips together with the flap
- Middle temporal artery flap—An axial superiorly based flap immediately deep to the temporalis muscle is used to reline the mastoid cavity
- Posteriosuperior temporalis muscle periosteal flap—The flap is raised and rotated in the mastoid cavity for resurfacing
- Inferiorly-based myoperiosteal flap—In most cases this flap is used together with cochal cartilage for cavity obliteration.

Often a combination of various techniques is used to obtain better results.

Technique chosen should be according to patient's status, intraoperative findings and surgeon's familiarity with the operations. Ultimate aim of surgery is to give a dry, safe and self-cleaning ear postoperatively.

Postoperative follow-up of mastoid surgery:

- Mastoid dressing is changed after 24 hours and patient is discharged with advice of antibiotics of 7days along with analgesic and antihistamine
- In close cavity—Dressing and suture are removed after one week of operation (first visit). Cotton balls in the ear are removed after 3 weeks of operation. Patient is advised to use topical antibiotics and steroid drops for three weeks (second visit). At the end of 6 weeks of operations ear canal is expected to heal completely (third visit)
- In open cavity—Postauricular suture and pack in EAC are removed after two weeks of operation and patient is advised to use topical antibiotics and steroid drop for 4 weeks more (first visit). After 6 weeks, cavity is cleaned with hydrogen peroxide and gentle suction (second visit). Cavity is expected to heal within 8–12 weeks of operation depending on the size of the cavity (third visit).

Illustration of Ossiculoplasty with PORP are shown in Figures 39Ato E.

Illustration of Ossiculoplasty with TORP are shown in Figures 40A to E.

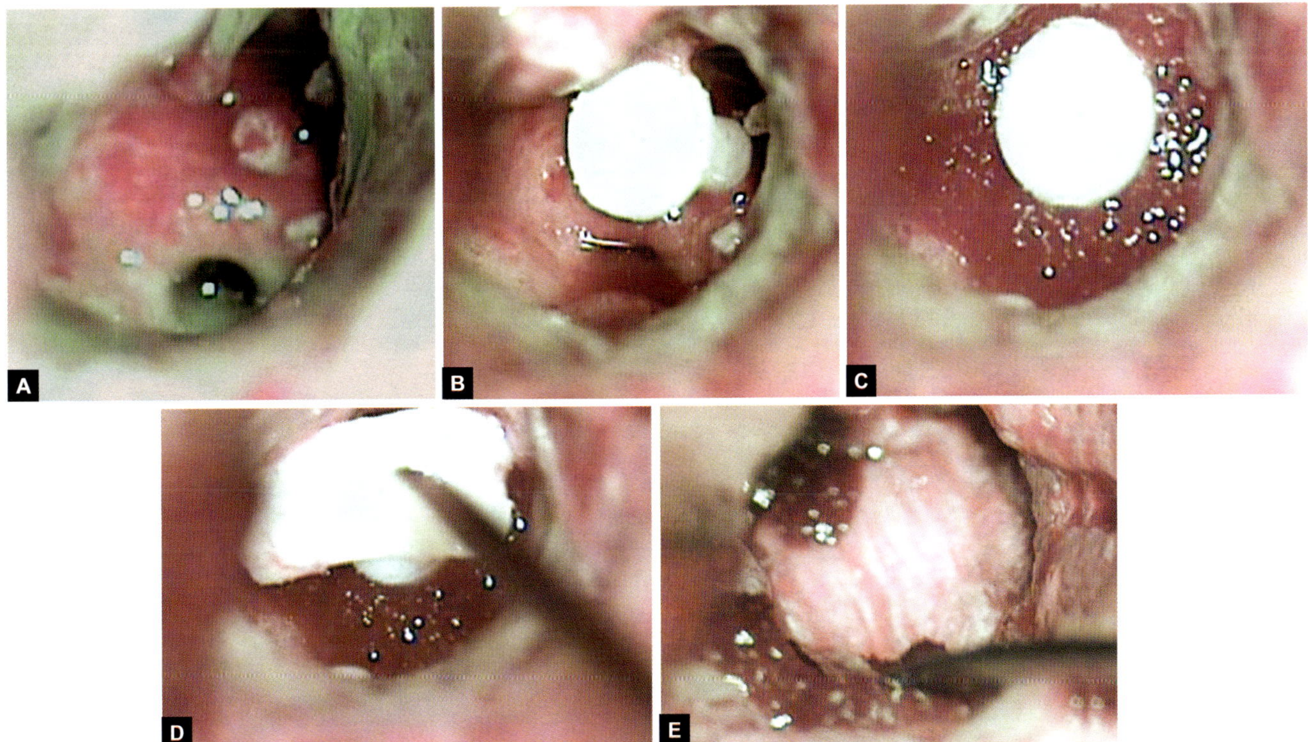

Figs 39A to E: Ossiculoplasty with PORP: (A) Incus is eroded and incudostapedial joints is dislocated; (B) Placement of teflon PORP; (C) PORP is secured by Gelfoam; (D) Placement of cartilage on PORP; (E) Placement of TFG with TM on cartilage

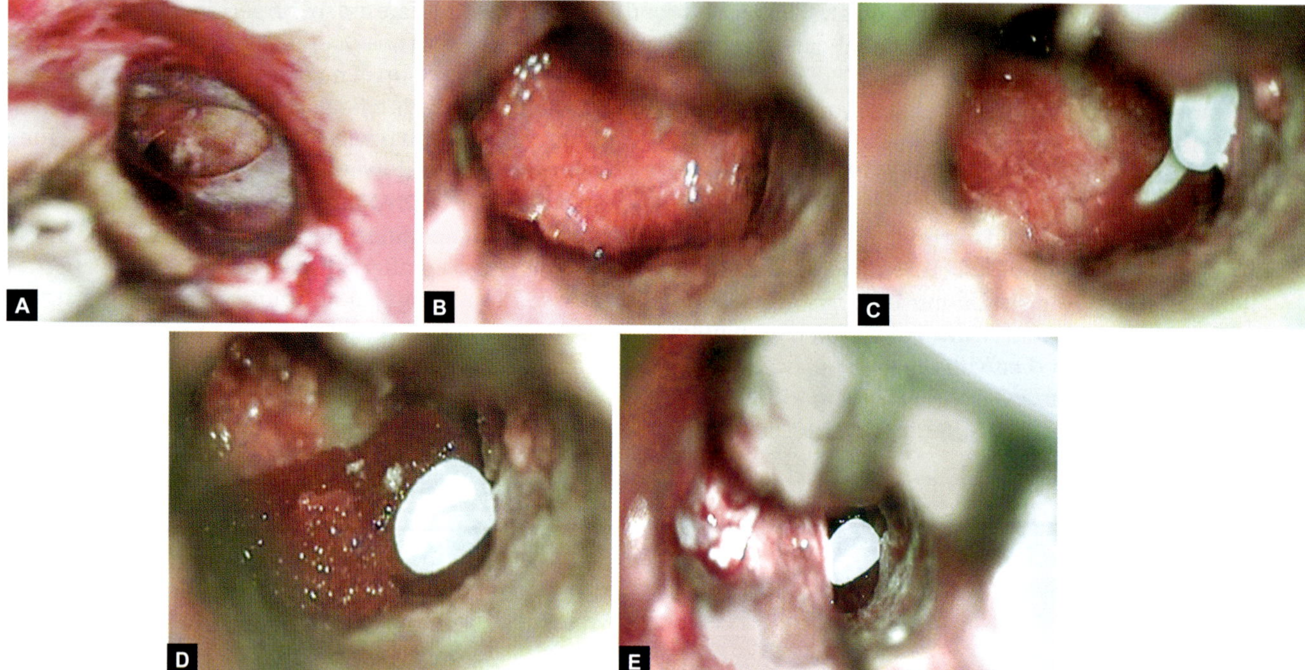

Figs 40A to E: Ossiculplasty with TORP: (A) Perforation of pars tensa; (B) Absence of ossicles except footplate of stapes. (C) Placement of TORP on the footplate; (D) Position of TORP is secured by Gelfoam; (E) Placement of TFG with TM flaps on TORP

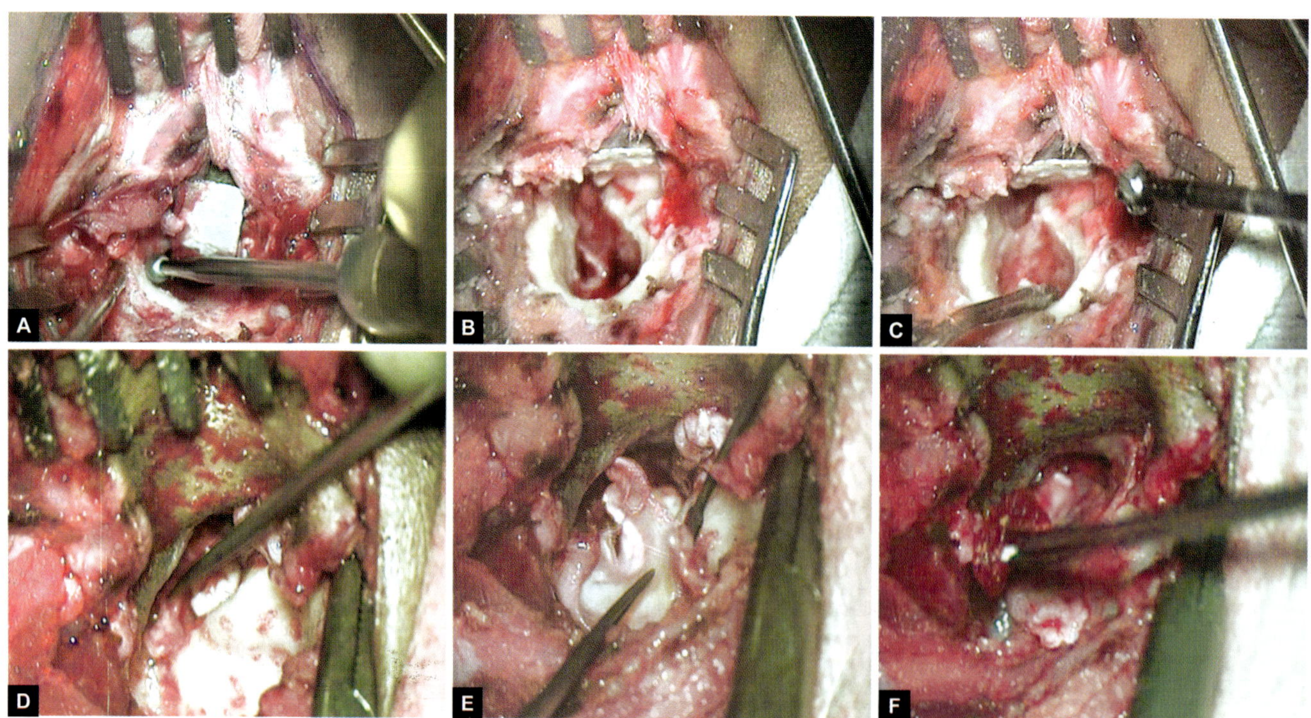

Figs 41A to F: Atticoantrostomy with cartilage tympanoplasty: (A) Atticotomy; (B) AtticoAntrostomy; (C) Removal of Posteriorsuperior canal wall; (D) Placement of cartilage on stapes superstructure; (E) Placement of TFG on cartilage; (F) TM Flap repositioned

Surgical steps of Atticoantrostomy with cartilage tympanoplasty are shown in Figures 41 A to F.

ENDOSCOPIC EAR SURGERY[21]

Conventional ear surgery is performed under operative microscope and often requires larger postoperative incision to approach the tiny structures of the ear. Use of endoscope for performing ear surgery provides surgeon better illumination and visualization of tiny complex structures of the ear through permeatal approach, avoiding any endaural or postauricular incision with less painful recovery from surgery. The procedure is done with 4 mm wide angle 0° and 30° Hopkins II telescopes of 18 cm length, video camera and a monitor. Smaller endoscope of size 2.7 mm giving similar field of view is being used. Patients with chronic ear diseases suffering from TM perforation or cholesteatoma are taken for endoscopic ear surgery. Endoscopes are used as an adjuvant of microscope or a full surgical technique. View of operations under microscope via permeatal approach is limited by narrowest segment of the ear canal and postauricular approach is performed to overcome the limited view. Use of endoscope permeatal helps to bypass the narrowest segment and provides wide view for anterior part of attic, hypotympanum and sinus tympani as well as better visualization of ligaments and folds of middle ear with precise understanding of ventilation of these spaces (Figs 42 and 43).

Permeatal Endoscopic View of Tympanum

With the use of permeatal endoscope facial recess is clearly visible and looks like shallow depression in the posterior wall of mesotympanum. Pyramidal eminence and vertical segment of facial nerve form the medial wall of facial recess. Bony annulus forms the lateral wall of the recess (Fig. 44).

Retro tympanum—Precise knowledge of anatomy of retro tympanum is essential. Oval window is located superiorly within posterior sinus. Round window is located inferiorly within sinus subtympanicum. Sinus tympani lies between this two sinuses by ponticulus above and sobiculum below. Hypotympanum is separated from sinus subtympanicum by finiculus (Fig. 45).

Lateral part of attic is separated from mesotympanum by a lateral incudomalleolar and lateral malleolar folds. This mucosal folds act as a barrier to ventilate attic from mesotympanum laterally. Anterior part of attic is separated from anterior mesotympanum and the Eustachian tube by tensor tympani fold. The tensor tympani has two segments—a vertical segment that attaches to COG and a horizontal segment that makes the part of the floor of supratubal recess (STR). Therefore, tensor fold prevents

direct ventilation between anterior attic and the Eustachian tube (Figs 46 and 47).

Illustration of transcanal endoscopic nuyringoplasty underlay technique is shown (Figs 48A to I).

There is a fully formed tympanic diaphragm which separates the mesotympanum from attic. The diaphragm is formed by

- Lateral and medial incudal folds
- Anterior and lateral malleolar folds

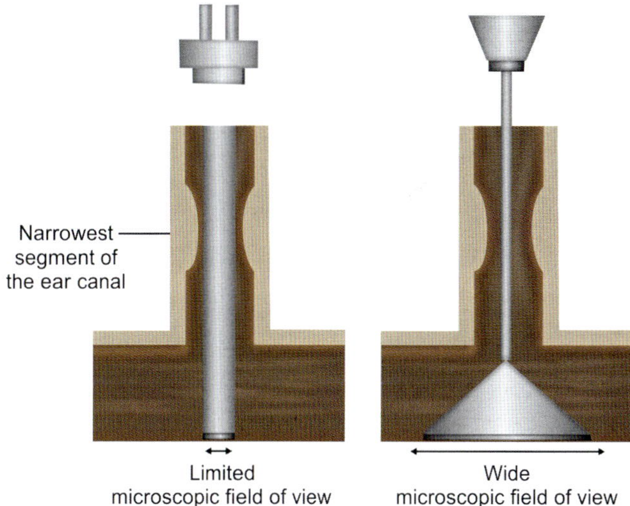

Fig. 42: View from microscope during permeatal surgery is limited by the narrowest segment of EAC. Whereas transcanal endoscope bypasses this narrowest segment and gives a wide view[21]

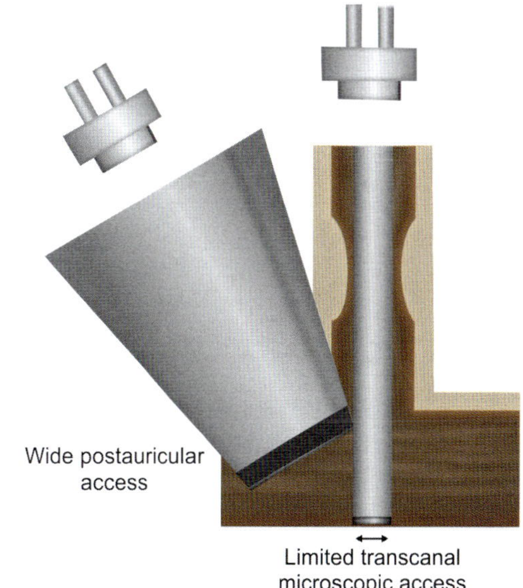

Fig. 43: Permeatal use of microscope gives limited view for which post auricular approach is adopted to provide a port parallel to attic following removal of healthy bone and enables much better access to attic[21]

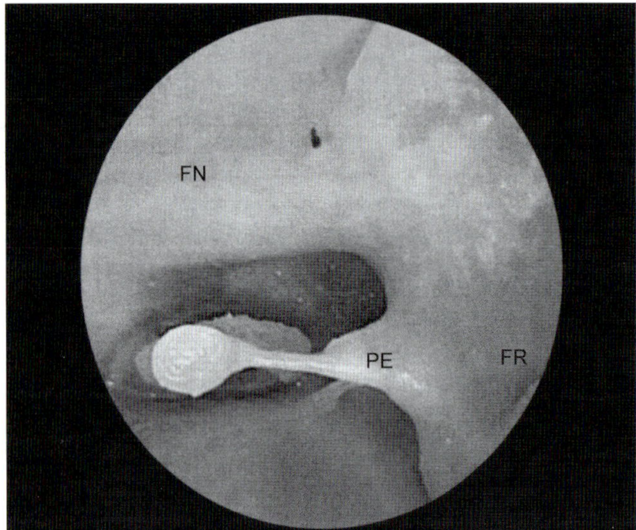

Fig. 44: Permeatal endoscopic view of left ear.
Abbreviations: FR, facial recess; PE, pyramidal eminence; FN, vertical segment of facial nerve[21]

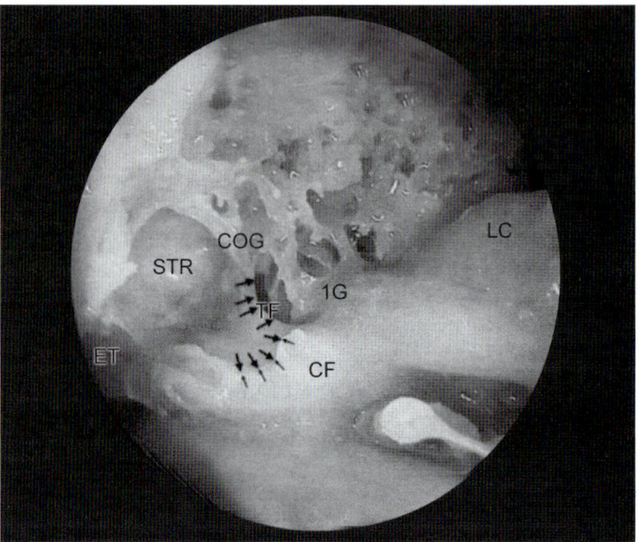

Fig. 46: Endoscopic view of tensor tympani fold (Left Ear). Single arrows, insertion of vertical segment of tensor fold; double arrows, insertion of horizontal segment of tensor fold.
Abbreviations: TF, tensor tympani fold; STR, supra tubal recess; ET, eustachian tube; CF, cochleari form process; 1G, 1st genu of facial nerve and surrounding geniculate ganglion; LC, lateral semicircular canal; COG, Sheehy's COG[21]

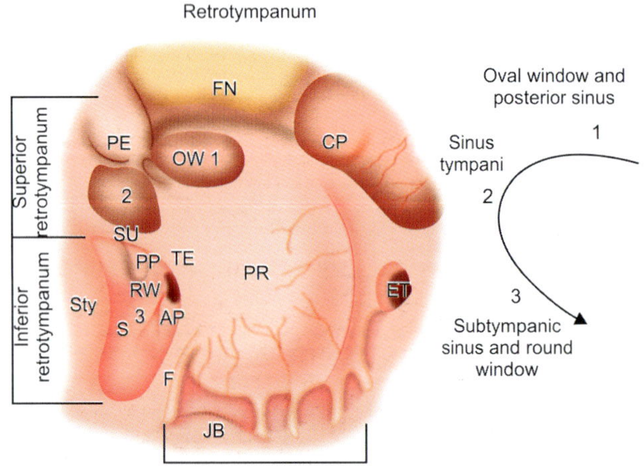

Fig. 45: Schematic diagram of retro tympanum.
Abbreviations: FN, facial nerve; PR, promontory; PE, pyramidal eminence; OW, oval window; P, ponticulus; SU, subiculum; RW, round window; JB, jugular bulb; ET, eustachian tube; F, finiculus[21]

Fig. 47: Endoscopic view of anterior isthmus tympani (left ear).
Abbreviations: TT, tensor tympani tendon; IM, anterior isthmus tympani; ISJ, incudostapedial joint[21]

- Tensor tympani fold

Only two narrow passages—Anterior and posterior tympanic isthmus breach this diaphragm and act as ventilation port between attic and mesotympanum.

Anterior isthmus tympani—The area lies medial to the body of incus and passes between incudostapedial joint and tensor tympani tendon. This is the main port of attic ventilation.

Posterior isthmus tympani—The area posterior to incudostapedial joint lies between medial incudal fold and posterior tympani wall. It is extremely narrow part for ventilation.

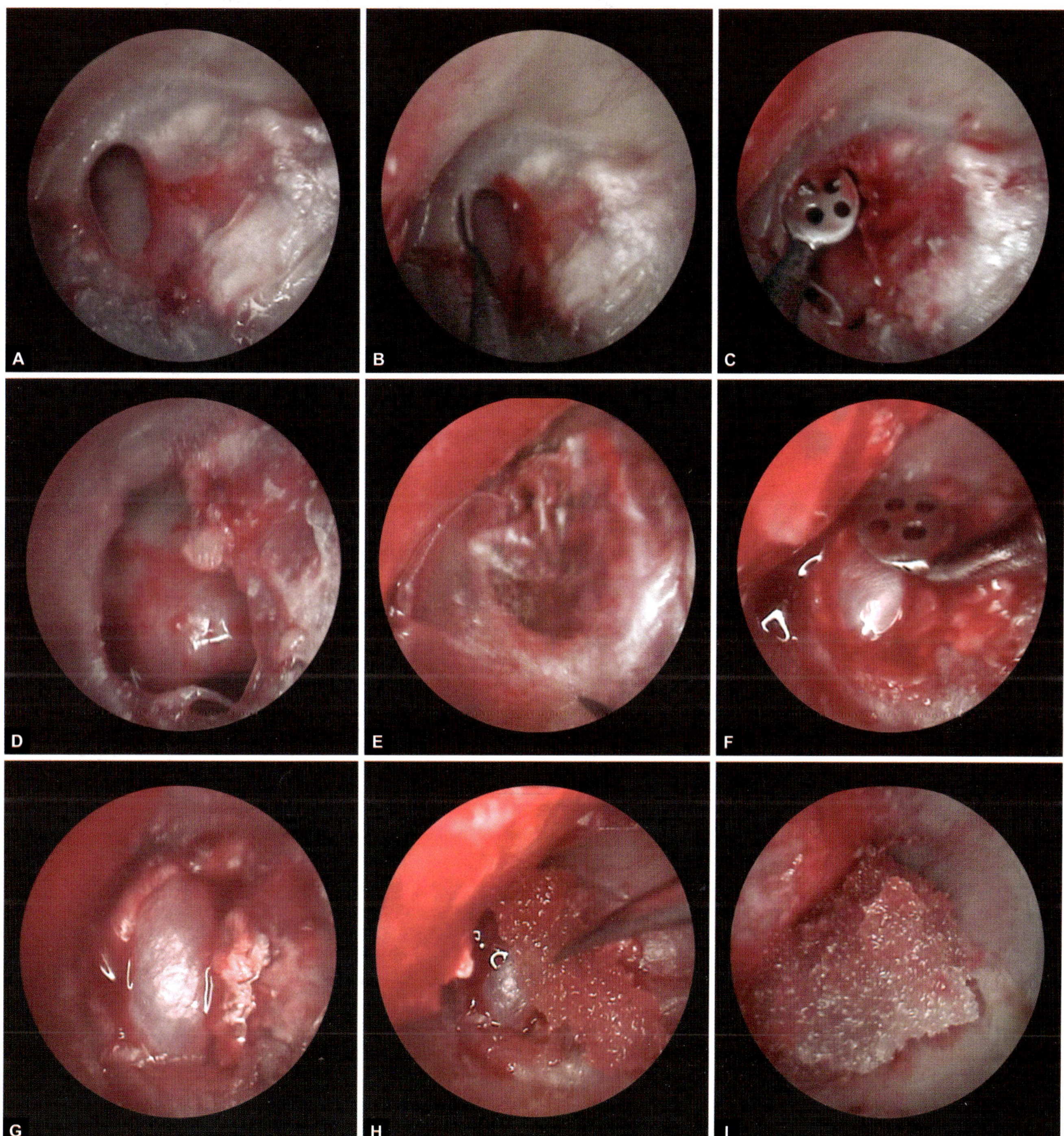

Figs 48A to I: Transcanal endoscopic myringoplasty (A) Central perforation in pars tensa; (B) freshening of the margin of perforation; (C) freshening of the under surface of the margin of perforation; (D) margin of perforation is freshened; (E) Placing of the temporalis fascia graft (TFG); (F) TFG is placed; (G) TFG is placed; (H) Placing of Gelfoam on the graft; (I) Gelfoam is placed on the graft

REFERENCES

1. Ballantyne JC, Morrison A. Surgical approaches to middle ear and mastoid – Rob and smith's operative surgery–Ear, 4th edition. 1983. P 47-50.
2. Shenoi PM. Surgical approaches to middle ear and mastoid – Rob and Smith's operative surgery – Ear. In: John C Ballantyne and Andrew Morrison (eds), 4th edition. 1983. P 51-4.
3. Bllantyne JC, Morrison A. Surgical approach to middle ear and mastoid. Rob & Smith's operative surgery – Ear, 4th edition. 1983. P 55-8.
4. Mastoid. Atlas of ear surgery. 4th edition. 1986, P 188.
5. Muller C, Gadre A. Tympanoplasty, university of texas medical branch. Galveston, Tx.
6. Sismanis A. Tympanoplasty- Glasscock – shambaugh, surgery of the ear, 5th edition. 2003. P 467-8.
7. Desai ABR, Desai AA. Tympanomastoid surgery to day – Principls and practice otolaryngology review, In: Shah VH, Karnik PP. 2000. P 54-67.
8. Fich U. chapter 2 Tympanoplasty, Mastoidectomy and steps sugery, 2nd edition. 2008. P 8-46.
9. Vijayandra H, Surandran K. Micro ear surgery–its purpose and procedure for tubotympanic pathology. A guide to ENT practice. 2002–2003, P 28-31.
10. Fisch U. Myringoplasty, Meatoplasty and canalplasty; tympanoplasty, Mastoidectomy and stapes surgery, 2nd edition. New York: Theime Stuttgart; 2008. P 11-36.
11. Bell HL. A technique of tympanoplasty (tympanomallear stapediopexy). Trans-actions of the American laryngological Rhinological and Otolaryngological society. 1958. P 572-67.
12. Hildyard VH. Transplant of incus homograft in the human. Archives of otolaryngology. 1967;86:294-7.
13. FrootKo NJ. Reconstruction of the ear. Scott Brown's Otolaryngology, 5th edition. Otology. 1987. P-238-59.
14. Fich U. Ossiculoplasty; tympanoplasty, Mastoidectomy and stepes surgery, 2nd edition. Georgetheme verlog; 2008. P58-83.
15. Tepan MG. Modified cat technique for cholesteatoma, otolaryngology review. In: Shah VH, Karnik PP. 2000. P 88-90.
16. Fisch U. Mastoidectomy and Epitympanectomy: Tympanoplasty Mastoidectomy and stapes surgery, 2nd edition. 2008. P 170-185.
17. Mahadevaiah A, Parikh B. Surgical anatomy of temporal bone, surgical technique in chronic otitis media and otosclerosis-text and atlas, 2nd edition. CBS; 2011. P 15.
18. Visvanathan PG, Visvanathan A. Current status of tympanomastoid surgery otolaryngology review 2000. In: Shah VH, Karnik PP. 2000. P 68-78.
19. Paparella MM, Meyerhoff WL, Michael S Morris and Sady S. Da Costa. Mastoidectomy and Tympanoplasty, Otolaryngology, Vol-II, Otology and Neuro-otology, 3rd edition. 1991. P-1422-27.
20. Ojala K, Palva A. Results of obliterative cholesteatoma surgery, Arch otolaryngol head neck surgery. 1982;108:1-3.
21. Tarabichi M, Marchioni D, Presutti L. Endoscopic Ear Surgery, Recent Advances in OTOLARYNGOLOGY Head and Neck Surgery. In: Lalwani AK, Pfister MHF. New Delhi: Jaypee Brothers Medical Publishers (P) Ltd. 2014;3:188-98.

B

C